CONGENITAL HEART DISEASE

A SURGICAL COLOR ATLAS

CONGENITAL HEART DISEASE

A SURGICAL COLOR ATLAS

AUTHORS

A. Sukru Mercan, MD, FETCS
Consultant Pediatric Cardiac Surgeon
Head, Pediatric Cardiovascular Services
Saad Specialist Hospital
Al Khobar, Saudi Arabia

Zakariya Hubail, BMedSc, MD, FAAP
Consultant Pediatric Cardiologist
Salmaniya Medical Complex, and
Arabian Gulf University
Manama, Bahrain

S. Yen Ho, PhD, FRCPath, FESC, FHEA
Professor of Cardiac Morphology
Consultant, Royal Brompton Hospital &
Harefield NHS Foundation Trust
Imperial College London
London, UK

cardiotext PUBLISHING
Minneapolis, Minnesota

Cardiotext Publishing, LLC
3405 W. 44th Street
Minneapolis, Minnesota 55410
USA

www.cardiotextpublishing.com

Any updates to this book may be found at: www.cardiotextpublishing.com/congenital-heart-disease-a-surgical-color-atlas/

Comments, inquiries, and requests for bulk sales can be directed to the publisher at: info@cardiotextpublishing.com.

Library of Congress Control Number: 2014957046

ISBN: 978-1-935395-90-4

eISBN: 978-1-935395-32-4

Printed in the United States of America

CONTENTS

ABOUT THE AUTHORS

A. Sukru Mercan, MD, FETCS, Consultant Pediatric Cardiac Surgeon, Head of Pediatric Cardiovascular Services, Saad Specialist Hospital, Al Khobar, Saudi Arabia

Dr. Mercan has operated on more than 3,000 cases in the field of congenital cardiac cardiology since 1996. He has established new pediatric cardiac centers in Istanbul, Turkey (2004), and in Al Khobar, Saudi Arabia (2007). He has been actively involved with digital photography and the capturing of intraoperative images of cardiac anomalies for the last 15 years. He is also the Deputy Chief of Cardiovascular Services at Saad Specialist Hospital.

Zakariya Hubail, BMedSc, MD, FAAP, Consultant Pediatric Cardiologist, Salmaniya Medical Complex and Arabian Gulf University, Manama, Bahrain

Dr. Hubail has trained and worked in Bahrain, the United States, and Saudi Arabia. He is currently a consultant pediatric cardiologist at the Salmaniya Medical Complex in Bahrain, and also holds a teaching post at the Department of Pediatrics, College of Medicine, Arabian Gulf University. He has published in local and international journals, and is also a referee for many local journals.

S. Yen Ho, PhD, FRCPath, FESC, FHEA, Professor of Cardiac Morphology, Consultant, Royal Brompton Hospital & Harefield NHS Foundation Trust, Imperial College London, London, UK

Professor Ho carries out research on the morphology and anatomy of normally structured hearts, hearts with conduction disturbance, and hearts with congenital malformations. She conducts regular courses on morphology of congenital heart defects and on cardiac anatomy for surgeons and interventionists.

FOREWORD

Modern medicine dawned with *De Humani Corporis Fabrica*, published in 1543 by Andreas Vesalius. The accurate anatomy based on direct observation began the new era of evidence-based medicine. Although Vesalius clearly described the anatomy of the human heart, it took nearly another century before the function of the heart was clarified by William Harvey in *De Motu Cordis* in 1628.

More recently, in the past 2 centuries, modern surgeons expanded their territory from the abdominal cavity to the thoracic and intracranial spaces and, finally, the inside of the human heart. The accurate knowledge of anatomy and the clear understanding of cardiovascular and pulmonary functions brought about the golden era of cardiovascular surgery and interventional cardiology practiced by medical professionals today.

In 1966, I was introduced to pediatric cardiac surgery at Children's Memorial Hospital (now Lurie Children's Hospital) in Chicago. The team, which was gathered by Dr. Willis J. Potts (1895–1963), was in full function, and I worked closely with Dr. Farouk S. Idriss (1928–1992), who was a pioneer in congenital heart surgery. Dr. Idriss shared an interest in the anatomy of congenital heart disease with Dr. Maurice Lev (1908–1994) of the Hektoen Institute in Chicago. Dr. Lev contributed immensely, as a pathologist, in the understanding of congenital heart disease.

Dr. Idriss began collecting surgical photographs of congenital heart defects, while I enjoyed my hobby of making line drawings of operative findings. We talked about making an album of these photographs with illustrations from a surgeon's point of view. After acquiring hundreds of photographs, I left Chicago at the end of 1977, and the project was abandoned. The need for such a book of anatomy for congenital heart defects remained real to this day.

This need and my dream are realized in this *Atlas* by the impressive work of 3 doctors: a surgeon, a cardiologist, and a pathologist. This *Atlas* includes a remarkably wide range of congenital heart disease with details of anatomy and clinical information. The beautiful pictures teach us much about surgical repair over and above the pathological anatomy. Understandably, congenital heart disease includes numerous variations, and even this *Atlas* cannot give totally comprehensive coverage. Yet, this *Atlas* may very well be the most accurate photographic description of congenital heart disease ever published.

We, the community of medical professionals, should be grateful to the authors, as I believe that this *Atlas* will help countless infants, children, and young adults by guiding their doctors, both surgeons and cardiologists, toward better understanding of the anatomic details of their heart defects.

The more we learn in medicine, the more we are amazed how "fearfully and wonderfully our bodies are made" (Psalm 139:14).

Hisashi Nikaidoh, MD, FACS, FAAP
Professor of Cardiothoracic Surgery (Retired)
University of Texas Southwestern Medical Center
Dallas, Texas

PREFACE

Congenital heart disease constitutes an important cause for morbidity and mortality in pediatrics. Interventional cardiology has made important strides over the past 2 decades, but despite this, many congenital malformations still require surgical treatment. Recent advances have made it possible to repair or palliate almost all types of congenital heart defects. This book is a pictorial illustration of congenital heart disease. The pictures in this *Atlas* represent real views as seen through the surgeon's eyes, from actual patients in the operating room. The old saying that "a picture is worth a thousand words" cannot be overemphasized.

The material was collected by one of the authors intraoperatively using a digital camera. The images were processed by computer software, and line drawings were made to clarify the anatomic and surgical details. Numbers and legends were used to mark areas of interest. We avoided the overuse of arrows because they may obscure views and, when numerous, make the pictures look overcrowded. The numbering starts from the top of the figure and continues in a clockwise direction. A brief clinical history is provided to keep the surgical procedure in context with the clinical status. Important surgical, anatomic, and pathologic points are highlighted. However, we kept the text to a minimum because this is primarily an atlas.

This book is intended for general pediatric surgeons, cardiac surgeons, pediatric cardiologists, cardiac pathologists, cardiac intensivists, and those interested in congenital heart disease. We hope this *Atlas* will complement the already existing textbooks of pediatric cardiology and cardiac surgery.

We are grateful to our patients, who are the material of this book; to our colleagues for help and encouragement; and to our families for their support and the time "sabbatical" they granted us to prepare this book.

A.S. Mercan
Z. Hubail
S. Yen Ho
2015

ACKNOWLEDGMENT

We would like to acknowledge the contribution of Professor Mehmet Salih Bilal, Istanbul, Turkey, and Professor Emin Tireli, Istanbul University, Istanbul, Turkey, who shared with us some of the photographs of their patients. Professor Bilal has graciously provided us with the following photographs.

Pulmonary Atresia: Figures 14.8 to 14.11, 14.14 to 14.23

Congenitally Corrected Transposition of the Great Arteries: Figures 16.24 to 16.39

Single Ventricle: Figures 17.7 to 17.14, 17.38 to 17.40

Aortic Valve: Figures 19.26 to 19.42

Valve Surgery: Figures 20.24 to 20.28

Coronary Artery Abnormalities: Figures 21.19 to 21.28

Professor Emin Tireli has provided us with the following photographs.

Transposition of the Great Arteries: Figures 15.23 to 15.37

ABBREVIATIONS

3D	three-dimensional
ALCAPA	anomalous left coronary artery from the pulmonary artery
APW	aortopulmonary window
ASD	atrial septal defect
AV	atrioventricular
AVSD	atrioventricular septal defect
BT shunt	Blalock-Taussig shunt
ccTGA	congenitally corrected transposition of the great arteries
CPB	cardiopulmonary bypass
CS	coronary sinus
DILV	double inlet left ventricle
DKS	Damus-Kaye-Stansel
DORV	double outlet right ventricle
d-TGA	*(see TGA)*
ePTFE	expanded polytetrafluoroethylene
HLHS	hypoplastic left heart syndrome
ICU	intensive care unit
IVC	inferior vena cava
LAA	left atrial appendage
LAD	left anterior descending (coronary artery)
l-TGA	L-transposition of the great arteries
LV	left ventricle; left ventricular
LVOT	left ventricular outflow tract
MAPCA	major aortopulmonary collateral artery
MPA	main pulmonary artery
PA	pulmonary artery
PDA	patent ductus arteriosus
PFO	patent foramen ovale
PTFE	polytetrafluoroethylene
PV	pulmonary vein
RAA	right atrial appendage
RV	right ventricle; right ventricular
RVOT	right ventricular outflow tract
SVC	superior vena cava
TAPVC	totally anomalous pulmonary venous connection
TAPVD	totally anomalous pulmonary venous drainage
TGA	transposition of the great arteries
TOF	tetralogy of Fallot
VATS	video-assisted thoracoscopic surgery
VSD	ventricular septal defect

CHAPTER 1

Introduction

Cardiac surgery effectively started with Robert Gross closing a patent ductus arteriosus (PDA) in 1938.[1] The next major advance was palliation of cyanotic heart disease by systemic-to-pulmonary shunt, performed by Alfred Blalock in 1944.[2] However, it was the cardiopulmonary bypass machine (1953) that ushered in modern cardiac surgery.[3] It enabled performing intracardiac repair under direct vision in a bloodless field. Coupled with accurate preoperative assessment and sophisticated postoperative intensive care, congenital heart surgery has made, and continues to make, significant strides. Nowadays even the most complex heart diseases can be palliated or repaired with low mortality and acceptable morbidity. In recent years, there has been a trend toward earlier repair for most lesions.

Interventional cardiac catheterization has also advanced significantly, and has changed the way we currently treat many congenital heart diseases. In due time, some of the techniques described in this book will be replaced by catheter-based interventions or hybrid procedures.

Although the outcomes of congenital heart disease have improved significantly, there are still a few lingering issues. With the growing population of survivors of CHD came the realization of important physical, neurodevelopmental, and psychosocial morbidities that may affect the overall quality of life.[4]

STERNOTOMY

A median sternotomy (Figures 1.1–1.10) is the approach most commonly utilized for the majority of congenital heart surgeries.

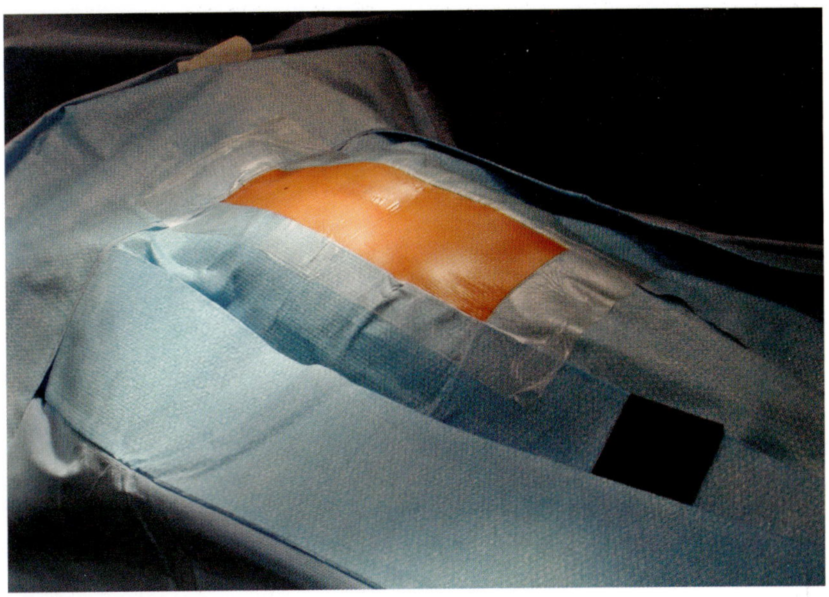

Figure 1.1. A child on the operating table, anesthetized, prepped, and draped, prior to skin incision for repair of congenital heart disease via a median sternotomy.

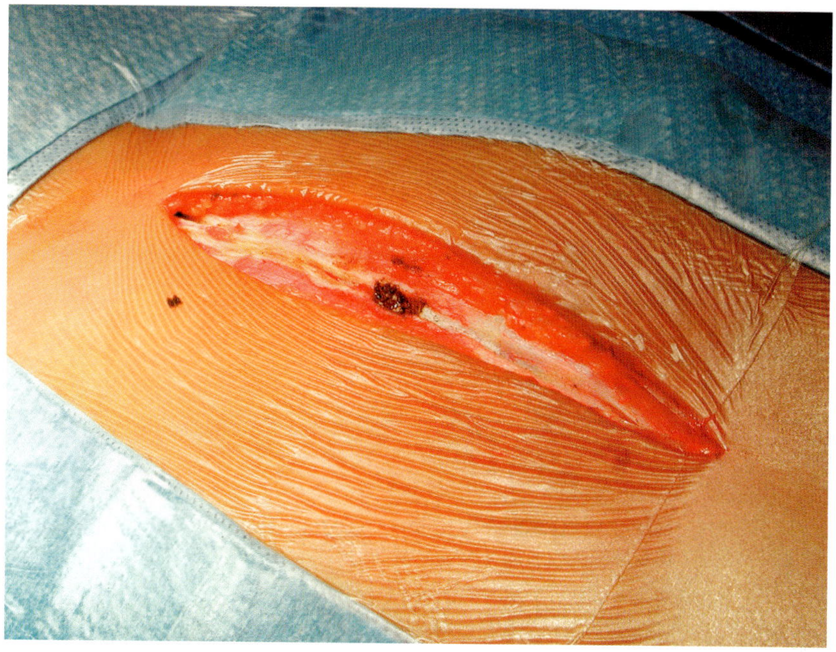

Figure 1.2. A skin incision has been made for a standard median sternotomy.

Upon opening the sternum, the anterior mediastinal structures come into view. The thymus is large in children and begins to involute at puberty. It is usually sub-totally excised to facilitate access (Figures 1.4–1.6). The heart and the proximal great vessels are wrapped by the pericardial sac. Cardiopulmonary bypass (CPB) is established by cannulating the superior vena cava (SVC) and inferior vena cava (IVC). The blood is oxygenated in the CPB machine and returned back through an arterial cannula to the ascending aorta. A cardioplegia catheter is inserted into the aorta proximal to the site of arterial cannula. Between these 2 catheters, an aortic cross-clamp is placed (Figure 1.7). The operative field is often small and crowded with instruments (Figure 1.8). Metal wires are usually used to close the sternum after the repair.

Occasionally a submammary incision is made, especially in females for cosmetic reasons (Figure 1.11). Through this incision a limited number of lesions, such as atrial septal defects (ASD), can be repaired.

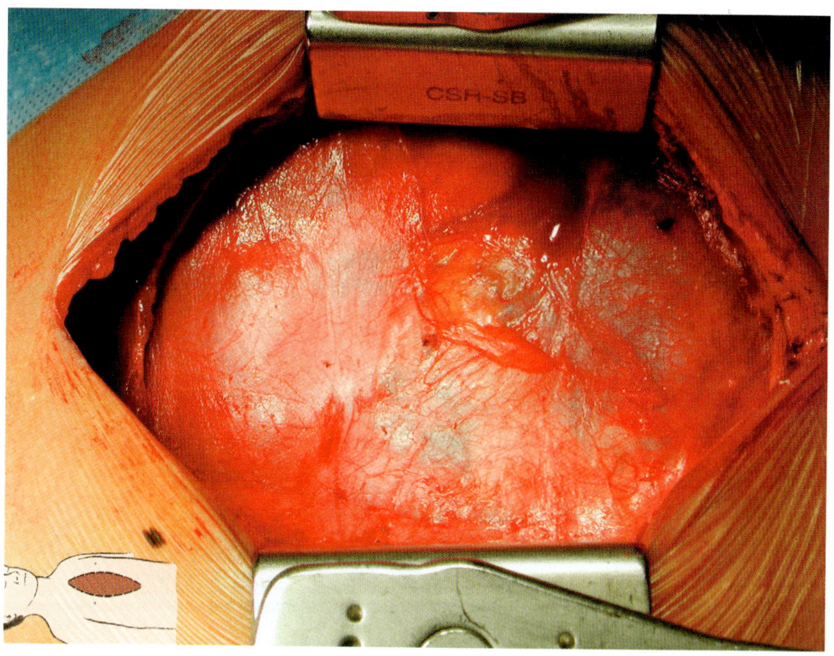

Figure 1.3. The sternal bone has been cut, and a pair of retractors placed. The anterior mediastinal structures are seen.

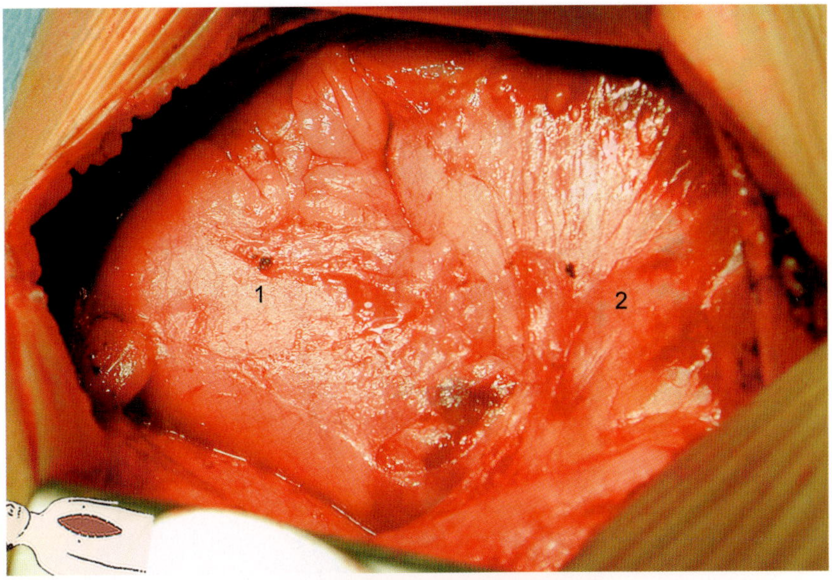

Figure 1.4. A median sternotomy view from another child undergoing heart surgery. The thymus gland is usually large in children.

1. Thymus gland
2. Pericardial sac

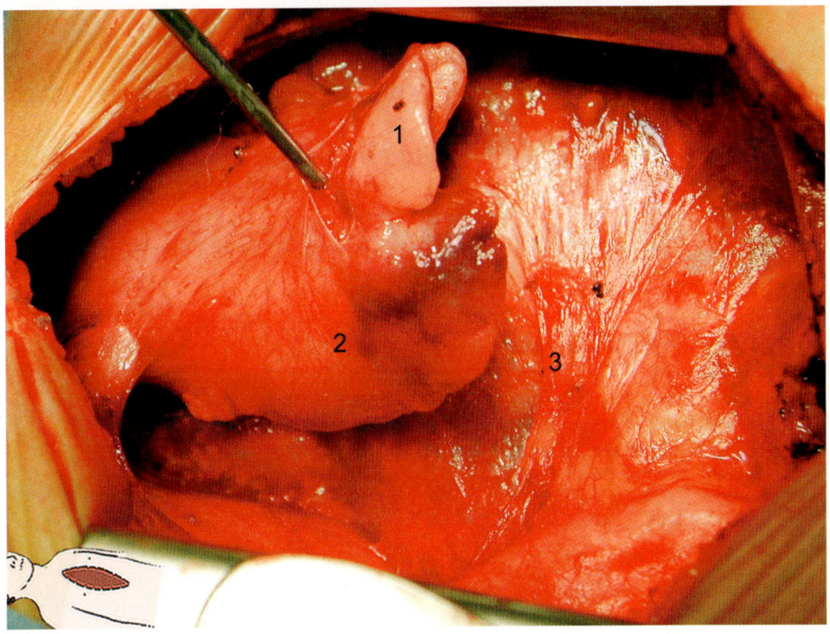

Figure 1.5. The thymus gland is mobilized prior to excision.

1. Left lobe of thymus
2. Right lobe of thymus
3. Heart

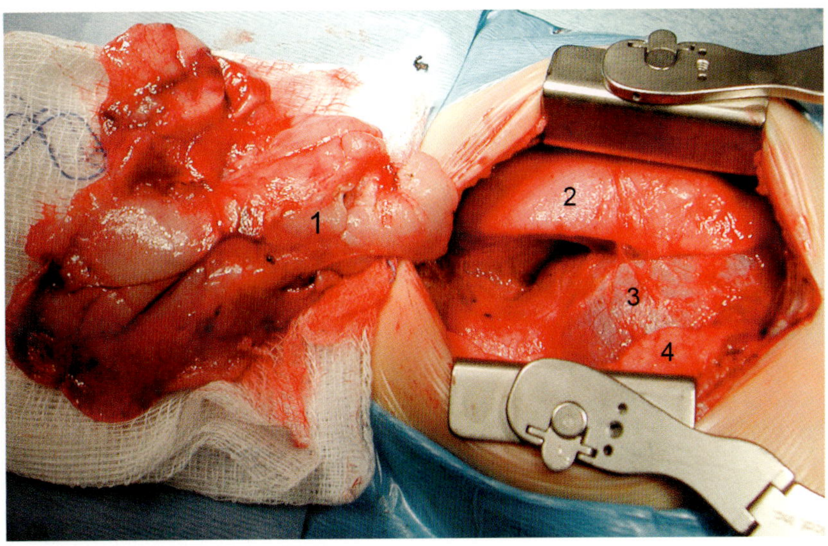

Figure 1.6. The thymus is excised to gain better access to the heart and great vessels for repair and cannulation.

1. Thymus
2. Left lung
3. Heart
4. Right lung

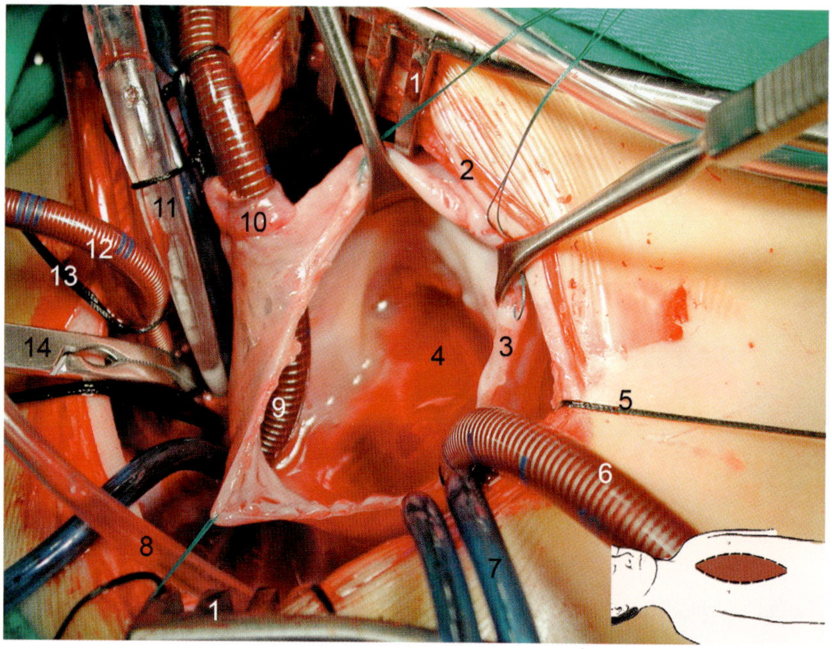

Figure 1.7. The operative field through a median sternotomy and right atriotomy in a 2-year-old child with an ASD.

1. Sternal retractor
2. Skin incision
3. Atriotomy incision
4. Blood in floor of opened right atrium
5. Stay suture for pericardium
6. IVC venous cannula
7. Tourniquet
8. Suction catheter
9. SVC venous cannula
10. Entry of SVC cannula through atrial appendage
11. Cardioplegia catheter
12. Aortic cannula
13. Stay suture isolating ascending aorta
14. Aortic cross-clamp

Figure 1.8. The operative field of another patient, an infant, undergoing cardiac surgery. The surgeons have to work through a small window cluttered with cannulas, catheters, tourniquets, retractors, and surgical instruments. Magnifying loops are indispensable for good visualization.

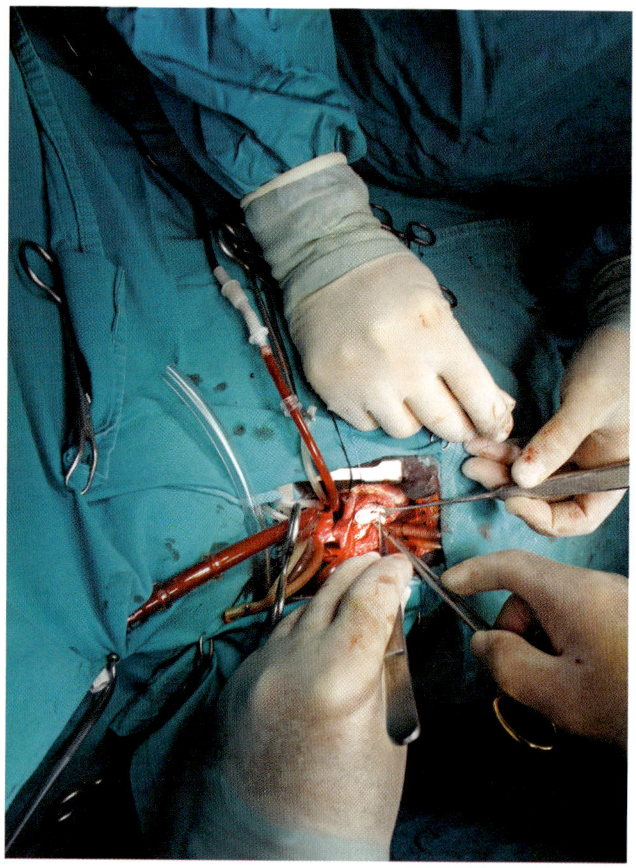

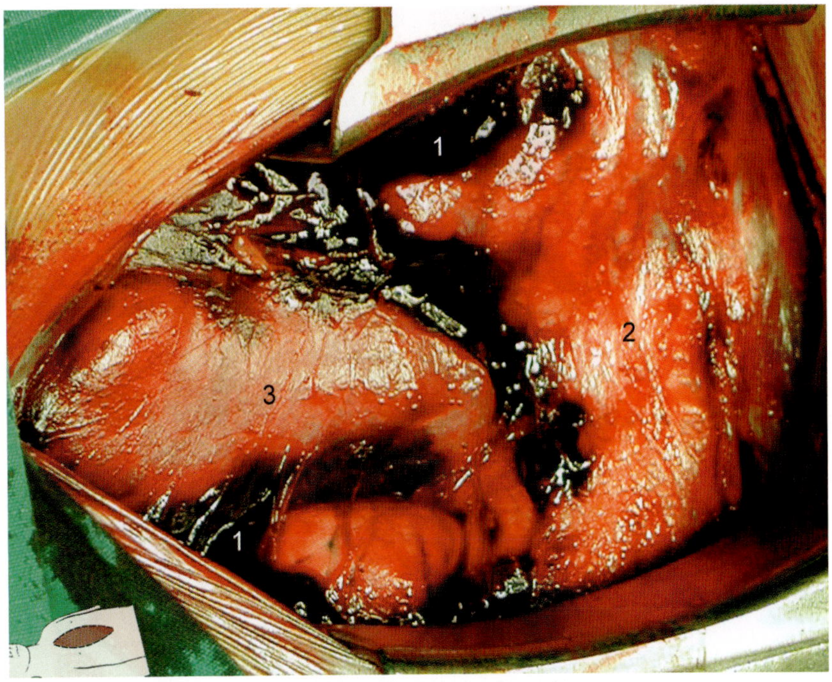

Figure 1.9. Median sternotomy view of a child undergoing heart surgery. Clotted blood is seen around the heart and thymus. It came from a vein inadvertently perforated during placement of a central venous catheter by the anesthesiologist.

1. Clotted blood
2. Heart
3. Thymus

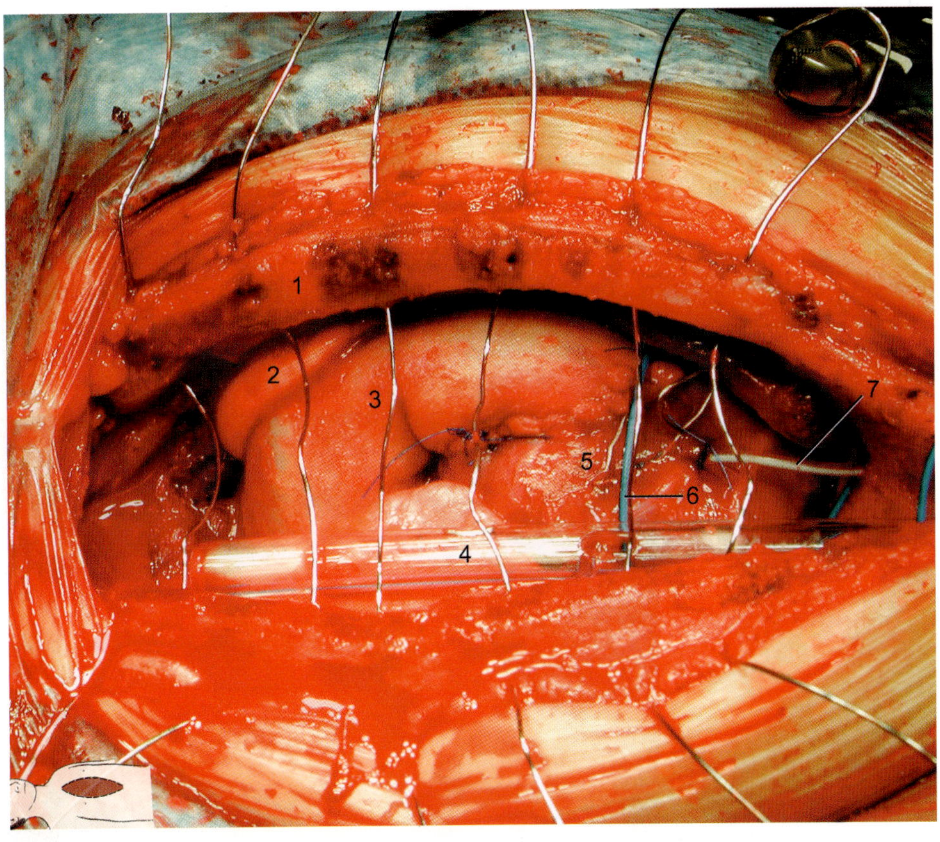

Figure 1.10. A median sternotomy view at the conclusion of a heart surgery, just prior to sternal closure. The patient, a 4-month-old infant with double outlet left ventricle (LV), underwent ventricular septal defect (VSD) closure and right ventricle–to–pulmonary artery (RV-to-PA) conduit implantation.

1. Sternum bone
2. Left lung
3. RV-to-PA conduit (Contegra)
4. Mediastinal chest tube
5. RV
6. Temporary pacing wire
7. Pulmonary artery catheter

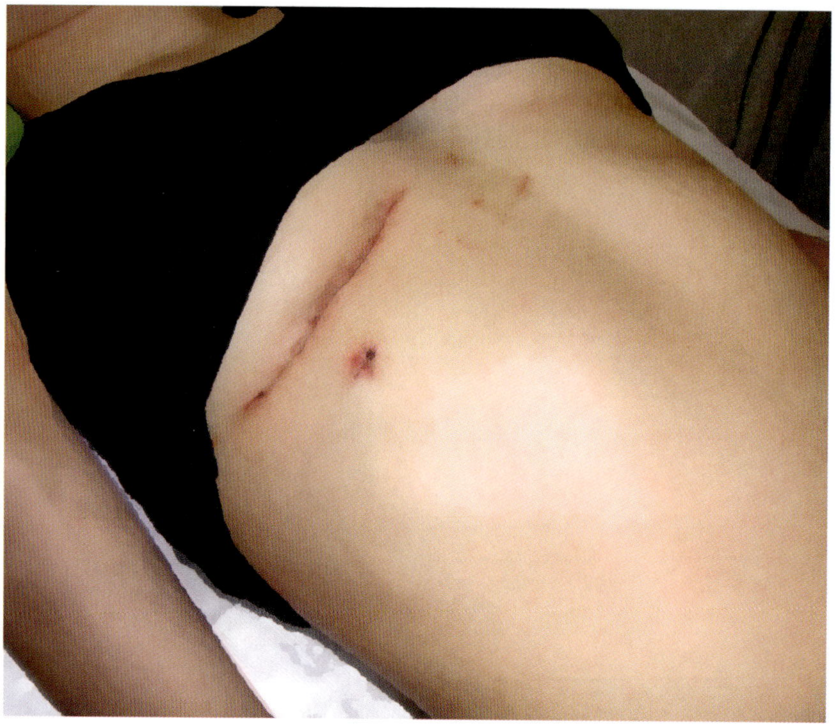

Figure 1.11. A submammary incision may alternatively be used for cosmetic reasons, as in this female patient with an ASD.

LATERAL THORACOTOMY

A lateral thoracotomy approach is utilized when performing surgeries on the distal aortic arch, descending thoracic aorta or ductus arteriosus, and for placement of modified Blalock-Taussig (BT) shunt (Figures 1.12 and 1.13). The fourth or fifth intercostal spaces are used. The lung is retracted to reveal the structures in the posterior mediastinum. In left thoracotomy, the superior intercostal vein (Figure 1.14) runs across the upper surgical field and is usually ligated. The left vagus nerve runs downward along the lateral border of the aorta. As it crosses the left pulmonary artery, it gives

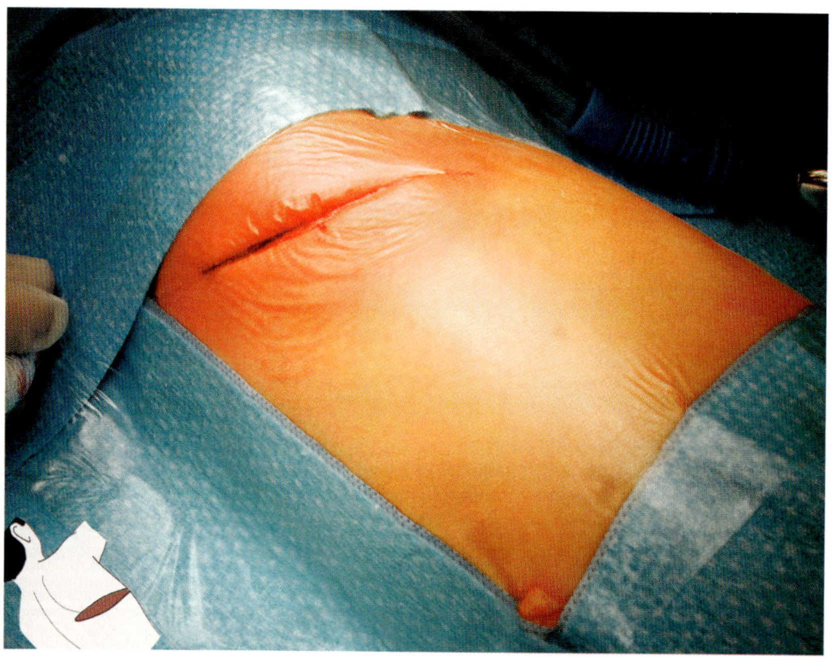

Figure 1.12. A right lateral thoracotomy incision for BT shunt in a 5-day-old neonate with tetralogy of Fallot (TOF) and severe pulmonary stenosis. Further images of this patient are shown in chapter 13 (Figures 13.1–13.8).

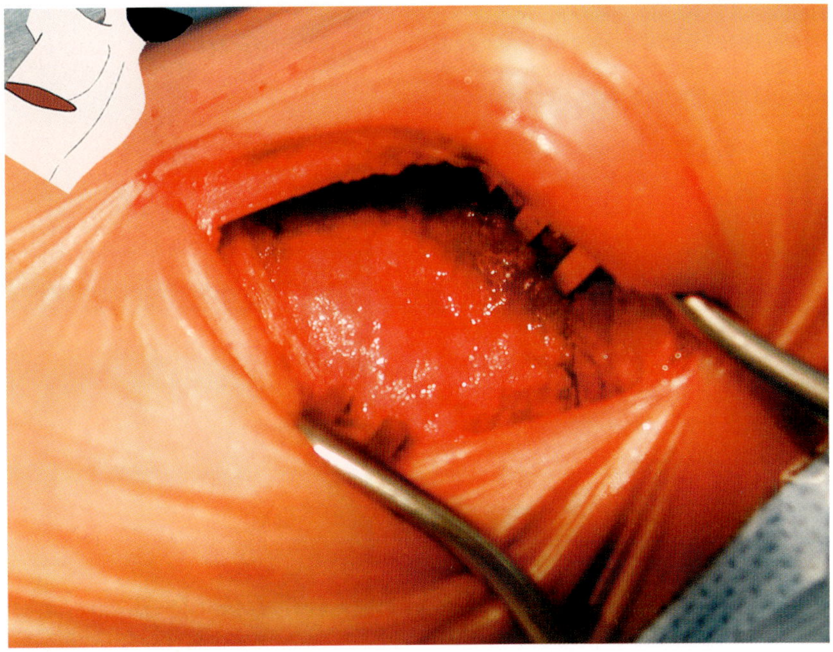

Figure 1.13. A left lateral thoracotomy incision for PDA ligation in a 3-month-old infant. This patient was born prematurely and has chronic lung disease. Note the emphysematous lung.

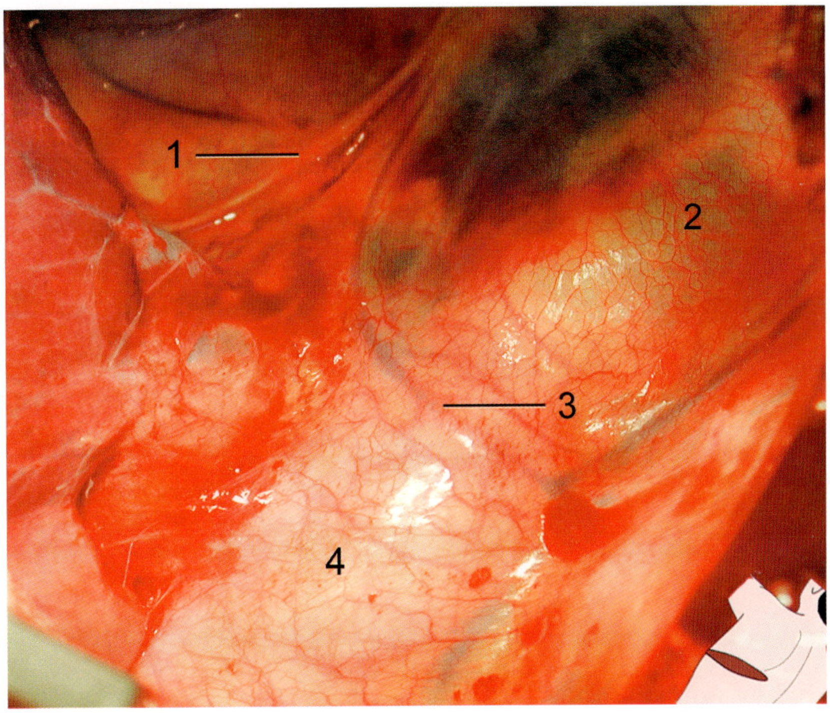

Figure 1.14. Left lateral thoracotomy view after retracting the left lung. The posterior mediastinum structures are seen, covered by parietal pleura.

1. Left vagus nerve
2. Distal end of aortic arch
3. Superior intercostal vein
4. Descending thoracic aorta

off the left recurrent laryngeal nerve that turns around the ductus arteriosus (or ligamentum arteriosum) and then ascends back toward the neck. The left phrenic nerve is located more medially, anterior to the hilum of the lung, and runs over the pericardial sac.

Some unexpected findings are shown in Figures 1.15 to 1.17. In right thoracotomy (Figure 1.18), the SVC is encountered, joined in its distal part by the azygos vein. Occasionally bilateral SVC is found.

POSTOPERATIVE CARE

Improved outcome of congenital heart surgeries is to a large part attributable to advanced postoperative

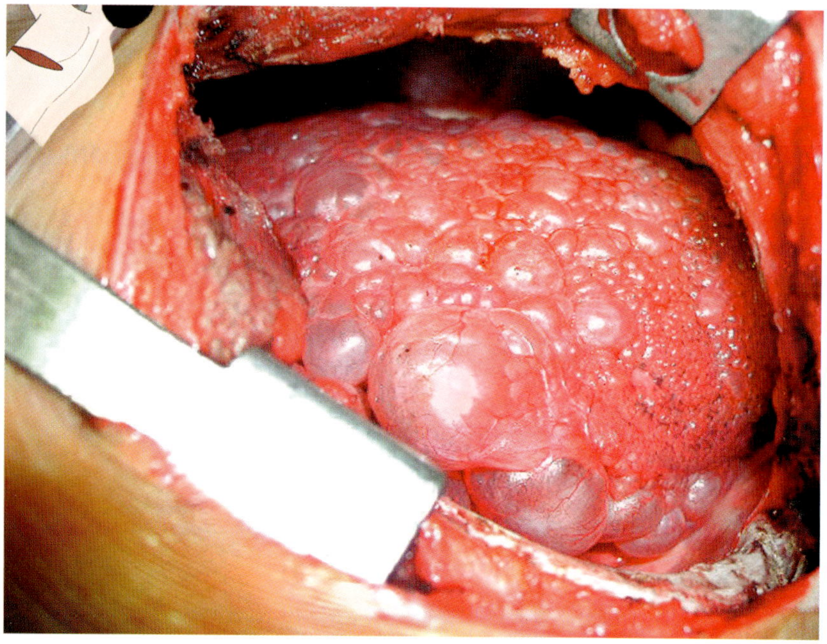

Figure 1.15. An abnormal lung as seen through a left lateral thoracotomy. The lung surface shows emphysematous bullae of various sizes, not diagnosed preoperatively.

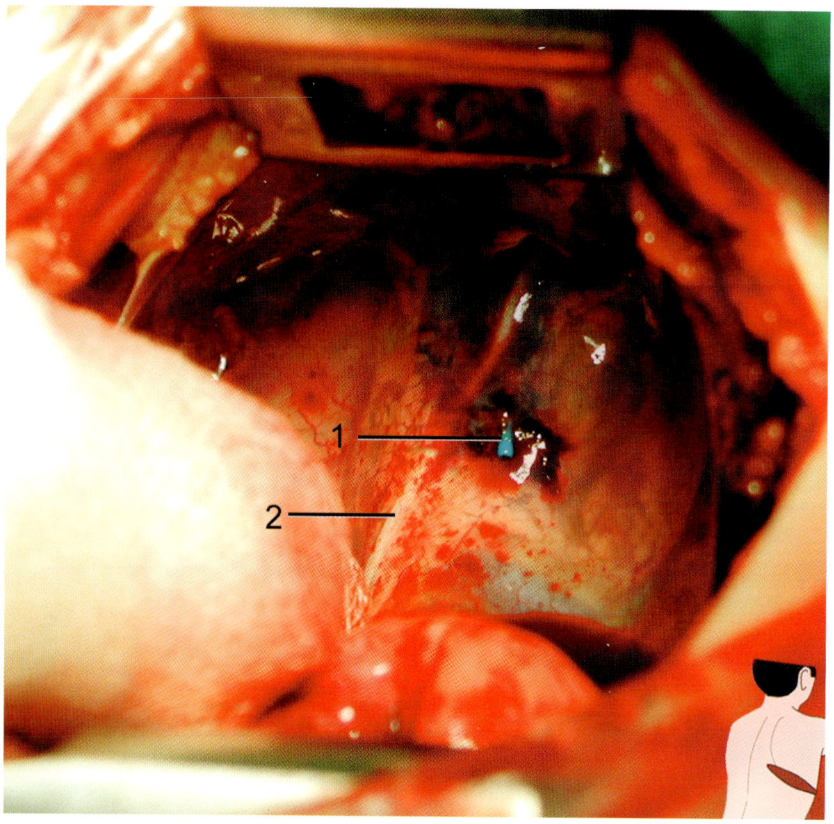

Figure 1.16. A right thoracotomy view in a child with congenital heart disease. Upon retracting the lung, the tip of a central venous catheter was seen, having perforated the wall of the SVC.

1. Tip of central venous catheter
2. Left vagus nerve

intensive care. Invasive monitoring, mechanical ventilation, inotropic, and even mechanical circulatory support are often required in the postoperative child. Figures 1.19 and 1.20 show a postoperative child in the intensive care unit (ICU) after cardiac surgery. The sternum may be left open and the surgical wound covered with silastic or Dacron (Figure 1.21). This is done after some complex surgeries to improve postoperative hemodynamics and ventricular relaxation and facilitate easier ventilation with lower positive pressures. It also gives more room when significant edema is present and provides ready access for reintervention or open cardiac massage. The sternum is usually closed in the ICU after 2 to 3 days.

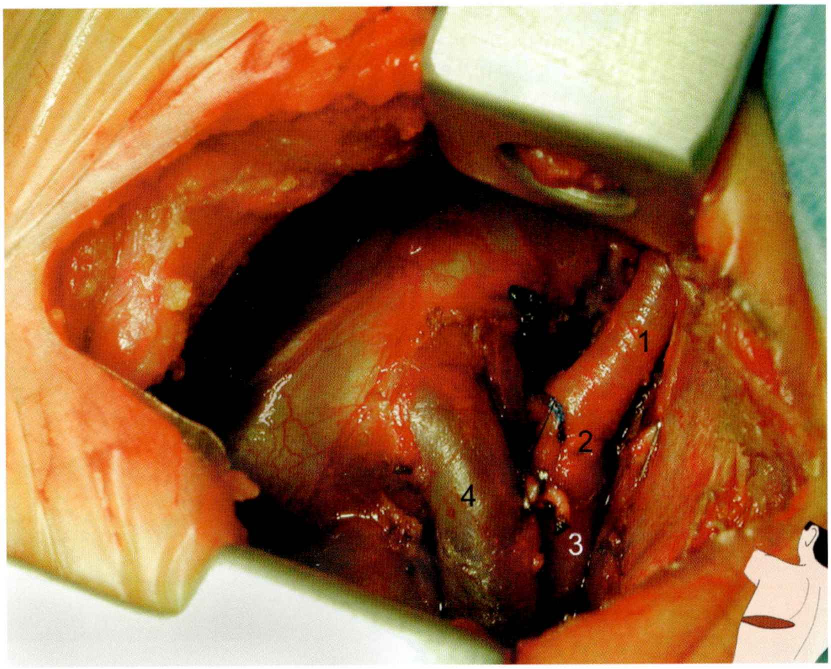

Figure 1.17. A surgical view through left thoracotomy in a 5-day-old neonate with coarctation of the aorta. A prominent anomalously draining hemiazygos vein is seen. The coarctation has already been repaired by resection and end-to-end anastomosis.

1. Left subclavian artery
2. Anastomosis site
3. Descending thoracic aorta
4. Hemiazygos vein

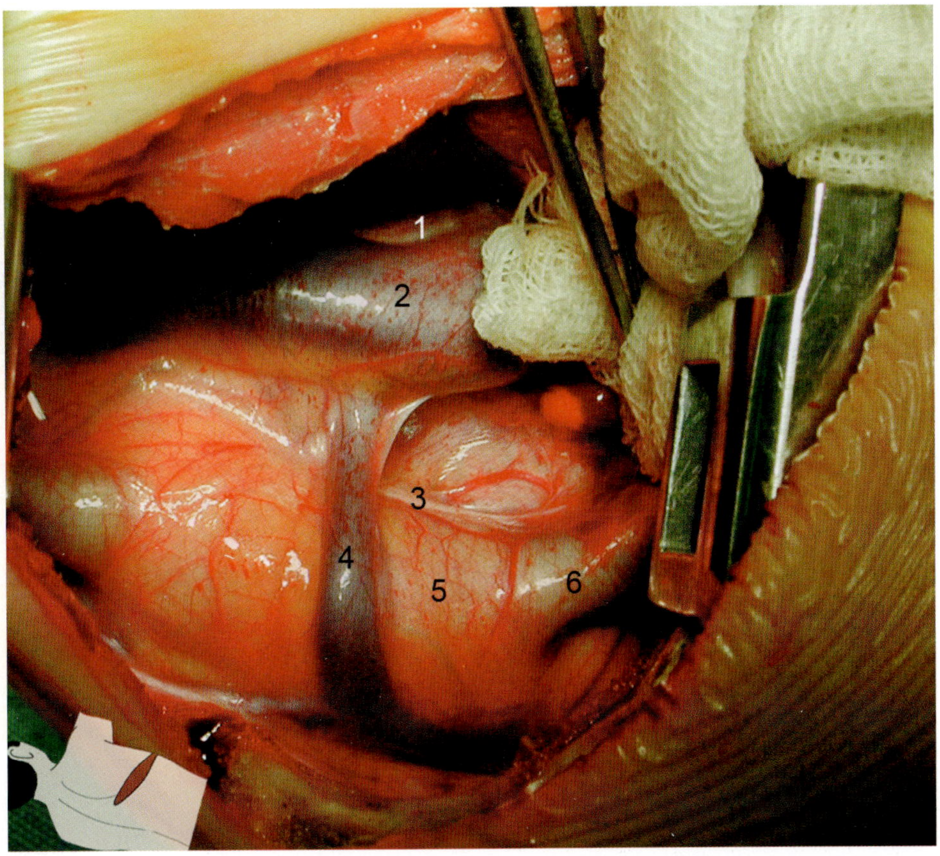

Figure 1.18. A right thoracotomy view of 9-month-old infant with PA/VSD and aortopulmonary collateral arteries. This patient has a right aortic arch, and the descending aorta is seen here on the right aspect of the posterior mediastinum.

1. Right phrenic nerve
2. SVC
3. Right vagus nerve
4. Azygos vein
5. Descending thoracic aorta
6. Aortopulmonary collateral artery

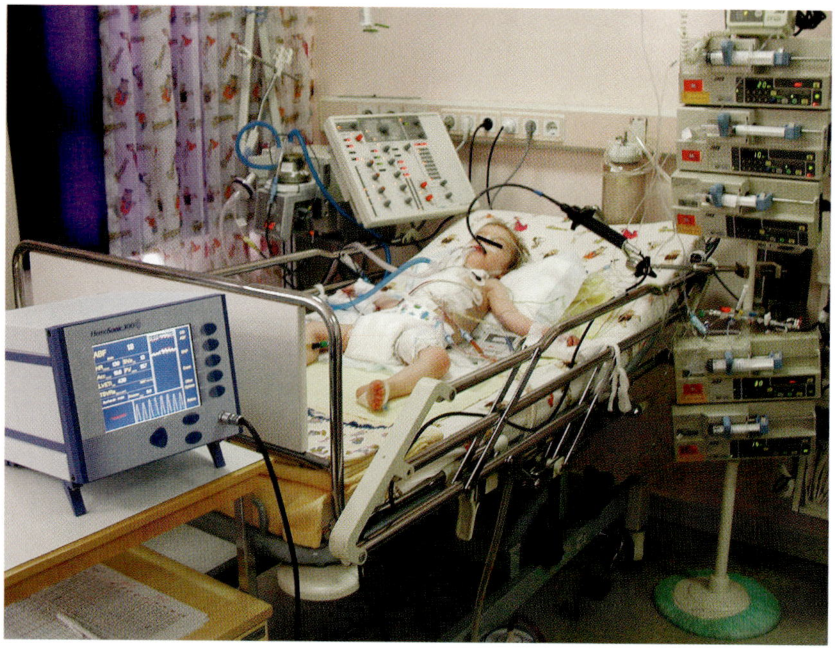

Figure 1.19. A postoperative cardiac patient in the pediatric cardiac ICU. The child is connected to various infusion pumps, invasive and noninvasive monitors, drains, and a mechanical ventilator. The patient is fitted with a transesophageal cardiac output hemodynamic monitor.

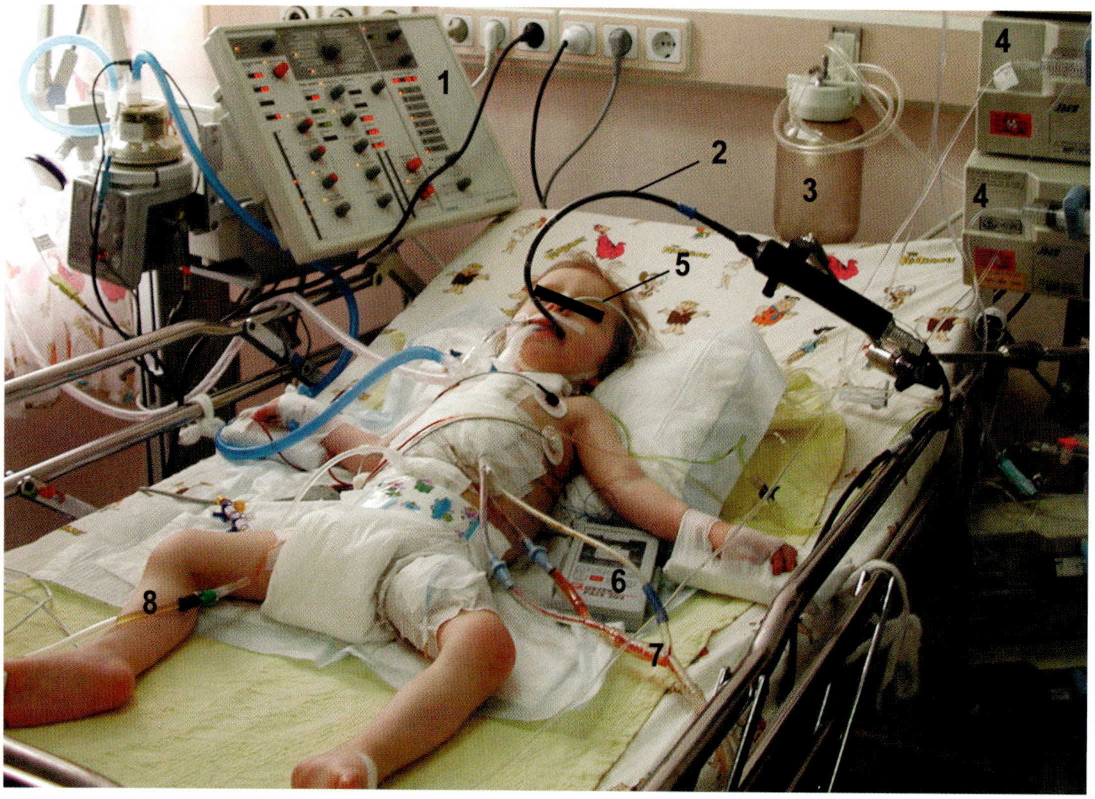

Figure 1.20. A close-up view of the same child shown in Figure 1.19.

1. Mechanical ventilator
2. Transeophageal probe
3. Suction apparatus
4. Intravenous infusion pumps
5. Nasogastric tube
6. Temporary pacemaker
7. Chest tube drains
8. Urinary catheter

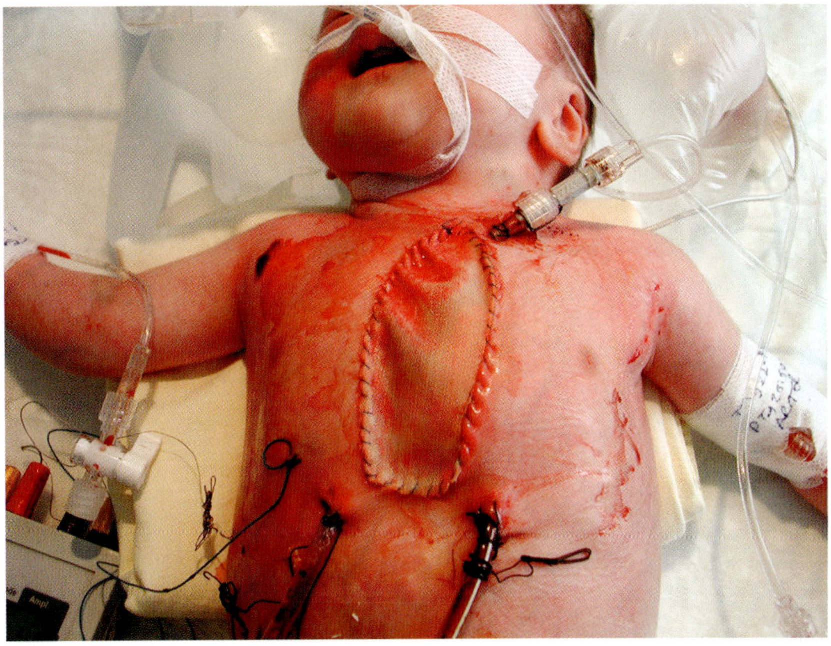

Figure 1.21. A postoperative cardiac patient, with open sternum, in the cardiac ICU. The sternal bone is left open, and the wound is covered with a piece of Dacron. The patient is connected to invasive monitors, temporary epicardial pacemaker, chest drains, and endotracheal tube.

REFERENCES

1. Gross RE, Hubbard JP. Surgical ligation of a patent ductus arteriosus. A report of first successful case. *JAMA*. 1939;112:729–731.
2. Blalock A, Taussig HB. The surgical treatment of malformations of the heart in which there is pulmonary stenosis or pulmonary atresia. *JAMA*. 1945;128:189–192.
3. Gibbon JH Jr. Application of a mechanical heart and lung apparatus to cardiac surgery. *Minn Med*. 1954;37:171–185.
4. Marino BS, Tomlinson RS, Drotar D. Quality-of-life concerns differ among patients, parents, and medical providers in children and adolescents with congenital and acquired heart disease. *Pediatrics*. 2009; 123:e708–e715.

CHAPTER 2

Ventricular Septal Defect

Ventricular septal defect (VSD) is one of the most common congenital heart defects (second only to bicuspid aortic valve).[1] The ventricular septum is a complex three-dimensional (3D) structure that can be broadly divided into 4 parts for the purpose of localizing defects: inlet, trabecular muscular, outlet, and membranous (Figure 2.1A and B). Defects in and around the membranous area are the most common.[2]

Diagnosis of VSD is often made in early infancy because of its distinctive murmur, which leads to echocardiography, the diagnostic tool. Symptomatic patients are treated initially with anticongestive medications.

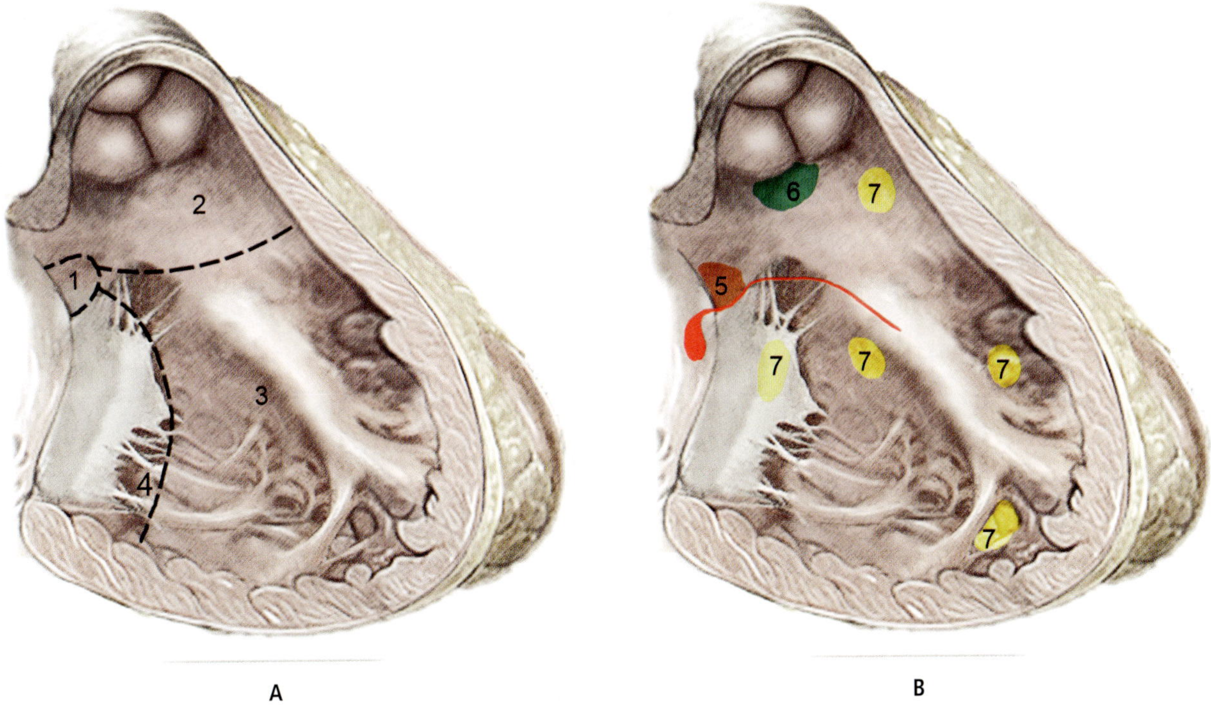

Figure 2.1. A: Schematic diagrams of the interventricular septum viewed from the right ventricular (RV) aspect. The RV can be considered as having 3 portions. **Panel B** shows the common locations of the septal defects and their relationship to the conduction system, the membranous septum, and the muscular septum.

1. Membranous septum
2. Outlet
3. Trabecular
4. Inlet
5. Perimembranous defect
6. Doubly committed/juxtaarterial defect
7. Muscular defects

For some defects, closure can be achieved percutaneously in the catheterization laboratory. Overall, only a minority of VSDs that come to medical attention will require surgical intervention.

Surgical repair is performed through a median sternotomy on cardiopulmonary bypass. The majority of defects are accessible through a right atriotomy. Most commonly, knitted Dacron velour is used, sutured in place using mattress suture with Teflon pledgets. Other techniques include using a Gore-Tex patch, usually with continuous sutures, and, rarely, primary suturing of the edges of the VSD.

PERIMEMBRANOUS DEFECTS

A perimembranous VSD is in the membranous area involving also the surrounding muscular septum, and may extend to parts of the ventricular septum corresponding to the inlet, trabecular, or outlet portions of the RV. The defect is in contact with the tricuspid and aortic valves, usually at the fibrous remnant of the membranous septum, and the leaflets of these valves may attach to, or protrude through, the defect.

Figure 2.2 shows the operative field in a 1-year-old child operated on for closure of a perimembranous VSD. Figure 2.3 is a close-up view of the VSD. Spontaneous closure is common; Figure 2.4 shows an attempt at spontaneous closure by fibrous tissue formation. Another mechanism of spontaneous closure is by accessory tissue from the tricuspid valve. Figures 2.5 and 2.6 are from a 4-month-old infant with a perimembranous VSD extending to the outlet septum. Various degrees of prolapse of aortic valve leaflets through the defect are not uncommon (Figures 2.7 and 2.8).

Subaortic membrane with left ventricular (LV) outflow obstruction is another complication of perimembranous defects (Figures 2.9–2.11). Another example of subaortic membrane is shown in Figure 2.12, along with posterior malalignment of the outlet septum. More examples of subaortic membranes are shown in chapter 19. Double-chambered RV occasionally develops as a complication of VSD. In this condition, anomalous muscle bundles divide the RV cavity into a proximal inflow part and a distal outflow part. In Figures 2.13 and 2.14, the VSD is seen opening into the proximal part of a double-chambered RV. Another example of a double-chambered RV is shown in Figure 2.15.

Figures 2.16 to 2.18 show placement of Teflon on the contralateral aspect of the tricuspid valve, and sutures are passed through the tricuspid septal leaflet.

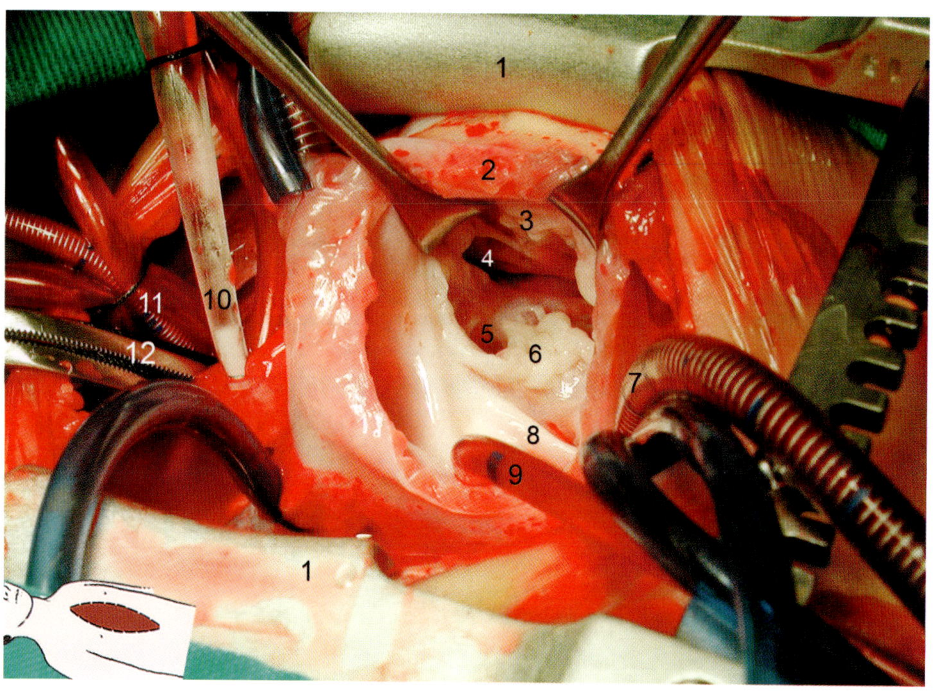

Figure 2.2. Operative field in a 1-year-old child operated on for closure of a perimembranous VSD.

1. Sternal retractor
2. Right atrial wall
3. Anterior leaflet of tricuspid valve
4. Right ventricular outflow tract (RVOT)
5. VSD
6. Septal leaflet of tricuspid valve
7. Inferior vena cava (IVC) venous cannula
8. Tendon of Todaro
9. Suction catheter going to foramen ovale
10. Cardioplegia catheter
11. Aortic cannula
12. Aortic cross-clamp

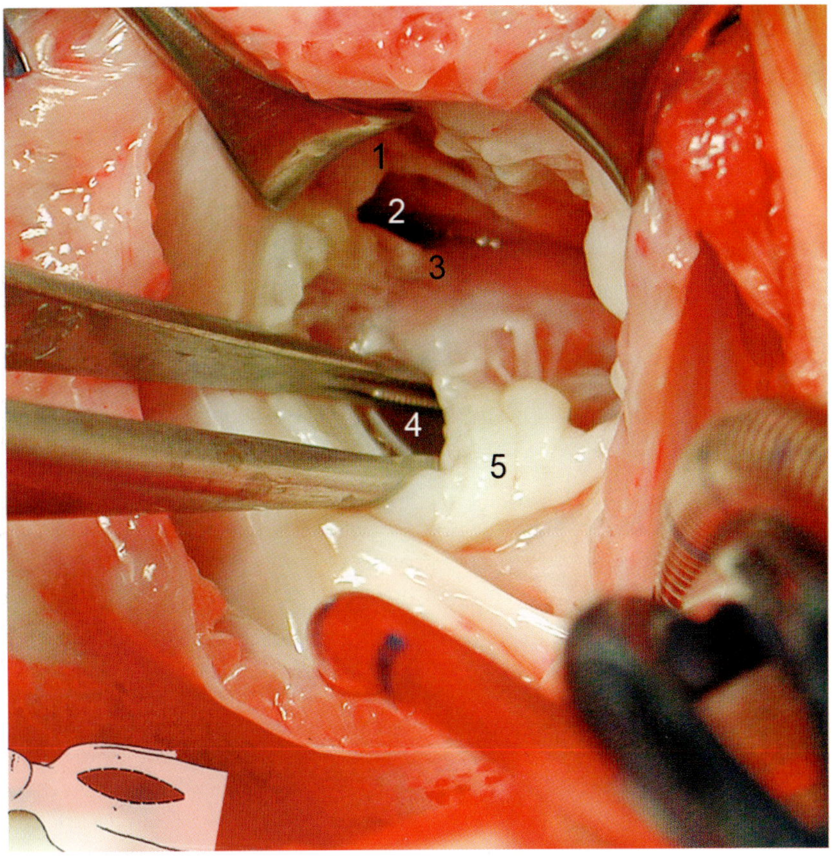

Figure 2.3. Close-up view of the VSD in the same patient shown in Figure 2.2. A pair of forceps is passed through the VSD (4).

1. Anterior leaflet of tricuspid valve
2. RVOT
3. Outlet septum
4. VSD
5. Septal leaflet of tricuspid valve

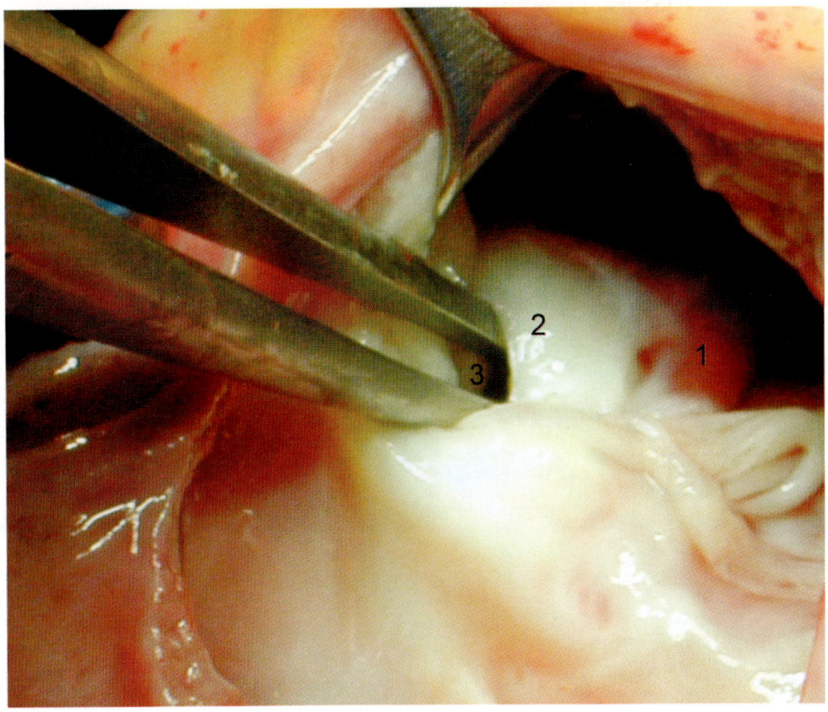

Figure 2.4. A perimembranous VSD with outlet extension in a 6-year-old child seen through a right atriotomy. Notice the fibrous tissue formation at the margin of the defect, which represents an attempt at spontaneous closure.

1. Muscular septum
2. Fibrous tissue formation
3. VSD

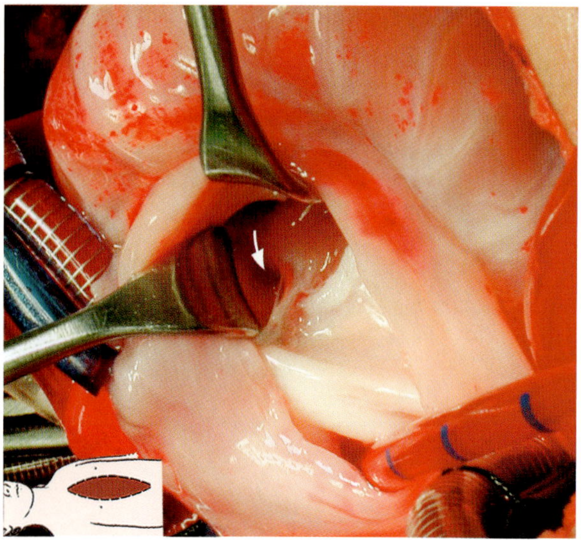

Figure 2.5

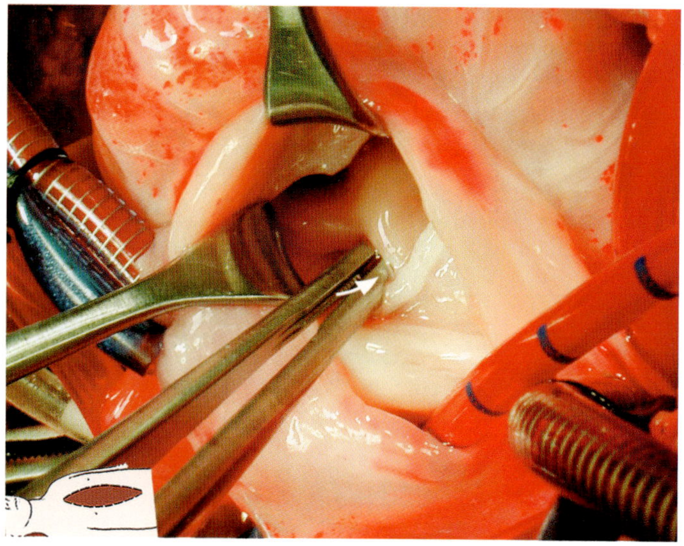

Figure 2.6

A perimembranous VSD with outlet extension in a 4-month-old child. The arrow points to the VSD, which is probed in Figure 2.6 by forceps. This is a large VSD, the extent of which is not well seen because of tricuspid valve leaflet attachment.

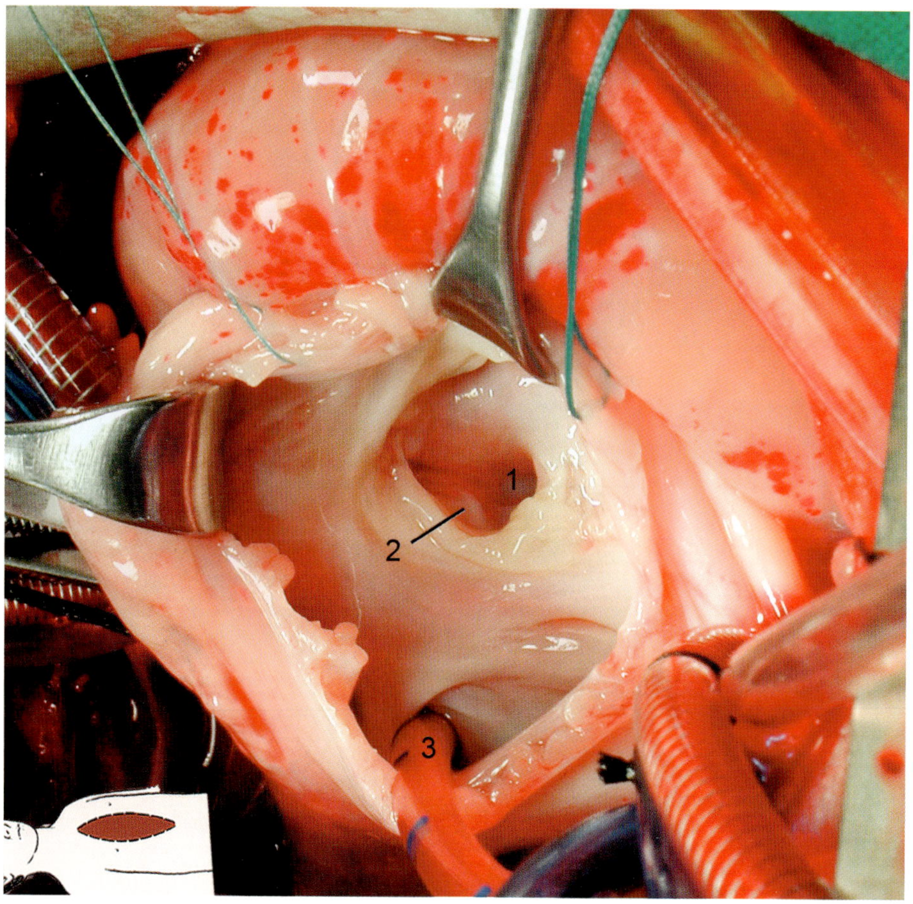

Figure 2.7. A large perimembranous VSD extending to the outlet septum as seen through right atriotomy in a 4-month-old infant. Aortic valve leaflet is seen through VSD. The defect was closed with a Dacron patch (not shown).

1. VSD
2. Aortic valve leaflet
3. Suction catheter draining left atrium through foramen ovale

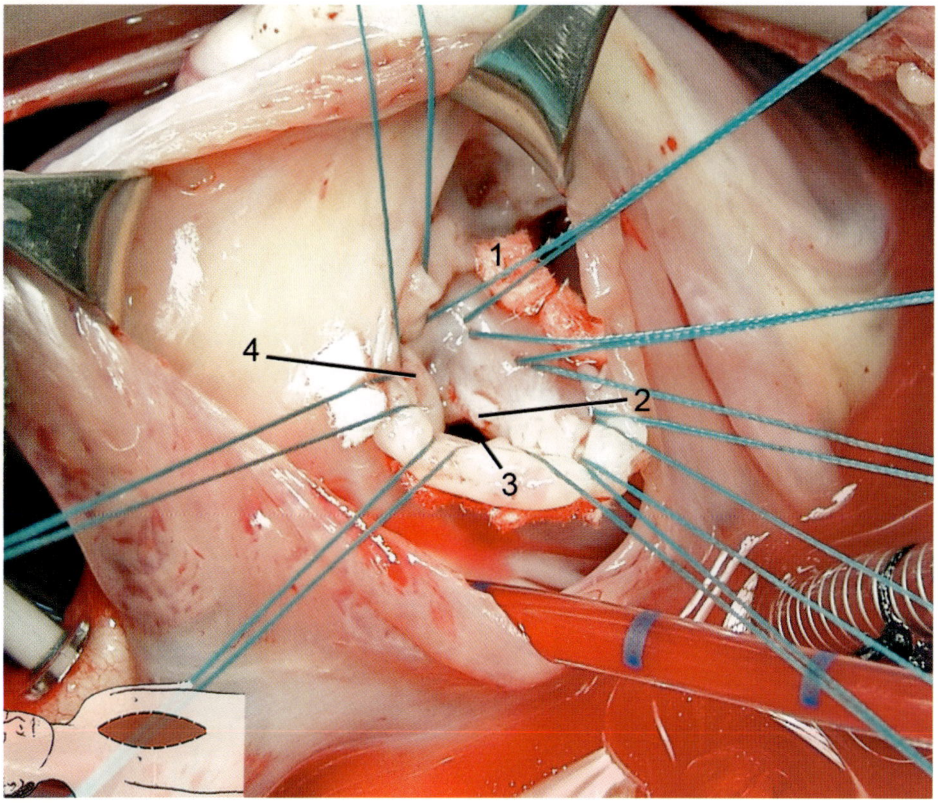

Figure 2.8. A perimembranous VSD in a 9-month-old infant as seen through right atriotomy. Notice the prolapsed aortic valve leaflet. Fibrous tissue is seen at the lower margin of the VSD, which makes a subaortic membrane. Pledgeted mattress sutures have been placed around the defect and through the septal leaflet of tricuspid valve.

1. Teflon pledget
2. Subaortic membrane, visible through VSD
3. VSD
4. Prolapsed aortic valve leaflet

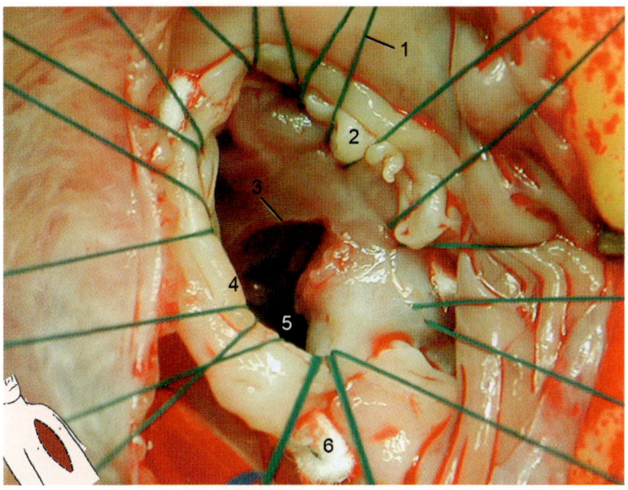

Figure 2.9

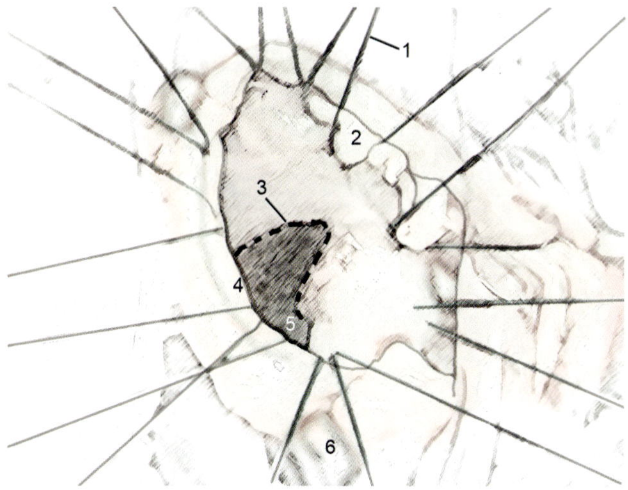

Figure 2.10

Right atriotomy view of a 3-year-old infant with a large perimembranous VSD complicated by a discrete subaortic membrane. The edges (3) of the resected membrane are shown. Pledgets have been placed around the margin of the VSD in preparation for patch closure.

1. Mattress suture
2. Anterior tricuspid valve leaflet
3. Edge of resected subaortic membrane
4. Septal tricuspid valve leaflet
5. VSD
6. Teflon pledget

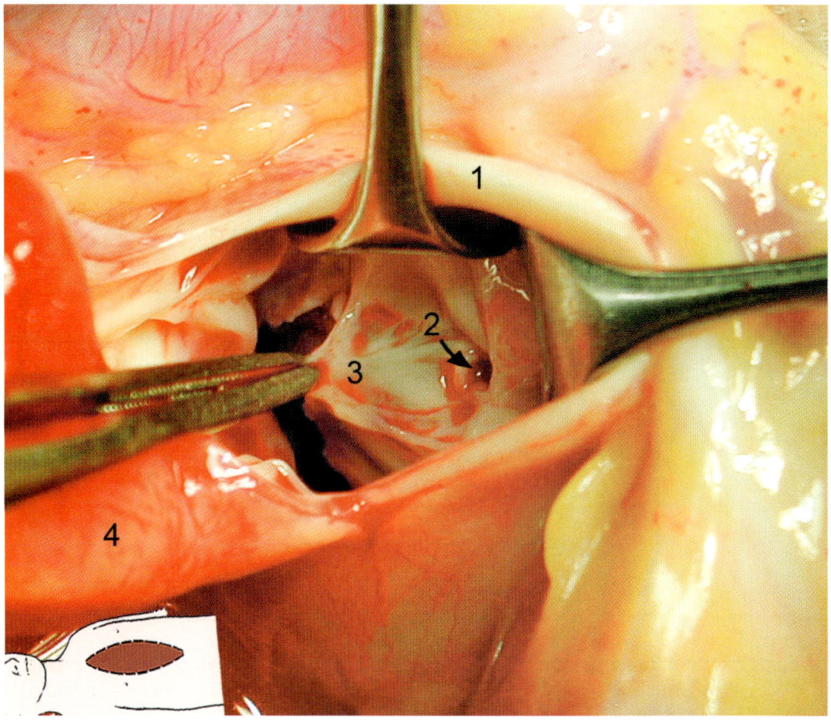

Figure 2.11. A perimembranous/outlet VSD in a 13-year-old child as seen through transverse aortotomy. A subaortic membrane is seen as a shelf in the left ventricular outflow tract (LVOT).

1. Transverse aortotomy
2. VSD
3. Subaortic membrane
4. Ascending aorta

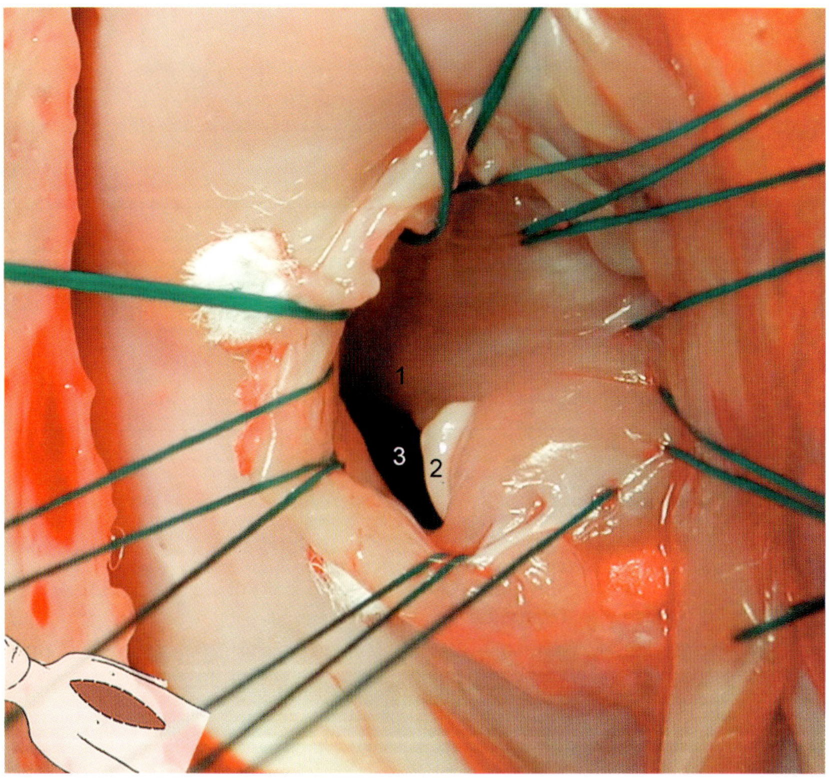

Figure 2.12. Right atriotomy view of a large perimembranous defect extending to the outlet portion. On the LV side, there is a discrete subaortic membrane, part of which (2) is seen at the edge of the VSD. The outlet septum in this patient was malaligned, deviating to the left and posteriorly.

1. Outlet septum
2. Subaortic membrane
3. VSD

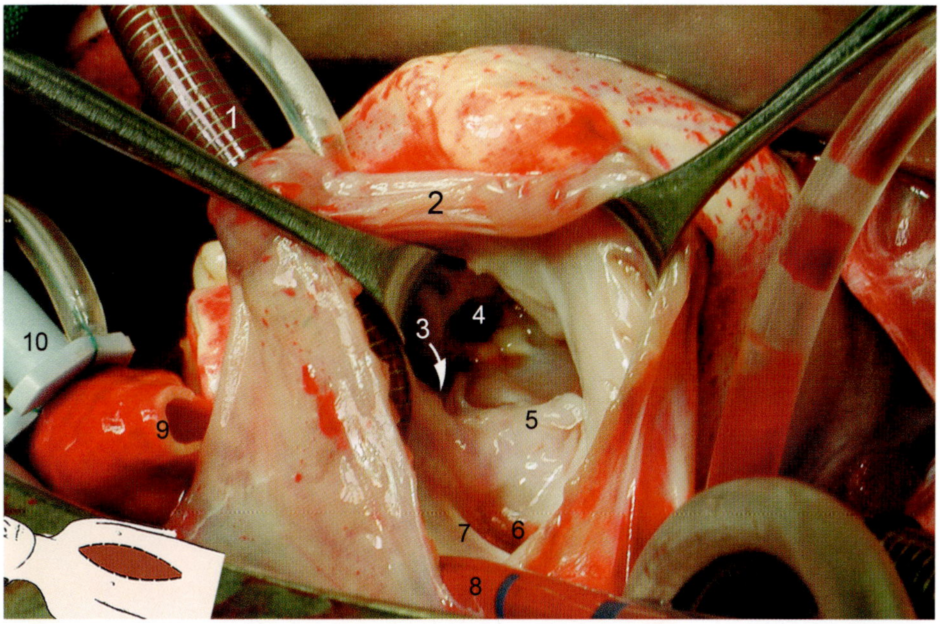

Figure 2.13. Right atriotomy view of a perimembranous VSD and double-chambered RV. The VSD opens proximal to the obstructing muscle bundles at the infundibular os (4). This patient also had a subaortic membrane (not shown), for which a transverse aortotomy (9) was performed.

1. Superior vena cava (SVC) cannula
2. Right atriotomy incision
3. VSD
4. Infundibular os
5. Septal leaflet of tricuspid valve
6. Blood pooled at coronary sinus (CS) opening
7. Tendon of Todaro
8. Suction catheter draining left atrium through foramen ovale
9. Transverse aortotomy incision
10. Cardioplegia catheter

Figure 2.14. Same patient as in Figure 2.13. Notice the RVOT obstruction caused by a fibromuscular ring.

1. Infundibular os
2. Fibromuscular ring
3. Septal leaflet of tricuspid valve
4. Forceps passing through VSD

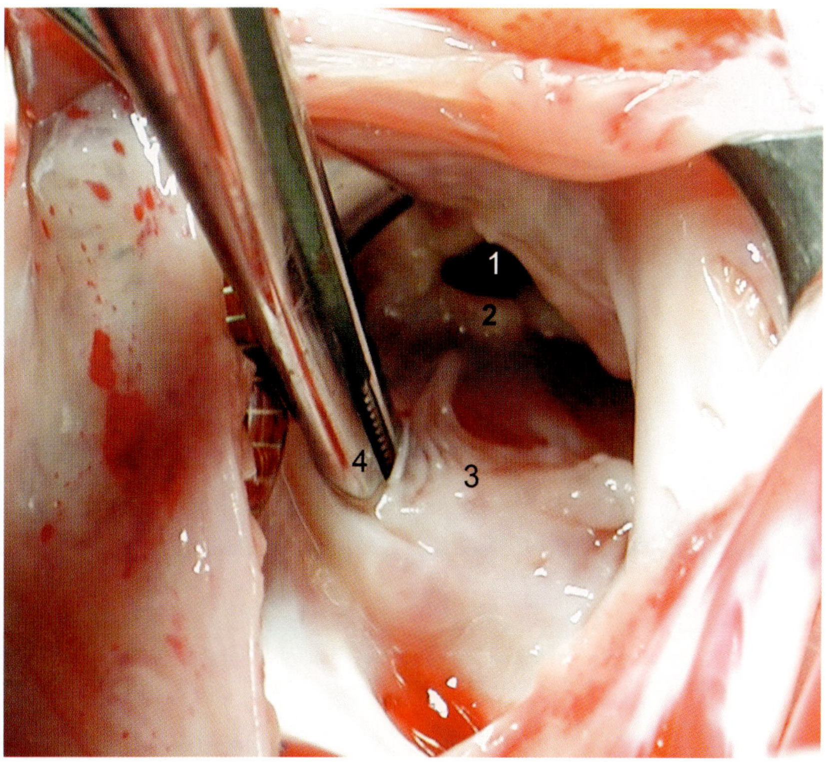

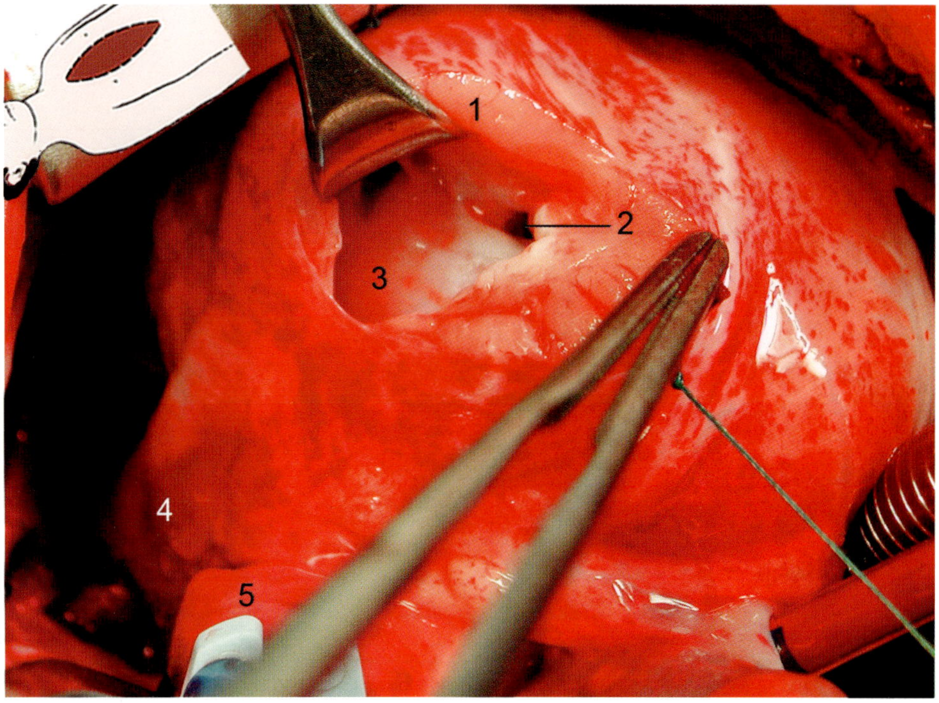

Figure 2.15. Right ventriculotomy view in a 1-year-old infant with VSD and double-chambered RV. The outflow chamber is revealed in this picture. Note the narrow orifice (2) between inlet and outlet portions of the RV.

1. Ventriculotomy incision
2. Orifice between inlet and outlet portions of the RV
3. Outflow (distal) chamber of the RV
4. Main pulmonary artery (MPA)
5. Aorta

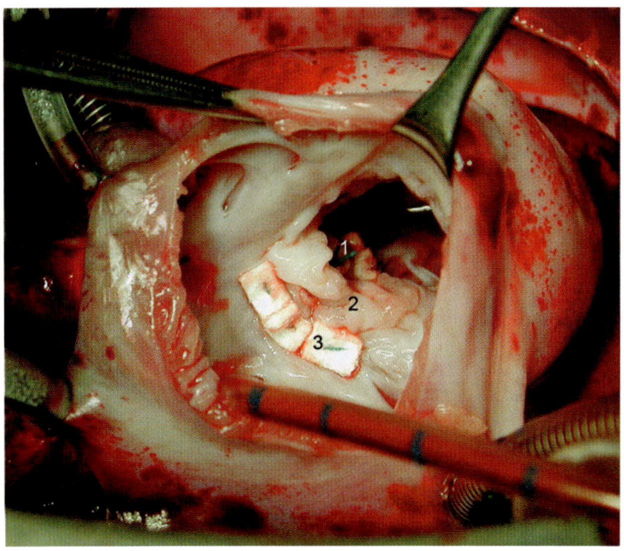

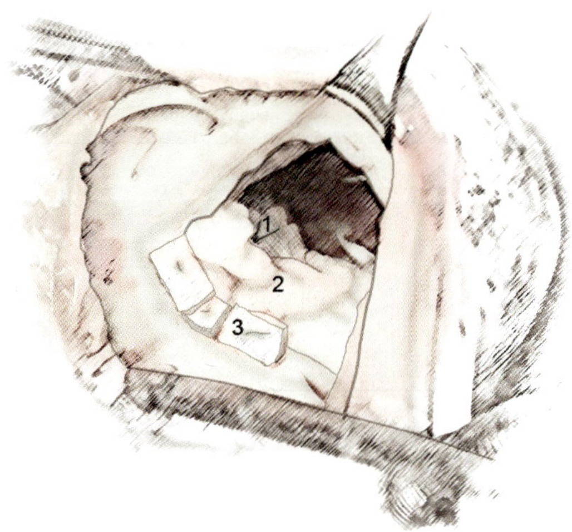

Figure 2.16 **Figure 2.17**

Perimembranous VSD after closure using a Dacron patch and interrupted pledget-supported mattress sutures. Some of the pledgets are placed on the contralateral aspect of the tricuspid valve, and sutures are passed through tricuspid septal leaflet. The Dacron patch and other Teflon pledgets are partly seen beneath the septal leaflet.

1. Dacron patch
2. Septal leaflet of tricuspid valve
3. Teflon pledgets placed across tricuspid valve

Figure 2.18. Schematic drawing showing placement of Teflon pledgets across the tricuspid valve. The other pledgets are placed around the VSD along the dotted line (1), and the free ends of the sutures are passed through the patch, which is then lowered down and the sutures tightened.

1. Outline of where the pledgets will be placed around the VSD
2. VSD
3. Septal leaflet of tricuspid valve
4. Teflon pledgets

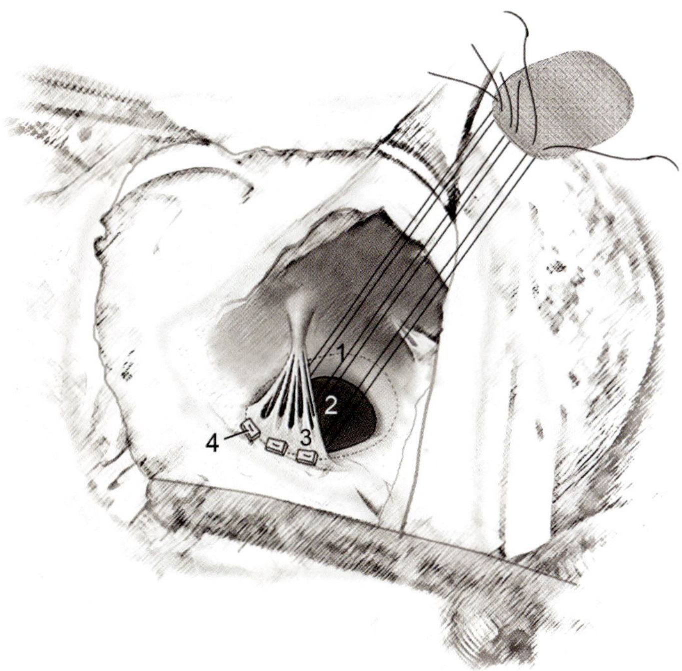

OUTLET DEFECTS

Outlet defects are also called supracristal, doubly committed juxtaarterial, infundibular, and conal defects. Surgical approach is usually through pulmonary arteriotomy. Figure 2.19 shows the surgical field of a median sternotomy and pulmonary arteriotomy in a child with an outlet defect. Figure 2.20 is a close-up of the VSD. Figures 2.21 to 2.26 are other examples of outlet defects closed via pulmonary arteriotomy using knitted Dacron.

An outlet defect can occasionally be accessed via right atriotomy as shown in Figures 2.27 and 2.28.

Rarely a right ventriculotomy may be used to access the defect (Figures 2.29 and 2.30).

Figure 2.19. The operative field setup during surgery for a doubly committed juxtaarterial outlet VSD, as seen through a median sternotomy and pulmonary arteriotomy.

1. Pericardium
2. MPA
3. Pulmonary valve
4. VSD
5. IVC cannula
6. SVC cannula
7. Cardioplegia catheter
8. Aortic cross-clamp
9. Aortic cannula

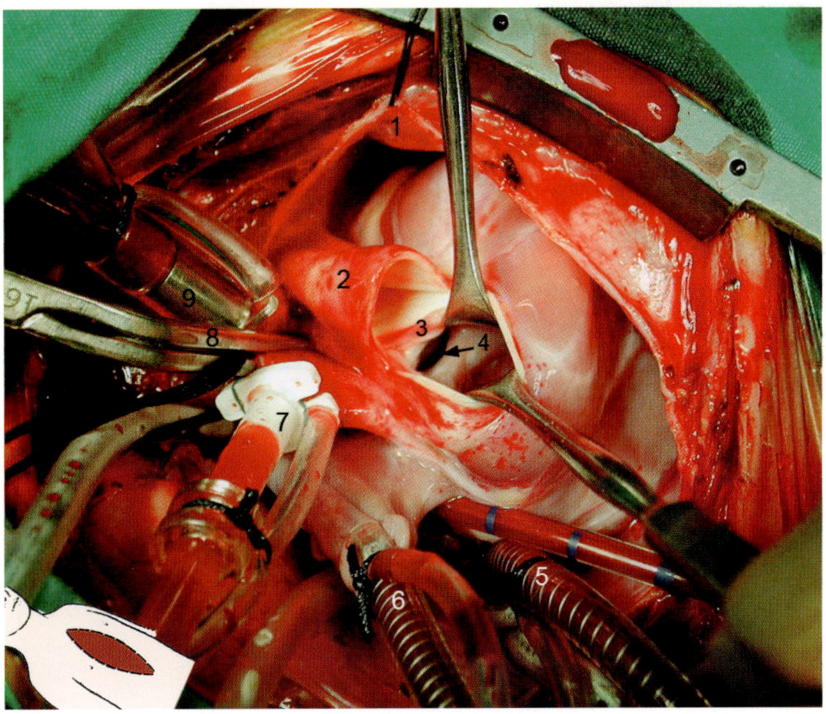

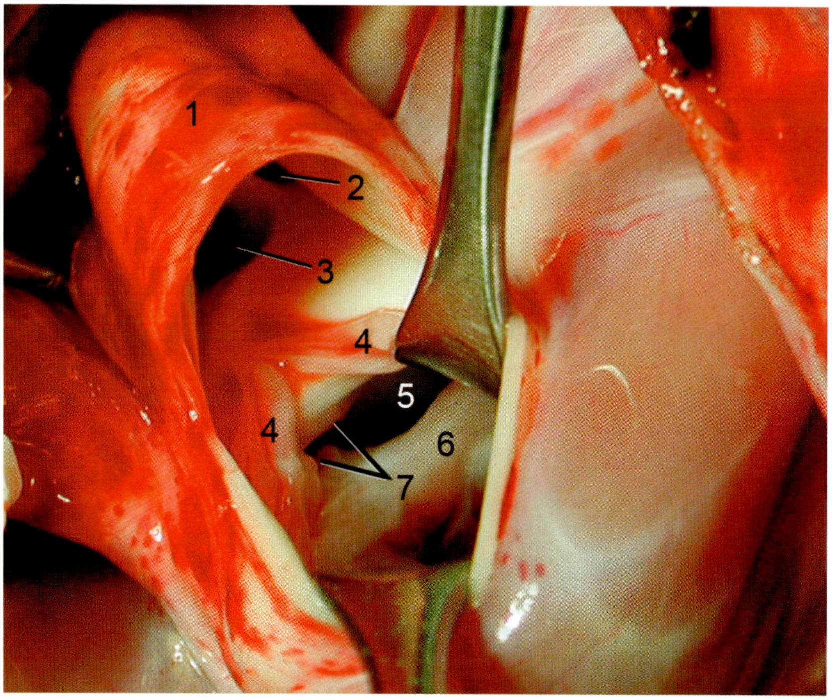

Figure 2.20. Close-up view of the VSD in the patient shown in Figure 2.19. The right and noncoronary aortic leaflets (7) are visible through the defects.

1. MPA
2. Origin of left pulmonary artery
3. Origin of right pulmonary artery
4. Pulmonary valve
5. VSD
6. Crest of ventricular septum
7. Right and noncoronary aortic leaflets

Sinus of Valsalva aneurysm is a rare complication of VSD, and is seen more commonly in adults. The right aortic sinus is most commonly involved.[3] Figures 2.31 to 2.38 are from a 19-year-old patient with an outlet VSD and ruptured sinus of Valsalva aneurysm. The VSD was closed with a Dacron patch through pulmonary arteriotomy, and the prolapsed sac was obliterated by passing the VSD sutures through the base of the aneurysm.

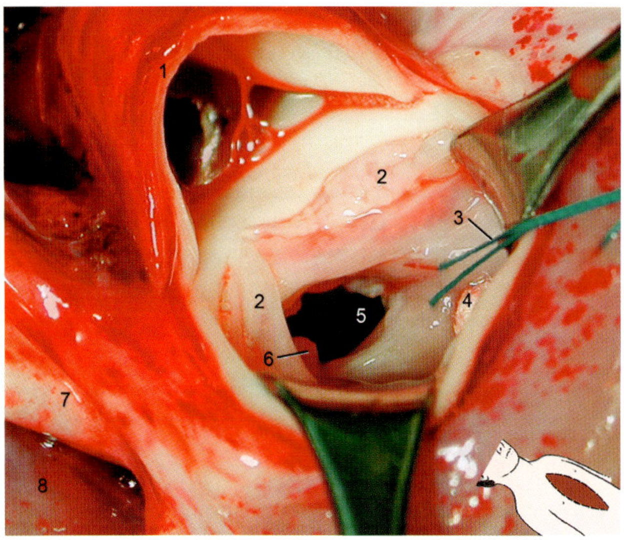

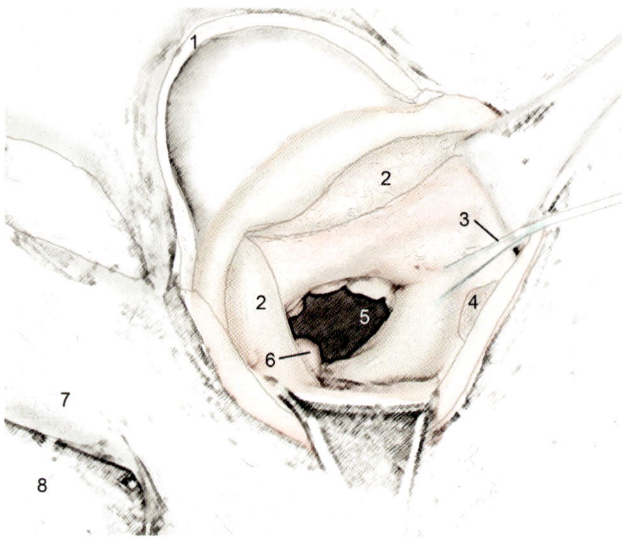

Figure 2.21 **Figure 2.22**

Doubly committed outlet VSD in a 7-month-old infant as seen through transverse pulmonary arteriotomy. Notice the prolapsed aortic valve leaflet (6). The defect was closed using a Dacron patch; its first pledget-supported suture (3) is shown.

1. Pulmonary arteriotomy incision
2. Pulmonary valve leaflet
3. First suture of VSD
4. Teflon pledget
5. VSD
6. Prolapsed aortic valve leaflet
7. Ascending aorta
8. SVC

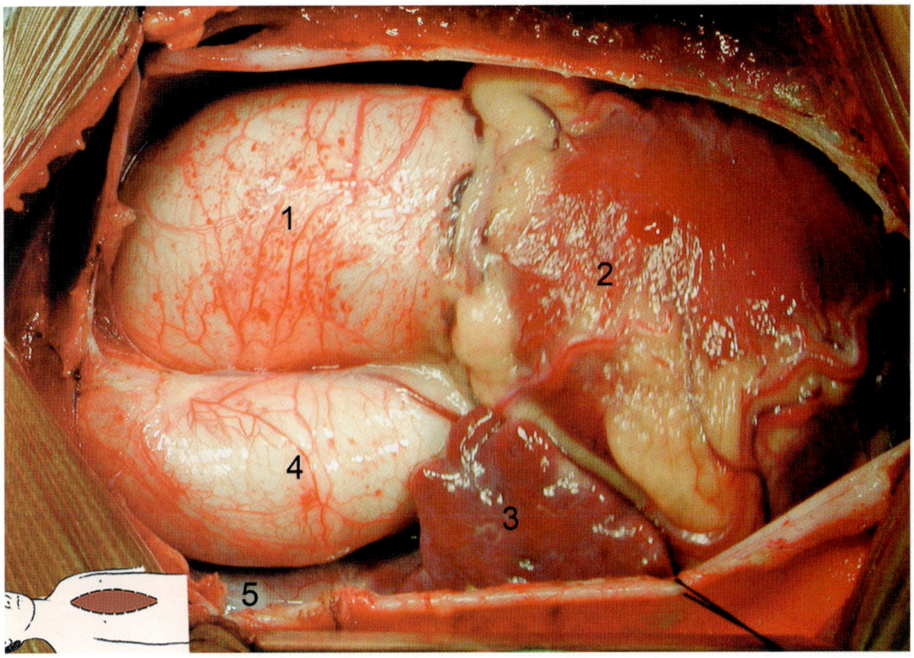

Figure 2.23. Median sternotomy view of a 2-year-old child with an outlet VSD. The pulmonary artery is markedly dilated.

1. MPA
2. RV
3. Right atrial appendage (RAA)
4. Ascending aorta
5. SVC

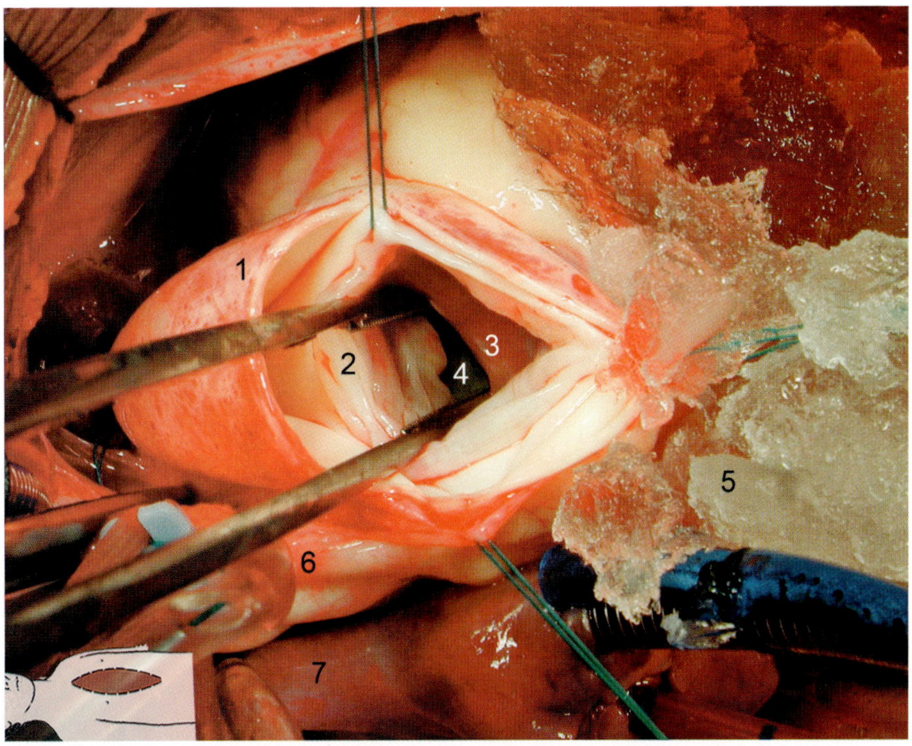

Figure 2.24. Same patient as in Figure 2.23 after pulmonary arteriotomy. Both right and noncoronary aortic cusps are visible through the VSD.

1. MPA
2. Pulmonary valve
3. Crest of ventricular septum
4. VSD
5. Ice used for cooling
6. Ascending aorta
7. SVC

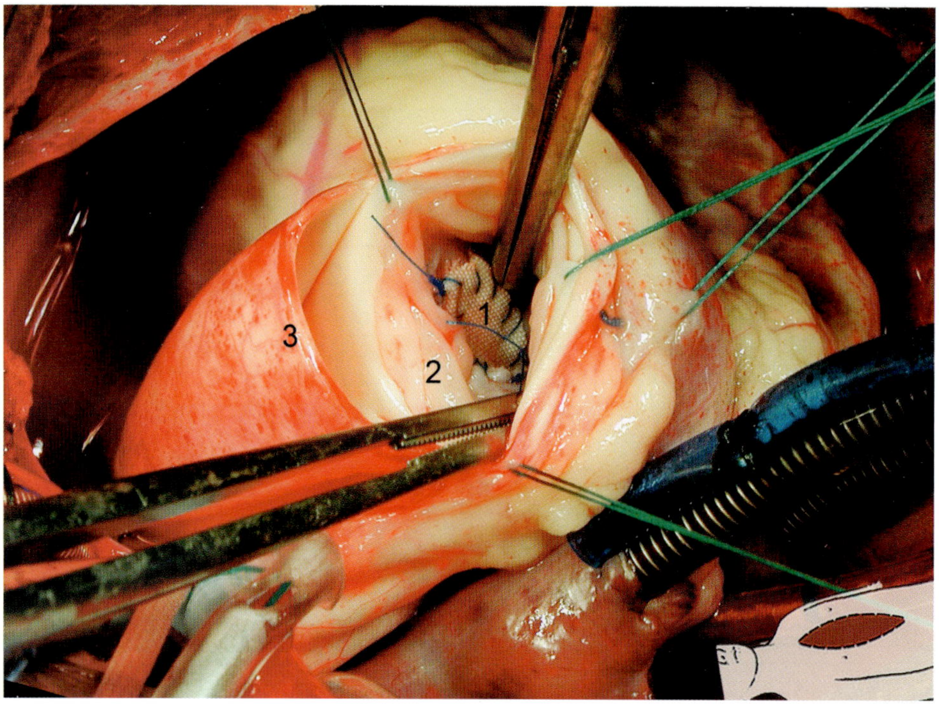

Figure 2.25. Same patient as in Figures 2.23 and 2.24 after closure of the VSD using a knitted Dacron patch and continuous sutures.

1. Dacron patch
2. Pulmonary valve
3. MPA

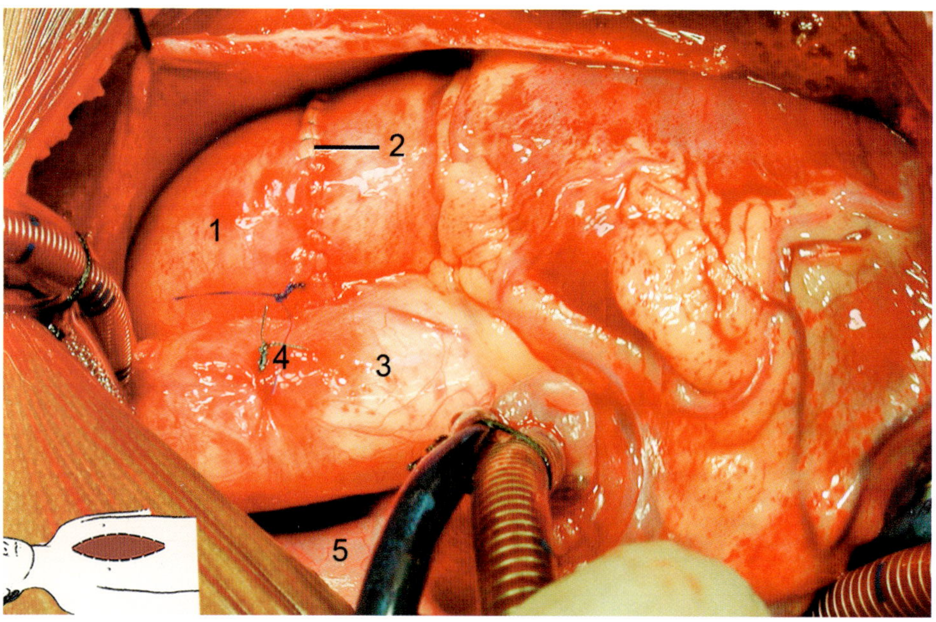

Figure 2.26. Same patient as in Figures 2.23 to 2.25 after repair and closure of pulmonary arteriotomy.

1. MPA
2. Arteriotomy incision closed with continuous sutures
3. Ascending aorta
4. Stitch at site of entry of cardioplegia catheter
5. SVC

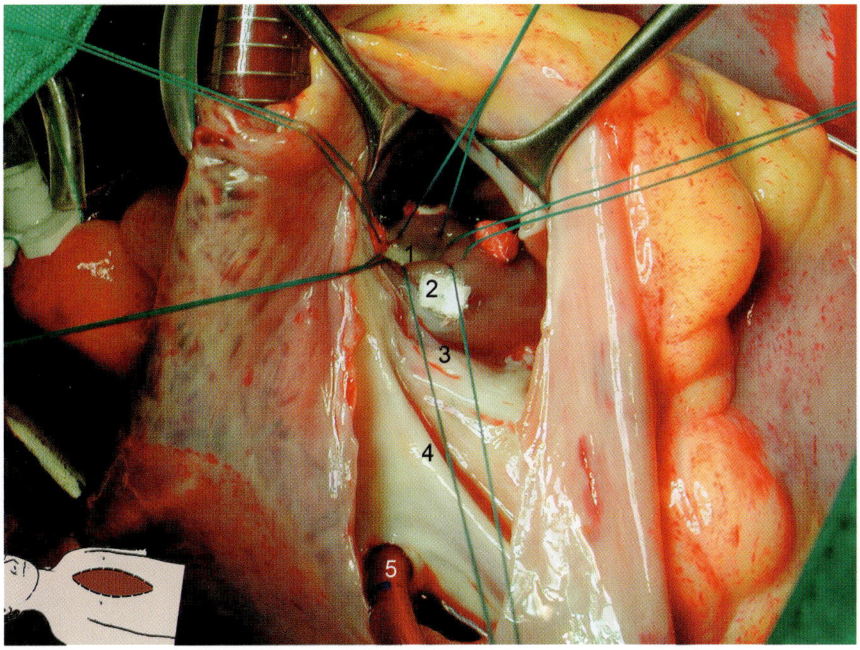

Figure 2.27. An outlet VSD in a 12-year-old child as seen through a right atriotomy.

1. VSD
2. Teflon pledget
3. Septal leaflet of tricuspid valve
4. Tendon of Todaro
5. Catheter in PFO

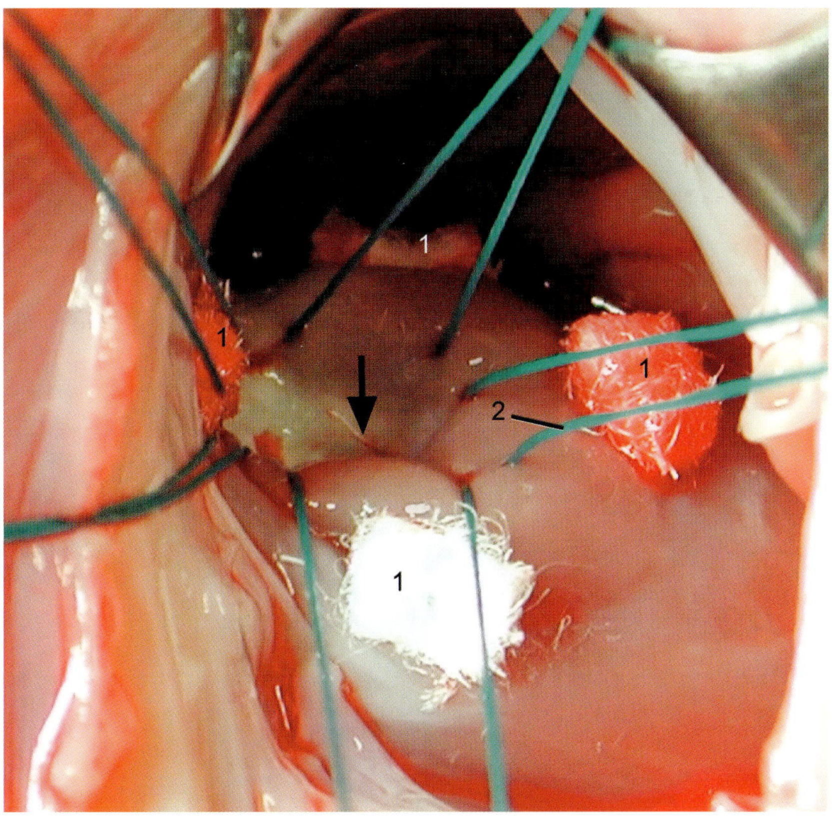

Figure 2.28. Same patient as in Figure 2.27. The arrow points to the VSD. Note that the defect has muscular borders, which makes it a muscular outlet defect.

1. Teflon pledgets placed around the VSD
2. Interrupted mattress sutures

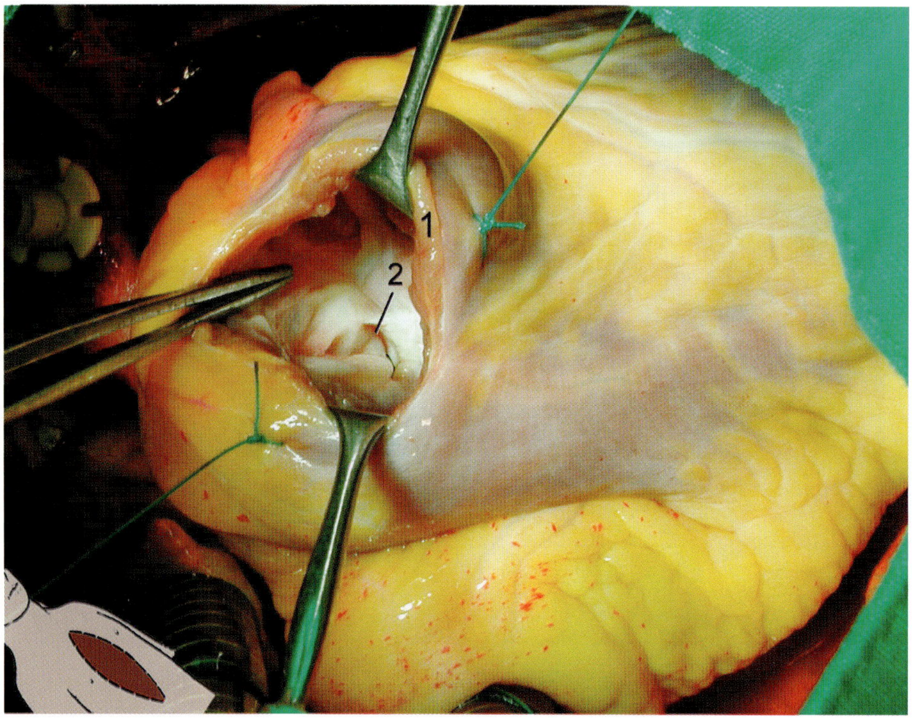

Figure 2.29. An outlet doubly committed juxtaarterial VSD as seen through a right ventriculotomy in a 24-year-old patient. This patient also had aortic regurgitation; aortic valve leaflets are seen prolapsing through the VSD. Note that the defect has no upper muscular margin.

1. Right ventriculotomy
2. VSD

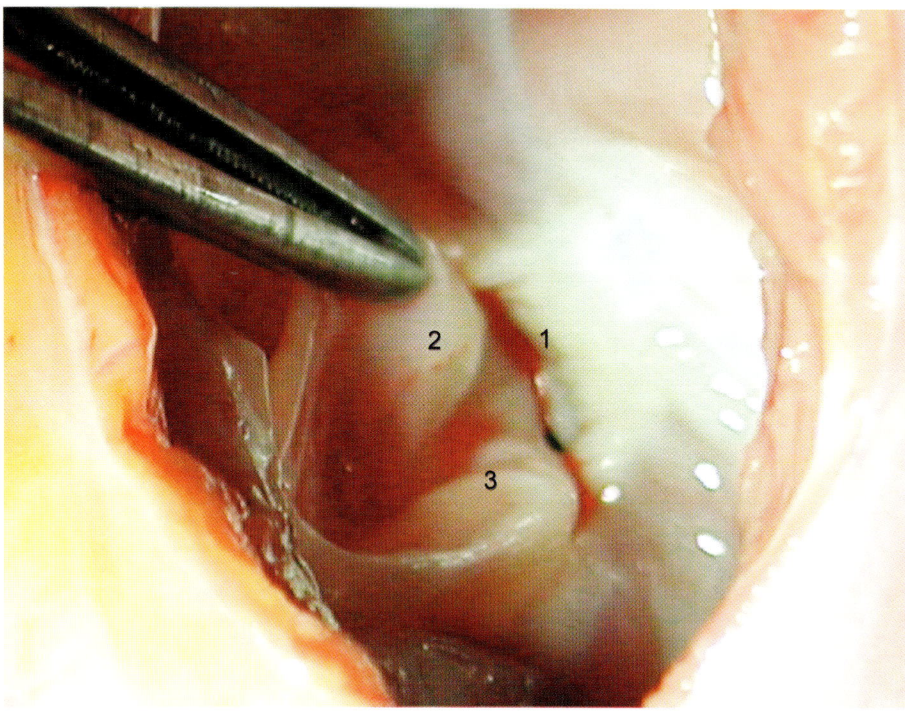

Figure 2.30. Close-up view of the VSD in the same patient shown in Figure 2.29. Notice the prolapsed aortic valve leaflets.

1. Edge of the VSD
2. Right coronary leaflet
3. Noncoronary leaflet

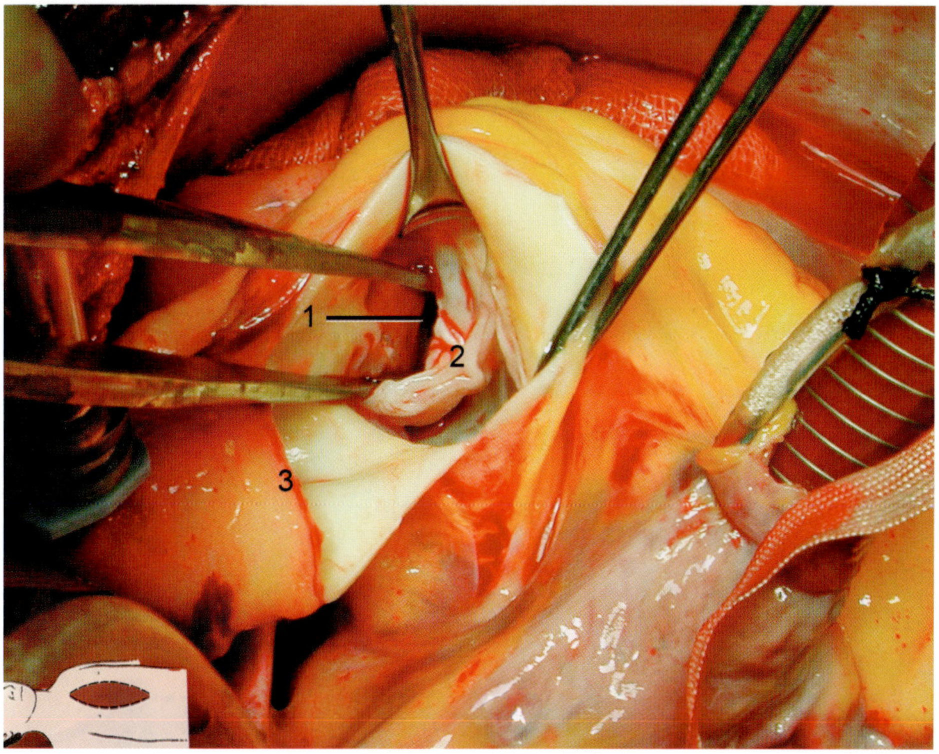

Figure 2.31. Surgical view through an aortotomy in a 19-year-old patient with a sinus of Valsalva aneurysm associated with an outlet VSD (shown in Figure 2.32).

1. Opening of the aneurysm of sinus of Valsalva of right coronary leaflet
2. Right coronary leaflet
3. Aortotomy incision

Figure 2.32. The same patient as in Figure 2.31. The right coronary leaflet is retracted by forceps to reveal a juxtaarterial outlet VSD.

1. Aortotomy incision
2. Opening of the aneurysm of sinus of Valsalva
3. Right coronary leaflet
4. VSD

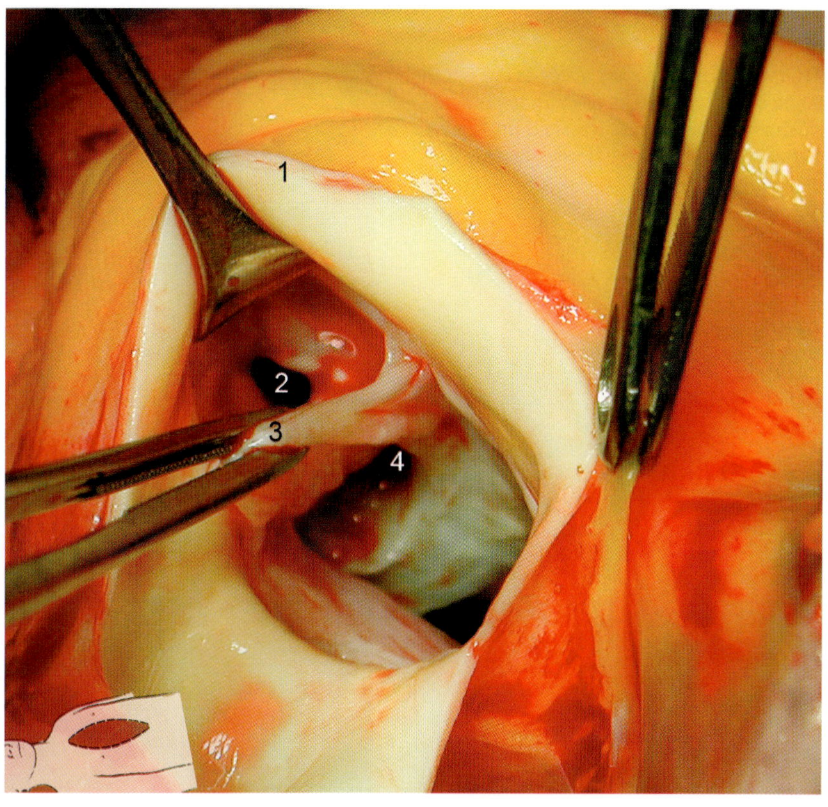

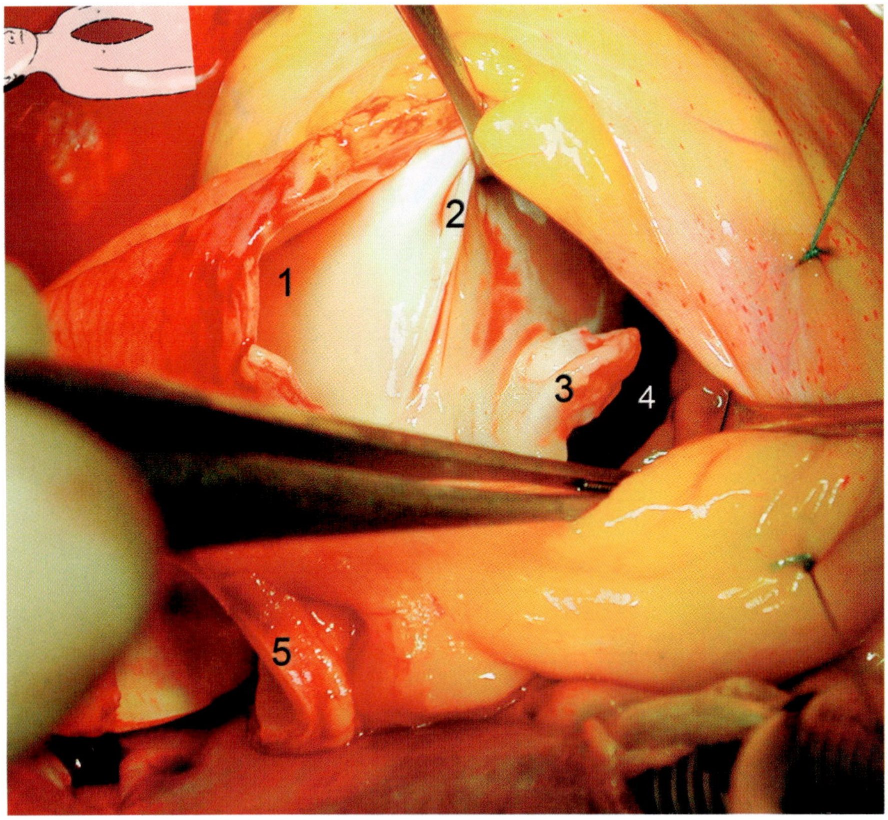

Figure 2.33. The same patient as in Figures 2.31 and 2.32, now viewed through a pulmonary arteriotomy. Notice the windsock appearance of the sinus of Valsalva aneurysm as it protrudes into the RVOT. The VSD lies posterior to the aneurysm (as shown in Figure 2.34).

1. Lumen of MPA
2. Pulmonary valve
3. Sinus of Valsalva aneurysm
4. RVOT
5. Aortotomy incision

Figure 2.34. The same patient as in Figures 2.31 to 2.33, as viewed through pulmonary arteriotomy. The sinus of Valsalva aneurysm is retracted superiorly to show the VSD.

1. Lumen of MPA
2. Pulmonary valve
3. Sinus of Valsalva aneurysm
4. VSD
5. Aortotomy

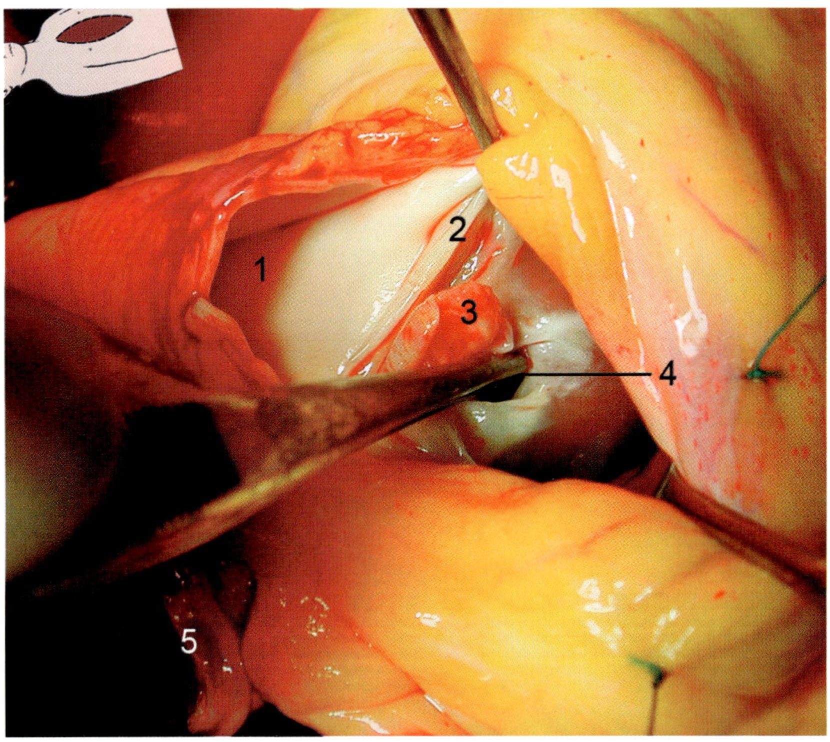

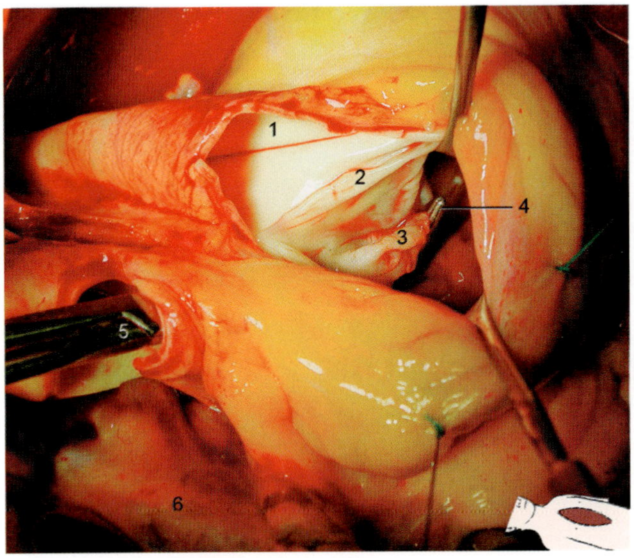

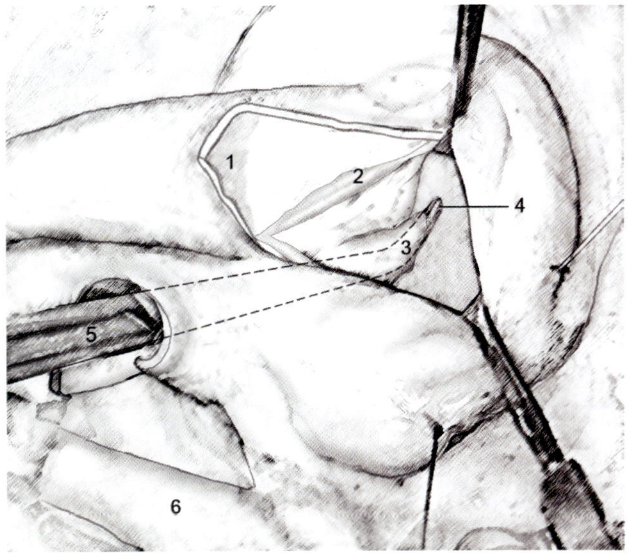

Figure 2.35 **Figure 2.36**

The same patient as in Figures 2.31 to 2.34, with forceps inserted into the aorta and passed through the ruptured sinus of Valsalva into the RVOT.

1. Pulmonary artery
2. Pulmonary valve
3. Sinus of Valsalva aneurysm
4. Tip of forceps
5. Forceps inserted through aortotomy
6. SVC

Figure 2.37. The same patient as in Figures 2.31 to 2.36. Pledget-supported mattress sutures have been placed around the defect and through the base of the aneurysm of sinus of Valsalva. These sutures will be used to close the defect using a Dacron patch.

1. Pulmonary valve
2. Teflon pledget
3. Sinus of Valsalva aneurysm
4. VSD
5. MPA
6. Aortotomy incision

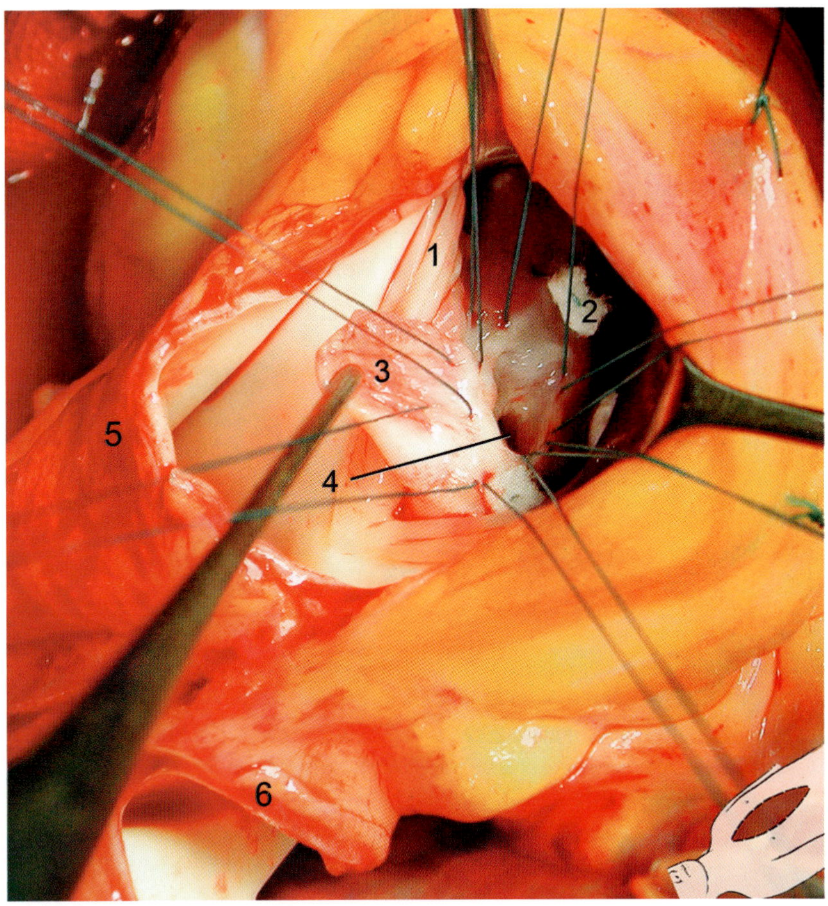

Figure 2.38. The same patient as in Figures 2.31 to 2.37 after repair. The VSD has been closed by a Dacron patch; the sutures have been passed through the base of the aneurysm, effectively obliterating its communication with the aorta.

1. Lumen of MPA
2. Pulmonary valve
3. Sinus of Valsalva aneurysm
4. Dacron patch

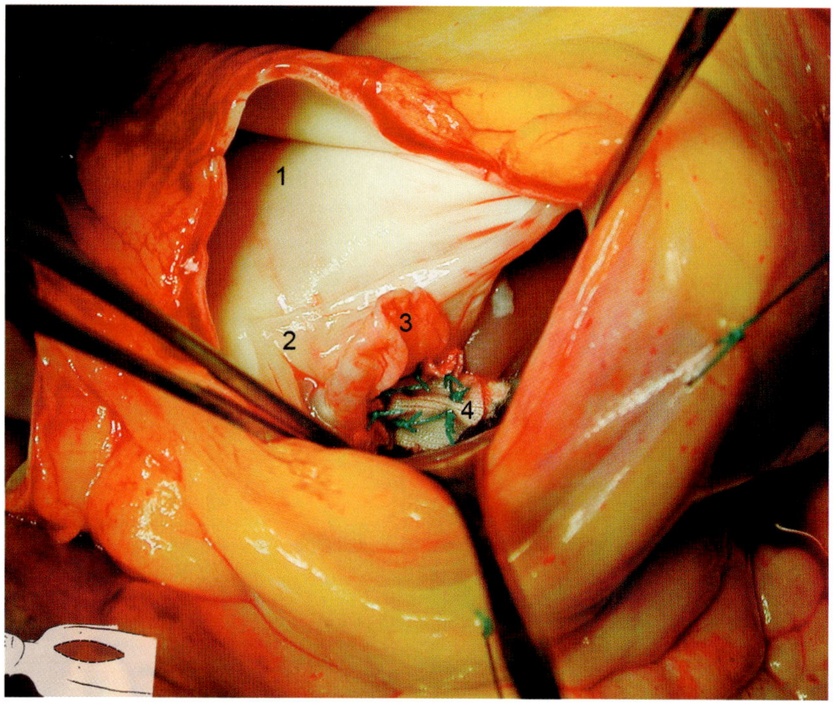

TRABECULAR MUSCULAR DEFECTS

These defects are located within the trabecular muscular septum and may be single or multiple. Most defects can be closed via right atriotomy. Defects close to the apex are particularly difficult to visualize because of the heavily trabeculated nature of the right surface of the ventricular septum.

Muscle bundles often overlie or cross the defect (Figures 2.39–2.41) and may need to be divided to

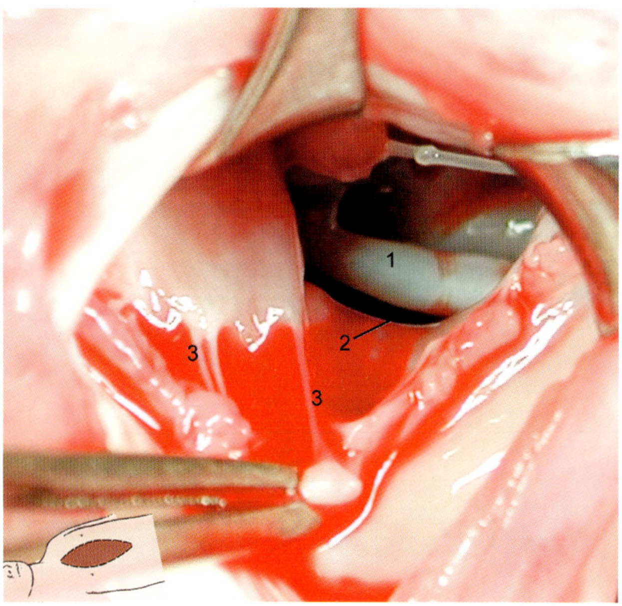

Figure 2.39

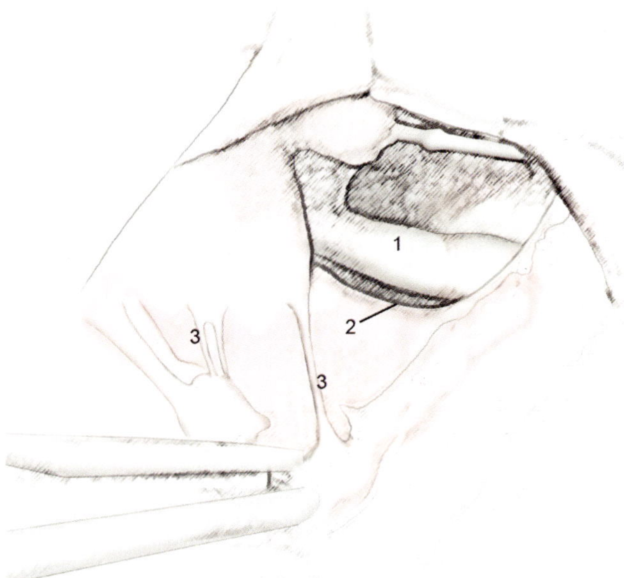

Figure 2.40

Right atriotomy view of large trabecular muscular VSD in a 2-month-old infant. A prominent muscle bundle (1) is seen crossing the defect.

1. Muscle bundle
2. Edge of the VSD
3. Chordal attachment of septal leaflet of tricuspid valve

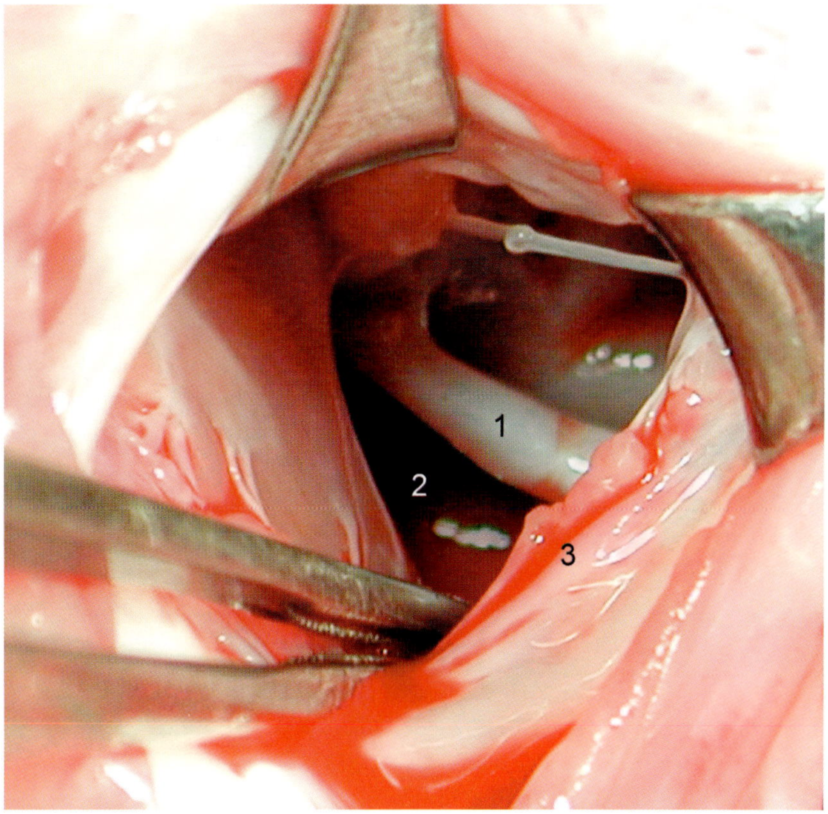

Figure 2.41. The same patient as in Figure 2.39, with the edge of the VSD retracted. The defect was closed with a double velour Dacron patch with continuous sutures (not shown).

1. Muscle bundle
2. VSD
3. Tricuspid valve

facilitate access (Figure 2.45). A defect may be closed using Gore-Tex with continuous sutures or by using double-knitted Dacron and pledget-supported interrupted mattress sutures (Figures 2.42–2.46).

INLET DEFECTS

These defects are located in the inlet part of the muscular septum behind the septal leaflet of the tricuspid valve. Repair is achieved through right atriotomy. The

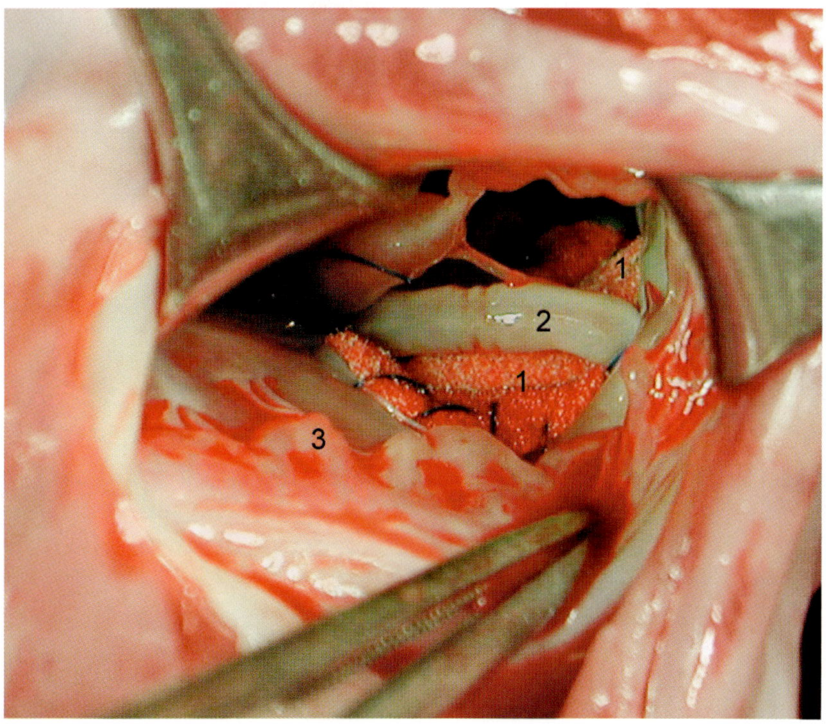

Figure 2.42. The same patient as in Figures 2.39 to 2.41. A Dacron patch has been sewn in place to close the defect.

1. Dacron patch
2. Muscle bundle
3. Tricuspid valve

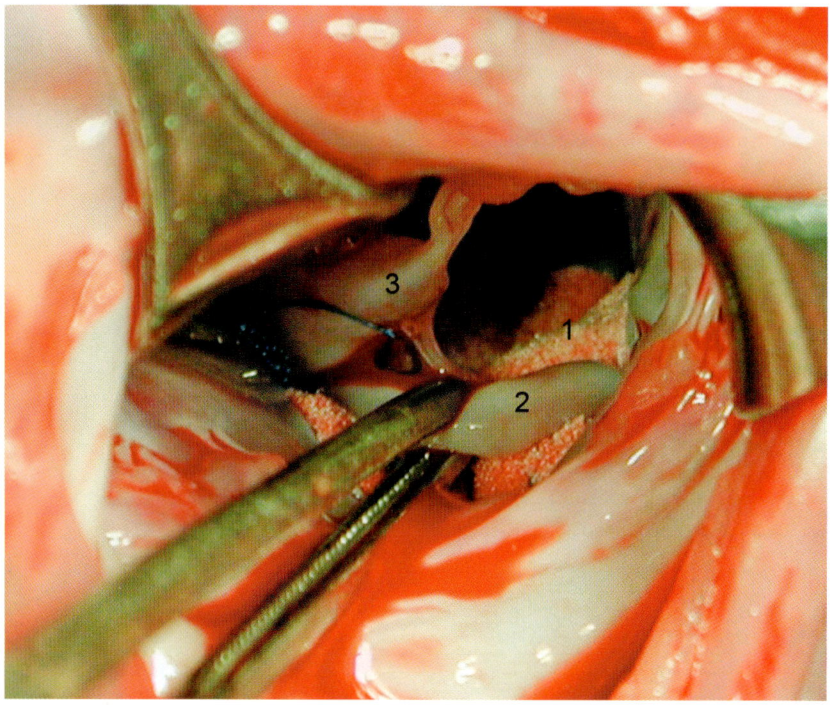

Figure 2.43. The same patient as in Figures 2.39 to 2.42; the muscle bundle is retracted to better show the Dacron patch.

1. Dacron patch
2. Muscle bundle
3. Papillary muscle

septal leaflet may need to be detached to facilitate access.

Figures 2.47 to 2.51 show examples of inlet defects. Tricuspid valve straddling is not uncommon, especially when the defect is juxtatricuspid, hence the designation "canal-type" defects (Figure 2.51). It should be noted that when straddling tricuspid valve is associated with rightward malalignment of

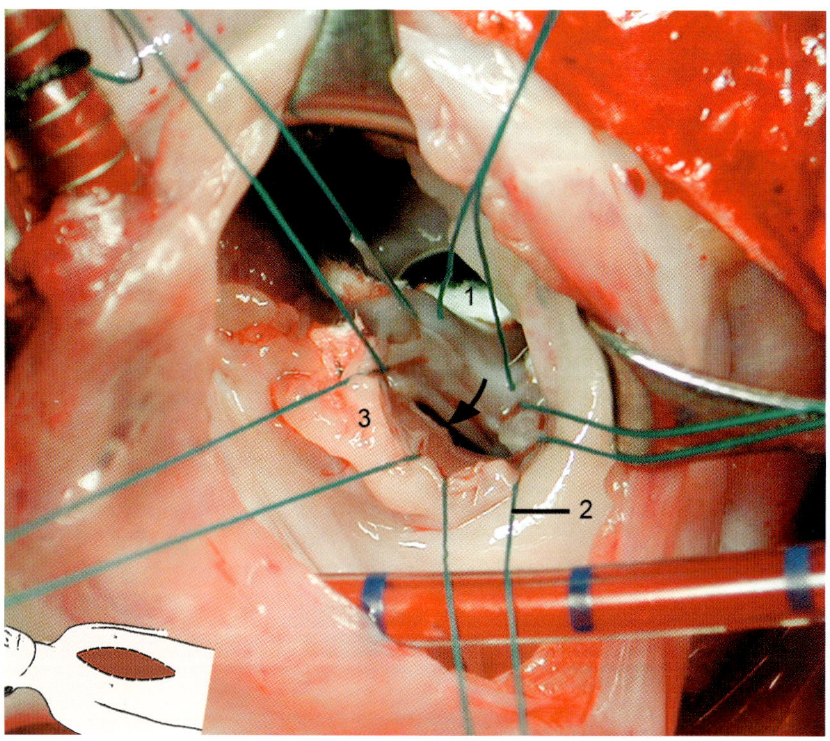

Figure 2.44. A trabecular muscular VSD as seen through a right atriotomy incision in a 10-month-old infant. The arrow points to the defect. Pledget-supported mattress sutures have already been placed around the defect.

1. Teflon pledget
2. VSD suture
3. Tricuspid valve septal leaflet

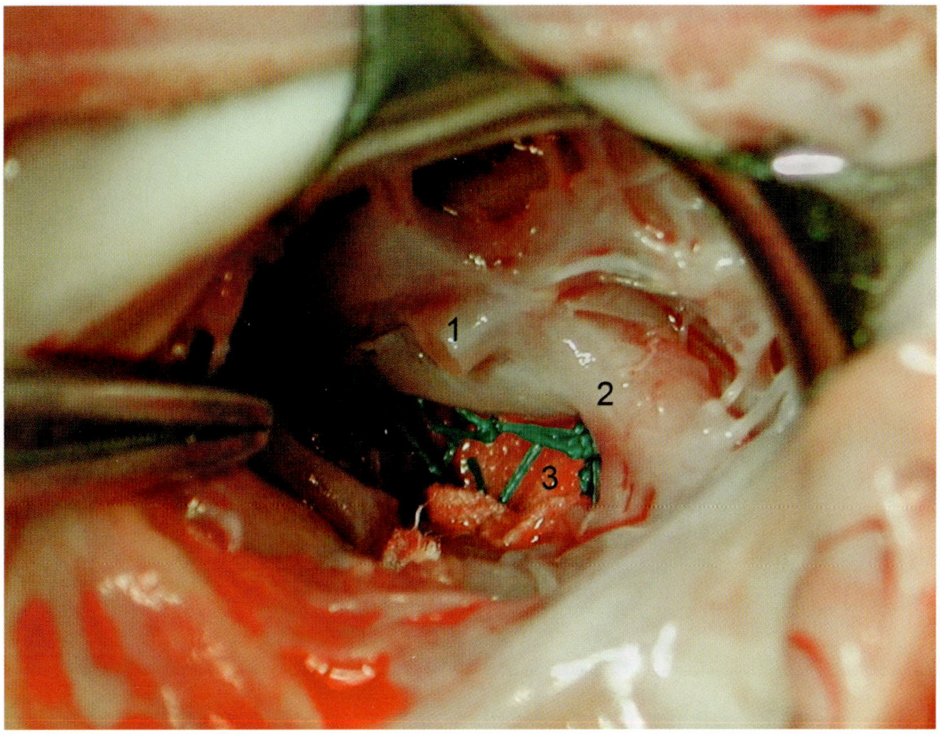

Figure 2.45. Right atriotomy view of a 5-month-old infant with 2 muscular VSDs. The defects have already been closed using a single Dacron patch. Notice that some of the muscle bundles (1) had to be cut to facilitate access to the defects.

1. Transected muscle bundle
2. Moderator band
3. Dacron patch

the ventricular septum, the atrioventricular node and conduction bundle are abnormally located at the site where the displaced septum meets with the atrioventricular junction.

The patient shown in Figures 2.52 to 2.55 illustrate the importance of thorough preoperative evaluation. An inlet VSD was missed on preoperative echocardiography, and the patient required a reoperation.

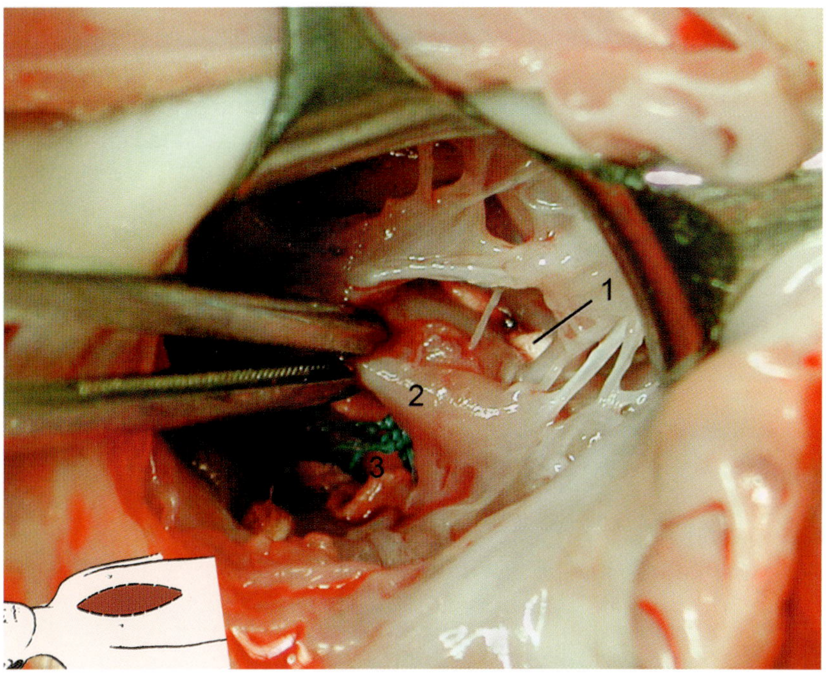

Figure 2.46. The same patient as in Figure 2.45. The moderator band is retracted to show the distal end of the apical end of the patch and Teflon pledgets.

1. Teflon pledget
2. Moderator band
3. Dacron patch

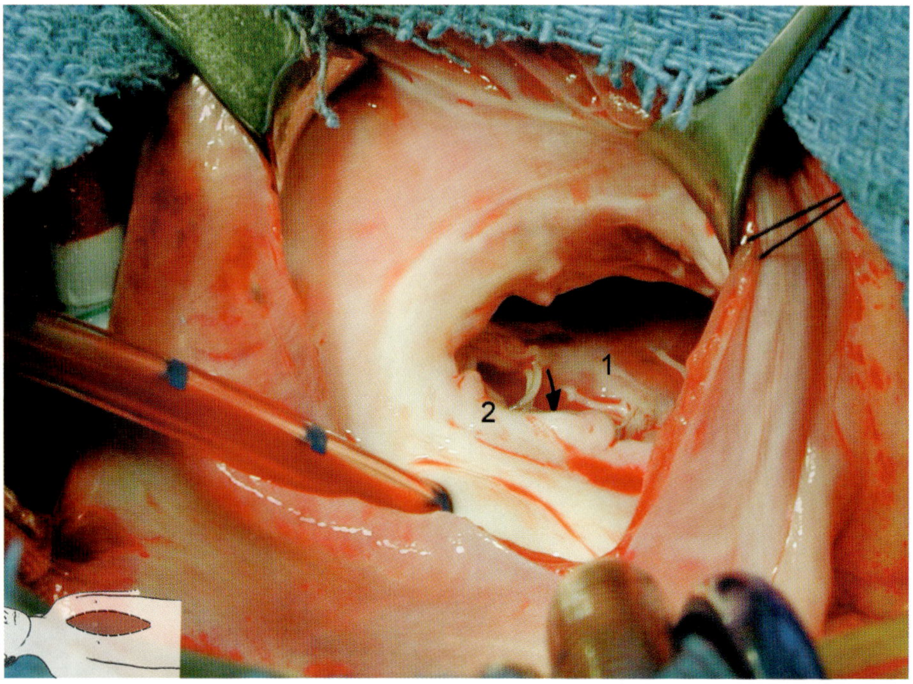

Figure 2.47. An inlet VSD as seen through a right atriotomy. The arrow points to the defect, which is largely hidden behind the septal leaflet of the tricuspid valve.

1. Ventricular septum
2. Septal leaflet of the tricuspid valve

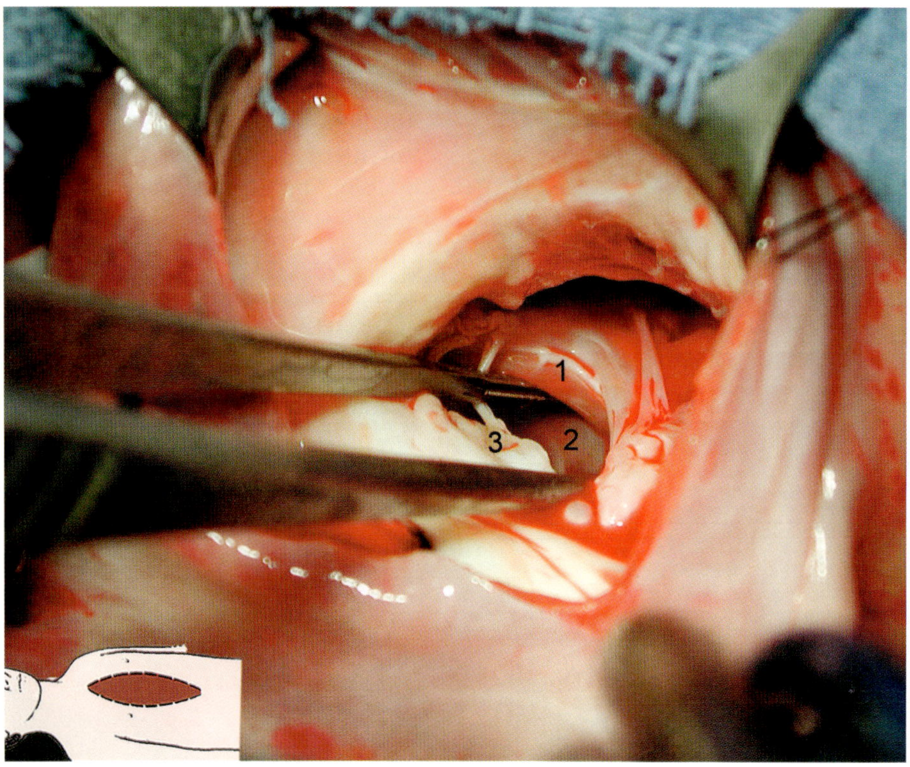

Figure 2.48. The same patient as in Figure 2.47, with septal leaflet of the tricuspid valve retracted to reveal the inlet VSD.

1. Crest of the ventricular septum
2. VSD
3. Septal leaflet of the tricuspid valve

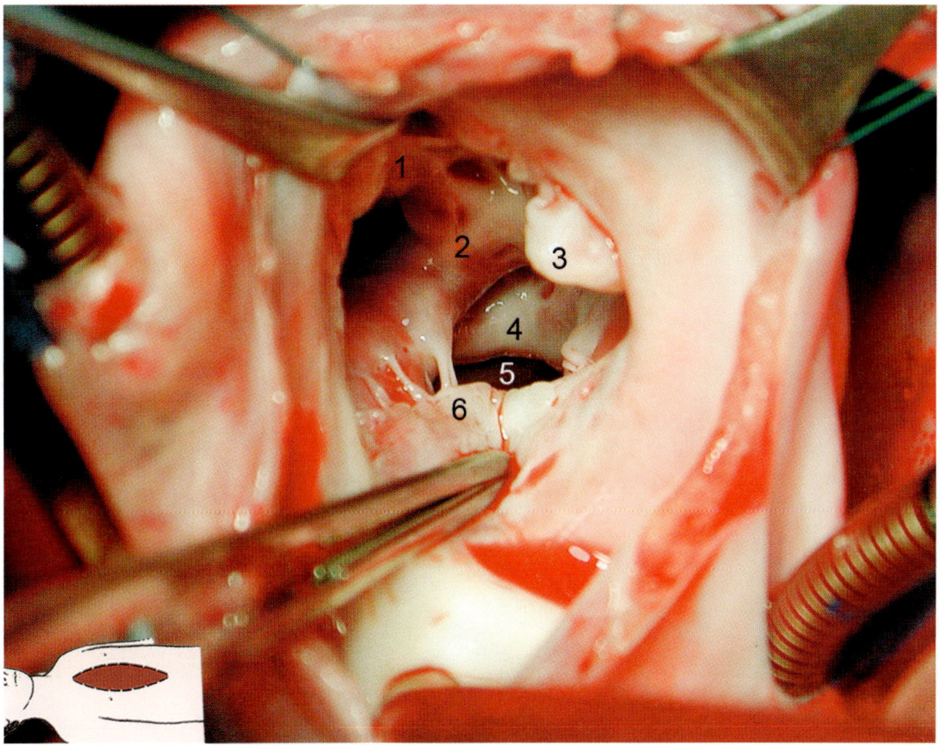

Figure 2.49. A large inlet VSD, seen through right atriotomy in a 1-year-old child. An abnormal muscle bundle (2) is seen covering part of the VSD.

1. Anterior leaflet of the tricuspid valve
2. Abnormal muscle bundle
3. Posterior leaflet of the tricuspid valve
4. Ventricular septum
5. VSD
6. Septal leaflet of the tricuspid valve

Figure 2.50. The same patient as in Figure 2.49 after closure of the VSD using a Gore-Tex patch and continuous sutures.

1. Right atriotomy incision
2. Gore-Tex patch closing the VSD
3. Septal leaflet of the tricuspid valve
4. VC cannula
5. Suction catheter draining left atrium via foramen ovale

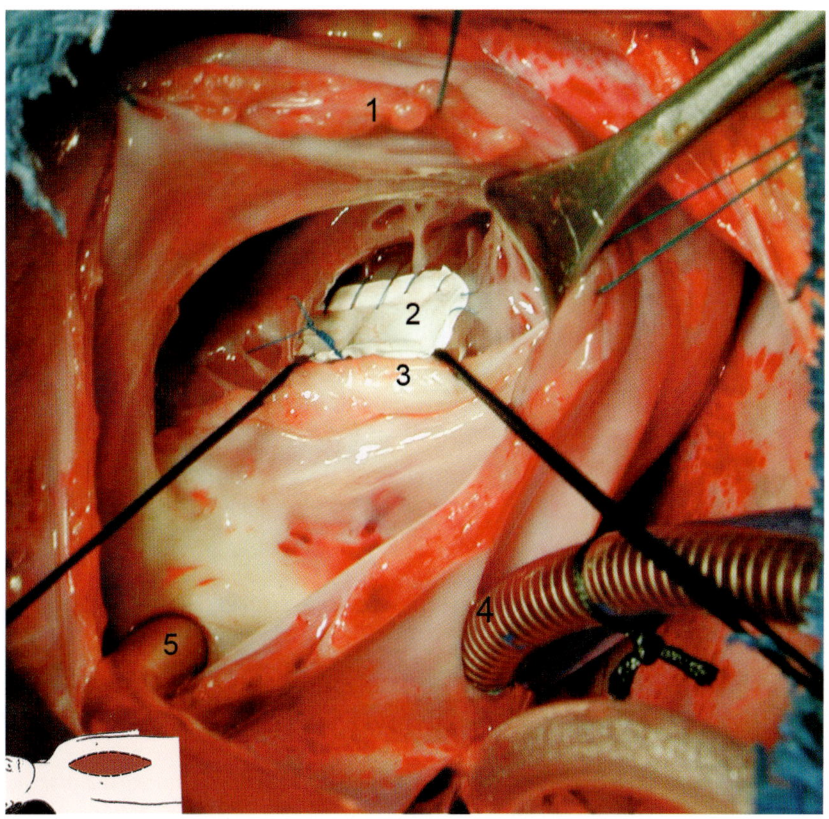

Figure 2.51. An inlet VSD in a 6-month-old infant associated with straddling of tricuspid septal leaflet. The VSD was closed with a Dacron patch (not shown), leaving tricuspid septal leaflet on the left side.

1. Ventricular septum
2. Ventricular septal defect
3. Septal leaflet of the tricuspid valve

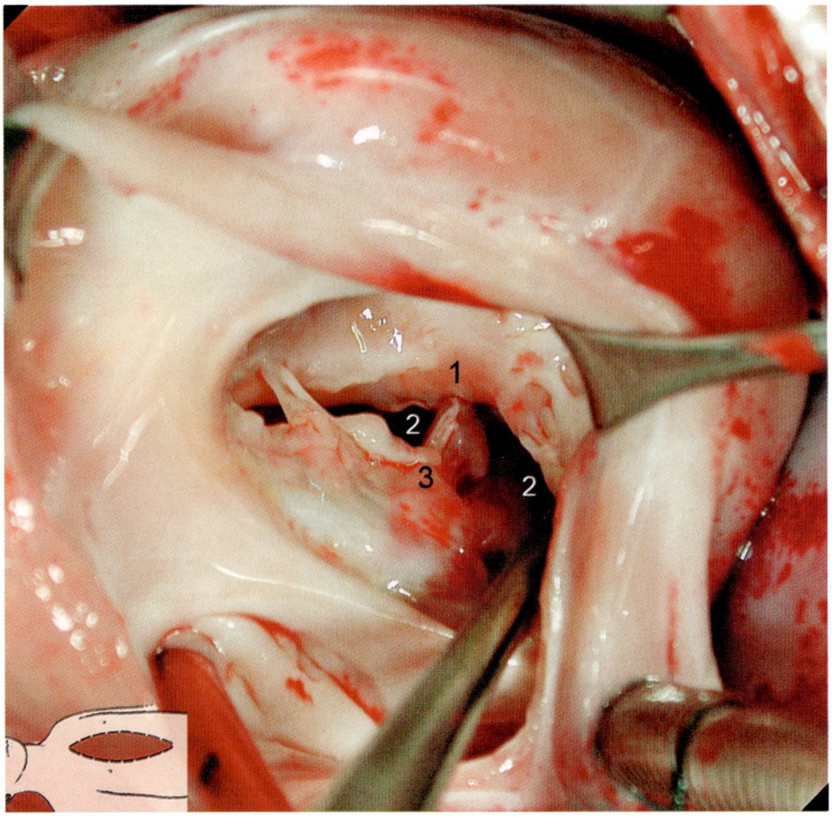

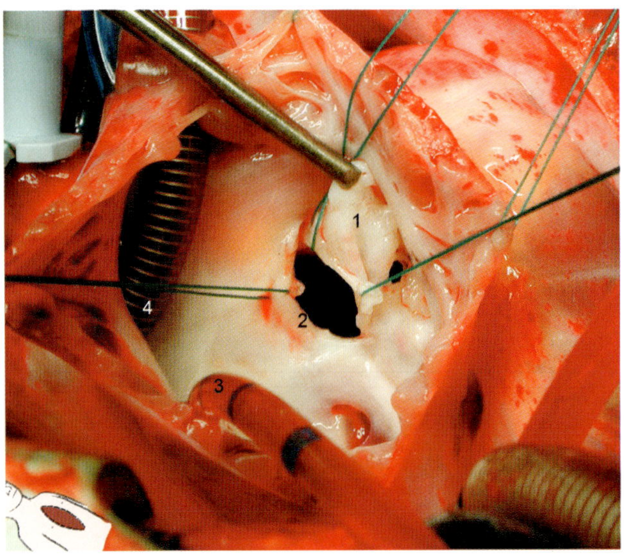

Figure 2.52

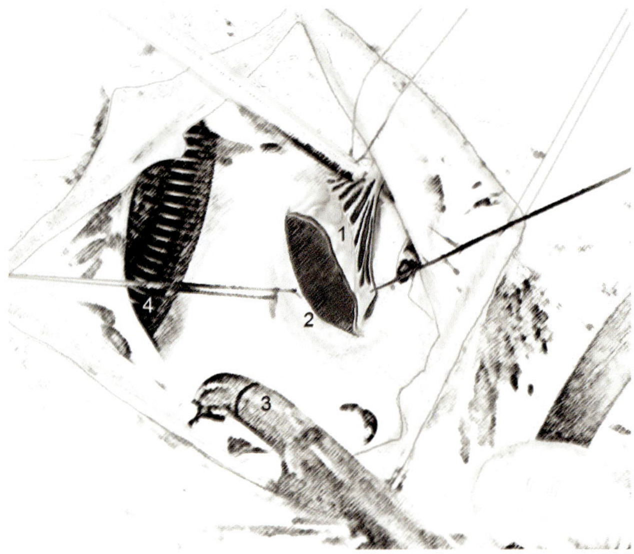

Figure 2.53

Perimembranous VSD in a 2-year-old child approached through right atriotomy. To facilitate access, the septal leaflet of the tricuspid valve was detached from the annulus of the valve. The defects were closed using a Dacron patch (partly shown in Figure 2.54).

1. Detached septal leaflet of tricuspid valve
2. Annulus of tricuspid valve
3. Suction catheter draining left atrium through foramen ovale
4. SVC cannula

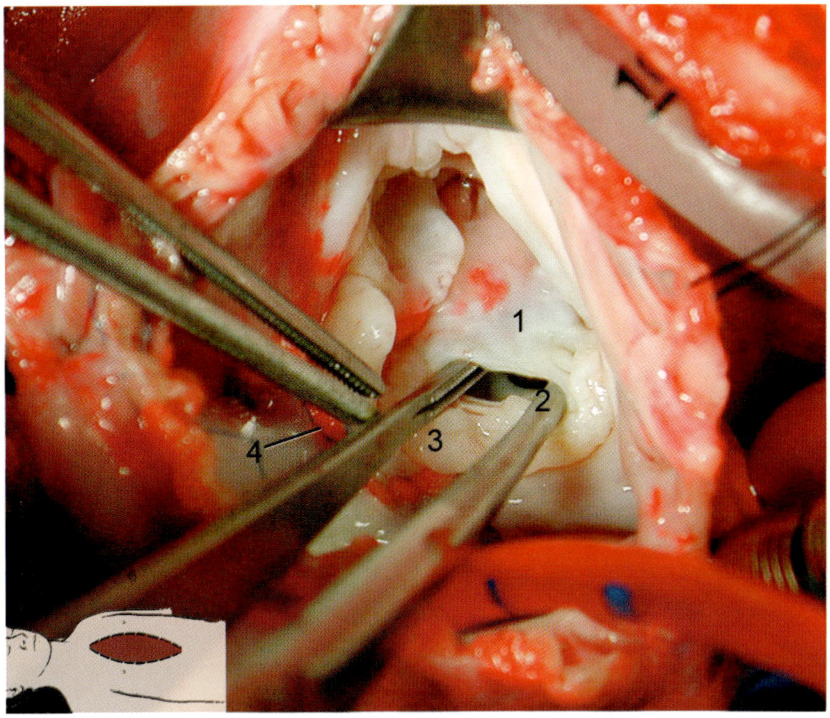

Figure 2.54. The same patient as in Figure 2.52. Postoperative echocardiogram showed a "residual VSD." On reoperation the next day, an inlet VSD was found, which was not diagnosed preoperatively.

1. Interventricular septum
2. Forceps passed through the VSD
3. Septal leaflet of the tricuspid valve
4. Dacron patch that was used to close the perimembranous VSD

GERBODE DEFECTS

True Gerbode defects are in the atrioventricular (AV) part of the membranous septum, and thus result in communication between the left ventricle and right atrium (Figure 2.56). This is a rare defect; the more common Gerbode-like defects result from communication between the left ventricle and right atrium through a perimembranous defect associated with deficiency in the tricuspid valve leaflets, or through the commissures between the leaflets[4] (Figure 2.57). Diagnosis may be difficult, as the lesion may simulate tricuspid regurgitation on echocardiography.

Figures 2.58 and 2.59 show a Gerbode defect that resulted from attachment of septal leaflet to

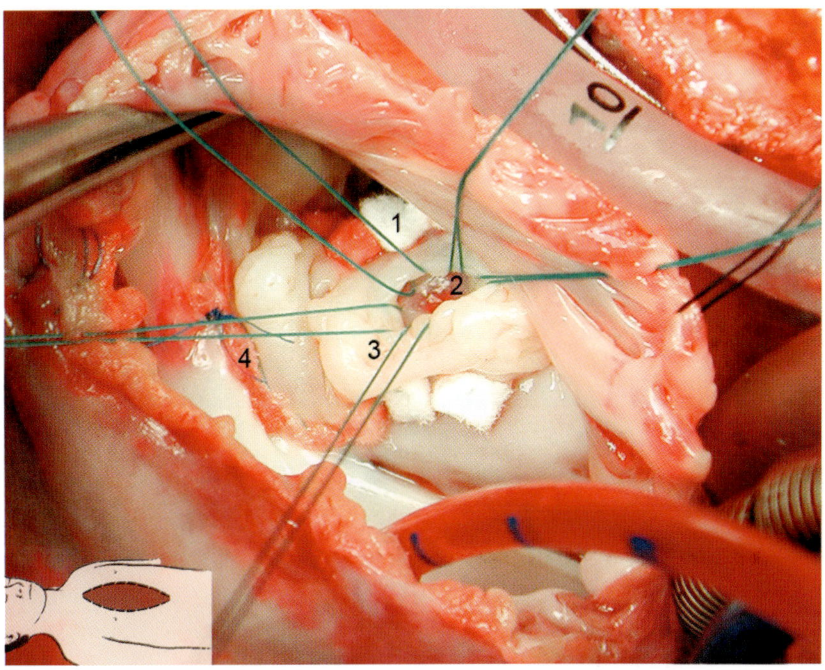

Figure 2.55. The same patient as in Figures 2.52 to 2.54. Teflon pledgets and interrupted mattress sutures have been placed around the inlet VSD. Notice the Dacron patch (4) that was used to close the perimembranous defect, sutured to the annulus through the detached septal leaflet (3).

1. Teflon pledget
2. VSD
3. Septal leaflet of the tricuspid valve
4. Dacron patch that was used to close the perimembranous VSD

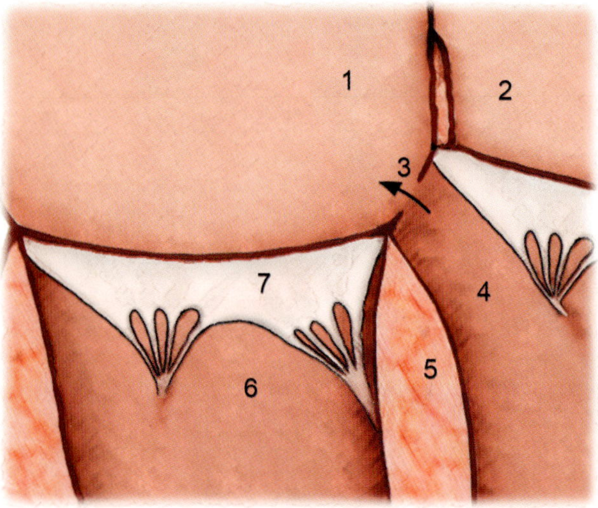

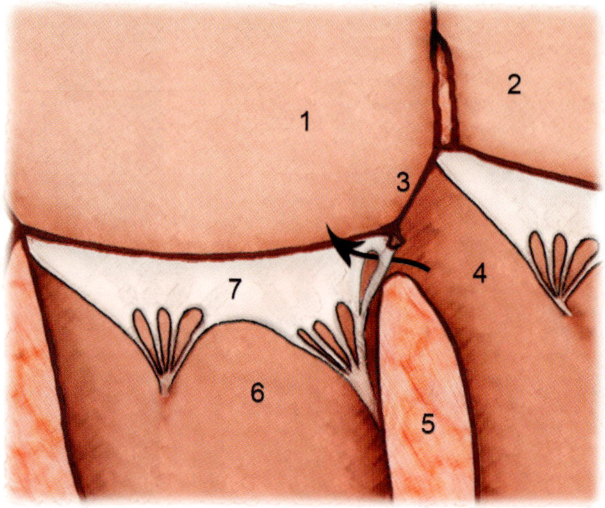

Figure 2.56 **Figure 2.57**

Schematic diagram of a left ventricle–to–right atrium communication. A true Gerbode defect will be in the atrioventricular part of the membranous septum (3). When viewed from the right atrium during surgery, the defect will be above the annulus of the tricuspid valve. Gerbode-like physiology results from communication between the left ventricle and the right atrium through a VSD and a defect in the tricuspid valve leaflets as indicated by the arrow in Figure 2.56, or through the commissures between the leaflets as indicated by the curved arrow in Figure 2.57.

1. Right atrium
2. Left atrium
3. AV membranous septum
4. Left ventricle
5. Ventricular septum
6. RV
7. Tricuspid valve

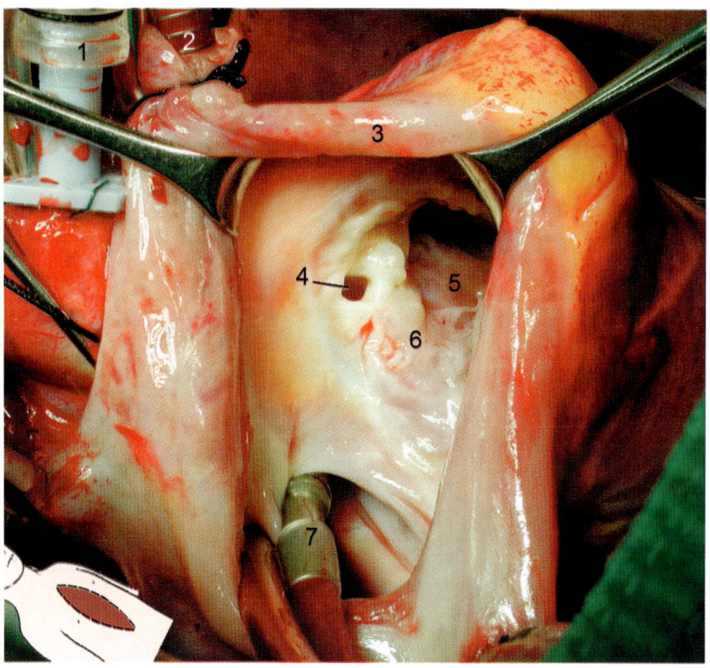

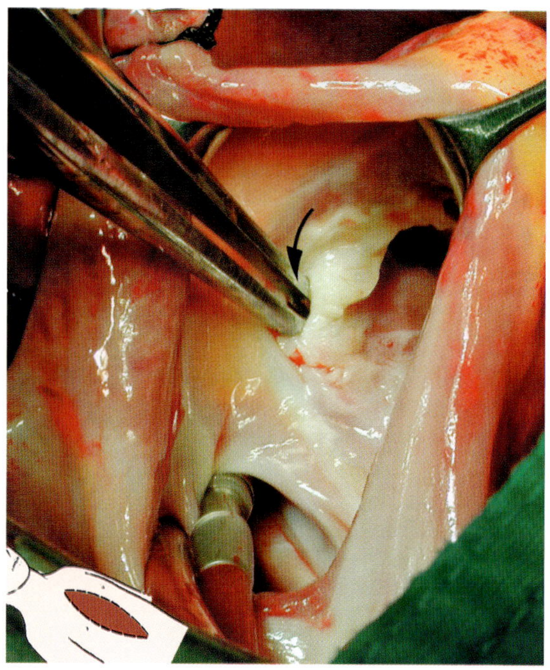

Figure 2.58 **Figure 2.59**

Left ventricular–right atrial communication (Gerbode defect) in a 5-year-old child. There is attachment of septal leaflet to the margin of the defect along with a defect in the leaflet itself, thus leading to shunting from the left ventricle to the right atrium during systole and tricuspid valve closure. The forceps (arrow in Figure 2.59) pass directly to the left ventricle. The CS is dilated because of the presence of a left SVC.

1. Cardioplegia catheter
2. SVC cannula
3. Right atriotomy
4. Gerbode defect
5. Ventricular septum
6. Septal leaflet of tricuspid valve
7. Suction catheter draining dilated CS

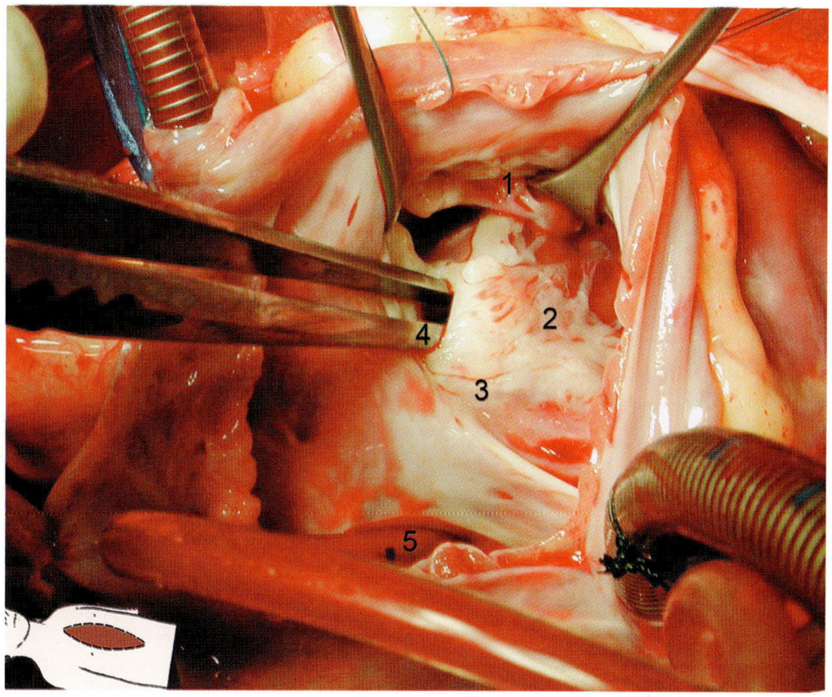

Figure 2.60. Perimembranous VSD with accessory tissue from tricuspid septal leaflet around the VSD. There is a communication from left ventricle to right atrium because of a defect in the septal leaflet. Notice that the defect is beneath the annulus of the tricuspid valve.

1. Anterior leaflet of tricuspid valve
2. Septal leaflet of tricuspid valve
3. Annulus of tricuspid valve
4. Forceps in the VSD
5. Suction catheter draining left atrium through foramen ovale

the margin of the VSD along with a defect in the leaflet itself, thus leading to shunting from the left ventricle to the right atrium during tricuspid valve closure in systole. Figure 2.60 is another example. Notice that the defect is caudal to the annulus of the tricuspid valve, which differentiates this from a true Gerbode defect.[5] A Gerbode-like defect may be iatrogenic because of perforation of the tricuspid leaflet by sutures placed across it as shown in Figure 2.61.

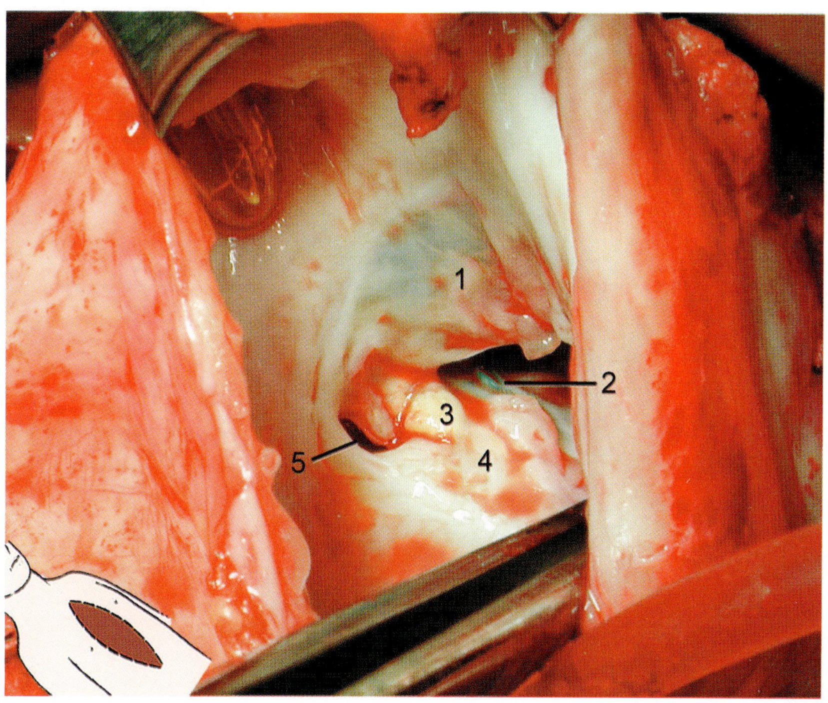

Figure 2.61. Recurrent VSD 6 months after initial repair. The septal leaflet of the tricuspid valve was torn by tension from the suture used to close the original VSD. The communication was from left ventricle to right atrium. Teflon pledgets (3) of the previous operation are seen on the septal leaflet.

1. Anterior leaflet of tricuspid valve
2. Sutures of previous surgery
3. Teflon pledget
4. Septal leaflet of tricuspid valve
5. Recurrent VSD

REFERENCES

1. Hoffman JE, Kaplan S. The incidence of congenital heart disease. *J Am Coll Cardiol.* 2002;39:1890–1900.
2. Soufflet V, Van de Bruaene A, Troost E, et al. Behavior of unrepaired perimembranous ventricular septal defect in young adults. *Am J Cardiol.* 2010;105:400–407.
3. Abe T, Komatsu S. Surgical repair and long-term results in ruptured sinus of Valsalva aneurysm. *Ann Thorac Surg.* 1988;46:520–525.
4. Burrows PE, Fellows KE, Keane JF. Cineangiography of the perimembranous ventricular septal defect with left ventricular-right atrial shunt. *J Am Coll Cardiol.* 1983;1:1129–1134.
5. Sinisalo JP, Sreeram N, Jokinen E, Qureshi SA. Acquired left ventricular-right atrium shunts. *Eur J Cardiothorac Surg.* 2011;39:500–506.

CHAPTER 3

Atrial Septal Defect

A defect allowing interatrial communication is relatively common.[1] Atrial septal defects (ASD) are classified based on their location in the perceived interatrial septum (Figure 3.1) viewed from the right atrium. The most common type is a secundum ASD, which is caused by deficiency in the valve of the foramen ovale. More than one type of defect may occur concomitantly, and they may be multiple. Sinus venosus defects are related to the superior vena cava (SVC) and occasionally the inferior vena cava (IVC). They are typically associated with partial anomalous venous drainage and will be discussed in chapter 12. Primum ASDs fall within the spectrum of "endocardial cushion defects" and will be discussed in chapter 5. A coronary sinus (CS) defect is at the site of the CS orifice, allowing direct communication between the atria. Usually associated with a persistent left SVC, it involves varying extents of "unroofing" of the CS.

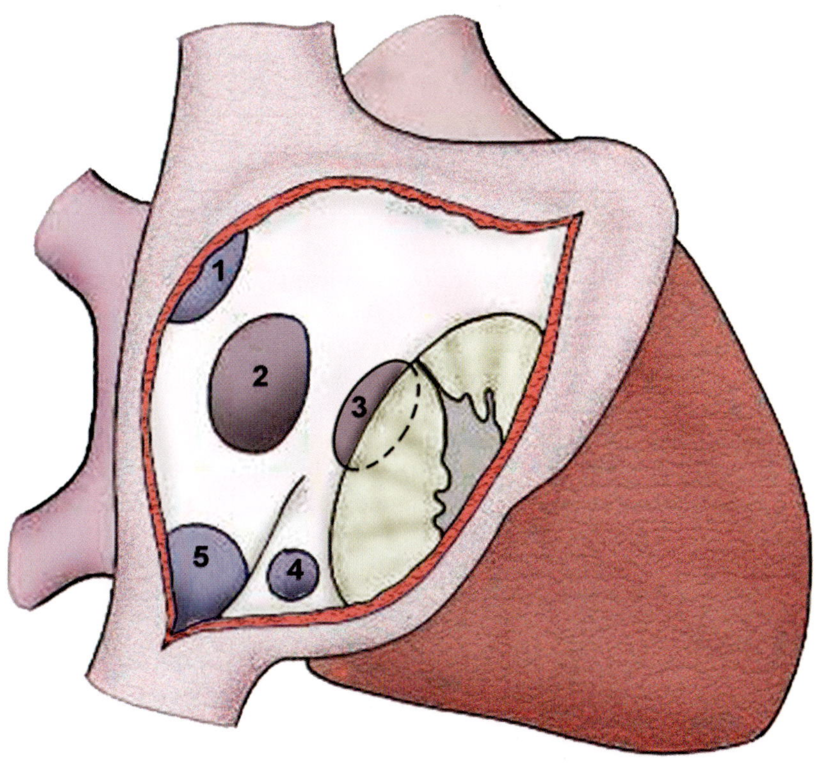

Figure 3.1. Classification of ASDs. See text.

1. Sinus venosus ASD, related to SVC
2. Secundum ASD
3. Primum ASD
4. CS ASD
5. Sinus venosus ASD, related to IVC

Congenital Heart Disease: A Surgical Color Atlas © 2015 A. Sukru Mercan, Zakariya Hubail, S. Yen Ho.
Cardiotext Publishing, ISBN: 978-1-935395-90-4.

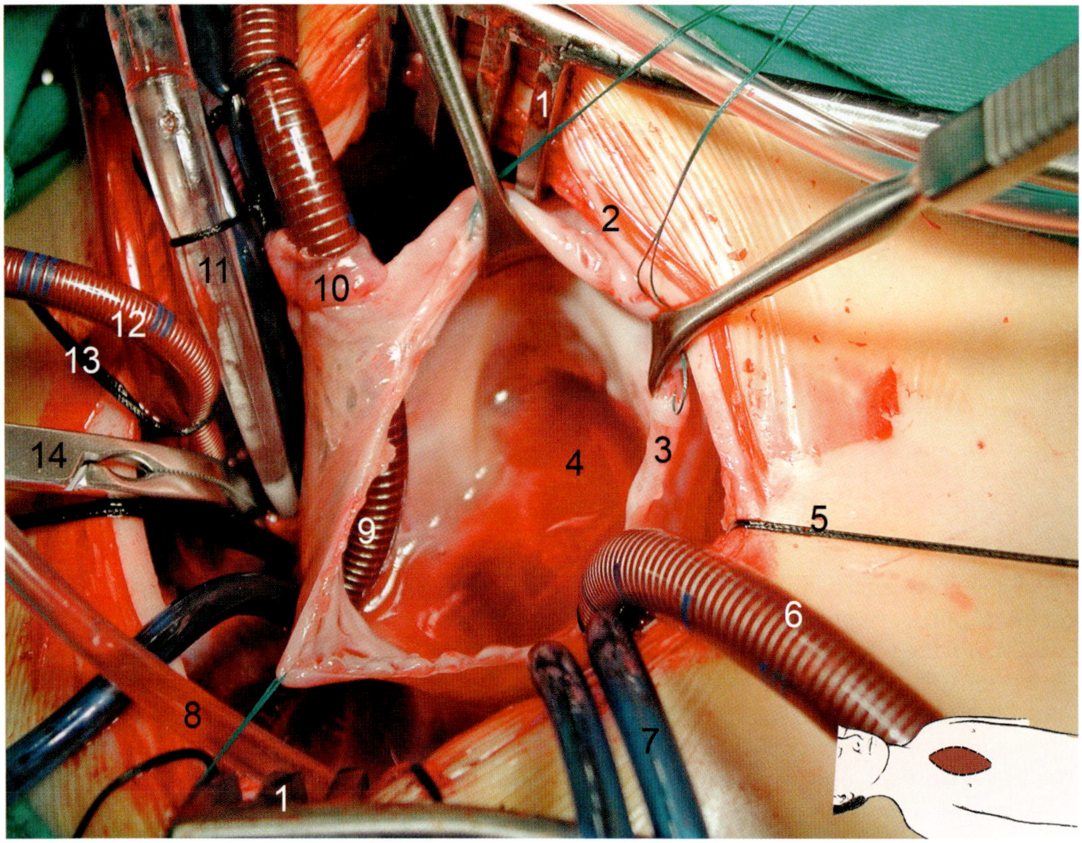

Figure 3.2. Operative field of a median sternotomy and a right atriotomy in a 2-year-old child with an ASD.

1. Sternal retractor
2. Skin incision
3. Atriotomy incision
4. Blood in floor of opened right atrium
5. Stay suture for pericardium
6. IVC venous cannula
7. Tourniquet
8. Suction catheter
9. SVC venous cannula
10. Entry of SVC cannula through atrial appendage
11. Cardioplegia catheter
12. Aortic cannula
13. Stay suture isolating ascending aorta
14. Aortic cross-clamp

Echocardiography has made it possible to easily diagnose small and asymptomatic defects. Most defects are not hemodynamically significant and do not require intervention.[2] When closure is indicated, however, the defects are often closed percutaneously in the catheterization laboratory, using devices such as the Amplatzer® septal occluder.[3] Surgery is reserved for patients who are not candidates for device closure because of the size, location, or number of defects. The most common approach is through a median sternotomy, or ministernotomy incision (Figure 3.2). A right submammary incision may occasionally be chosen for cosmetic reasons.

Figures 3.3 to 3.5 are from a 2-year-old child with a large secundum ASD. This patient also had a ventricular septal defect (VSD) that had closed spontaneously by tricuspid valve tissue. Note the dimple on septal leaflet of the tricuspid valve. The ASD was closed primarily by direct suturing.

Figures 3.6 to 3.10 are from an adult with a fenestrated atrial septum; the defects were also closed primarily. Figures 3.11 and 3.12 represent another example of multiple defects.

Figures 3.13 to 3.16 show a rather large secundum ASD that was, nonetheless, closed primarily without patching. A pericardial patch was used to close the defect in the patient shown in Figure 3.17.

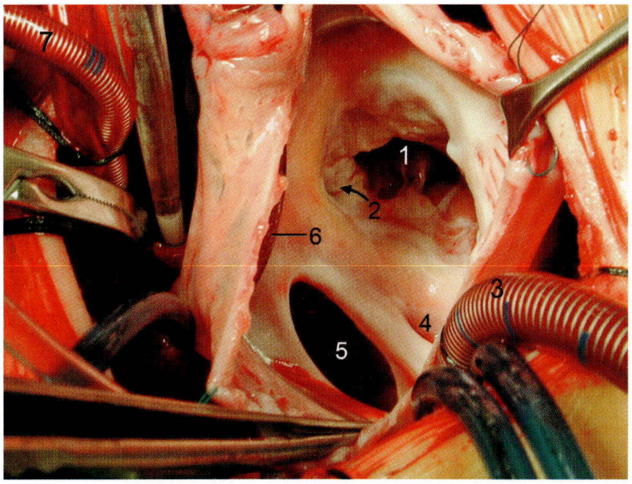

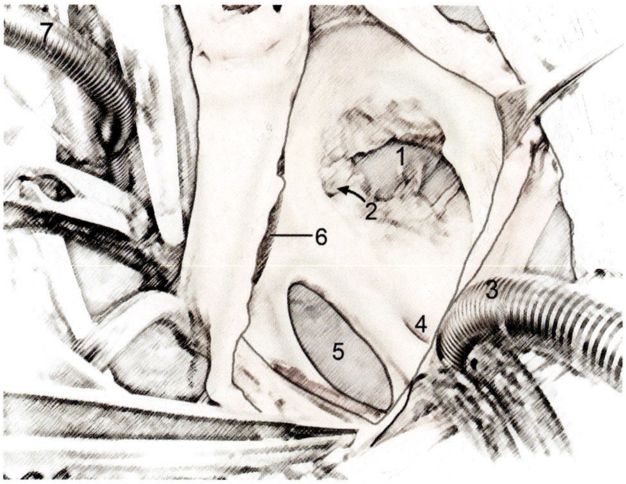

Figure 3.3 **Figure 3.4**

A secundum ASD in a 2-year-old child. This patient also had a VSD that closed spontaneously by tricuspid valve tissue, as indicated by the dimple on septal leaflet of the tricuspid valve (2).

1. Tricuspid valve
2. Dimple on septal leaflet caused by spontaneous closure of a VSD
3. IVC venous cannula
4. Opening of CS
5. ASD
6. SVC venous cannula
7. Aortic cannula

Figure 3.5. Same patient as in Figure 3.3. The ASD was closed primarily by direct suturing.

1. Tricuspid valve
2. Opening of CS
3. Suture line

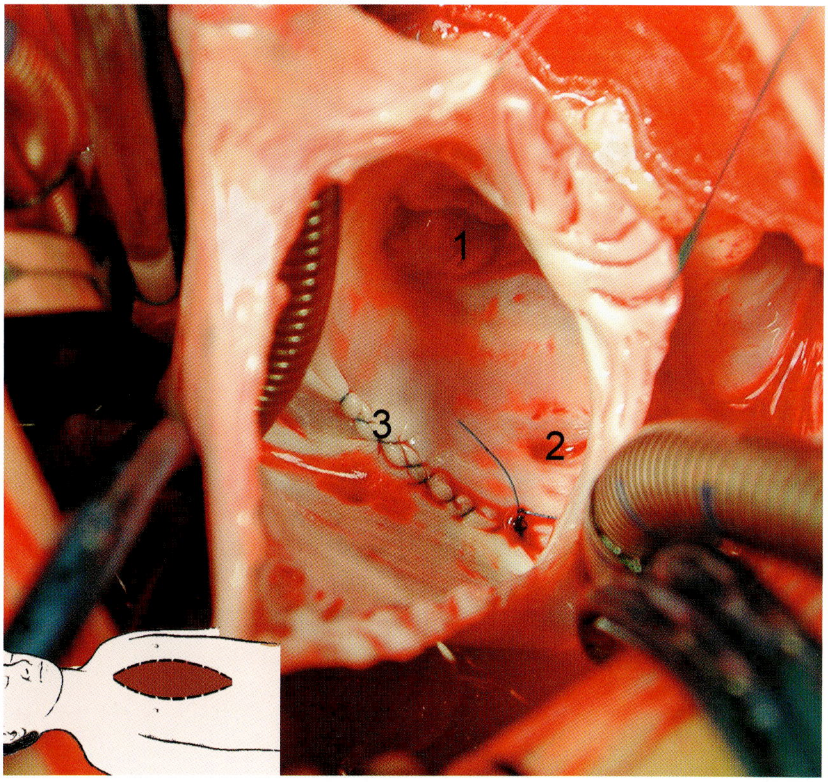

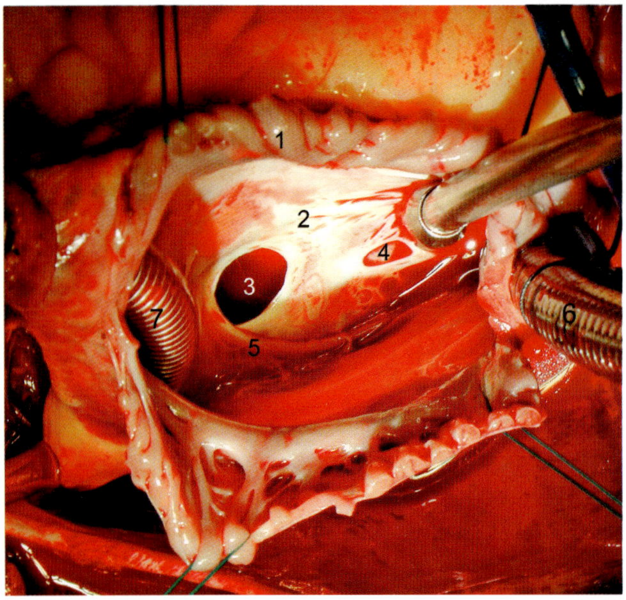

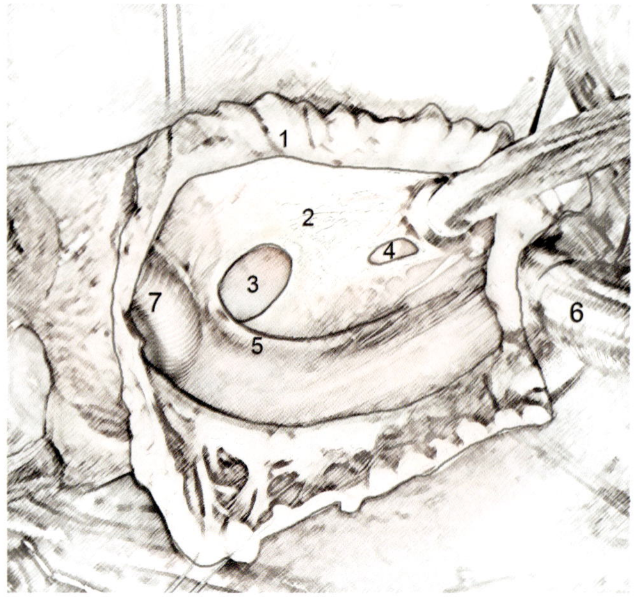

Figure 3.6 **Figure 3.7**

Intraoperative view of multiple secundum ASDs in an adult patient, seen through a right atriotomy.

1. Right atrial free wall (opened)
2. Interatrial septum
3. Defect at the site of foramen ovale
4. Secundum defect
5. Limbus of fossa ovalis
6. IVC venous cannula
7. SVC venous cannula

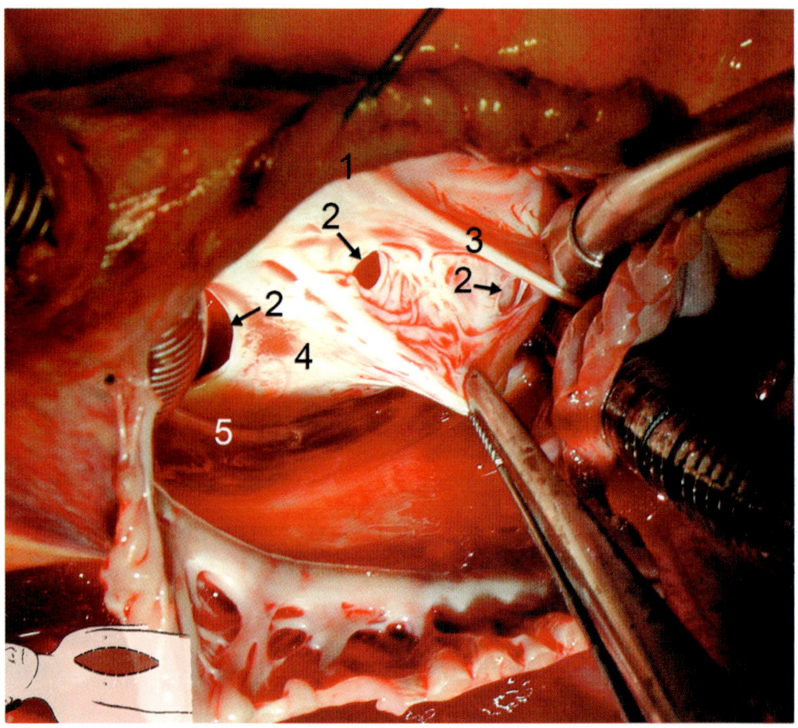

Figure 3.8. Same patient as in Figure 3.6, showing the inferior part of the septum where more defects existed.

1. Right atrial free wall (opened)
2. ASDs
3. Extension of Eustachian valve (tendon of Todaro)
4. Interatrial septum (septum primum)
5. Limbus of fossa ovalis (septum secundum)

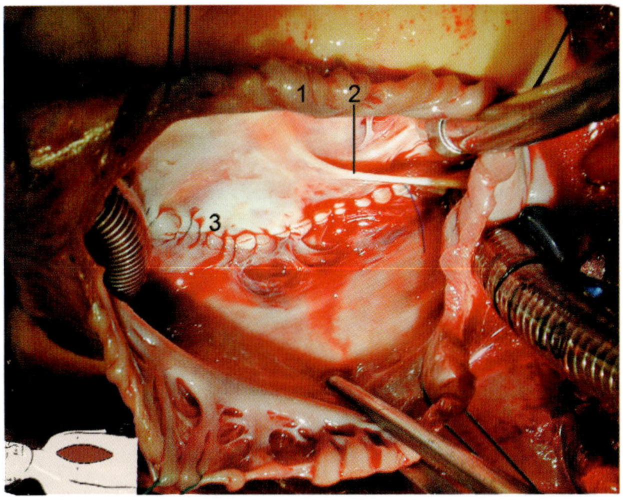

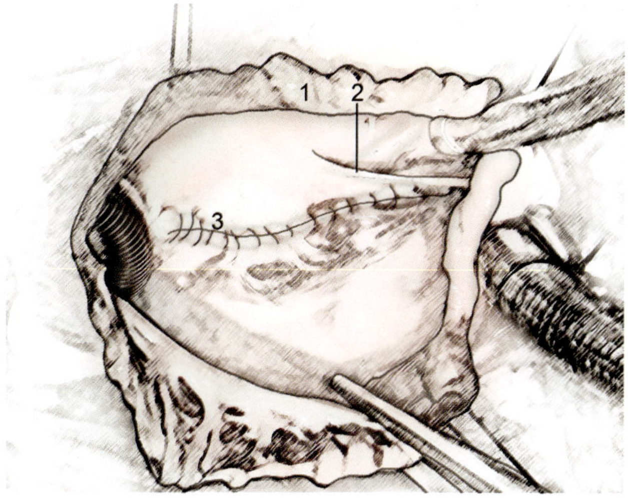

Figure 3.9 **Figure 3.10**

Same patient as in Figures 3.6 to 3.8. The defects were closed primarily by a single suture line.

1. Right atrial free wall (opened)
2. Extension of Eustachain valve (tendon of Todaro)
3. Suture line

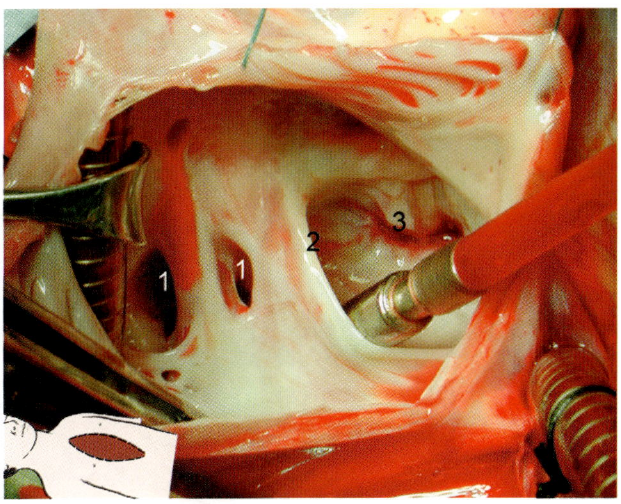

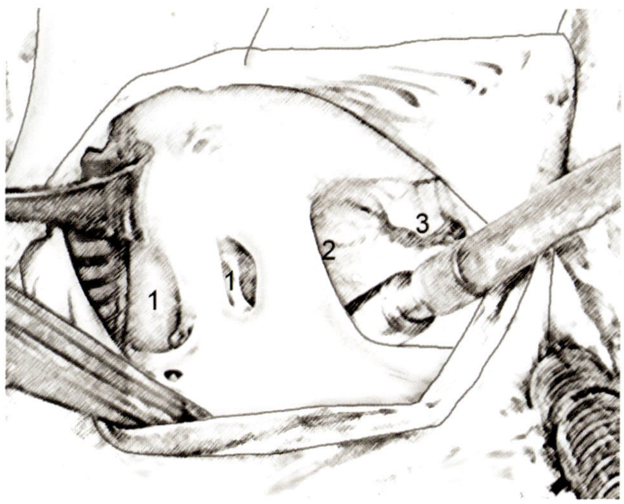

Figure 3.11 **Figure 3.12**

Multiple ASDs as seen through a right atriotomy. The mitral valve (3) is seen through the inferior defect.

1. Secundum ASDs
2. Edge of inferior sinus venosus ASD
3. Mitral valve

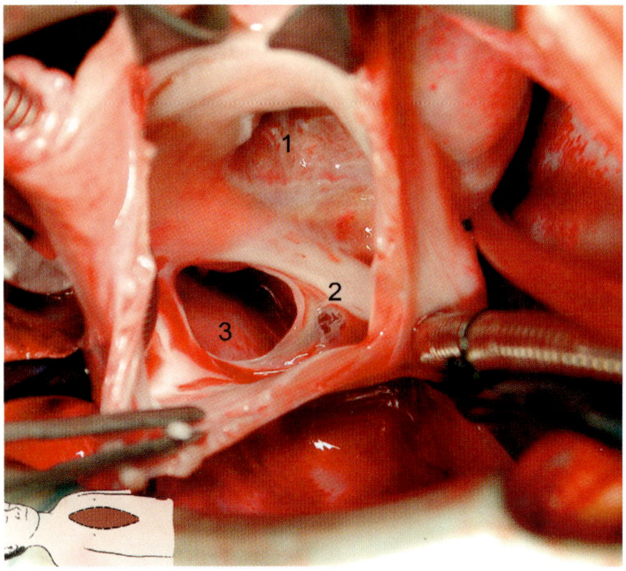

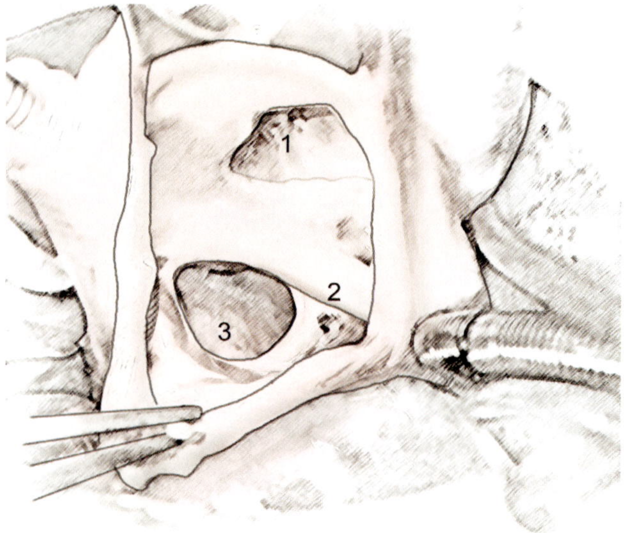

Figure 3.13 **Figure 3.14**

A secundum ASD in a 1-year-old child as seen through a median sternotomy and right atriotomy.

1. Tricuspid valve
2. Extension of Eustachian valve (tendon of Todaro)
3. Left atrial cavity seen through ASD

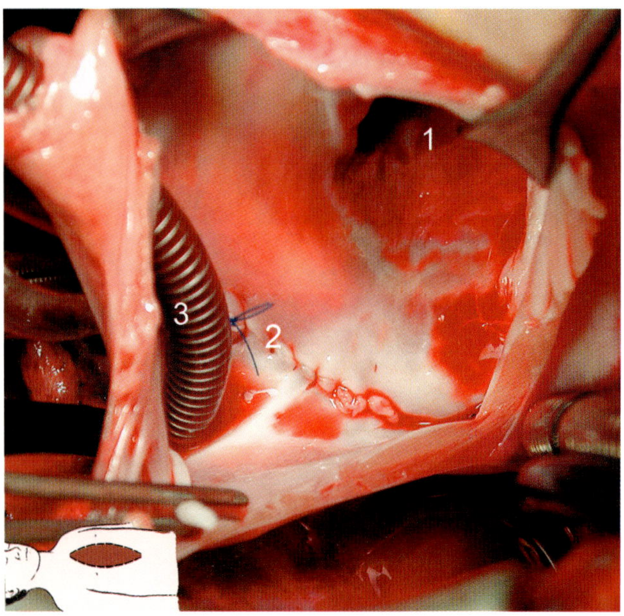

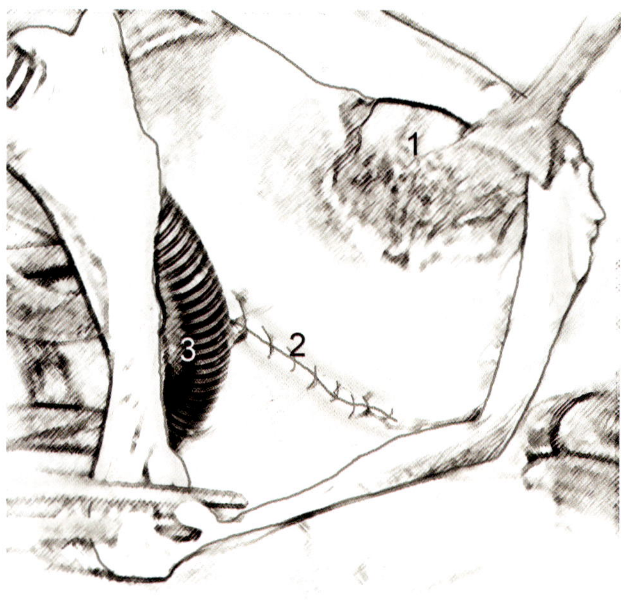

Figure 3.15 **Figure 3.16**

The same patient as in Figure 3.13 after closure of the ASD by primarily suturing together the edges of the defect.

1. Tricuspid valve
2. Suture line
3. SVC cannula

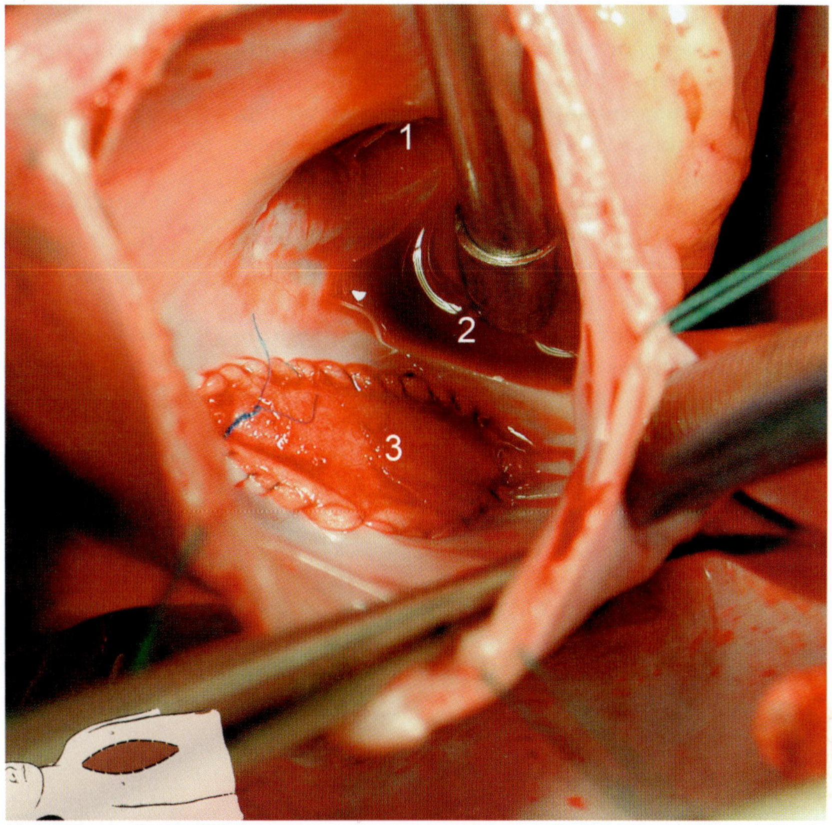

Figure 3.17. A large secundum ASD was closed by an autologous pericardial patch in this 7-year-old child.

1. Tricuspid valve
2. CS
3. An autologous pericardial patch closing the ASD

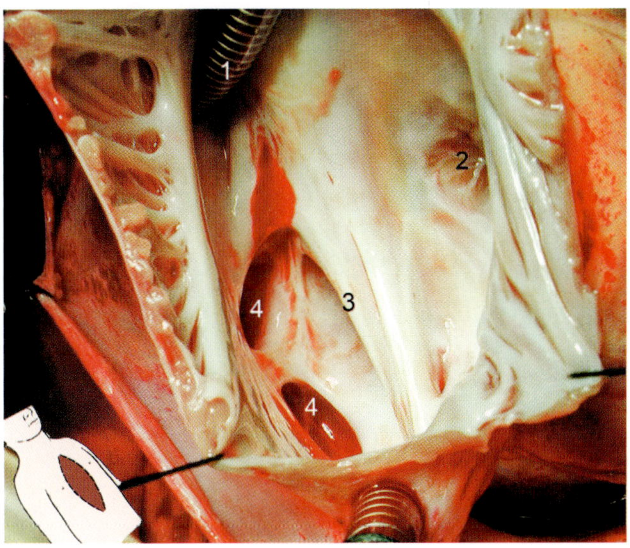

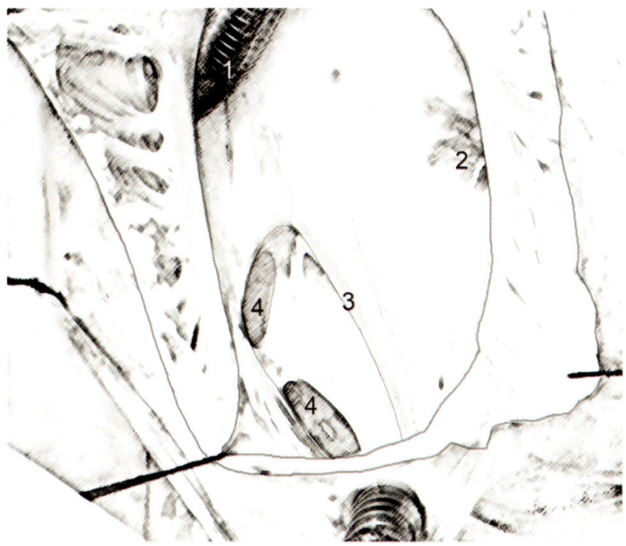

Figure 3.18 **Figure 3.19**

A large posterior–inferior ASD related to the IVC. Note that the right pulmonary veins are seen through the defect. The ASD was closed using an autologous pericardial patch.

1. SVC cannula
2. Tricuspid valve
3. Edge of the ASD
4. Right PVs

Figures 3.18 and 3.19 show a large defect with deficient posterior and inferior rims. The right pulmonary veins (PVs) can be seen through the defect, but are normally connected to the left atrium. Figures 3.20 and 3.21 are other examples of inferior sinus venosus defects related to the IVC. The septal defects in these patients were closed by autologous pericardial patches.

An ASD may be closed primarily by directly suturing together the edges of the defect. Some defects, however, because of their large size or location, cannot be closed in this manner. Various materials can be used for patching, but most commonly the patient's own pericardium is utilized. The ASDs in the patients represented in Figures 3.3, 3.6, and 3.13 were closed primarily by direct suturing. Figure 3.17 shows the postrepair view from a patient whose ASD was closed by an autologous pericardial patch.

Figures 3.22 to 3.26 are from a patient with the interesting findings of malposition of the great arteries, secundum ASD, left juxtaposition of the right atrial appendage (RAA), and unroofed CS. The latter is, in effect, a small CS ASD. Both septal defects were closed primarily (not shown).

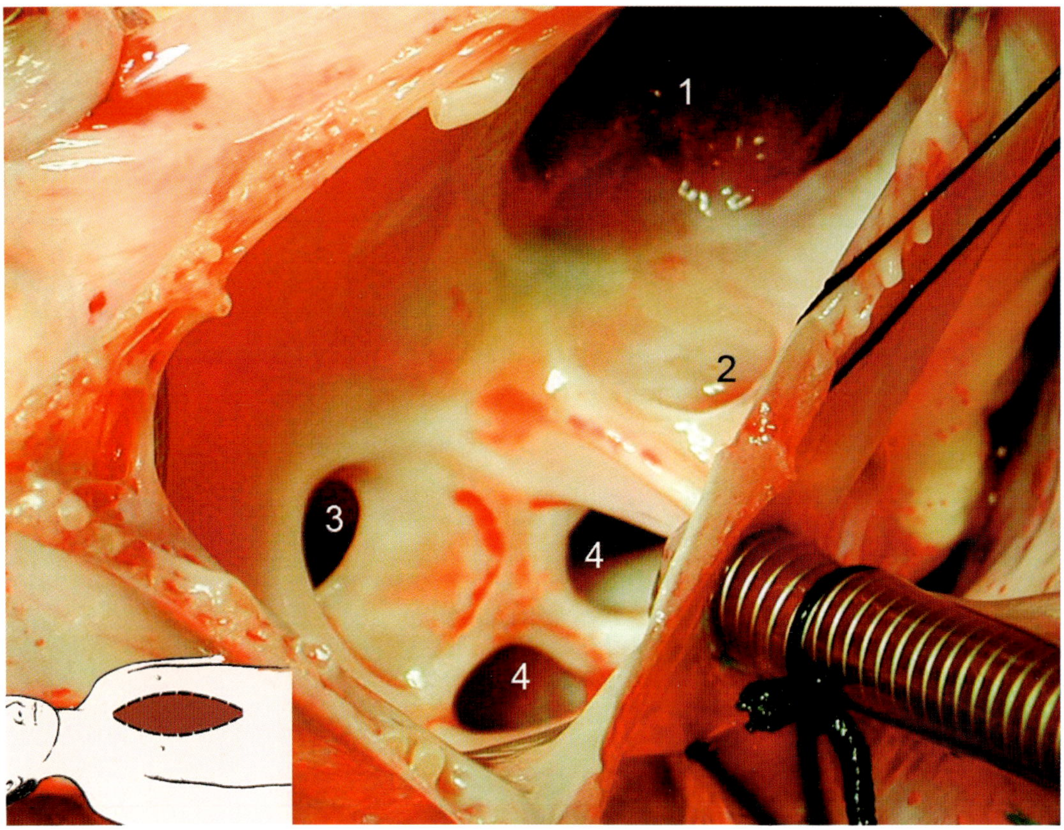

Figure 3.20. Multiple ASDs—one secundum and two IVC-related sinus venosus defects—in a 9-month-old infant. The secundum defect was closed primarily, but the other defects were closed by autologous pericardial patch.

1. Tricuspid valve
2. Opening of CS
3. Secundum defect
4. Sinus venosus defects

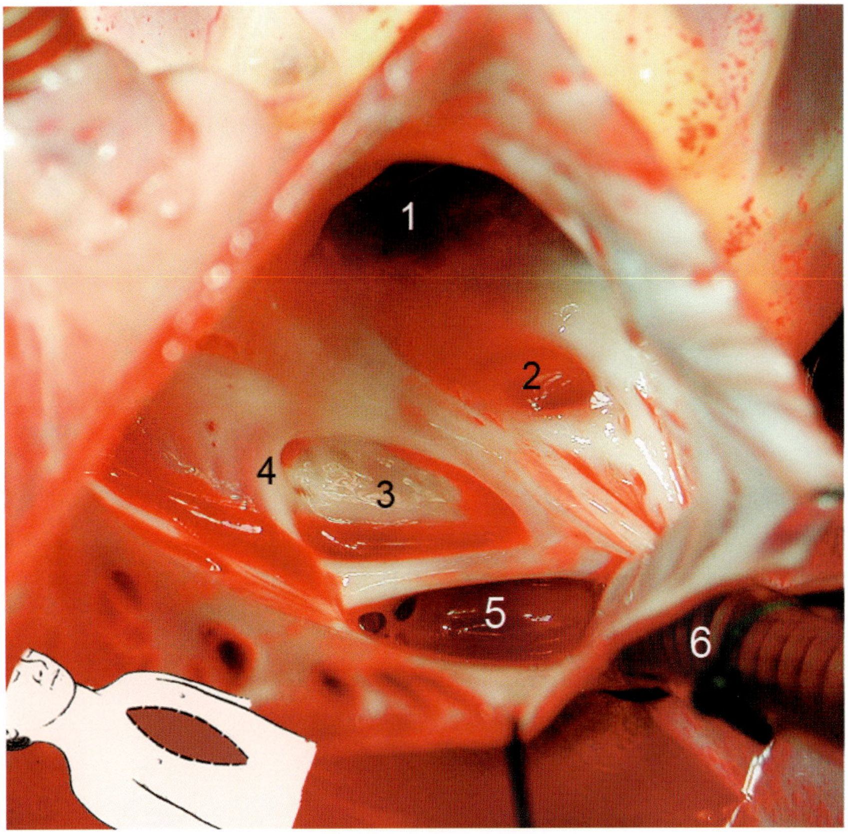

Figure 3.21. An IVC-related sinus venosus defect in a 30-month-old child. The defect was closed by an autologous pericardial patch.

1. Tricuspid valve
2. Opening of CS
3. Fossa ovalis
4. Limbus of septum secundum
5. Sinus venosus defect
6. IVC venous cannula

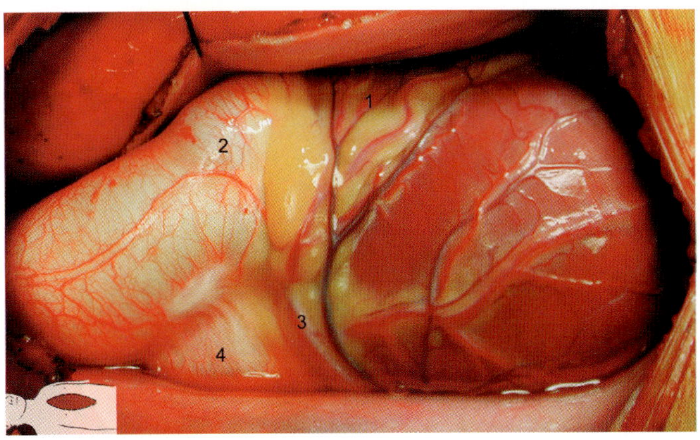

Figure 3.22

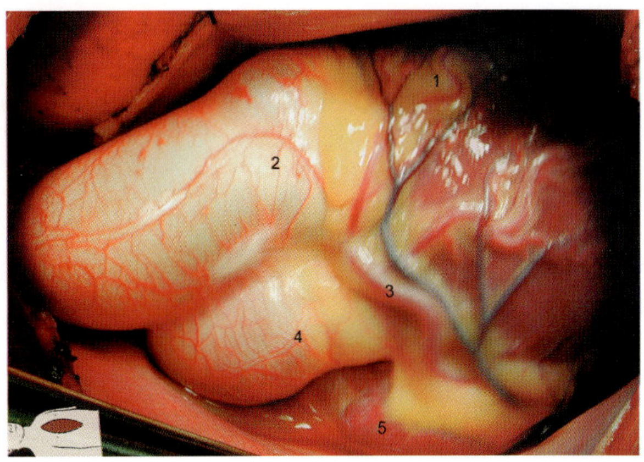

Figure 3.23

The gross appearance of the heart and great vessels in a 6-year-old child operated on for an ASD. The great arteries are malposed; the aorta arises from the left ventricle (LV) but is located left and anteriorly in relation to the pulmonary artery. Note that the RAA is not seen in its usual location.

1. LV
2. Ascending aorta
3. Right coronary artery
4. Main pulmonary artery (MPA)
5. Right atrium

Figure 3.24. The same patient as in Figures 3.22 and 3.23, with the heart retracted to the right. The left atrial appendage (LAA) comes to view as well as the juxtaposed RAA.

1. RAA
2. LAA
3. LV
4. Ascending aorta
5. Cardioplegia catheter

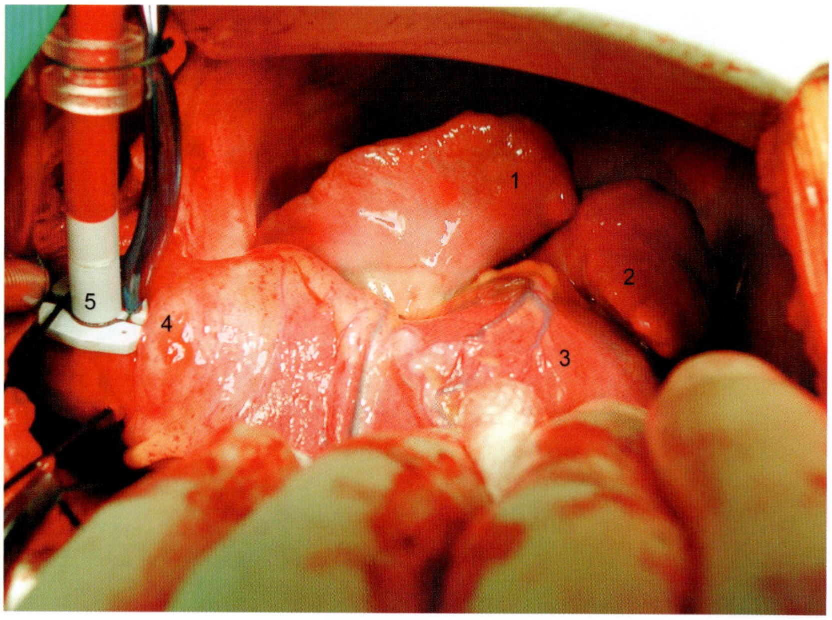

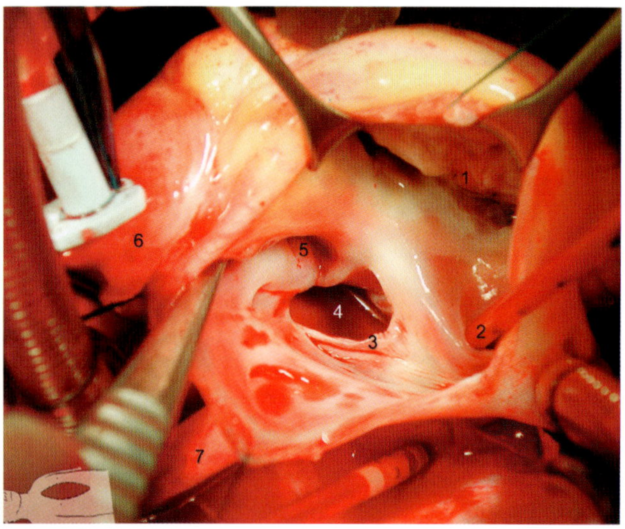

Figure 3.25

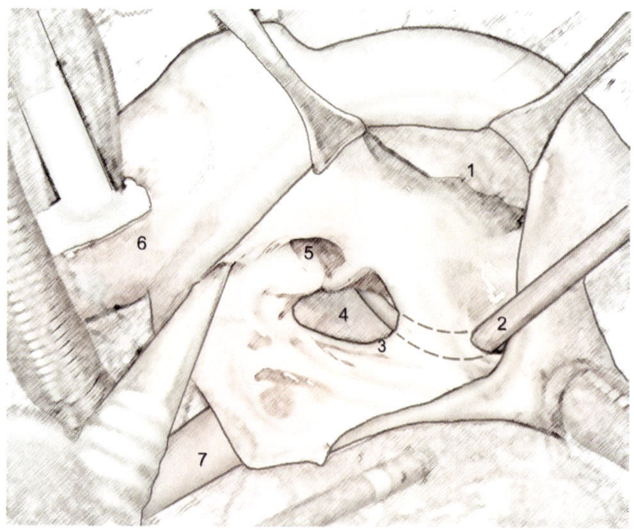

Figure 3.26

The same patient as in Figures 3.22 to 3.24. On cardiopulmonary bypass, the right atrium has been opened to reveal a large secundum ASD. A suction catheter is passed through the CS and is seen in the left atrial cavity, since the CS is unroofed. This, in effect, is a CS ASD. The secundum defect was closed by a patch, and the CS defect was closed primarily (not shown).

1. Tricuspid valve
2. Suction catheter in CS
3. Edge of secundum ASD
4. Left atrial cavity
5. Mouth of RAA
6. Ascending aorta
7. SVC

REFERENCES

1. Hoffman J, Kaplan S. The incidence of congenital heart disease. *J Am Coll Cardiol.* 2002;39:1890–1900.
2. Bostan OM, Cil E, Ercan I. The prospective follow-up of the natural course of interatrial communications diagnosed in 847 newborns. *Europ Heart J.* 2007; 28:2001–2005.
3. Rastogi N, Smeeton NC, Qureshi SA. Factors related to successful transcatheter closure of atrial septal defects using the Amplatzer Septal Occluder. *Pediatr Cardiol.* 2009;30:888–892.

CHAPTER 4

Patent Ductus Arteriosus

The ductus arteriosus is a normal component of fetal circulation. It is not required for postnatal circulation, and thus undergoes spontaneous closure within the first 2 days in the majority of term infants.[1] A persistently patent ductus arteriosus (PDA) results in left-to-right shunting and resembles a ventricular septal defect (VSD) from a hemodynamic point of view. Beyond early infancy, most PDAs are amenable to device closure percutaneously.

When surgery is indicated, the approach is through a lateral thoracotomy incision for isolated PDA or through median sternotomy when other intracardiac repair is being performed in the same session. Figures 4.1 and 4.2 show a surgical view of a PDA as seen through a left lateral thoracotomy; Figure 4.3, from another patient, shows a PDA as seen through a median sternotomy incision in a 4-month-old infant with a VSD, an atrial septal defect (ASD), and a PDA.

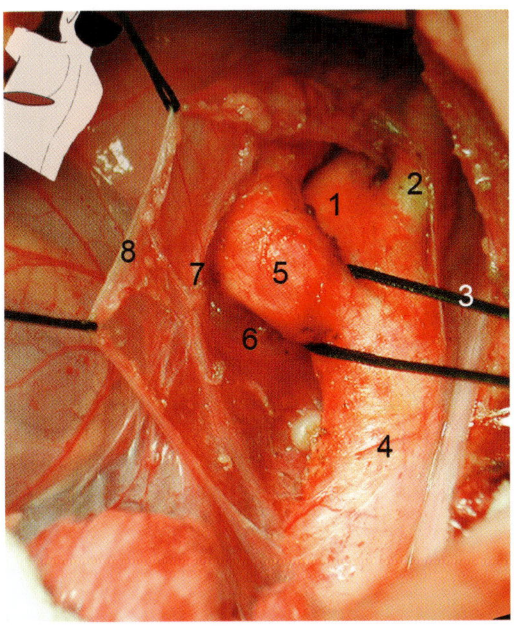

Figure 4.1

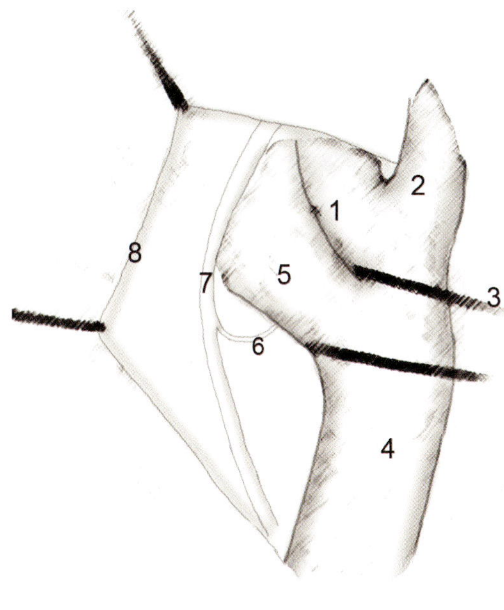

Figure 4.2

PDA in a 21-day-old term neonate weighing 4.3 kg. The ductus is somewhat aneurysmal. Minimal dissection is done, and the mediastinal pleura is retracted along with the left vagus nerve.

1. Transverse aortic arch
2. Left subclavian artery
3. Stay suture around PDA
4. Descending thoracic aorta
5. PDA
6. Recurrent laryngeal nerve
7. Left vagus nerve
8. Posterior mediastinal pleura

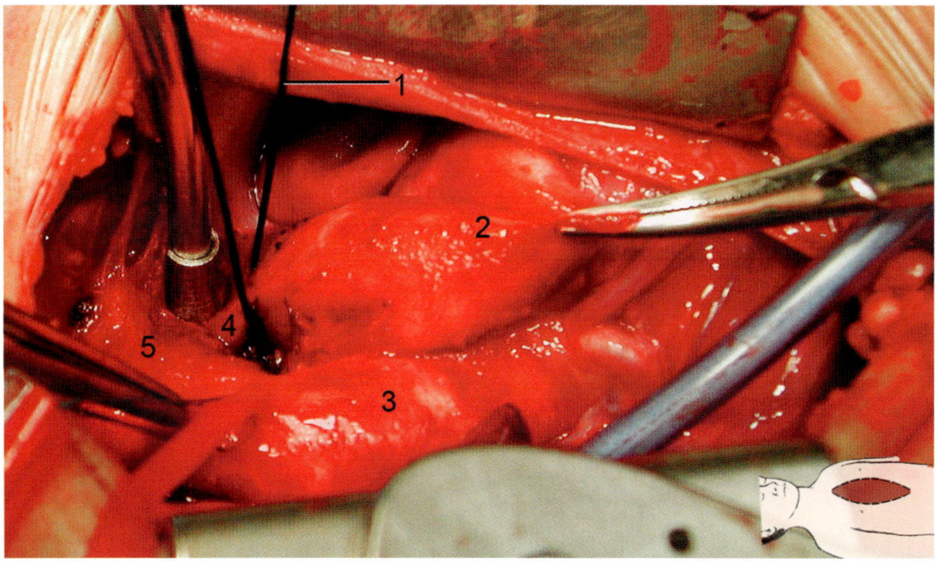

Figure 4.3. Median sternotomy view from a 4-month-old infant operated on for VSD, ASD (not shown), and PDA.

1. Stay suture around PDA
2. Main pulmonary artery (MPA)
3. Ascending aorta
4. PDA
5. Transverse arch

There are multiple techniques to close a PDA, including double ligature, division with oversewing, and closure with surgical clips. Video-assisted thoracoscopic surgery (VATS) is a relatively recent approach but is gaining popularity.

Figures 4.4 to 4.7 are from a 6-year-old child with a large ductus. Note that the diameter of the ductus is larger than the aortic arch. The ductus was divided and oversewn.

Figures 4.8 and 4.9 illustrate the technique of double ligation and transfixation in a 1-year-old infant with a PDA.

Figures 4.10 to 4.12 are from a 3-week-old infant with pulmonary atresia. Note the abnormal

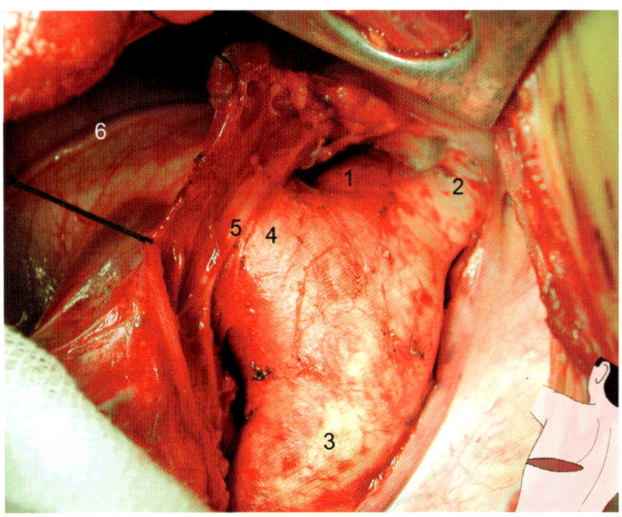

Figure 4.4

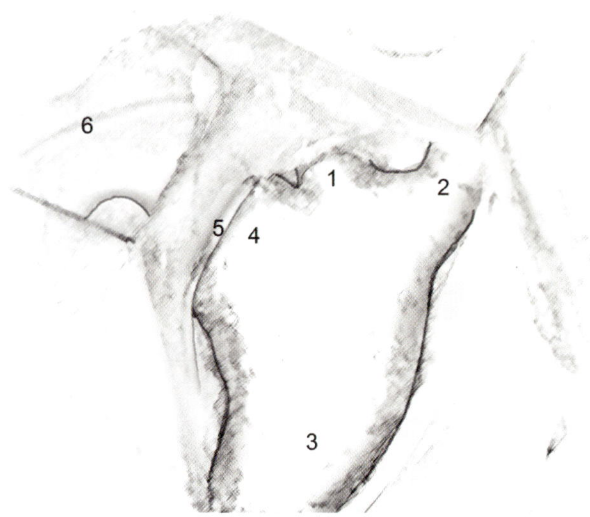

Figure 4.5

A large PDA in a 6-year-old boy as seen through a left lateral thoracotomy. Note that the size of the ductus is larger than the transverse aortic arch. The so-called ductal arch is distinguished from the true aortic arch by its relation to the left vagus and recurrent laryngeal nerves.

1. Transverse aortic arch
2. Left subclavian artery
3. Descending thoracic aorta
4. PDA
5. Left vagus nerve
6. Left phrenic nerve

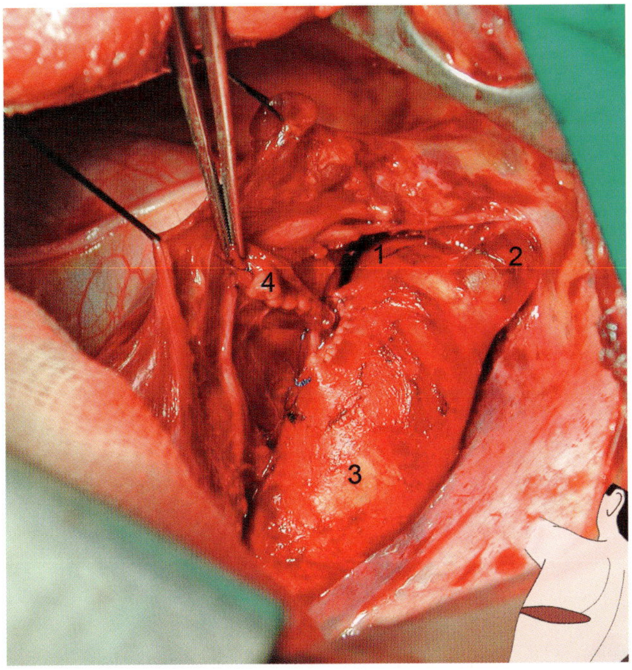

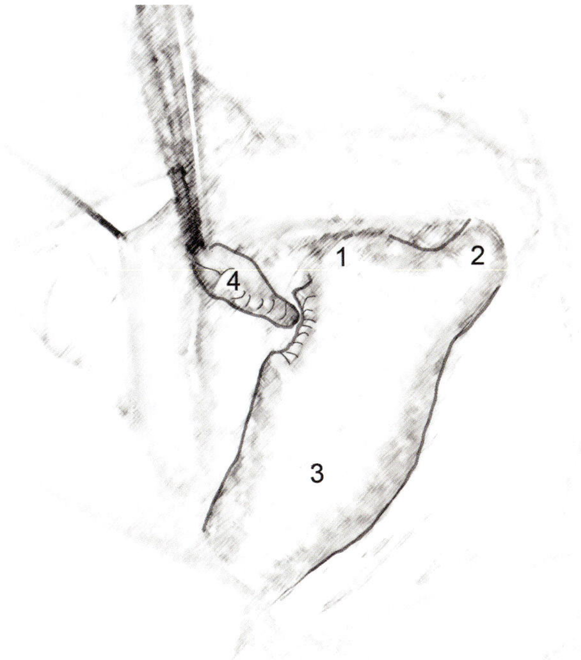

Figure 4.6 **Figure 4.7**

The same patient as in Figure 4.4 after division and oversewing of the ductus arteriosus.

1. Transverse aortic arch
2. Left subclavian artery
3. Descending aorta
4. Stump of divided ductus

Figure 4.8. A PDA in a 1-year-old infant as seen through a left lateral thoracotomy.

1. Left subclavian artery
2. Transverse aortic arch
3. PDA
4. Left vagus nerve
5. Descending aorta

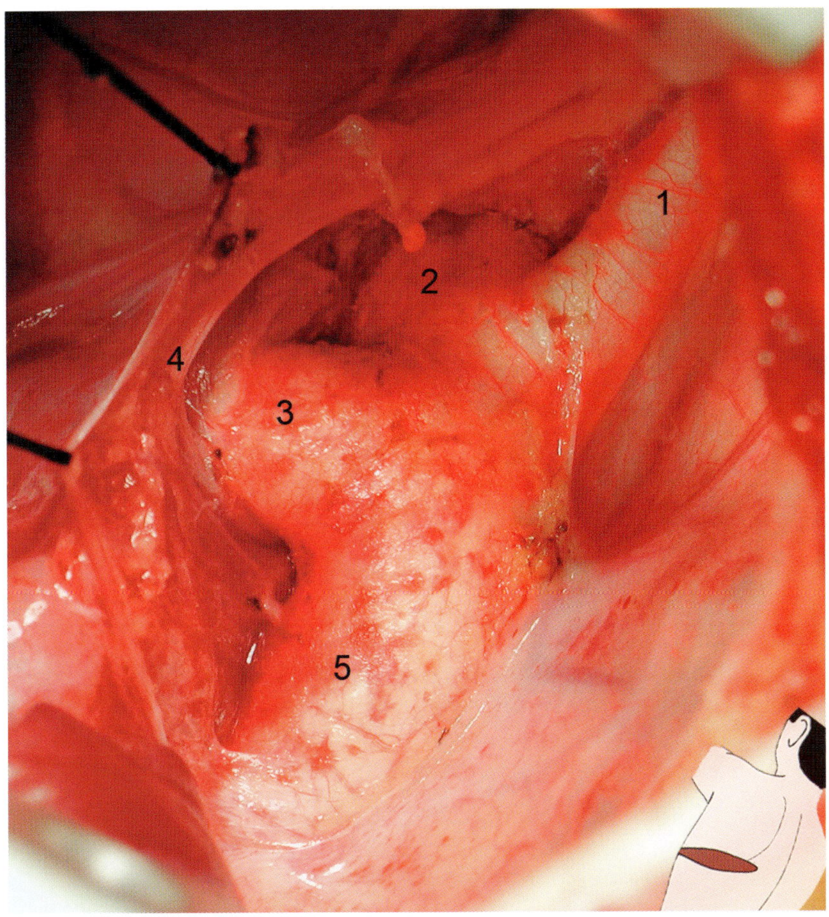

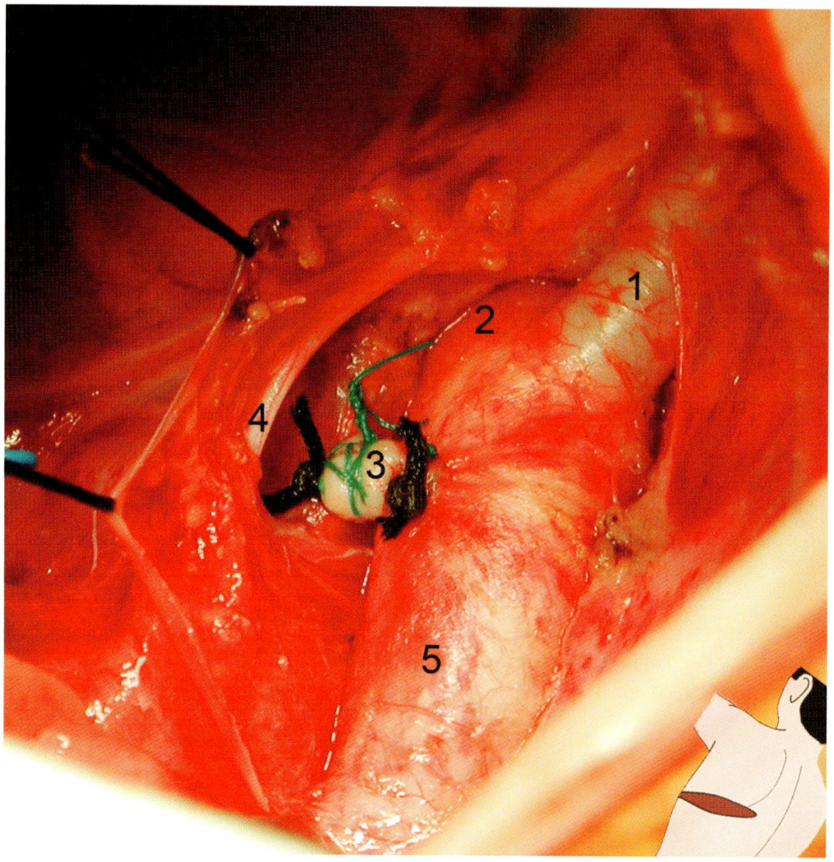

Figure 4.9. The same patient as in Figure 4.8. The PDA has been ligated with 2 ligatures and a transfixation suture placed (light green suture).

1. Left subclavian artery
2. Transverse aortic arch
3. Ligated PDA
4. Left vagus nerve
5. Descending aorta

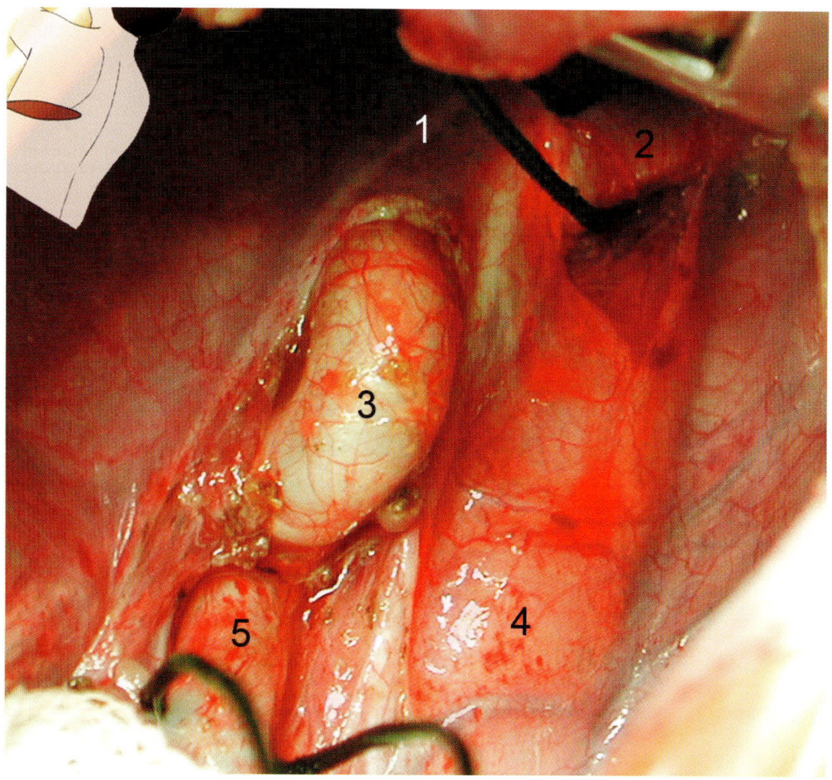

Figure 4.10. Left lateral thoracotomy view from a 3-week-old neonate with pulmonary atresia and a PDA. Note the unusual orientation and site of the ductus.

1. Left vagus nerve
2. Left subclavian artery
3. PDA
4. Descending aorta
5. Left pulmonary artery

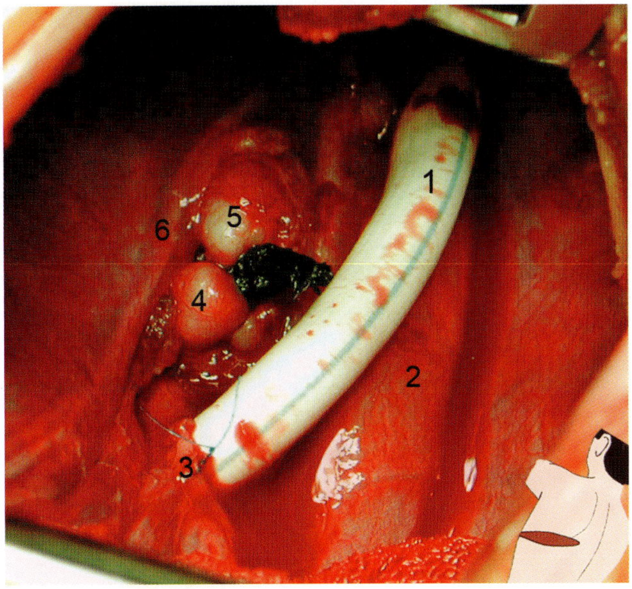

Figure 4.11

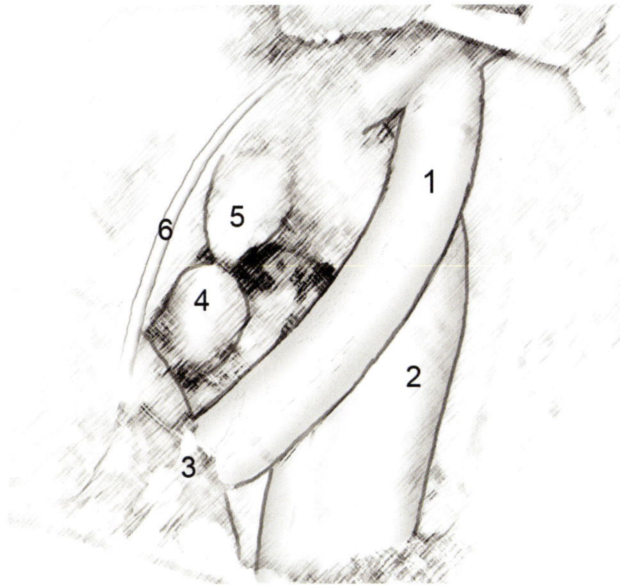

Figure 4.12

The same patient as in Figure 4.10. The ductus has been ligated and 4 mm modified Blalock-Taussig (BT) shunt placed between left subclavian and left pulmonary arteries.

1. Modified BT shunt (4 mm expanded PTFE)
2. Descending thoracic aorta
3. Left pulmonary artery
4. Pulmonary end of ductus
5. Aortic end of ductus
6. Left vagus nerve

orientation of the ductus, the so-called vertical ductus commonly seen in pulmonary atresia. A left modified BT shunt was placed between the left subclavian and left pulmonary arteries, and the ductus arteriosus was ligated. PDA in the prematurely born patient represents a special situation. Its incidence is inversely proportional to gestational age.[2] First-line treatment is with indomethacin or ibuprofen, which is effective in about 85% of cases.[3] When medical treatment is contraindicated or fails, surgical intervention is undertaken. Catheter-based interventions are not currently feasible. Figures 4.13 to 4.17 are from a 3-month-old infant born prematurely. He also has chronic lung disease of prematurity, and Figure 4.13

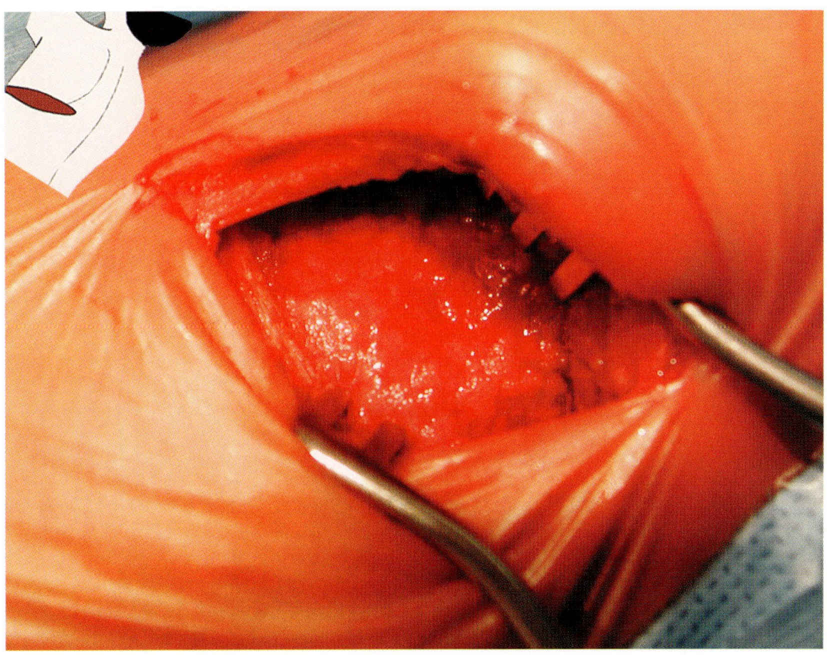

Figure 4.13. Left lateral thoracotomy view from a 3-month-old premature infant (born at 26 weeks gestation) with chronic lung disease and a PDA. Note the emphysematous left lung.

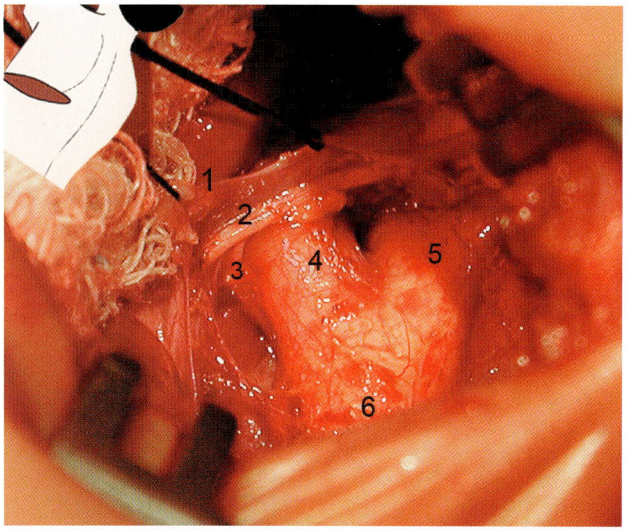

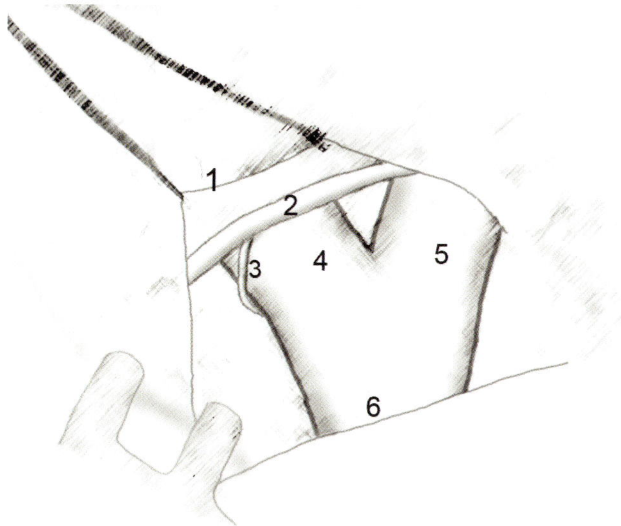

Figure 4.14 **Figure 4.15**

The same patient as in Figure 4.13. The lung has been retracted out of view. Minimal dissection is done. Note the large ductus.

1. Posterior mediastinal pleura
2. Left vagus nerve
3. Left recurrent laryngeal nerve
4. PDA
5. Isthmus part of aortic arch
6. Descending thoracic aorta

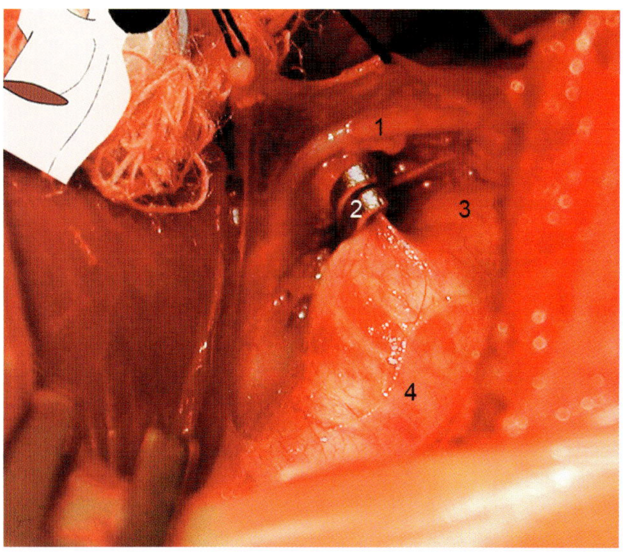

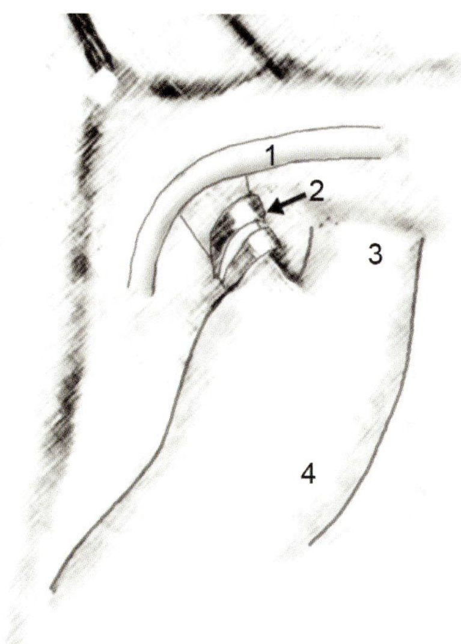

Figure 4.16 **Figure 4.17**

Same patient as in Figures 4.13 and 4.14. The ductus was closed by two metallic clips.

1. Left vagus nerve
2. Clips occluding the ductus
3. Isthmus part of aortic arch
4. Descending thoracic aorta

shows emphysematous lung. Ligation or clipping, rather than division, is used to close the ductus in such patients.

REFERENCES

1. Koch J, Hensley G, Roy L, et al. Prevalence of spontaneous closure of the ductus arteriosus in neonates at a birth weight of 1000 grams or less. *Pediatrics.* 2006;117:1113–1121.
2. Furzan JA, Reisch J, Tyson JE, Laird P, Rosenfeld CR. Incidence and risk factors for symptomatic patent ductus arteriosus among inborn very-low-birth-weight infants. *Early Hum Dev.* 1985;12:39–48.
3. Chemtobb S, Van Overmeirea B. The pharmacologic closure of the patent ductus arteriosus. *Semin Fetal Neonatal Med.* 2005;10:177–184.

CHAPTER 5

Atrioventricular Septal Defect

Atrioventricular septal defect (AVSD), also known as endocardial cushion defect and atrioventricular (AV) canal defect, refers to a group of disorders that include persistence of the embryonic ostium primum (primum atrial septal defect [ASD]), ventricular septal defect (VSD) at the inlet, and malformation of the AV valve. Various combinations of these defects give rise to a spectrum of different types of AVSD. This group of malformations is unified by its characteristic common AV junction, which results in displacement of the AV node postero-inferiorly (Figure 5.1) and the lack of wedging of the posterior great artery. Furthermore, the ventricular inlet length is shorter than the outlet length.

PARTIAL AVSD

There is an interatrial communication immediately above the AV valve,[1] representing persistence of the ostium primum. The crest of the ventricular septum is covered by adherent tissues of the bridging leaflets of the AV valve, which are shared by the 2 ventricles. Fusion of the bridging leaflets produces separate right and left valvar orifices at the AV junction. The valve on the right side has a 4-leaflet configuration, whereas the left-sided valve has 3 leaflets. The so-called cleft in the left-sided valve is the gap between the superior and inferior bridging leaflets, and the valve is not analogous to a mitral valve. Definitive treatment of

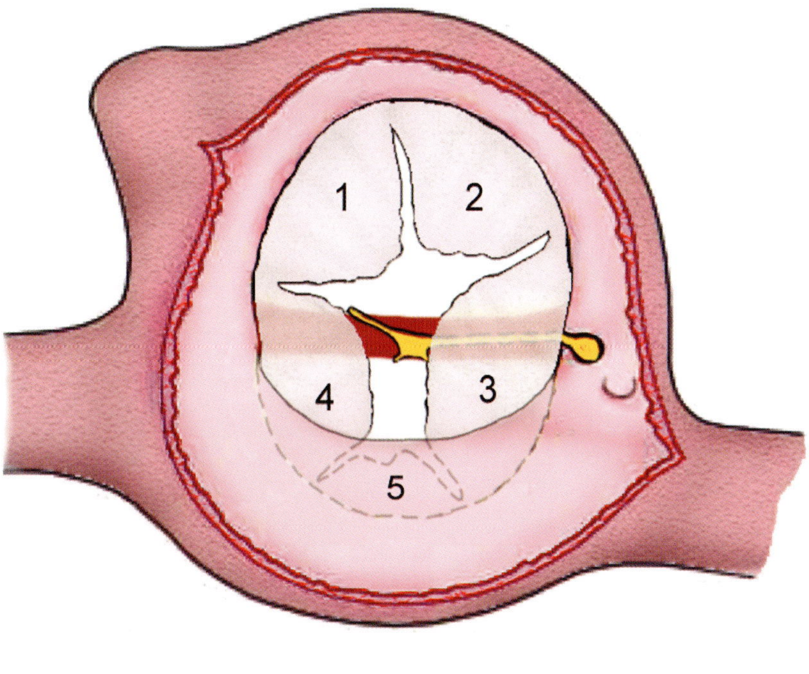

Figure 5.1. A schematic diagram of complete AVSD representing a right atriotomy surgical view. A 5-leaflet common AV valve characterized by 2 bridging leaflets that are inserted into both ventricles is depicted. The displaced AV node and AV conduction bundles (yellow) are shown. Note that the branching bundle is exposed on the septal crest in this example of a complete AVSD.

1. Right anterosuperior leaflet
2. Right inferior leaflet
3. Inferior bridging leaflet
4. Superior bridging leaflet
5. Left mural leaflet

Congenital Heart Disease: A Surgical Color Atlas © 2015 A. Sukru Mercan, Zakariya Hubail, S. Yen Ho.
Cardiotext Publishing, ISBN: 978-1-935395-90-4.

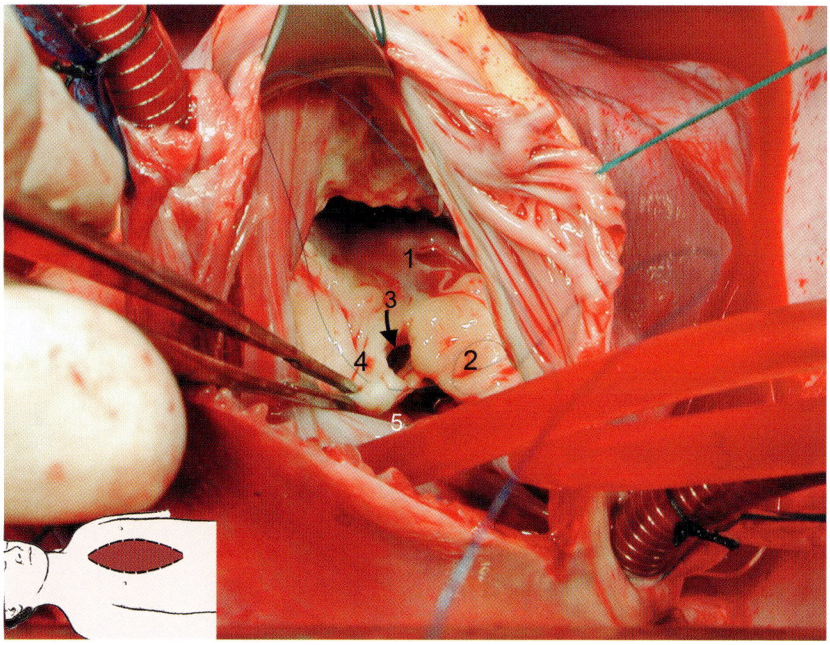

Figure 5.2. Partial AVSD in a 23-year-old patient, seen through a median sternotomy and right atriotomy. Note the "cleft" between the superior and inferior bridging leaflets in the left ventricle. The edges of these leaflets are approximated by a stay suture.

1. Ventricular septum
2. Inferior bridging leaflet
3. Cleft in left AV valve (arrow)
4. Superior bridging leaflet
5. Margin of primum ASD component

this anomaly is surgical and is performed on cardiopulmonary bypass through a right atriotomy incision.

Figure 5.2 shows a primum ASD as seen through a right atriotomy. Note the "cleft" in the left AV valve. The ASD was closed by an autologous pericardial patch, and the "cleft" in the valve was repaired by direct suturing (Figures 5.3 and 5.4). Another example is shown in Figures 5.5 to 5.10. When there is no left SVC, the patch is usually extended into the right atrium beyond the opening of the coronary sinus (CS) (see Figures 5.9 and 5.10). Thus, the CS is left to drain on the left of the pericardial patch into the left atrium. This is done to avoid placing sutures close to the AV node and bundle, thus minimizing

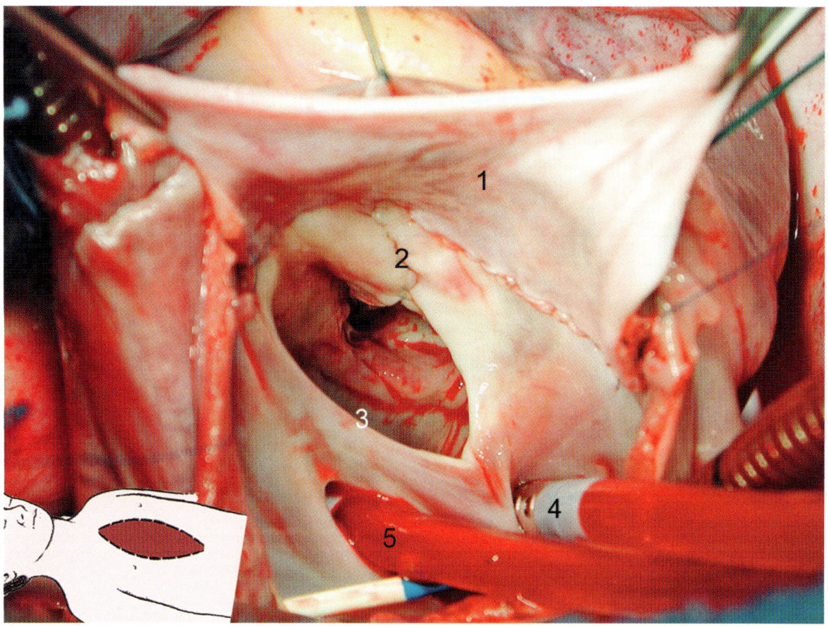

Figure 5.3. The same patient as in Figure 5.2. The "cleft" in the left AV valve has been repaired by direct suturing (2). A pericardial patch has been sutured to the base of the atrial septum and upper surface of the AV valves.

1. Pericardial patch
2. Site of "cleft" in AV valve
3. Border of ASD
4. Suction catheter in CS
5. Suction catheter in patent foramen ovale (PFO)

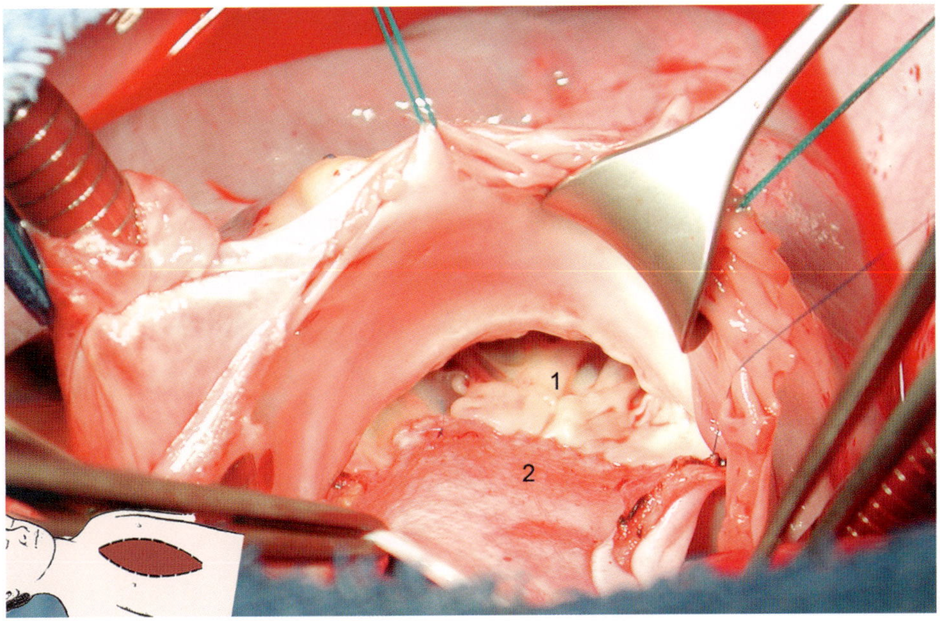

Figure 5.4. The same patient as in Figures 5.2 and 5.3. The pericardial patch is flipped to the left to reveal the right AV valve. The CS (see #4 in Figure 5.3) will drain to the left of the patch into the left atrium.

1. Right AV valve
2. Pericardial patch

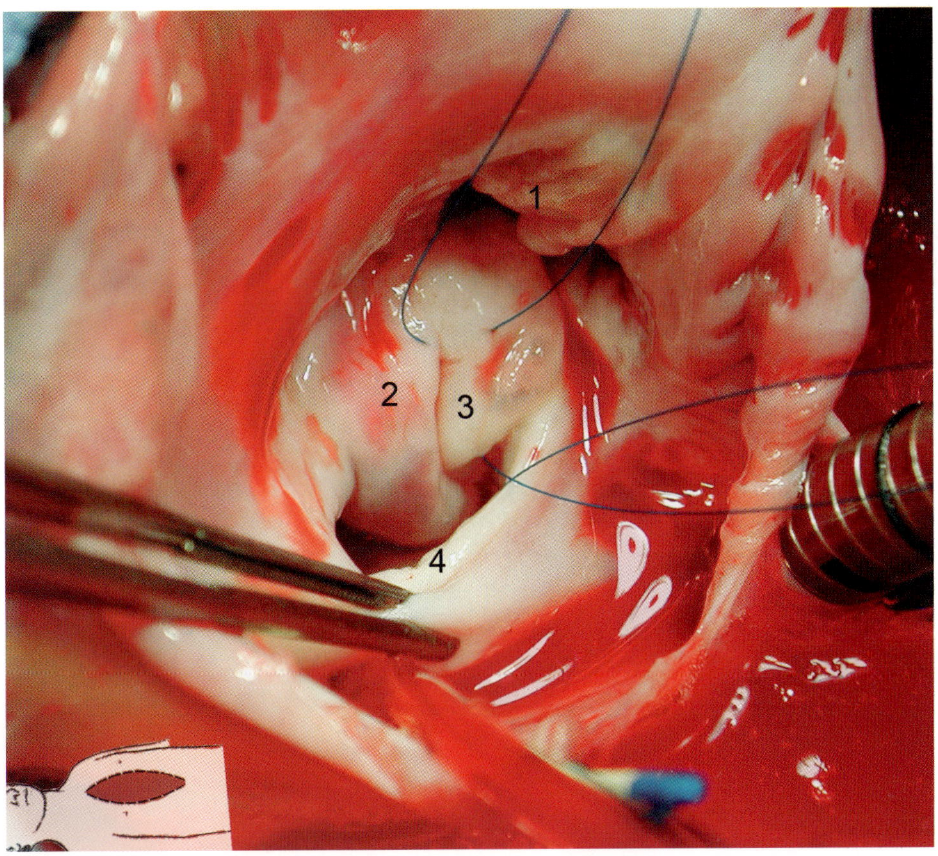

Figure 5.5. Partial AVSD in a child as seen through right atriotomy. Note the commissural "cleft" in the left component of the AV valve. An alignment suture has been placed just to the right of the "cleft."

1. Anterosuperior leaflet of right AV valve
2. Superior bridging leaflet
3. Inferior bridging leaflet
4. Edge of atrial septum (primum ASD)

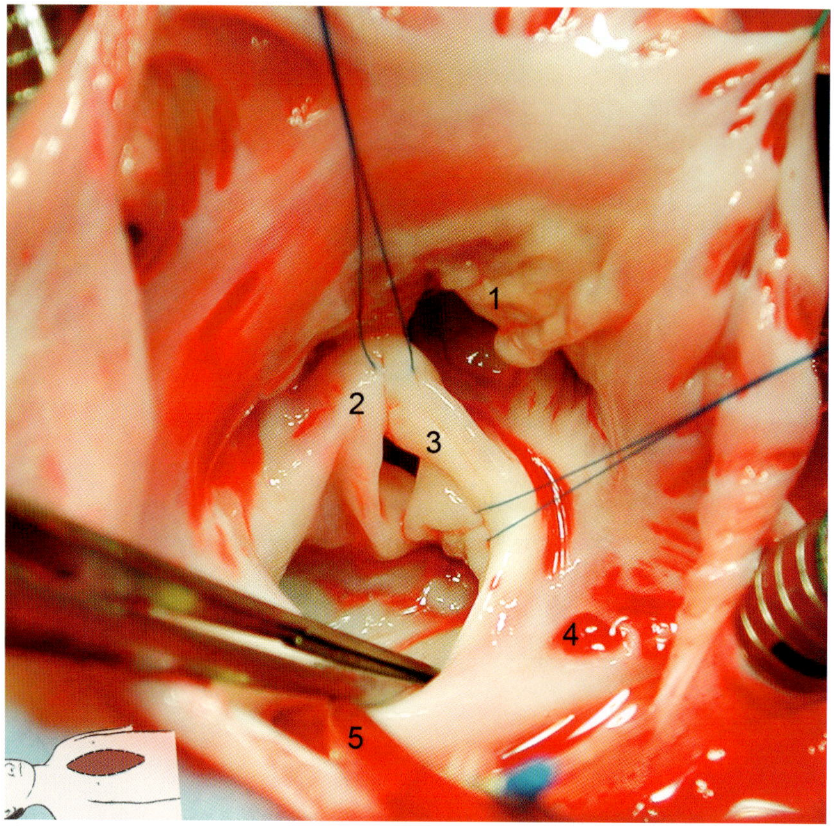

Figure 5.6. The same patient as in Figure 5.5 with bridging leaflets retracted up. The inferior leaflet has another cleft-like defect, and a suture has already been placed around it (further shown in Figure 5.8).

1. Anterosuperior leaflet of right AV valve
2. Superior bridging leaflet
3. Inferior bridging leaflet
4. Opening of CS
5. Catheter in PFO

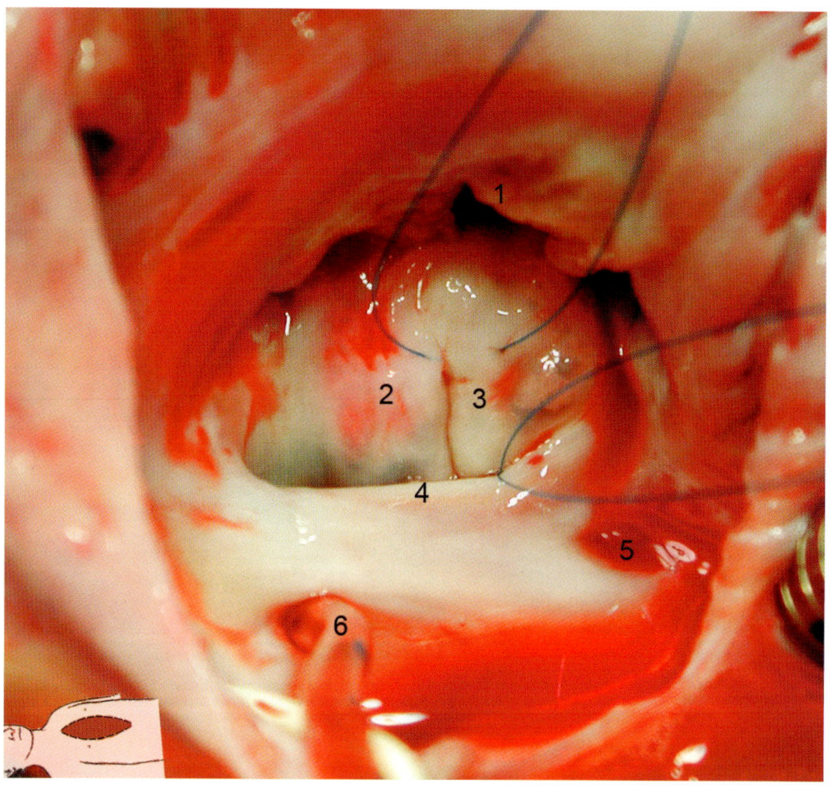

Figure 5.7. The same patient as in Figures 5.5 and 5.6 showing the AV valve in apposition.

1. Anterosuperior leaflet of right AV valve
2. Superior bridging leaflet
3. Inferior bridging leaflet
4. Edge of atrial septum (primum ASD)
5. Opening of CS
6. Catheter in PFO

Figure 5.8. The same patient as in Figures 5.5 to 5.7 after repair of the "clefts."

1. Anterosuperior leaflet of right AV valve
2. Superior bridging leaflet
3. Inferior bridging leaflet
4. Suture closing the cleft in inferior leaflet

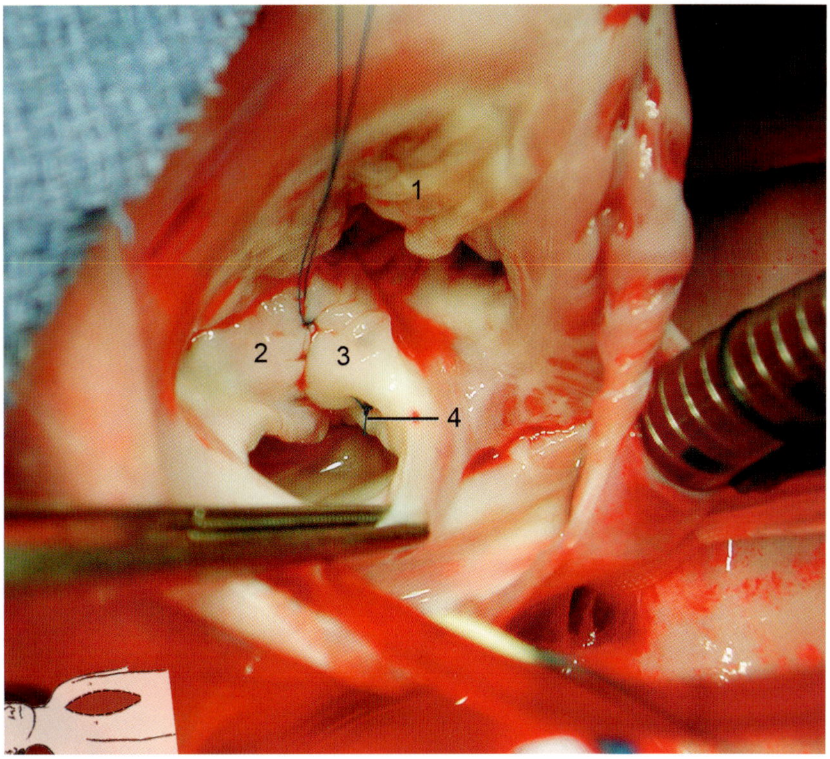

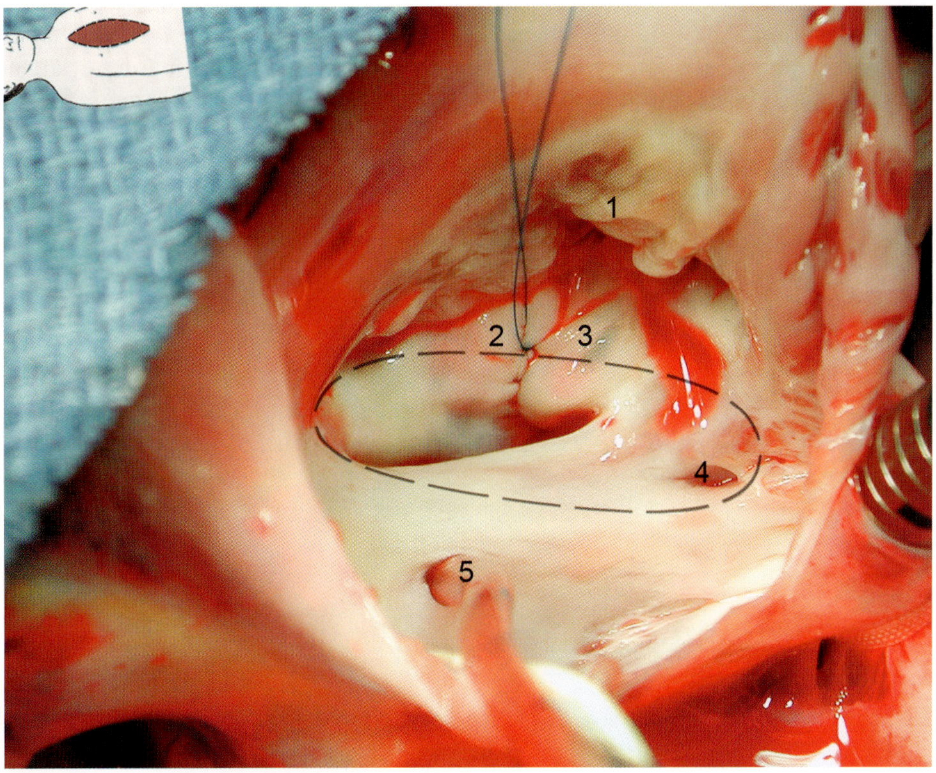

Figure 5.9. The same patient as in Figures 5.5 to 5.8 after repair of the clefts. The dashed line outlines the approximate location of the patch that will close the primum ASD. Note that the CS is incorporated into the new left atrium to avoid placing sutures in the vulnerable area of the conduction system.

1. Anterosuperior leaflet of right AV valve
2. Superior bridging leaflet
3. Inferior bridging leaflet
4. Opening of CS
5. Catheter in PFO

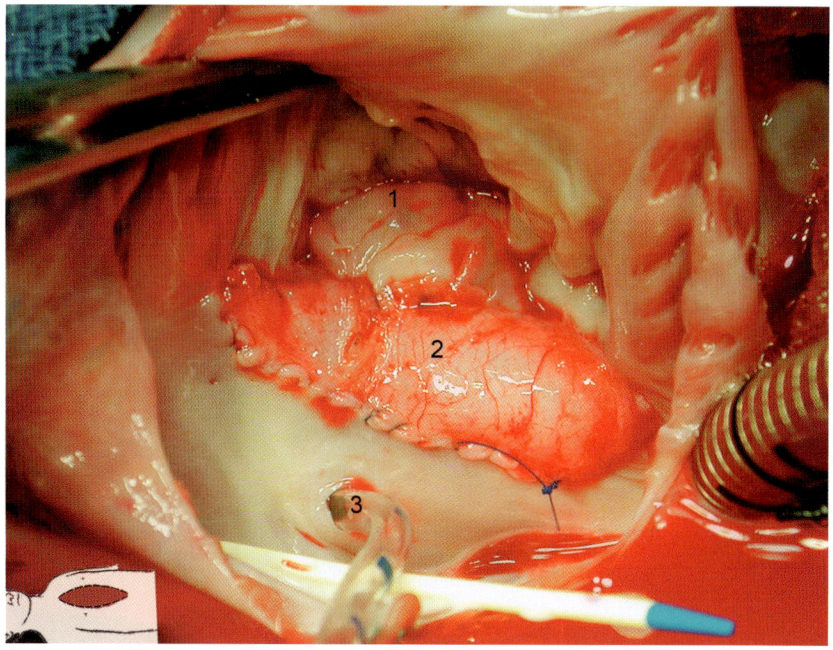

Figure 5.10. The same patient as in Figures 5.5 to 5.9 after completion of the intracardiac repair. An autologous pericardial patch has been used to close the ASD component.

1. Right AV valve
2. Pericardial patch closing the primum ASD
3. Catheter in PFO

the risk of AV heart block. When there is a left SVC draining to the CS, the blood flow may be directed to the right atrium by using a horseshoe-shaped patch, as illustrated in Figures 5.11 and 5.12.

Occasionally AVSD is associated with heterotaxy, particularly left atrial isomerism.[2] The abnormal venous connections often necessitate innovative atrial patching and baffling techniques (Figures 5.13–5.24).

COMPLETE AVSD

In the complete form (also known as AV canal defect), the shunt is at both the interatrial and interventricular levels since the bridging leaflets of the valve are not adherent to the crest of the ventricular septum and are usually not fused together. It is particularly common in patients who have Down syndrome.[3] The

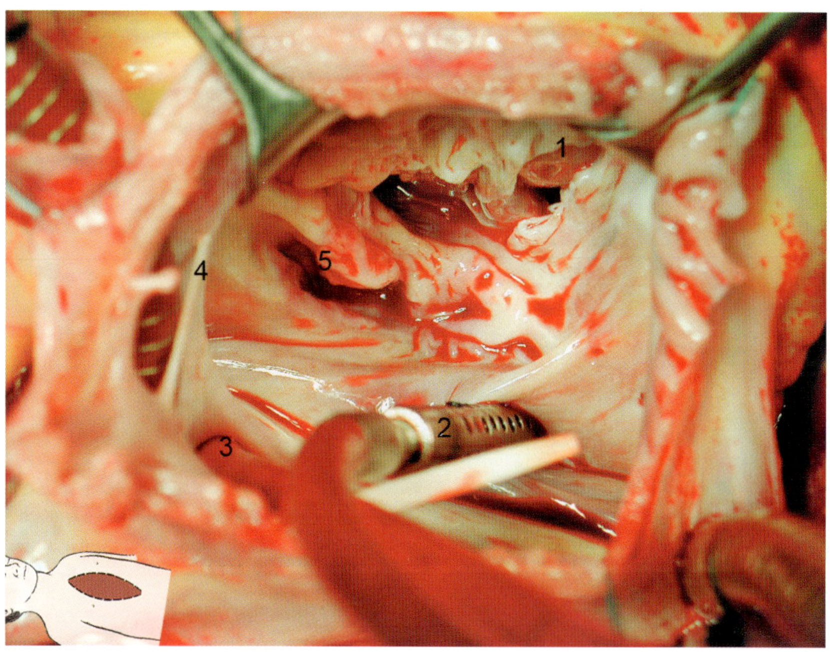

Figure 5.11. Partial AVSD, seen through a right atriotomy. The ASD is very large, amounting to almost a common atrium. This patient also had a left superior vena cava (SVC) (not shown) draining to the CS.

1. Right AV valve
2. Suction catheter in CS (draining left SVC)
3. Suction catheter in PFO
4. Superior border of ASD
5. Left AV valve

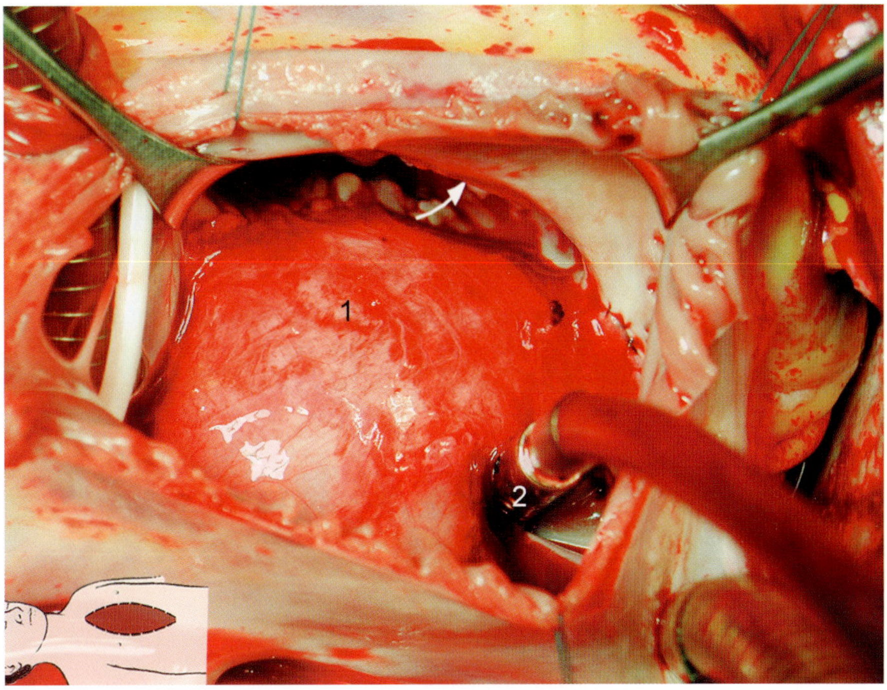

Figure 5.12. The same patient as in Figure 5.11. A horseshoe-shaped pericardial patch was used to close the ASD and baffle the CS flow to the right atrium. The white arrow points to the right AV valve.

1. Pericardial patch
2. Suction catheter in CS

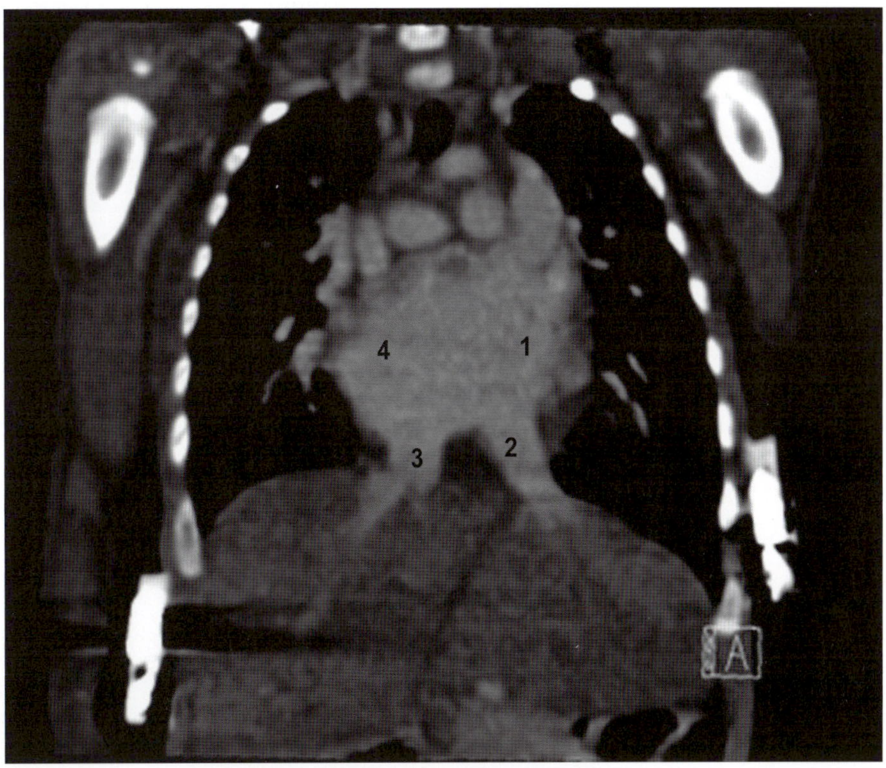

Figure 5.13. A computed tomography (CT) coronal image of 9-month-old infant with left atrial isomerism and partial AVSD. The ASD was huge with almost no septum (a common atrium). The inferior vena cava (IVC) is interrupted with azygos continuation to the left SVC, shown in Figure 5.15. The hepatic veins drain directly into the atrium.

1. Left-sided atrium
2. Left hepatic vein
3. Right hepatic vein
4. Right-sided atrium

Figure 5.14. Another CT image of the same patient in Figure 5.13. The cut is taken at a more posterior level. The 4 pulmonary veins (PVs) are seen draining into the middle part of the atrium.

1. Left upper PV
2. Left lower PV
3. Atrium
4. Right upper PV
5. Right lower PV
6. Descending thoracic aorta

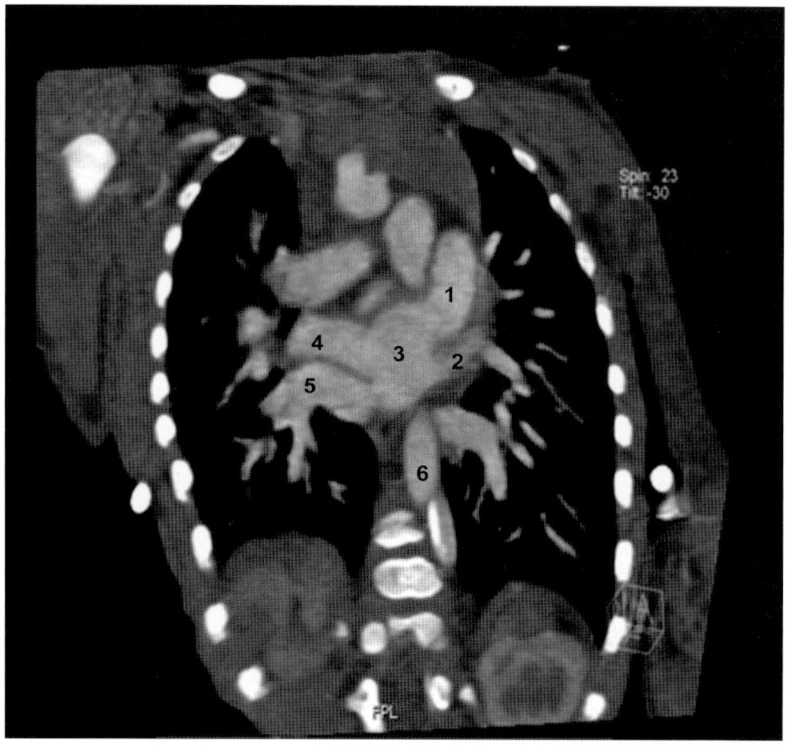

Figure 5.15. A sagittal CT image of the same patient in Figures 5.13 and 5.14. The lower body venous blood reaches the heart via the azygos vein and left SVC.

1. Azygos vein
2. Left SVC
3. Left side of atrium
4. Left hepatic vein

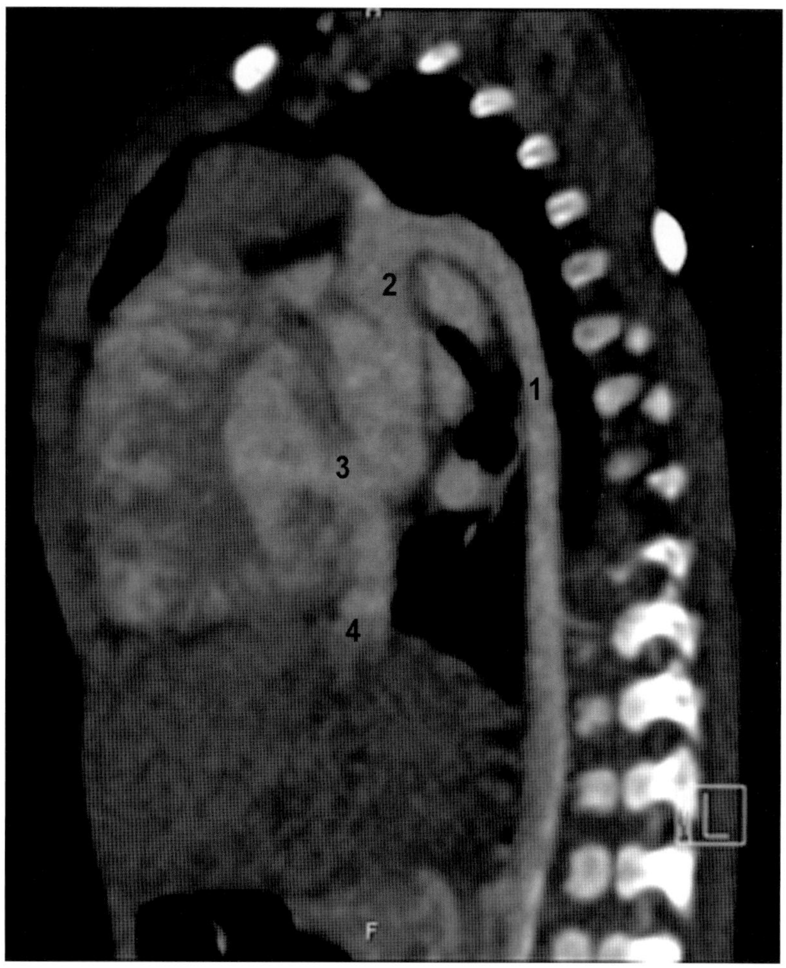

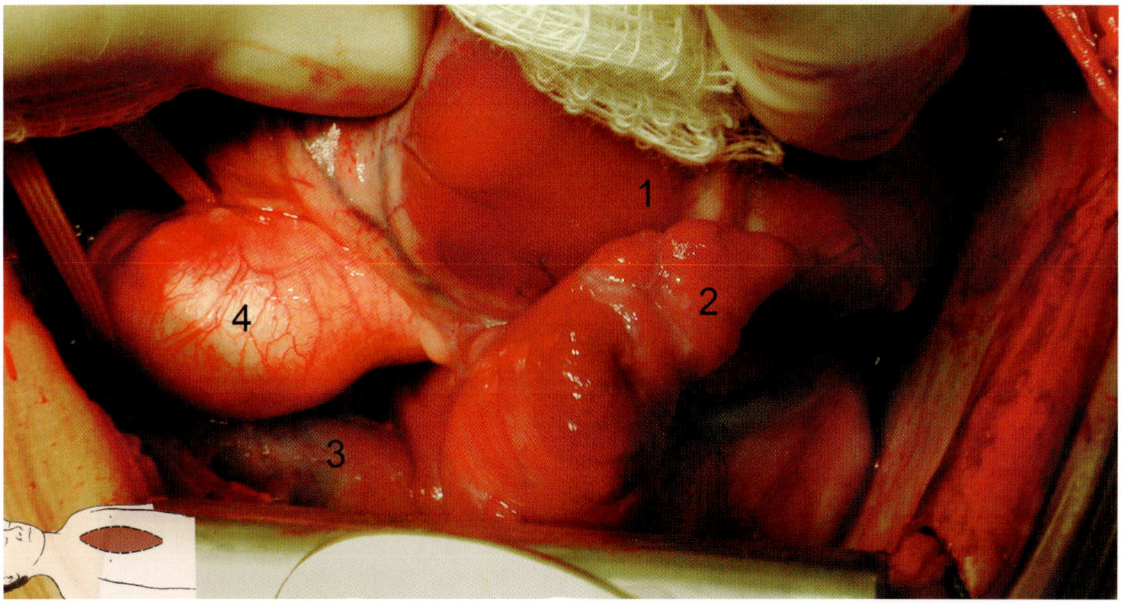

Figure 5.16. Median sternotomy view of the same patient whose CT images are shown in Figures 5.13 to 5.15. Both atria are morphologically left. The atrial appendage of the right-sided atrium is shown having left atria morphology.

1. Right ventricle (RV)
2. Atrial appendage
3. Right SVC
4. Ascending aorta

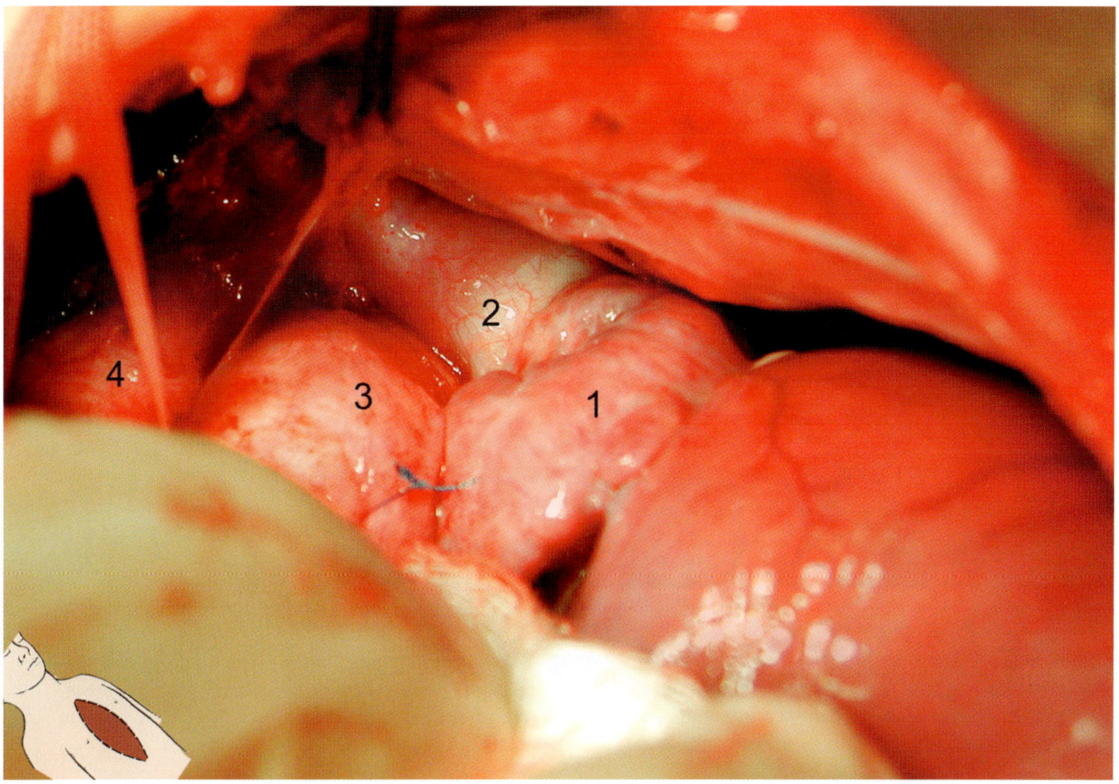

Figure 5.17. The left side of the mediastinum of the same patient as in Figures 5.13 to 5.16. The left SVC is shown.

1. Left atrial appendage
2. Left SVC
3. Main pulmonary artery (MPA)
4. Ascending aorta

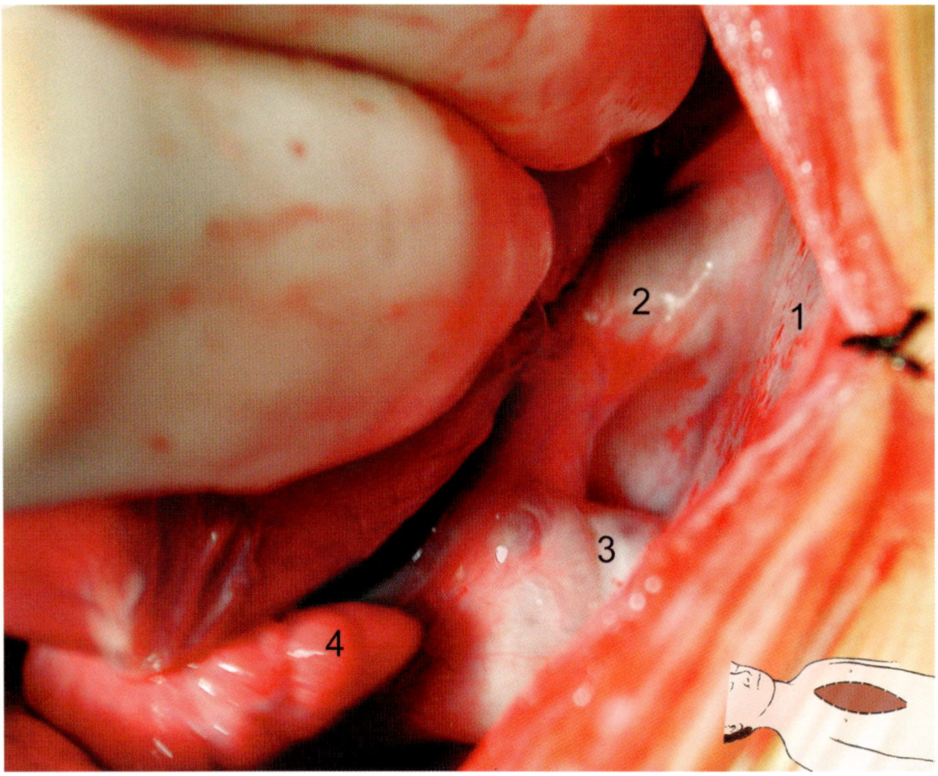

Figure 5.18. The hepatic veins of the same patient as in Figures 5.13 to 5.17. The left hepatic vein enters the left-sided atrium, and the right hepatic vein enters the right-sided atrium.

1. Parietal pericardium overlying the diaphragm
2. Left hepatic vein
3. Right hepatic vein
4. Atrial appendage (right sided, but morphologically left)

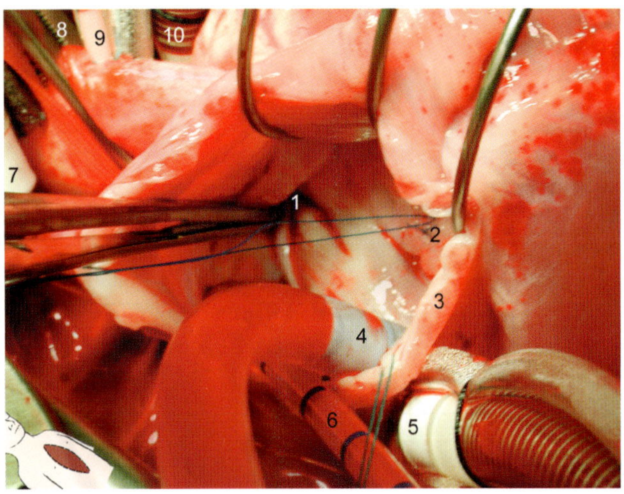

Figure 5.19

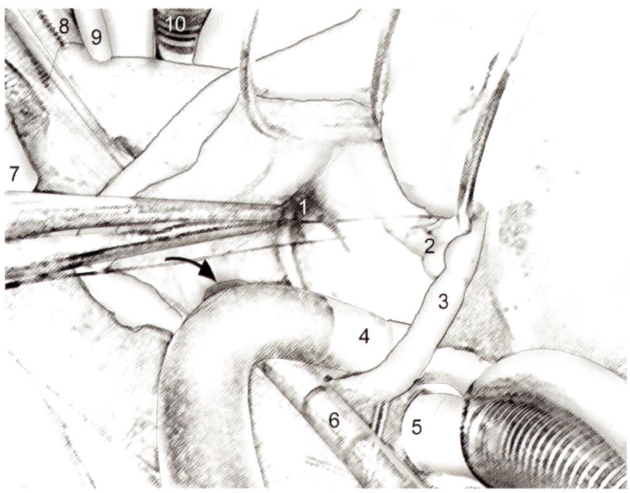

Figure 5.20

Right atriotomy view of the same patient as in Figures 5.13 to 5.18. Part of the cannulation setup is also shown. An alignment stay suture has been placed in the AV valve (2). The opening of the left SVC is seen in the left side of the atrium. The PVs drain to the central part of the atrium, in a more posterior location; a suction catheter (6) is draining one of the PVs, denoted by the arrow.

1. Opening of the left SVC
2. AV valve
3. Wall of right-sided atrium
4. Suction catheter (to left hepatic vein)
5. Venous cannula in right hepatic vein
6. Suction catheter (to a PV)
7. Venous cannula in right SVC
8. Aortic cross-clamp
9. Coronary perfusion catheter
10. Venous cannula in left SVC

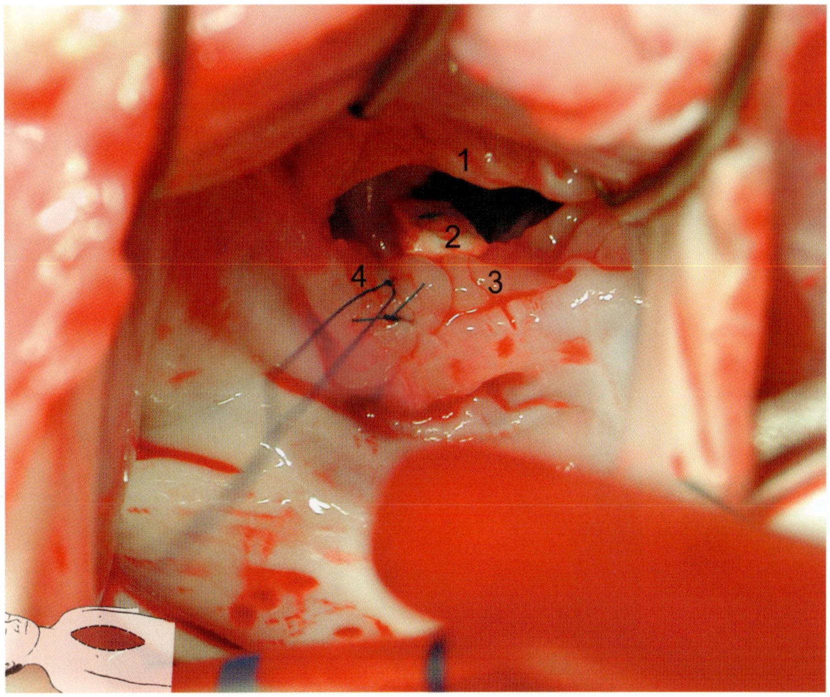

Figure 5.21. The same patient as in Figures 5.13 to 5.20. The AV valve is shown. A Teflon-supported suture is placed to help with coaptation. Another suture is used to close the median commissure ("cleft").

1. Right anterosuperior leaflet
2. Teflon pledget
3. Inferior bridging leaflet
4. Superior bridging leaflet

treatment is surgical and is undertaken during early infancy. Like the partial form, it is performed on cardiopulmonary bypass through a right atriotomy incision.

There are many techniques to repair this lesion.[4] A discussion of the merits of each technique is beyond the scope of this book. We usually use the double-patch technique.

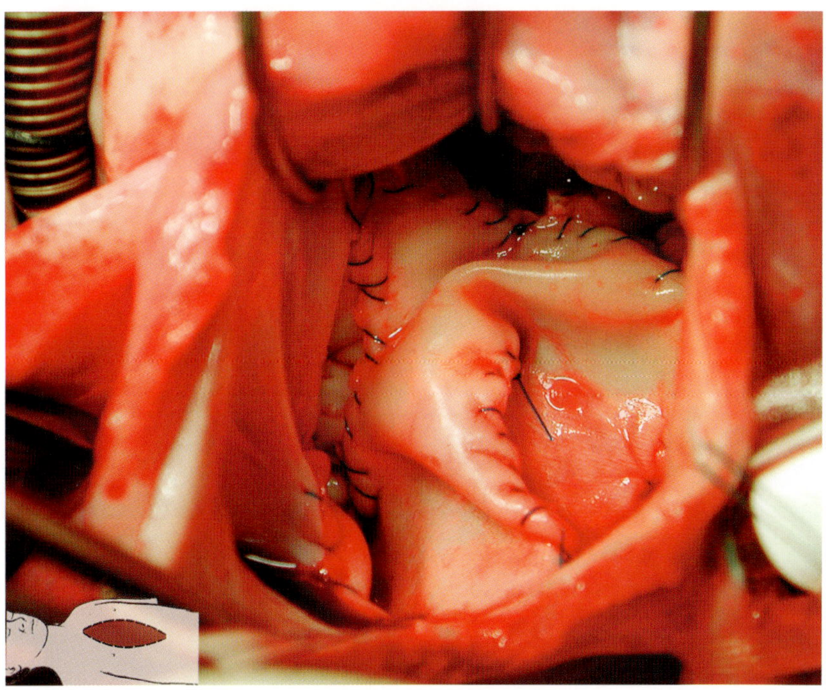

Figure 5.22. The same patient as in Figures 5.13 to 5.21 after repair. Systemic and pulmonary venous returns have been separated by an intra-atrial baffle, using a xenograft pericardial patch.

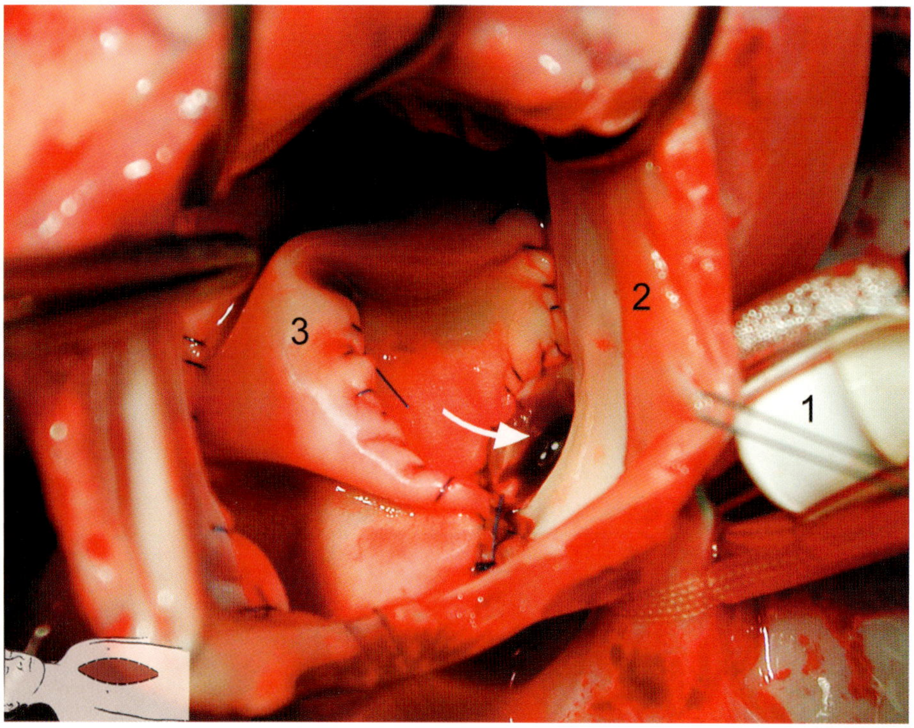

Figure 5.23. The same patient as in Figures 5.13 to 5.22. The arrow points to the opening of the left hepatic vein, draining into the new right atrium.

1. Venous cannula in right hepatic vein
2. Wall of right-sided atrium
3. Intra-atrial baffle (xenograft pericardium)

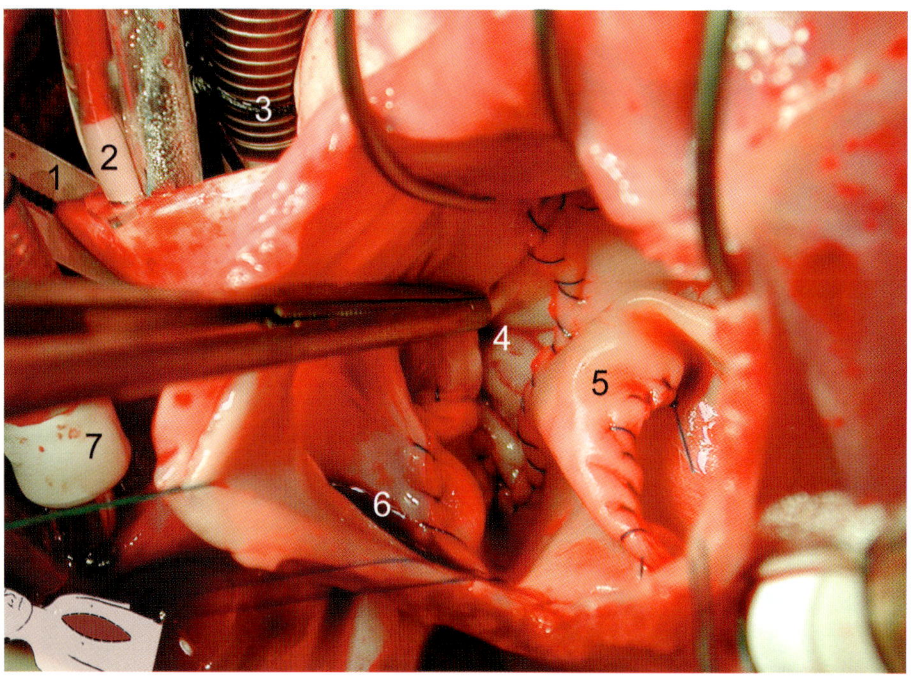

Figure 5.24. The same patient as in Figures 5.13 to 5.23. The openings of the left and right SVC into the new right atrium are shown. The PVs open into the new left atrium on the other side of xenograft baffle.

1. Aortic cross-clamp
2. Coronary perfusion catheter
3. Left SVC venous cannula
4. Opening of left SVC
5. Intra-atrial baffle (xenograft pericardium)
6. Opening of right SVC
7. Venous cannula in right SVC

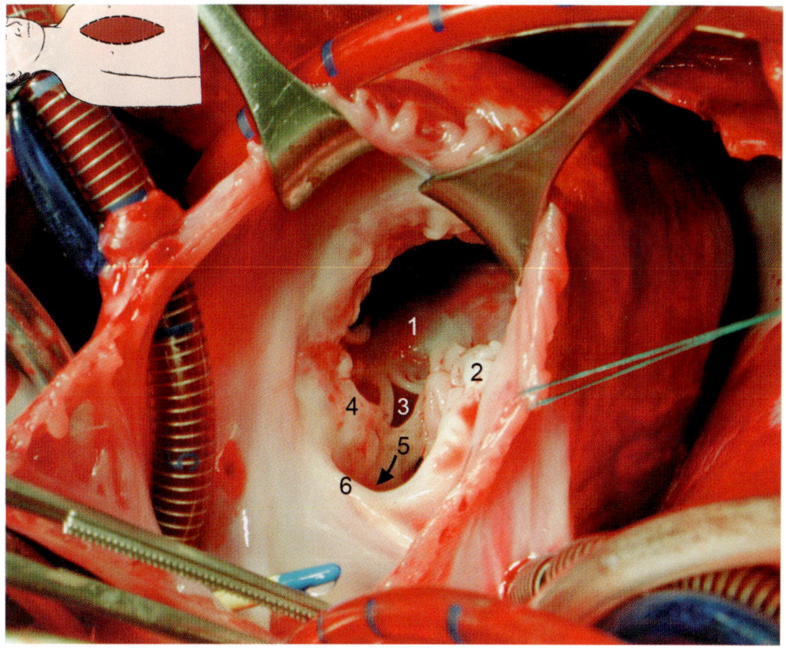

Figure 5.25. Complete AVSD in a 1-year-old child, as seen through a right atriotomy. Note the attachment of the superior bridging leaflet to the crest of the ventricular septum (Rastelli type A).

1. Ventricular septum
2. Inferior bridging leaflet
3. Ventricular septal defect component
4. Superior bridging leaflet
5. Primum ASD component (arrow)
6. Edge of atrial septum

Figures 5.25 and 5.26 show a surgical view through a median sternotomy and right atriotomy in a 1-year-old child with AVSD. The defect was repaired using double-patch technique (Figures 5.27–5.31). Figures 5.32 to 5.36 illustrate another example of AVSD repaired using the same technique, but with a different patching material.

AVSD WITH VENTRICULAR COMPONENT ONLY

Shunting only at the ventricular level is the least common pattern and can be mistaken for an inlet VSD. Nevertheless, this form has the distinctive

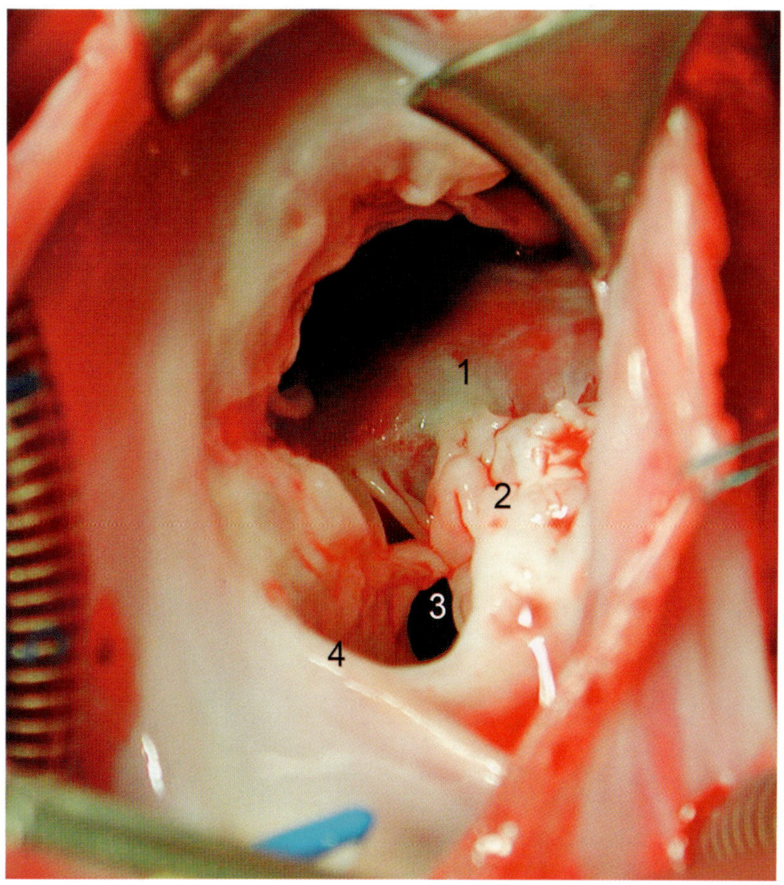

Figure 5.26. Zoomed-out view of the anatomy of the heart shown in Figure 5.25. Note the zone of apposition between the superior and inferior bridging leaflets, and the resultant "cleft" in the left component of the AV valve.

1. Ventricular septum
2. Inferior bridging leaflet
3. "Cleft" in left component of the AV valve
4. Edge of atrial septum

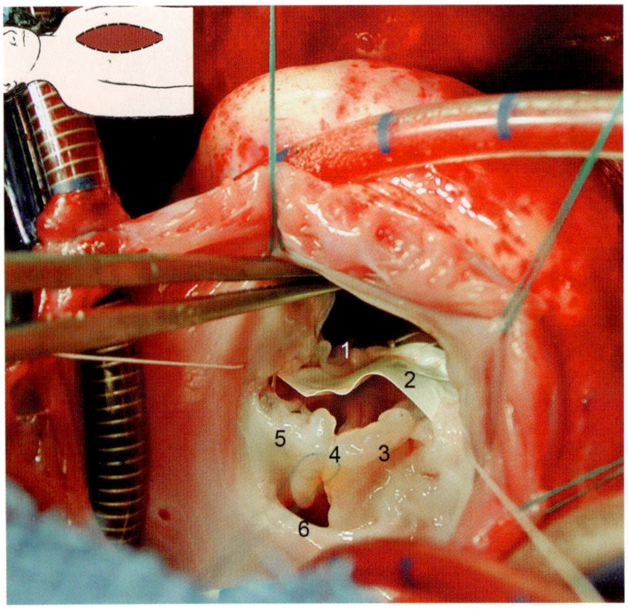

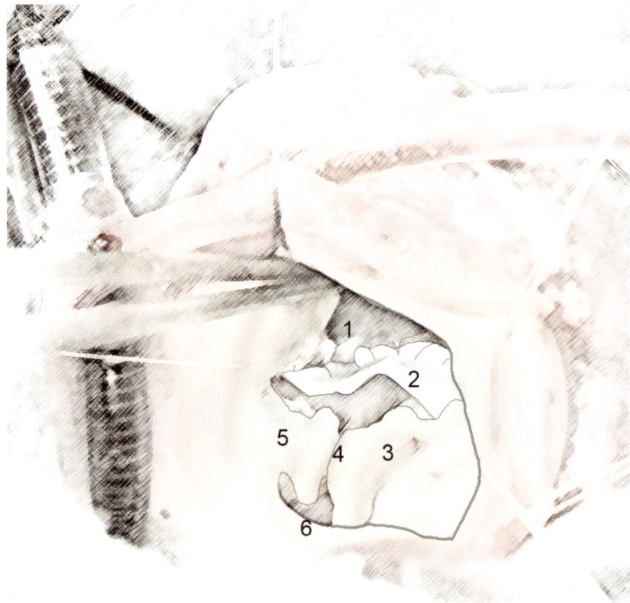

Figure 5.27 **Figure 5.28**

Same patient as in Figures 5.25 and 5.26. A stay suture (light green) has been placed in the zone of apposition of the superior and inferior bridging leaflets. A Gore-Tex patch is being sutured in place to close the VSD component.

1. Ventricular septum where the Gore-Tex patch is sutured
2. Upper margin of the Gore-Tex patch that will be sutured to the valve
3. Inferior bridging leaflet
4. Stay suture in the zone of apposition of the superior and inferior bridging leaflets
5. Superior bridging leaflet
6. Superior border of ASD component

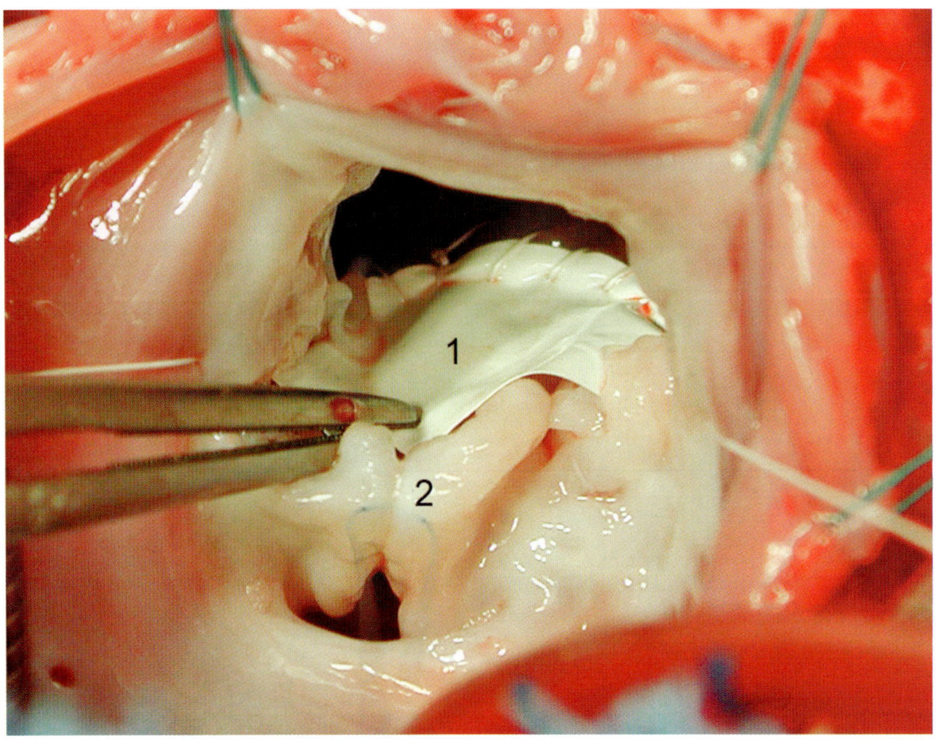

Figure 5.29. The same patient as in Figures 5.25 to 5.27. The Gore-Tex patch is positioned in the location where it will eventually be sutured to the AV valve.

1. Gore-Tex patch
2. Inferior bridging leaflet

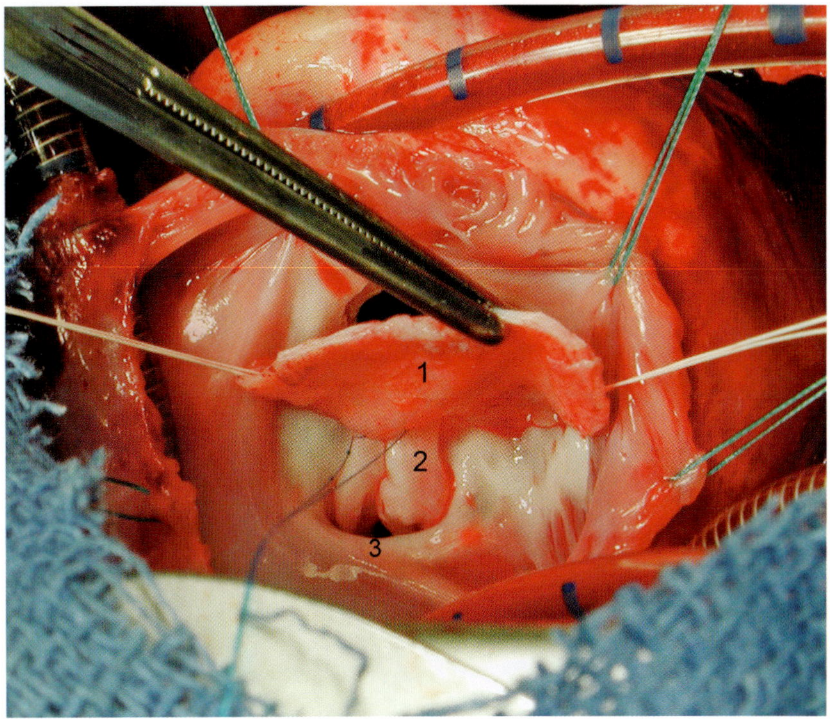

Figure 5.30. The same patient as in Figures 5.25 to 5.29. A pericardial patch is being placed to close the ASD. The inferior edge of the patch has already been sutured to the upper surface of the AV valve, immediately to the right of the stay suture.

1. Pericardial patch
2. Inferior bridging leaflet
3. Edge of atrial septum

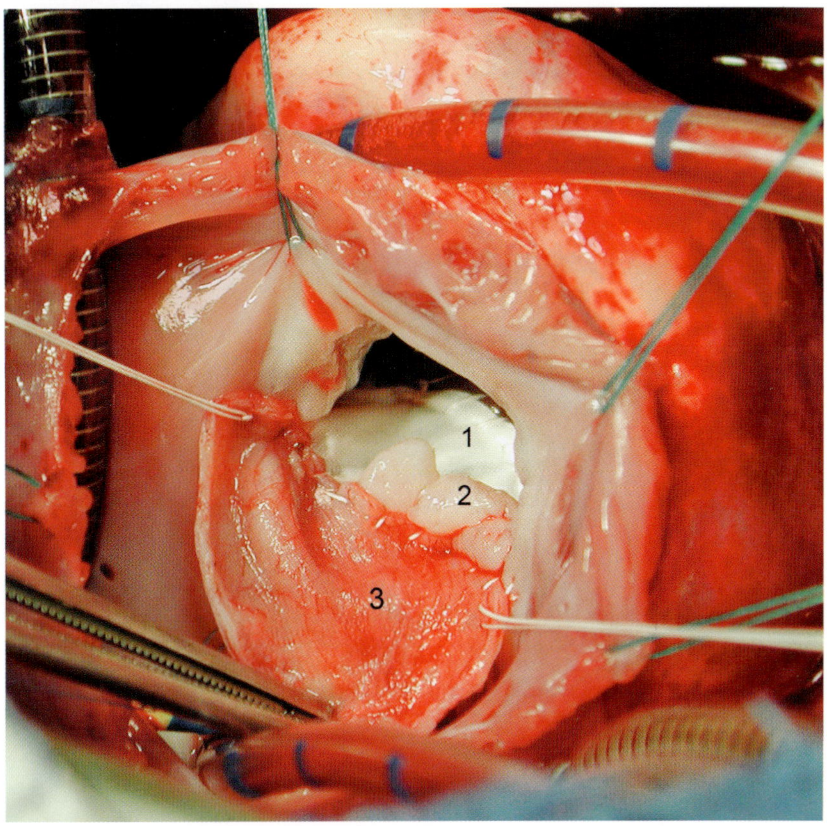

Figure 5.31. The same patient as in Figures 5.25 to 5.30. The pericardial patch is flipped leftward to show the right atrial aspect. Note that a larger share of the bridging leaflets is being incorporated into the left component of the AV valve.

1. Gore-Tex patch (closing the VSD)
2. Right side of inferior bridging leaflet
3. Pericardial patch

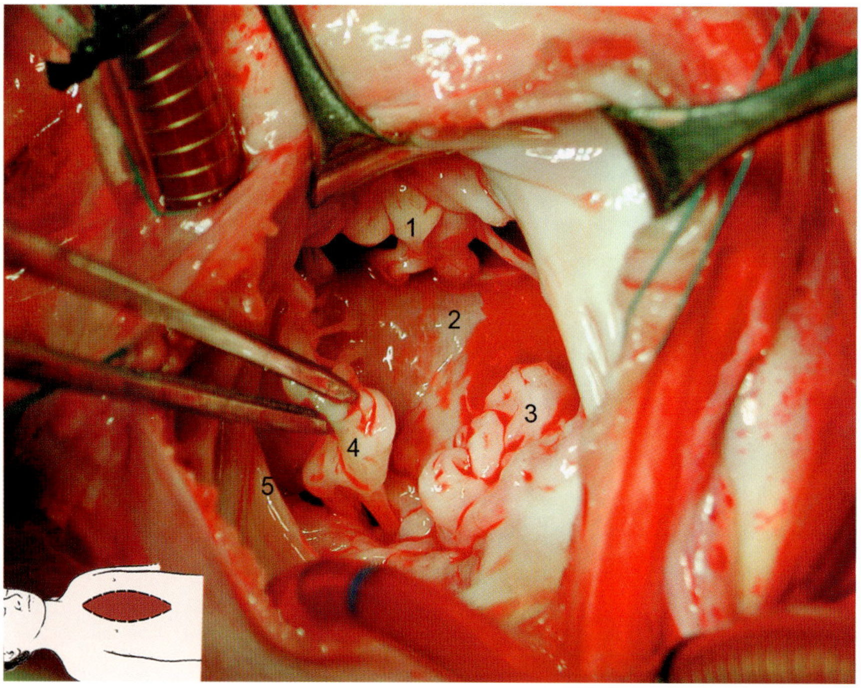

Figure 5.32. Complete AVSD as seen through a right atriotomy incision. Note the attachment of the superior bridging leaflet to the interventricular septum.

1. Anterosuperior leaflet
2. Ventricular septum
3. Inferior bridging leaflet
4. Superior bridging leaflet
5. Upper border of primum ASD component

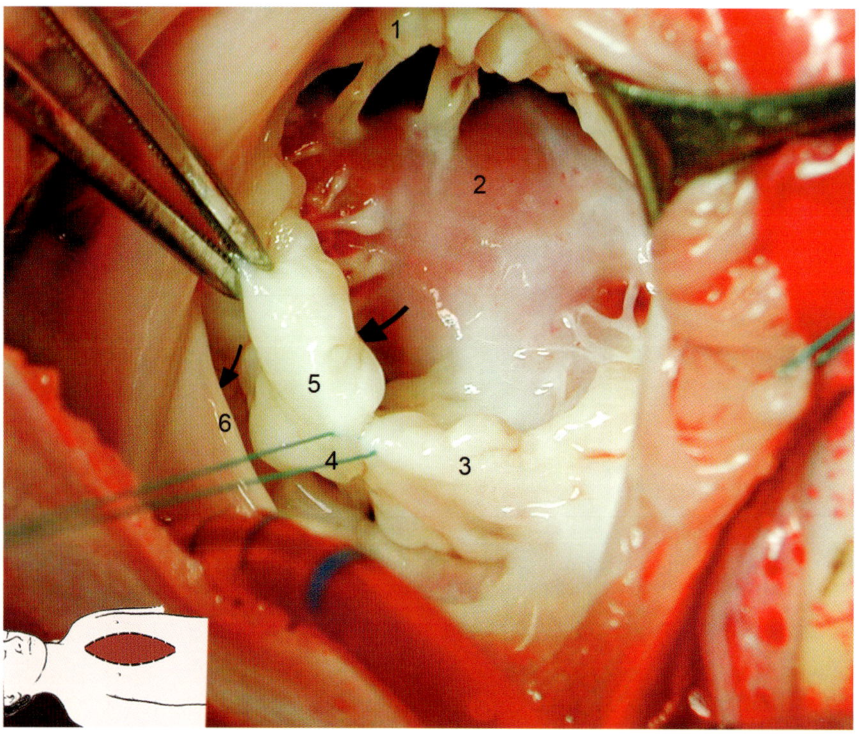

Figure 5.33. Same patient as in Figure 5.32. A stay suture has been placed at zone of apposition of the superior and inferior bridging leaflets. The large arrow points to the VSD component directly beneath the valve, whereas the small arrow points to the ASD component above the valve.

1. Anterosuperior leaflet
2. Ventricular septum
3. Inferior bridging leaflet
4. Stay suture bringing together the bridging leaflets
5. Superior bridging leaflet
6. Upper rim of primum ASD

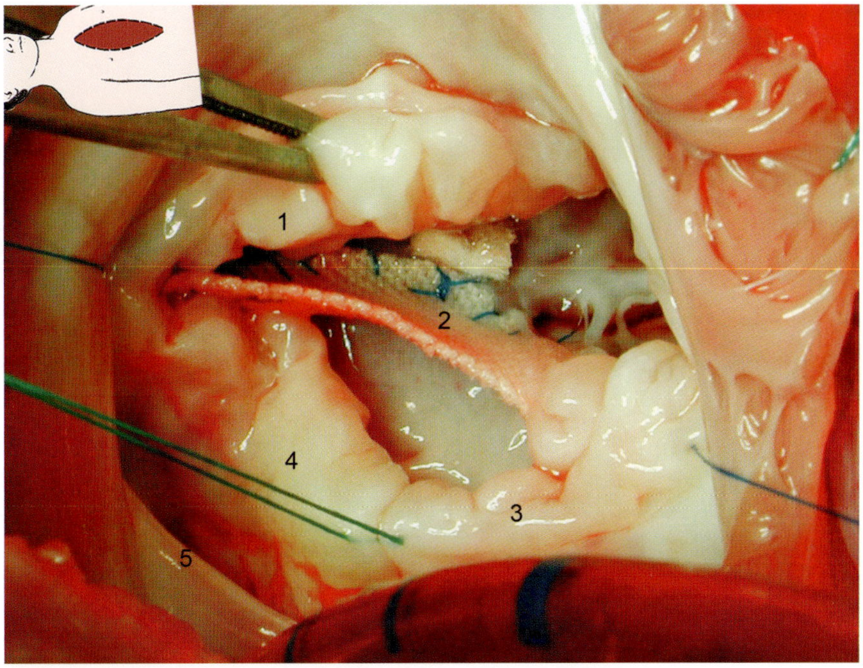

Figure 5.34. Same patient as in Figures 5.32 and 5.33. A Dacron patch is being used to close the VSD component. The inferior border of the patch has already been sutured to the ventricular septum; the superior edge will be sutured to the AV valve to completely close the VSD.

1. Anterosuperior leaflet
2. Dacron patch
3. Inferior bridging leaflet
4. Superior bridging leaflet
5. Upper rim of primum ASD

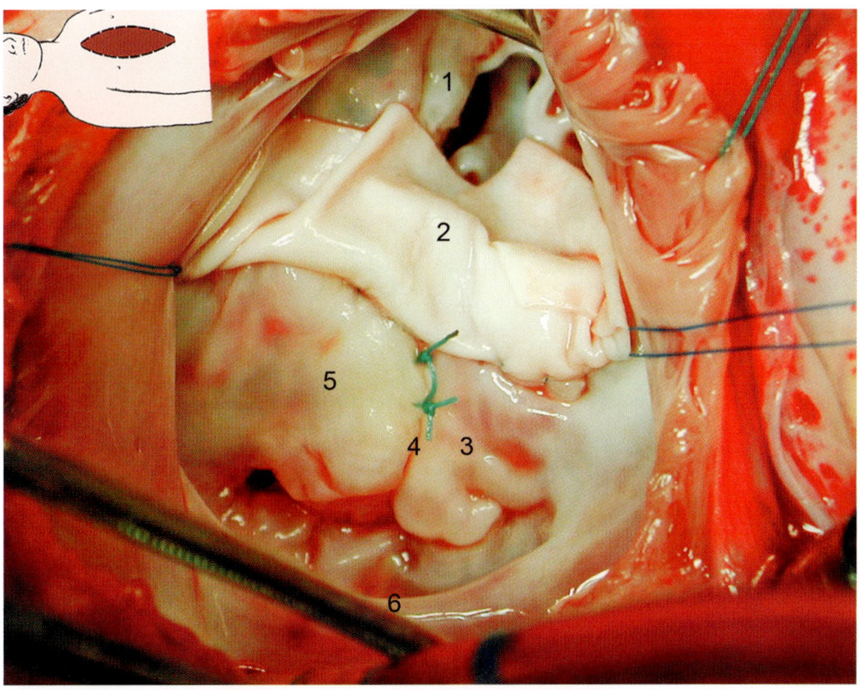

Figure 5.35. The same patient as in Figures 5.32 to 5.34. A xenograft pericardial patch is being placed to close the ASD. The inferior edge of the patch has already been sutured to the upper surface of the AV valve, immediately to the right of the stay suture.

1. Anterosuperior leaflet
2. Pericardial patch
3. Inferior bridging leaflet
4. "Cleft" in left AV valve
5. Superior bridging leaflet
6. Border of primum ASD

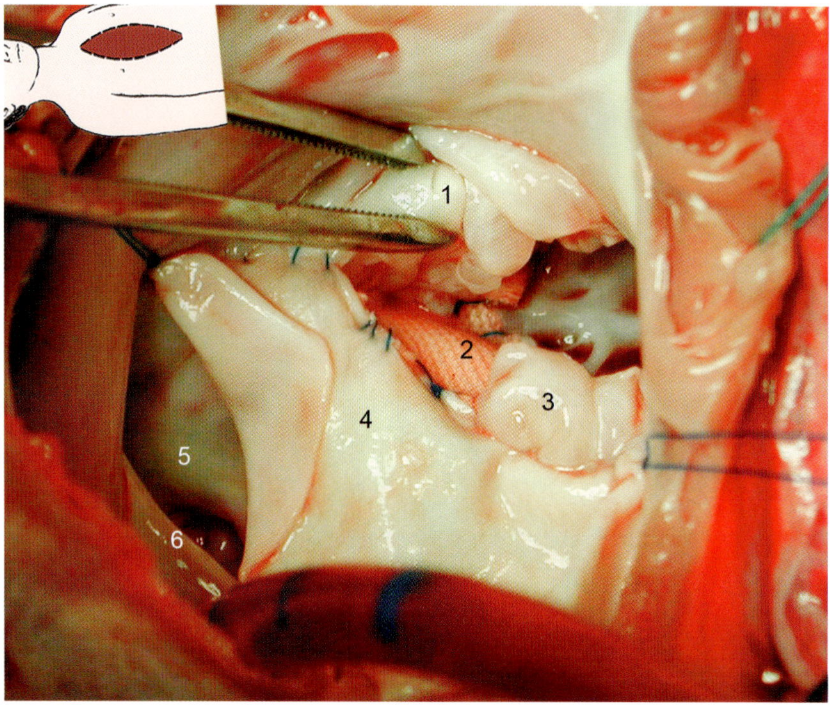

Figure 5.36. The same patient as in Figures 5.32 to 5.35. The pericardial patch is flipped leftward to show the right atrial aspect.

1. Anterosuperior leaflet
2. Dacron patch (closing the VSD)
3. Right part of inferior bridging leaflet
4. Pericardial patch
5. Left component of AV valve visible through the ASD
6. Border of the ASD

phenotypes of AVSD in having a common AV valve junction and disproportion between ventricular inlet and outlet lengths. Figures 5.37 to 5.40 show this variant having a VSD component in the inlet portion and AV valve morphology typical of AVSD but with no primum ASD communication because the bridging valvar leaflets are attached to the underside of the atrial septum. Note the superior bridging leaflet straddling the crest of the ventricular septum.

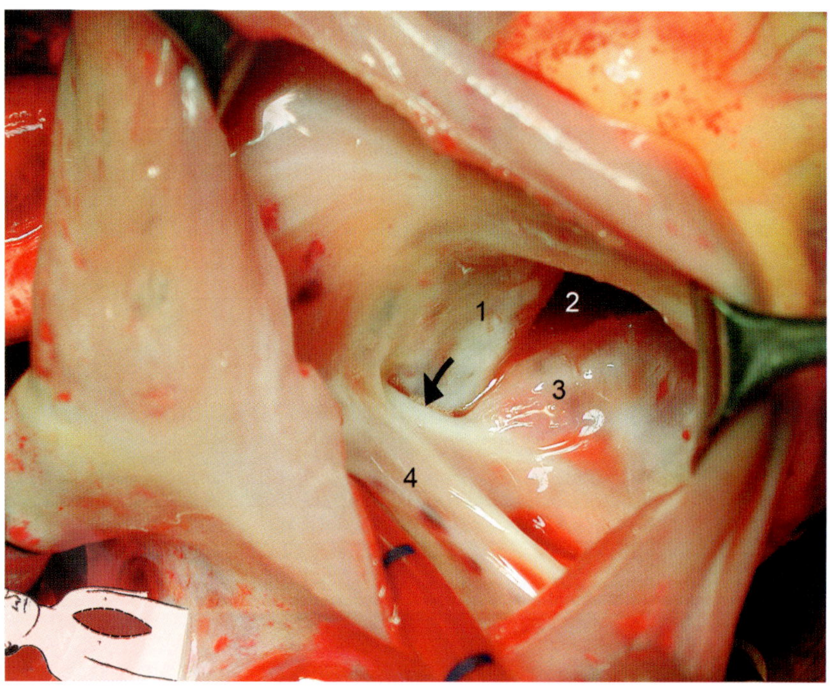

Figure 5.37. An AVSD with only the VSD component and no primum ASD owing to the attachment of the bridging leaflets to the under edge of the atrial septum. The gross appearance is seen through a right atriotomy. The arrow points to the location of the VSD.

1. Superior bridging leaflet
2. RV cavity
3. Inferior bridging leaflet
4. Atrial septum (intact)

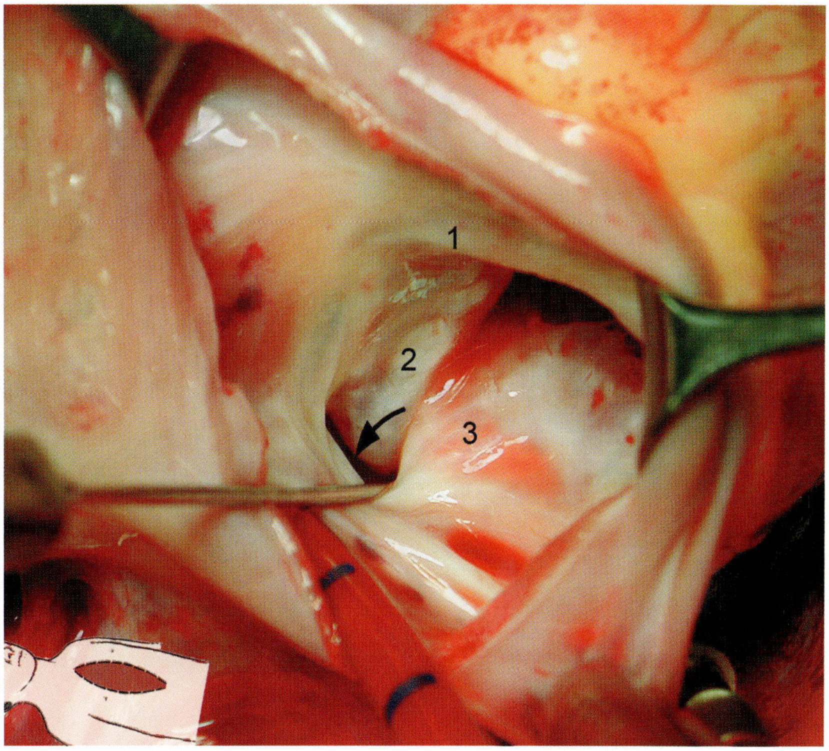

Figure 5.38. The same patient as in Figure 5.37. The bridging leaflets are retracted to show the VSD component.

1. Parietal annulus of right AV valve
2. Superior bridging leaflet
3. Inferior bridging leaflet

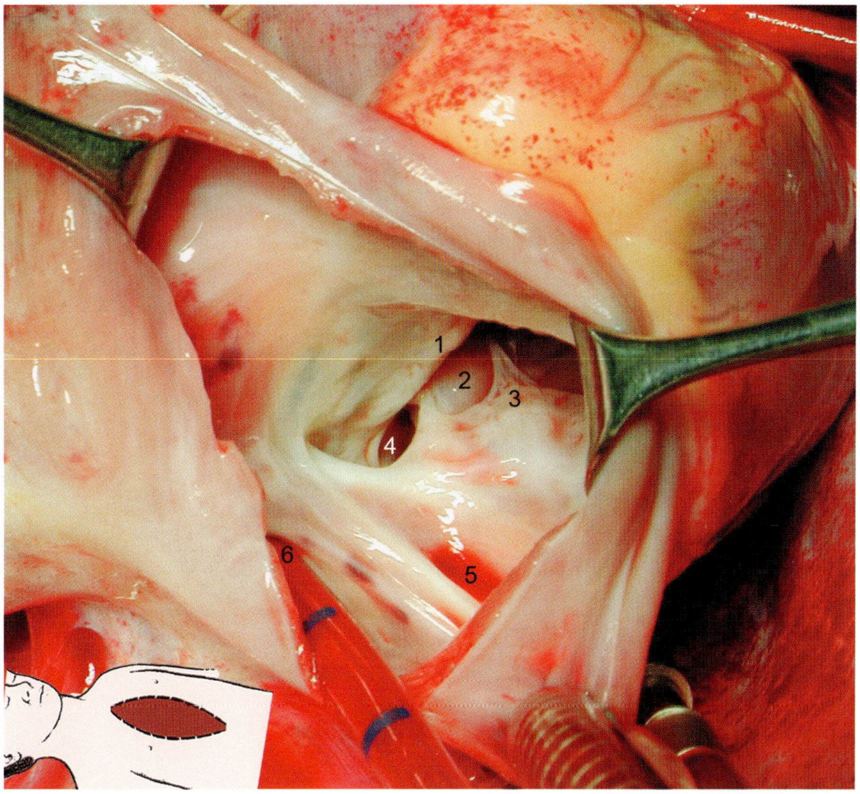

Figure 5.39. The same patient as in Figures 5.37 and 5.38. The AV valve has abnormal morphology with the atrial surfaces of the superior and inferior bridging leaflets lying close together or even adjoining at the atrial septum.

1. Superior bridging leaflet
2. Ventricular septum
3. Inferior bridging leaflet
4. Inlet VSD component
5. Blood pooling at the mouth of CS
6. Suction catheter in PFO

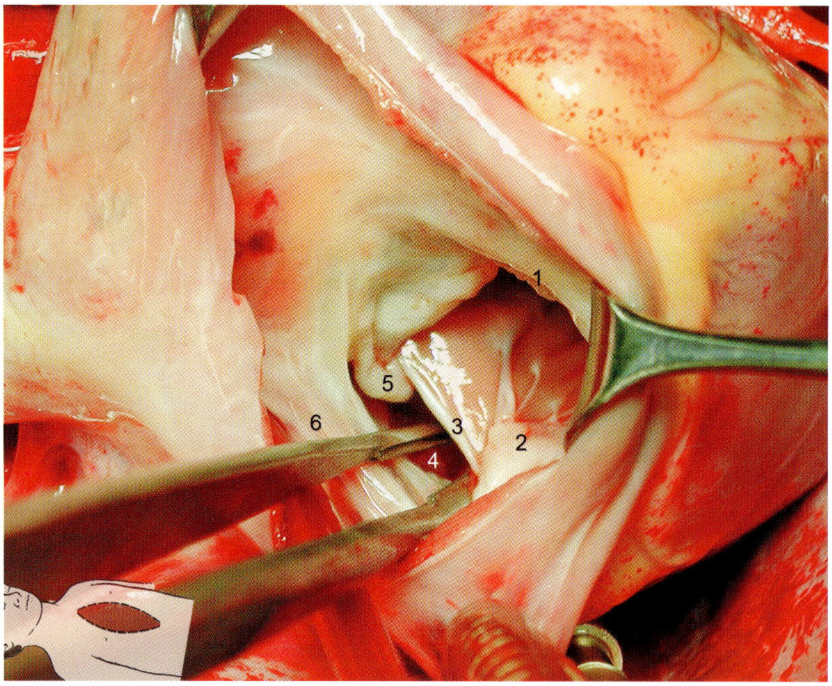

Figure 5.40. The same patient as in Figures 5.37 to 5.39. The right AV valve has been retracted to better show the VSD component and bridging leaflets.

1. Parietal annulus of right AV valve
2. Inferior bridging leaflet
3. Crest of ventricular septum
4. VSD component
5. Superior bridging leaflet
6. Atrial septum

REFERENCES

1. Ebels T, Anderson RH, Devine WA, et al. Anomalies of the left atrioventricular valve and related ventricular septal morphology in atrioventricular septal defects. *J Thorac Cardiovasc Surg.* 1990;99(2):299–307.
2. Prendiville T, Barton L, Fink D, et al. Heterotaxy syndrome: defining contemporary disease trends. *Pediatr Cardiol.* 2010;31:1052–1058.
3. Tubman TRJ, Shields MD, Craig BG, Mulholland HC, Nevin NC. Congenital heart disease in Down's syndrome: two year prospective early screening study. *BMJ.* 1991;302:1425–1427.
4. Daebritz S, del Nido P. Surgical management of common atrioventricular canal. *Prog Pediatr Cardiol.* 1999;10:161–171.

CHAPTER 6

Coarctation of the Aorta

Coarctation of the aorta accounts for about 4% to 7% of all congenital heart diseases.[1,2] It may occur in isolation or be associated with other cardiac defects. The narrowest area of the arch is usually in the vicinity of the ductus arteriosus.[3] The narrowing may be tubular (long segment) or discrete. The surgical approach to coarctation of the aorta is most commonly through a lateral thoracotomy. The area of coarctation may be quite obvious from outside inspection, but at times, it can only be fully appreciated upon opening the lumen of the aorta.

When the arch hypoplasia is more proximal, a median sternotomy approach may be more appropriate. A median sternotomy is also chosen when concomitant intracardiac repair for associated anomalies is to be performed.

Coarctation located proximal to the left subclavian artery can be repaired using patch augmentation, reverse subclavian flap, or extended end-to-end anastomosis. Figure 6.1 is an illustration of some of the techniques used in surgical repair of coarctation.

Figures 6.2 and 6.3 show the surgical view through a lateral thoracotomy. Upon retracting the lung anteriorly and downward, the posterior mediastinal pleura come to view. After further dissection, the aortic arch, the descending aorta, and the ductus arteriosus (or ligamentum arteriosum) can be clearly seen. Some variation in anatomy is to be expected.

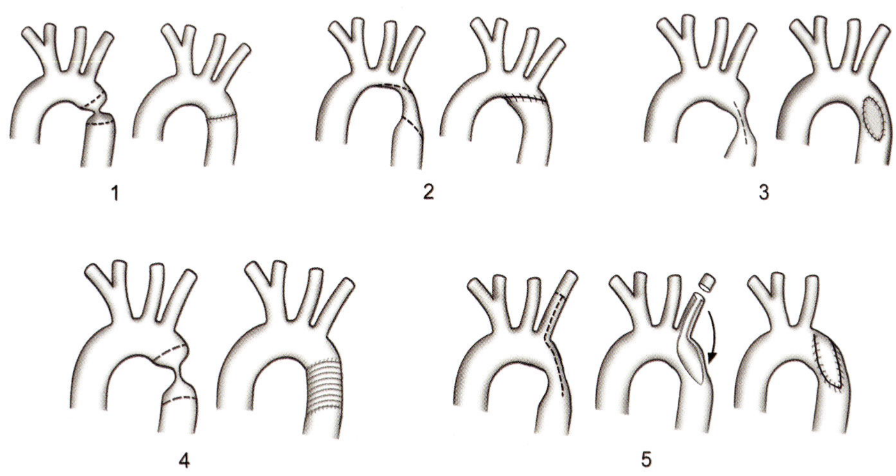

Figure 6.1. Diagrammatic illustration of some of the techniques used in surgical repair of coarctation of the aorta.

1. Resection and end-to-end anastomosis
2. Resection and extended end-to-end anastomosis
3. Patch angioplasty
4. Resection and placement of interposition graft
5. Subclavian flap technique

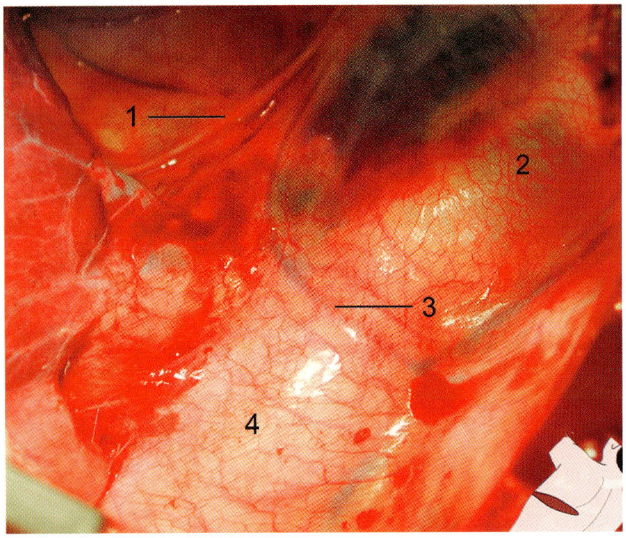

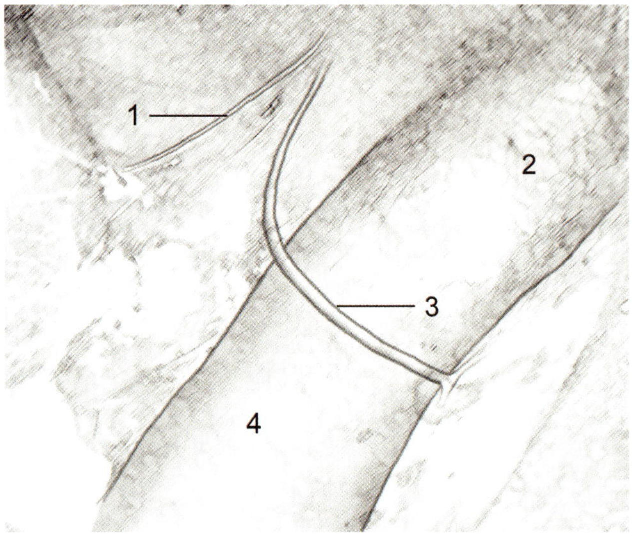

Figure 6.2 **Figure 6.3**

Left lateral thoracotomy view after retracting the left lung. The posterior mediastinum structures are seen covered by parietal pleura.

1. Left vagus nerve
2. Distal end of aortic arch
3. Superior intercostal vein
4. Descending thoracic aorta

Figure 6.4 shows a prominent anomalously draining hemiazygos vein, and Figures 6.5 and 6.6 show an aberrant origin of vertebral artery.

END-TO-END ANASTOMOSIS

Resection of the narrow segment and end-to-end anastomosis is the preferred technique in most infants. Figures 6.7 through 6.11 show a 2-month-old infant with coarctation repaired using this technique. Figures 6.12 and 6.13 represent another example of a similar case, but younger (2 weeks old). Note the tortuousity of the descending aorta. Extended end-to-end anastomosis (see Figure 6.1) is a modification to this technique that is used for long-segment coarctation. Figures 6.14 and 6.15 show an example of

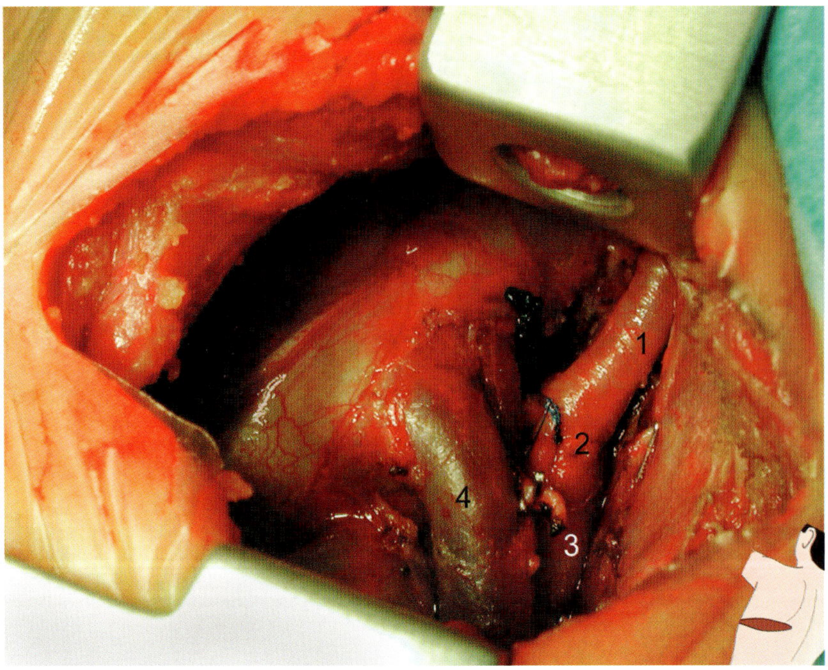

Figure 6.4. A surgical view through left thoracotomy for a 5-day-old neonate. A prominent anomalously draining hemiazygos vein is seen. The coarctation has been repaired by resection and end-to-end anastomosis.

1. Left subclavian artery
2. Anastomosis site
3. Descending thoracic aorta
4. Hemiazygos vein

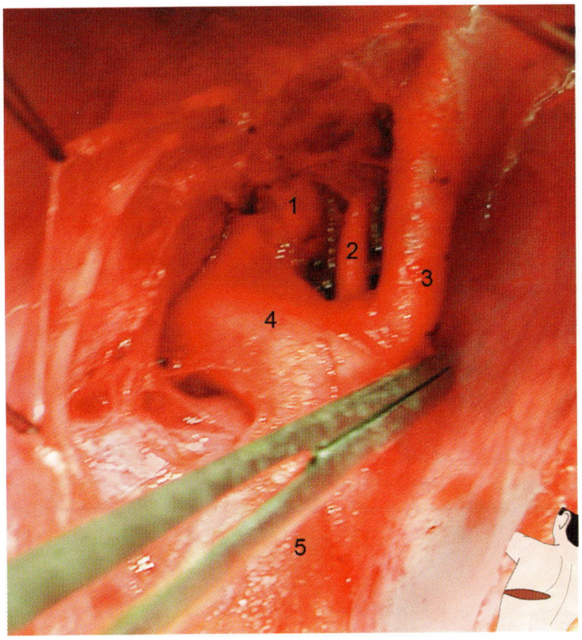

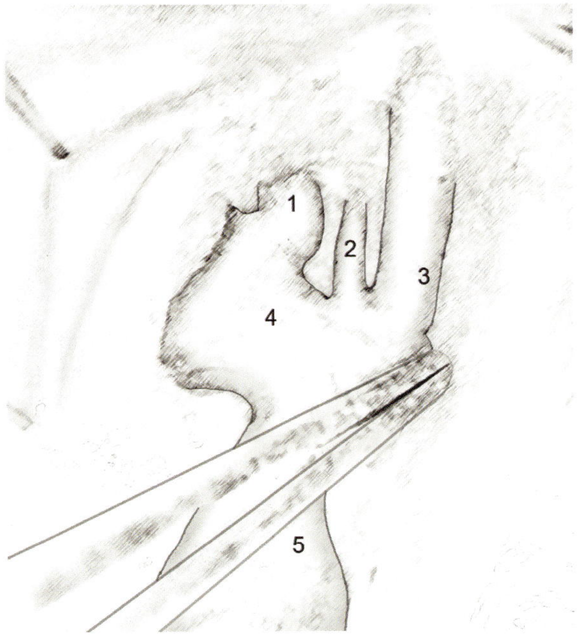

Figure 6.5 **Figure 6.6**

A lateral thoracotomy view of a 7-month-old infant with coarctation of aorta. An aberrant arterial branch (vertebral) originates from the aortic arch just proximal to the left subclavian artery.

1. Left common carotid artery
2. Vertebral artery
3. Left subclavian artery
4. Transverse arch
5. Descending thoracic aorta

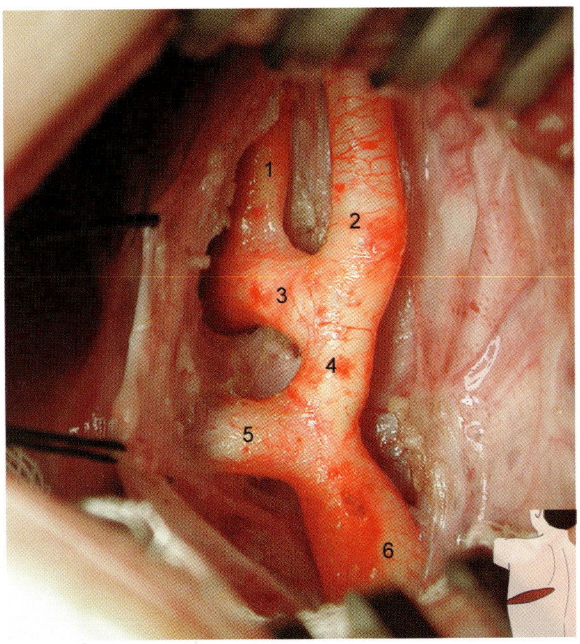

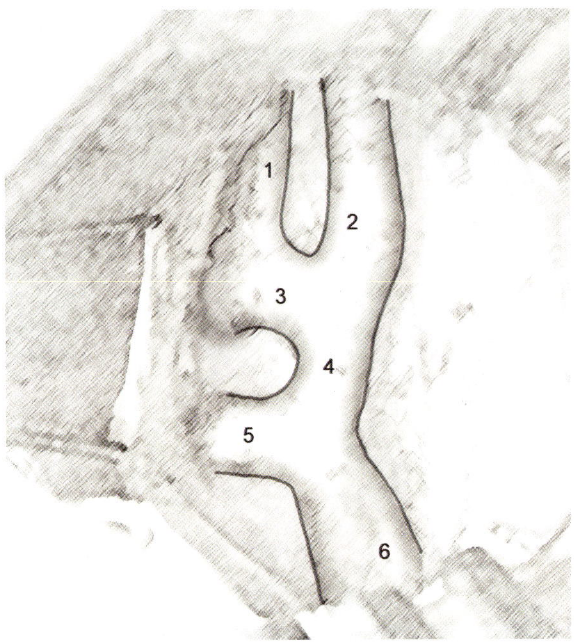

Figure 6.7 **Figure 6.8**

Coarctation of the aorta as seen through a left lateral thoracotomy in a 2-month-old infant. In Figure 6.7, the contrast and saturation have been modified to make the structures of interest stand out. The sketch in Figure 6.8 outlines the vessels after being dissected from the surrounding tissues.

1. Left common carotid artery
2. Left subclavian artery
3. Transverse arch
4. Coarctation area
5. Ductus arteriosus
6. Descending thoracic aorta

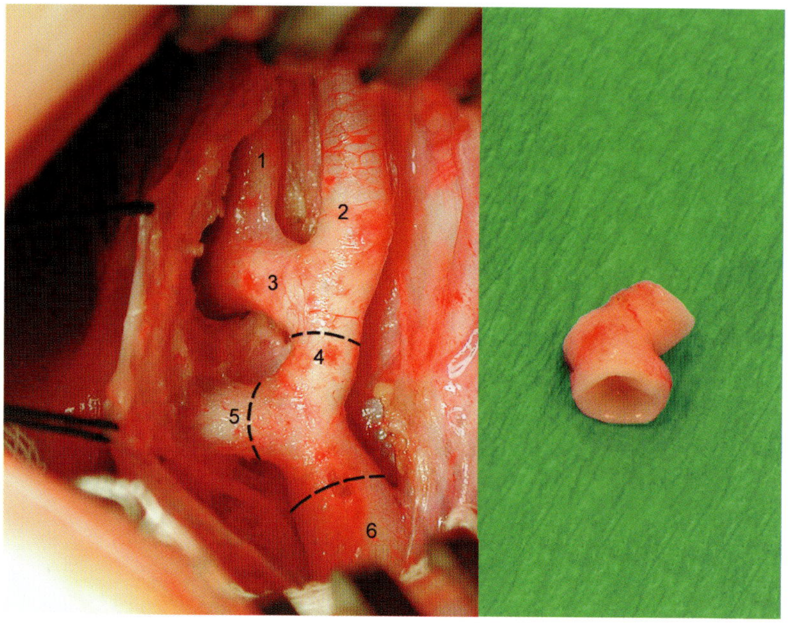

Figure 6.9. The same patient as in Figure 6.7. The area of coarctation is outlined. The lumen inside this portion of the arch is quite narrow, which is evident when inspected after excision (specimen on the right), a finding that corresponds to the image findings from CT and echocardiography (Figure 6.43).

1. Left common carotid artery
2. Left subclavian artery
3. Transverse arch
4. Coarctation area
5. Ductus arteriosus
6. Descending thoracic aorta

this technique. This case also illustrates the feasibility of coarctation repair using a sternotomy approach.

SUBCLAVIAN FLAP

The subclavian flap technique is an alternative technique that can be used to repair long-segment hypoplasia (Figure 6.16) of the distal arch.

Figures 6.17 through 6.22 are of an 8-month-old infant with long-segment distal arch hypoplasia. It was repaired through a lateral thoracotomy using a subclavian flap.

A reversed subclavian flap utilizes the same concept, but the flap is turned proximally. This will augment the hypoplastic segment when it is located between the left common carotid and left subclavian

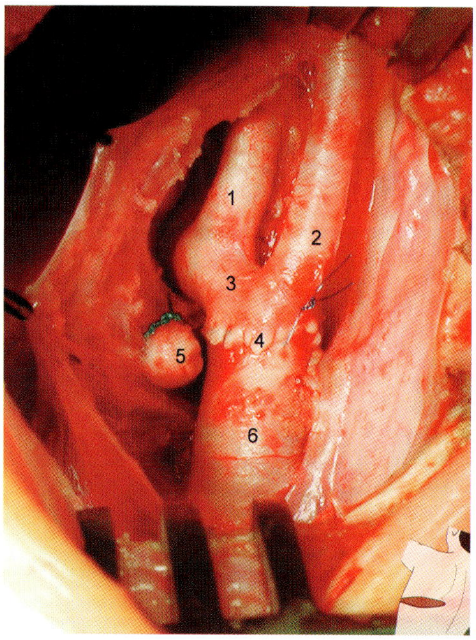

Figure 6.10

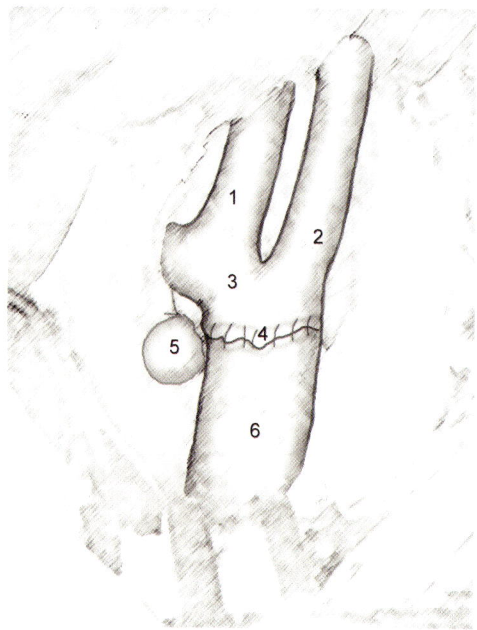

Figure 6.11

The same patient as in Figures 6.7 to 6.9 after completion of the repair by resection and end-to-end anastomosis using continuous suture. The stump of the ligated ductus arteriosus (5) is also shown.

1. Left common carotid artery
2. Left subclavian artery
3. Transverse arch
4. Anastomosis site
5. Ductus stump
6. Descending thoracic aorta

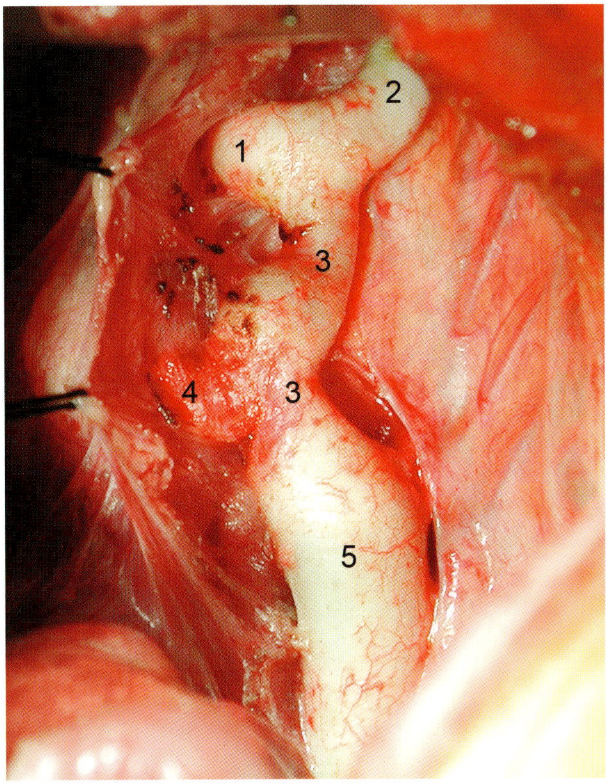

Figure 6.12. Coarctation of the aorta in a 2-week-old neonate, as seen through a left lateral thoracotomy. Note the tortuousity of the narrow segment.

1. Transverse arch
2. Left subclavian artery
3. Coarctation area
4. Ductus arteriosus
5. Descending thoracic aorta

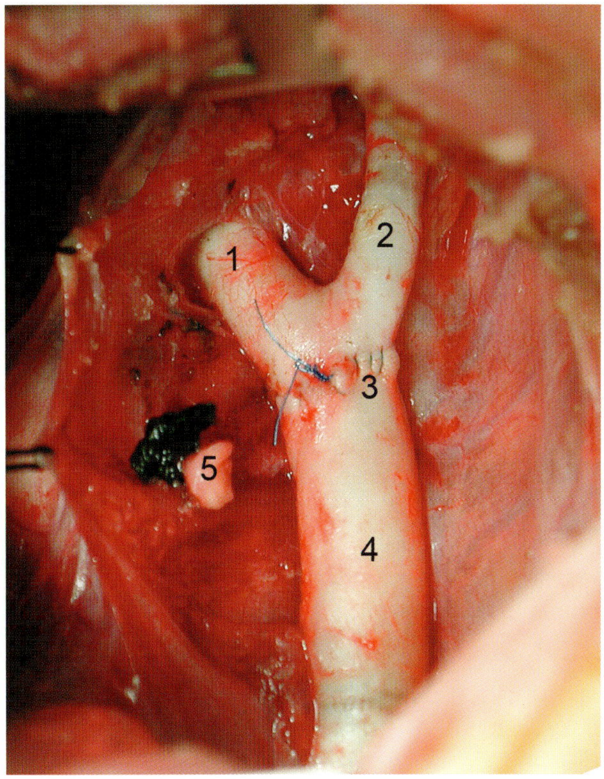

Figure 6.13. The same patient as in Figure 6.12 after resection and end-to-end anastomosis.

1. Transverse arch
2. Left subclavian artery
3. Anastomosis site
4. Descending thoracic aorta
5. Ductus stump

Figure 6.14. A median sternotomy view of a child with coarctation of the aorta. A sternotomy approach was chosen because the patient had intracardiac lesions that needed repair. At this stage of surgery, the patient is on total circulatory arrest. The narrow segment has been resected. The incision has been extended to the underside of the transverse arch up to the level of origin of the innominate artery.

1. Transverse arch
2. Descending thoracic aorta
3. Clamp
4. Ascending aorta
5. Right atrial appendage (RAA)

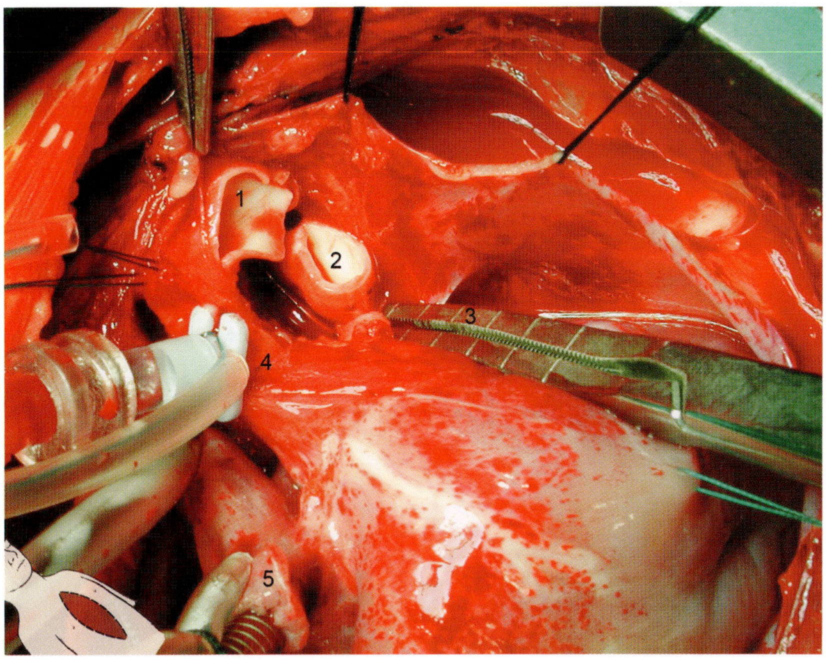

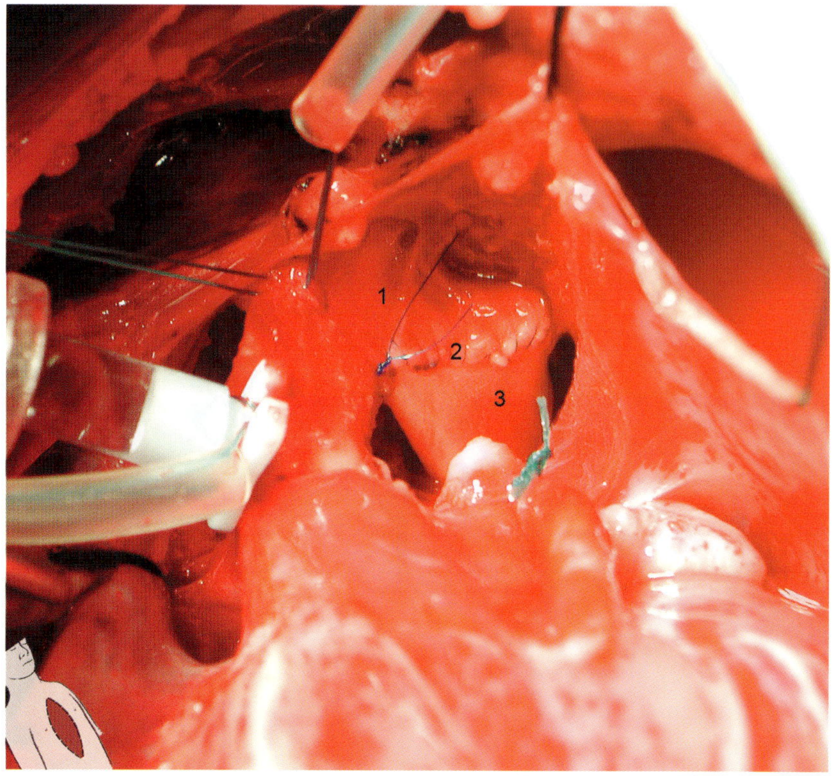

Figure 6.15. The same patient as in Figure 6.14 after repair. An extended end-to-end anastomosis has been performed.

1. Transverse arch
2. Anastomosis site
3. Descending thoracic aorta

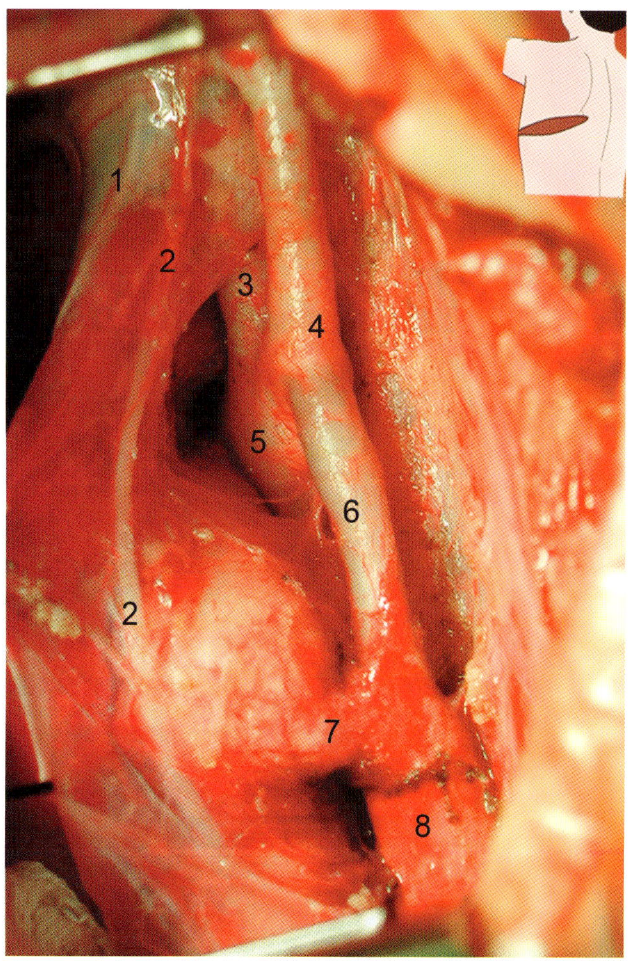

Figure 6.16. The aortic arch of a 4-month-old infant. Note the long, narrow segment of the aorta between the left subclavian artery and the insertion of the ductus.

1. Left phrenic nerve
2. Left vagus nerve
3. Left common carotid artery
4. Left subclavian artery
5. Transverse arch
6. Hypoplastic segment
7. Ductus arteriosus
8. Descending thoracic aorta

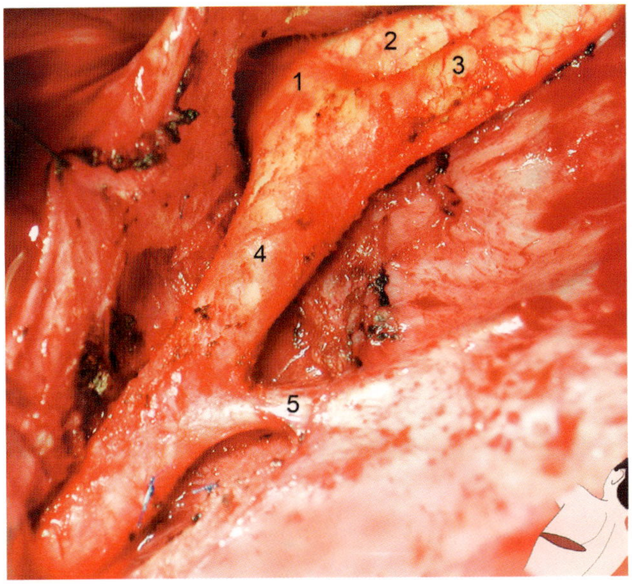

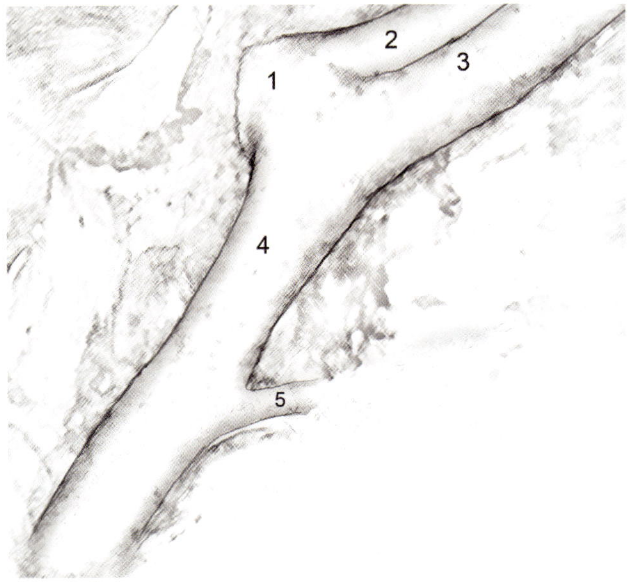

Figure 6.17 **Figure 6.18**

Long-segment coarctation in an 8-month-old infant. Note the prominent intercostal artery.

1. Transverse arch
2. Left common carotid artery
3. Left subclavian artery
4. Hypoplastic aortic segment
5. Intercostal artery

arteries. An example of this technique is illustrated in Figures 6.23 to 6.28 from a 9-month-old infant whose coarctation was between the left common carotid and left subclavian arteries.

PATCH ANGIOPLASTY

This is a relatively simple operation that does not require extensive dissection. It is used when other techniques are not suitable. Late aneurysm formation

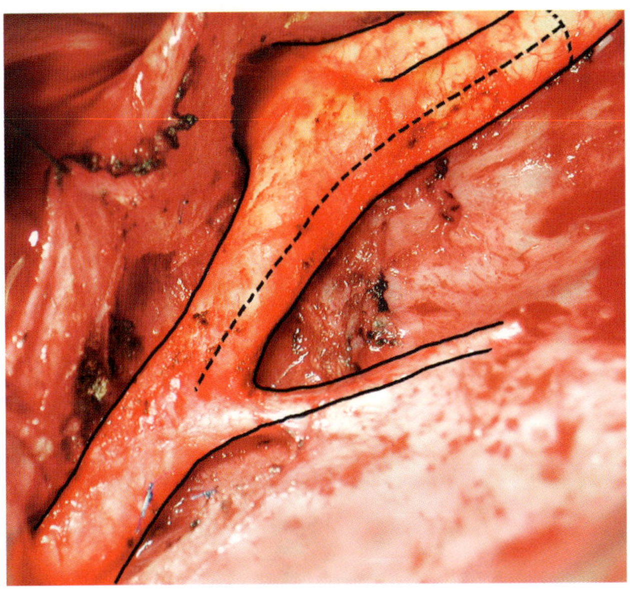

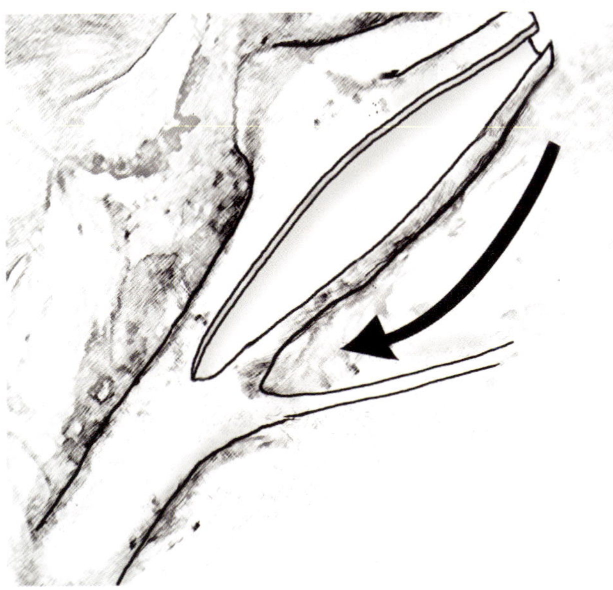

Figure 6.19 **Figure 6.20**

Same patient as in Figure 6.17. The dashed line represents where the incision is made in the subclavian artery and descending aorta. The subclavian artery is transected, the aorta and subclavian artery are opened, and the artery is inverted downward as a flap to augment the hypoplastic aortic segment.

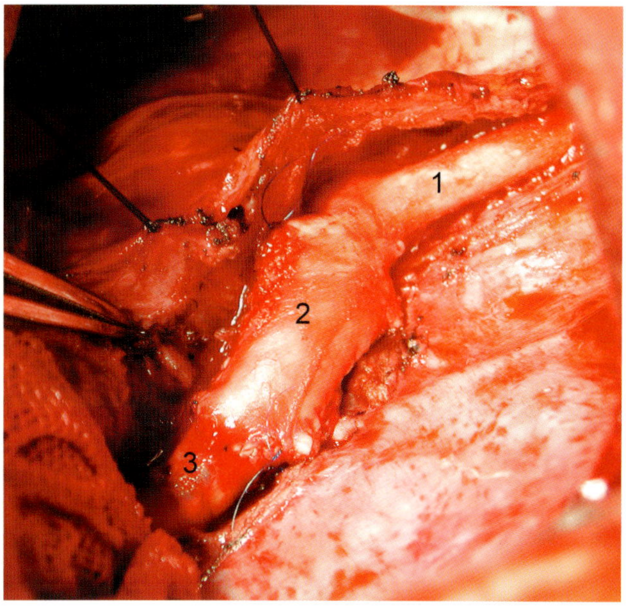

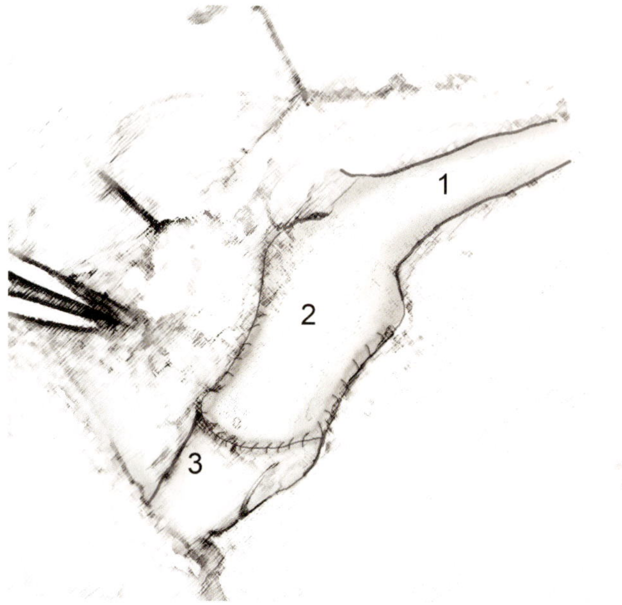

Figure 6.21 **Figure 6.22**

Same patient as in Figures 6.17 to 6.20 after completion of the repair using subclavian flap technique. The downturned subclavian artery flap (2) is now a part of the descending thoracic aorta. The dashed line in Figure 6.19 outlines the margins of the flap.

1. Left common carotid artery
2. Downturned flap of the left subclavian artery
3. Descending thoracic aorta

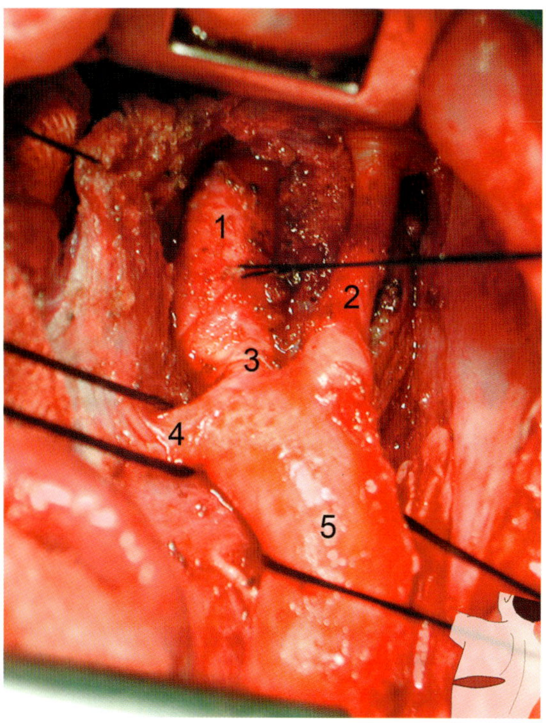

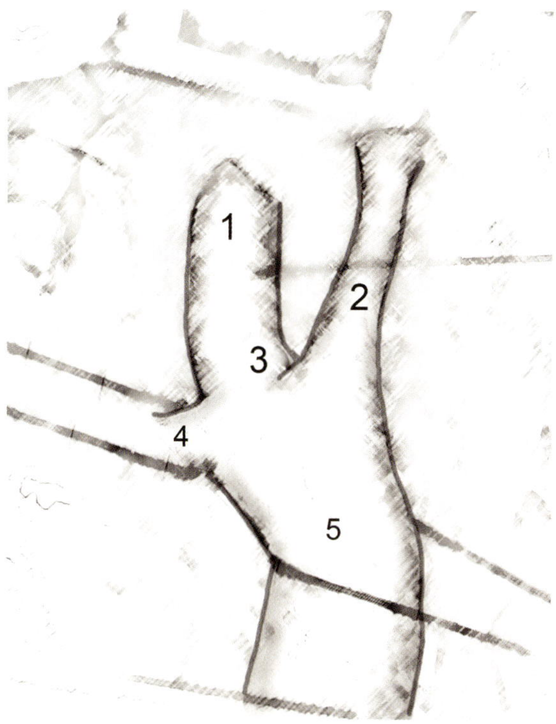

Figure 6.23 **Figure 6.24**

A 9-month-old infant. The narrow area of the arch (3) is between the left common carotid and left subclavian arteries.

1. Left common carotid artery
2. Left subclavian artery
3. Coarctation area
4. Ductus arteriosus
5. Descending thoracic aorta

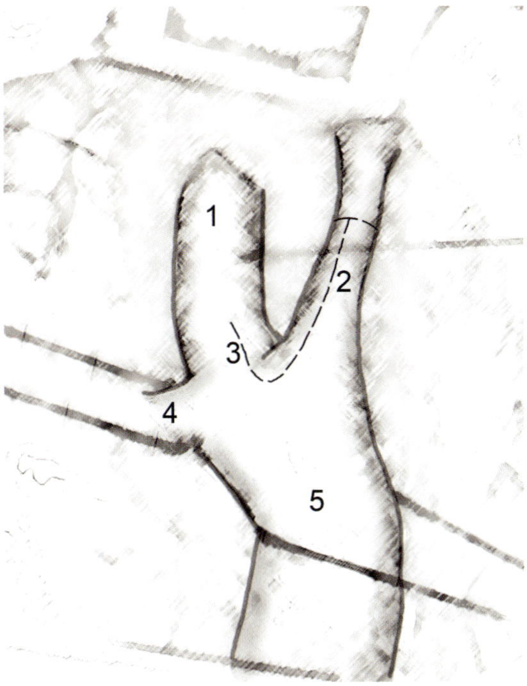

Figure 6.25

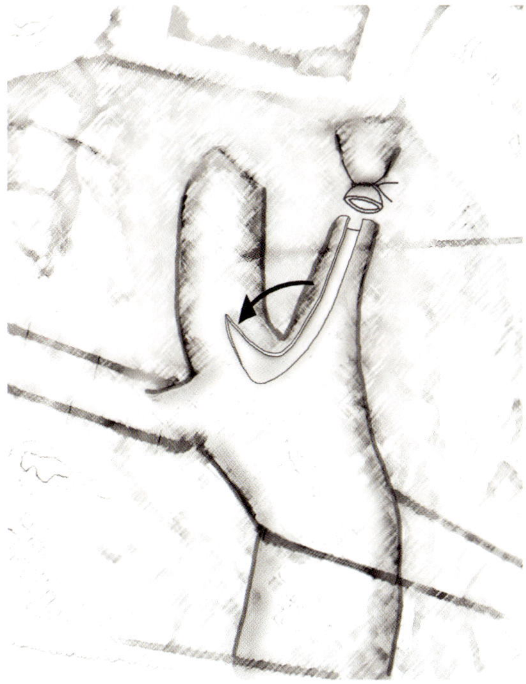

Figure 6.26

Same patient as in Figure 6.23. Reverse subclavian flap technique: The left subclavian artery is transected distally. The artery is opened along the dashed line, and the flap made thereof is turned proximally to augment the narrow area of the arch.

1. Left common carotid artery
2. Left subclavian artery
3. Coarctation area
4. Ductus arteriosus
5. Descending thoracic aorta

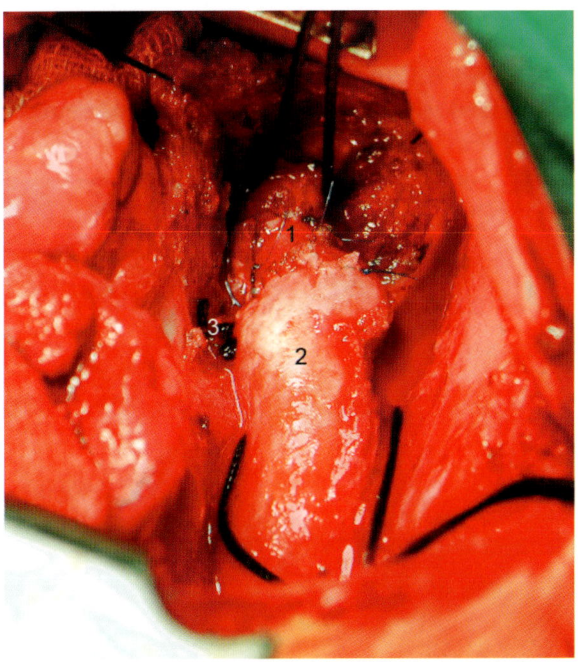

Figure 6.27

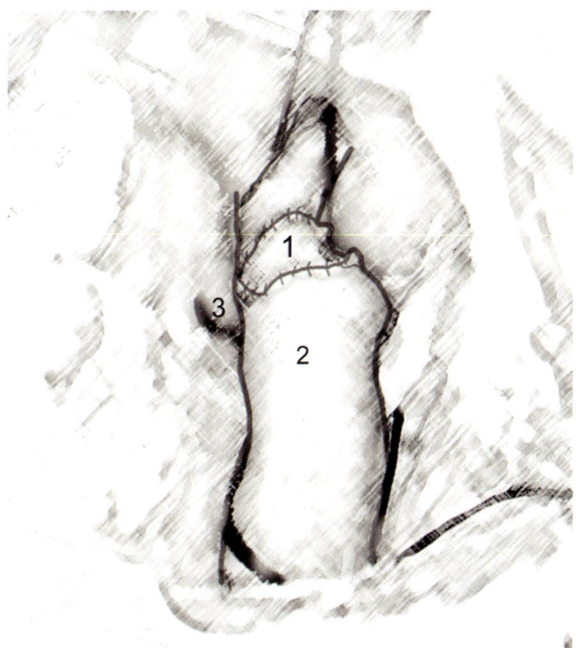

Figure 6.28

Same patient as in Figure 6.23 after completion of the repair using reversed subclavian flap technique. The subclavian artery flap (1) is now a part of the aortic arch.

1. Subclavian artery flap sutured to the arch
2. Descending thoracic aorta
3. Ductus arteriosus

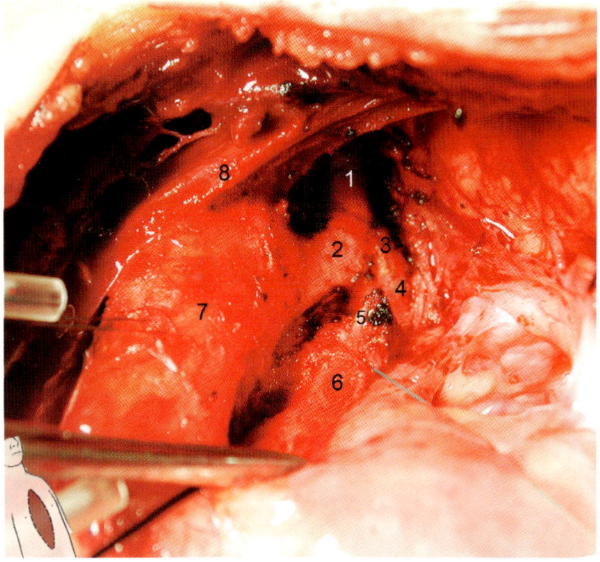

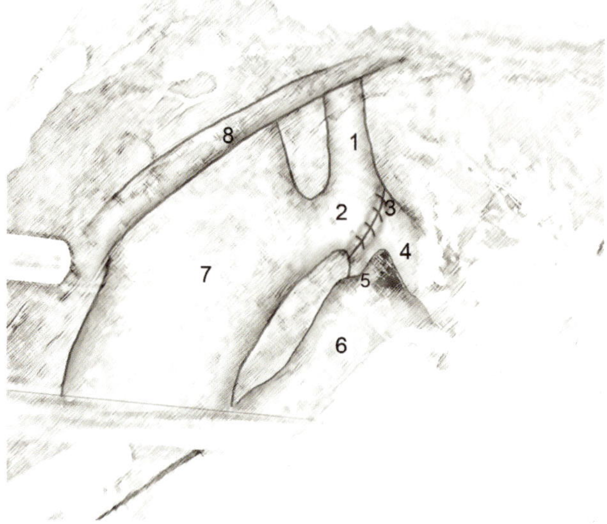

Figure 6.29 **Figure 6.30**

A 3-year-old child who had previous coarctation repair, end-to-end technique, viewed through a median sternotomy. Note the hypoplastic segment (2) between the left carotid and left subclavian arteries.

1. Left subclavian artery
2. Coarctation area
3. Previous end-to-end anastomosis
4. Descending thoracic aorta
5. Ductus arteriosus stump
6. Pulmonary artery (PA)
7. Ascending aorta
8. Innominate vein

has been described as a complication.[4] Biologic or synthetic material (Dacron) may be used.

Figures 6.29 to 6.34 are from a 3-year-old child who had previous coarctation repair using the end-to-end technique. This redo operation was carried out through a median sternotomy. Xenograft pericardium was used to augment the transverse arch.

Figures 6.35 to 6.38 are from a neonate with combined arch augmentation and end-to-end anastomosis.

An interposition tube graft may be placed in the older child or adult, as illustrated in Figures 6.39 and 6.40.

Figures 6.41 to 6.43 are pathological specimens of excised segments of coarctation. Aneurysmal

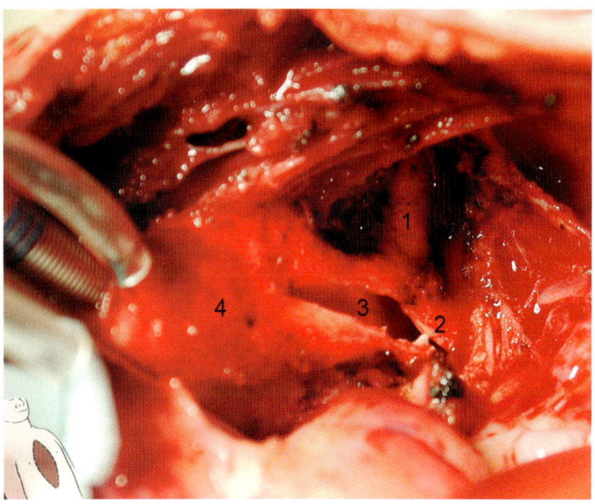

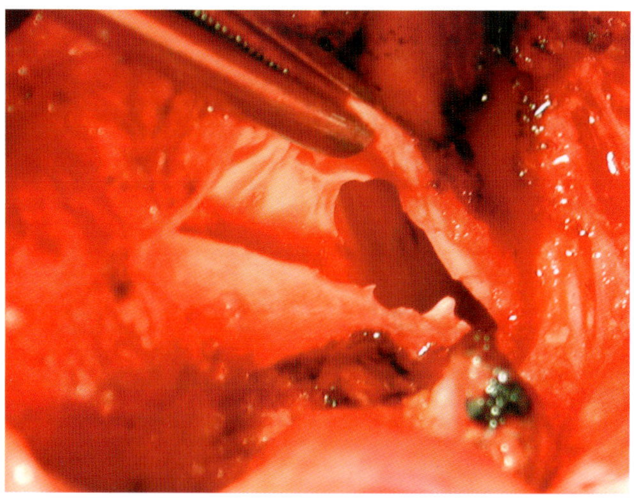

Figure 6.31 **Figure 6.32**

The same patient as in Figure 6.29. Now under circulatory arrest, the transverse arch has been opened. Figure 6.31 is a zoomed-in view of the arch.

1. Left subclavian artery
2. Descending aorta
3. The hypoplastic segment slit open
4. Ascending aorta

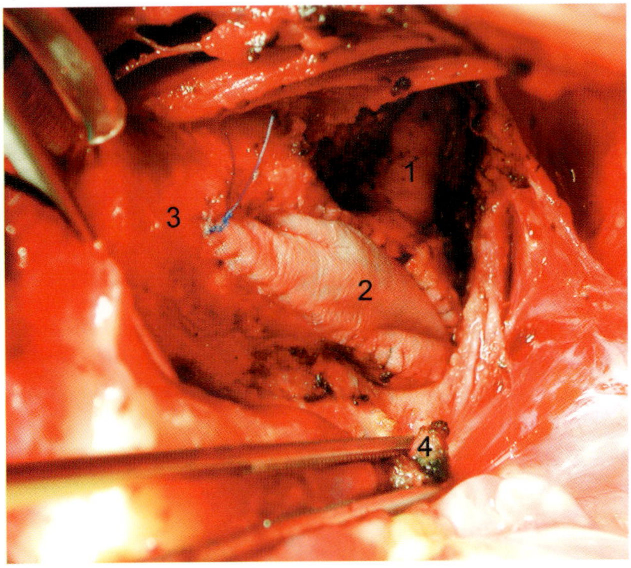

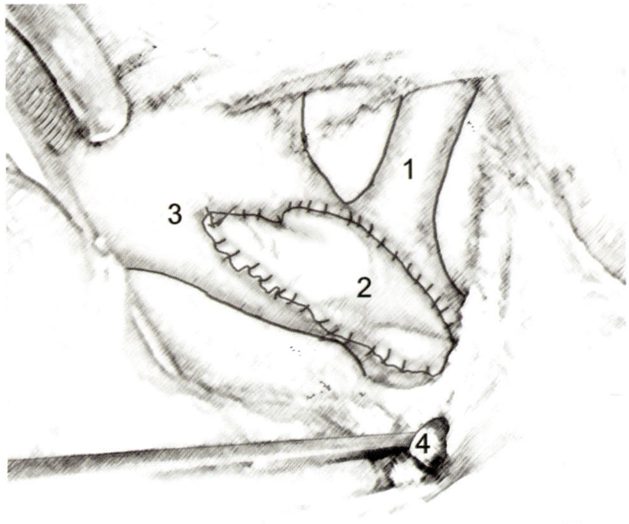

Figure 6.33 **Figure 6.34**

The same patient as in Figures 6.29 to 6.32. The arch has been augmented by a patch of xenograft pericardium.

1. Left subclavian artery
2. Xenograft patch
3. Ascending aorta and proximal arch
4. Ductus stump

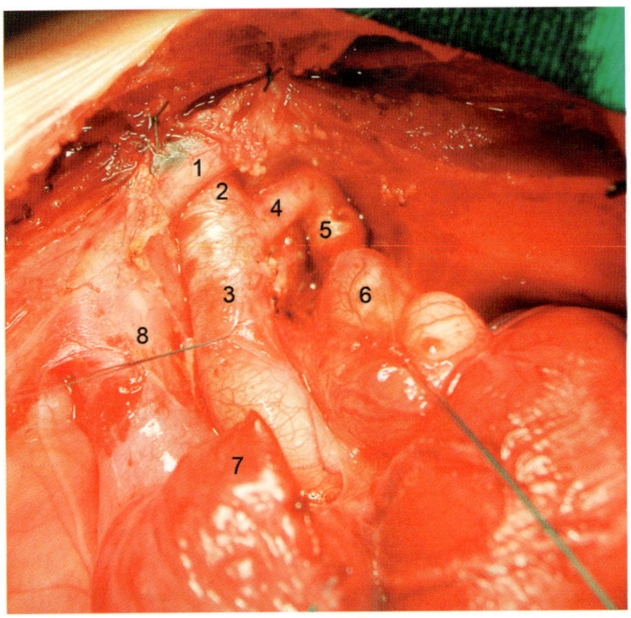

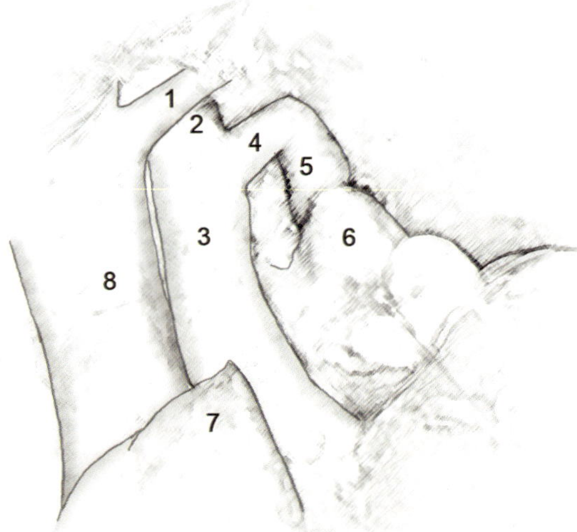

Figure 6.35 **Figure 6.36**

Surgical view through a median sternotomy in a 24-day-old neonate with coarctation. Note the hypoplastic transverse arch (4).

1. Left brachiocephalic (innominate) vein
2. Brachiocephalic artery
3. Ascending aorta
4. Transverse arch
5. Descending aorta
6. Main pulmonary artery
7. RAA
8. Superior vena cava (SVC)

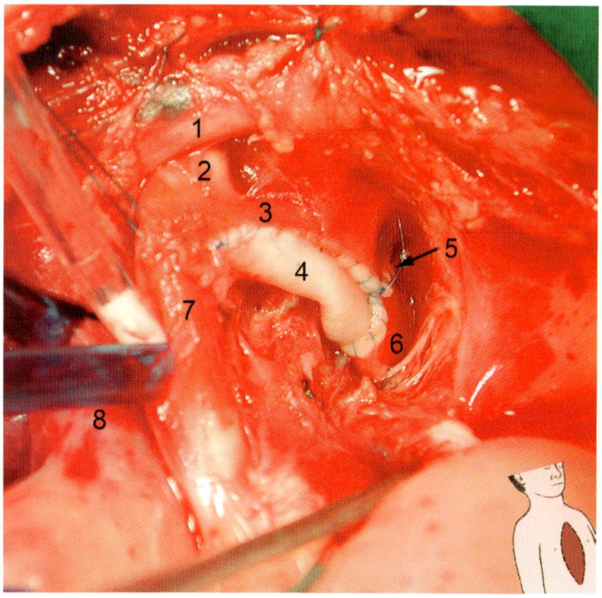

Figure 6.37

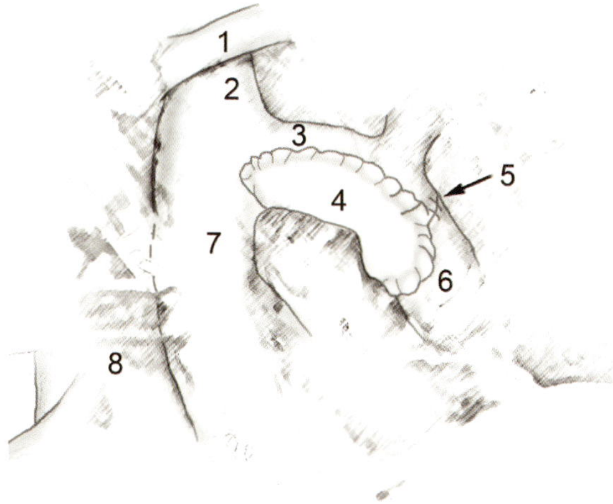

Figure 6.38

The same patient as in Figure 6.35 after repair of coarctation. Arch augmentation angioplasty was achieved using a xenograft pericardial patch (4), combined with end-to-end anastomosis (5).

1. Innominate vein
2. Brachiocephalic artery
3. Transverse arch
4. Xenograft pericardial patch
5. End-to-end anastomosis
6. Descending aorta
7. Ascending aorta
8. SVC

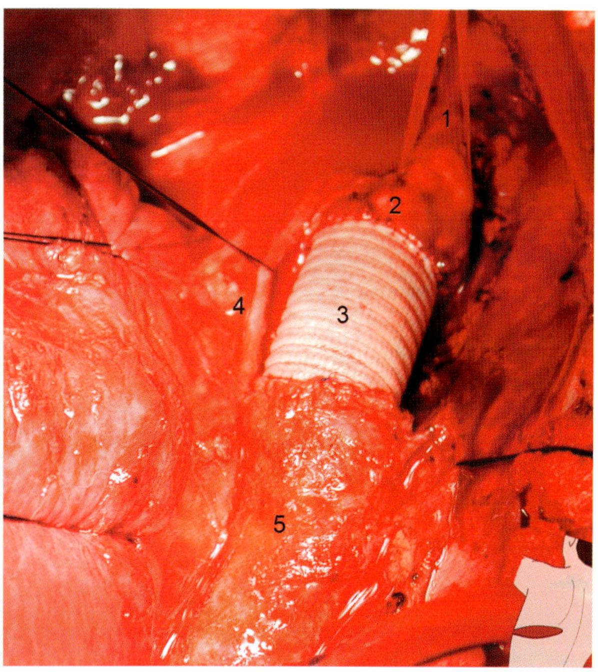

Figure 6.39

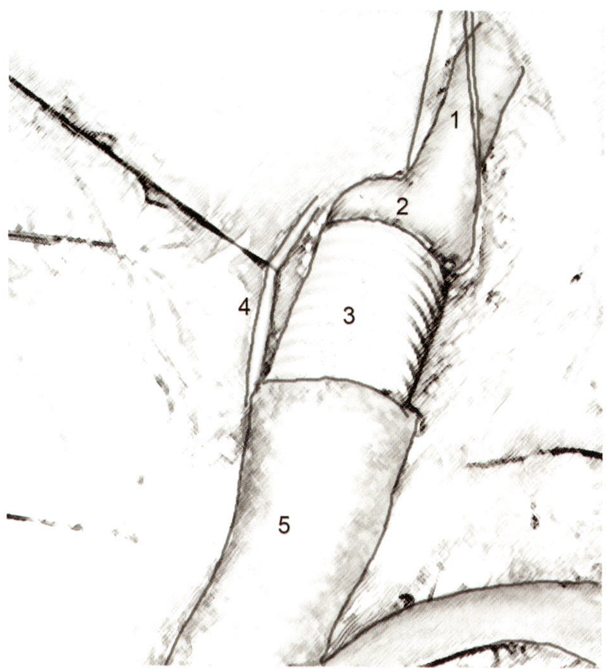

Figure 6.40

Lateral thoracotomy view of a 15-year-old patient, redo coarctation repair. The surgery was carried out on partial cardiopulmonary bypass from left atrium to descending aorta. A 20 mm Hemashield Dacron tubular graft was used for the angioplasty.

1. Left subclavian artery
2. Transverse arch
3. Interposition Dacron graft
4. Vagus nerve
5. Descending thoracic aorta

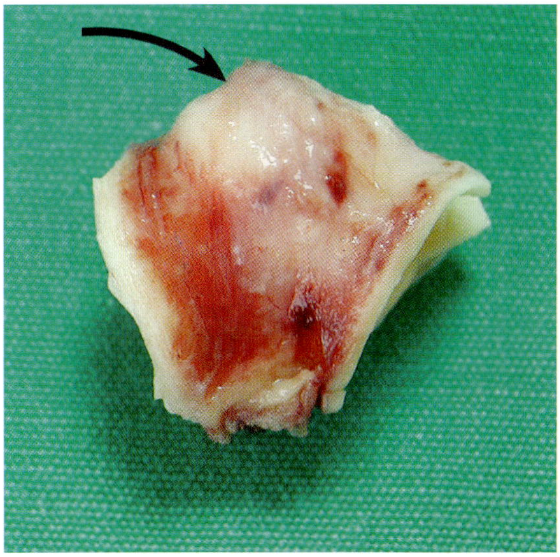

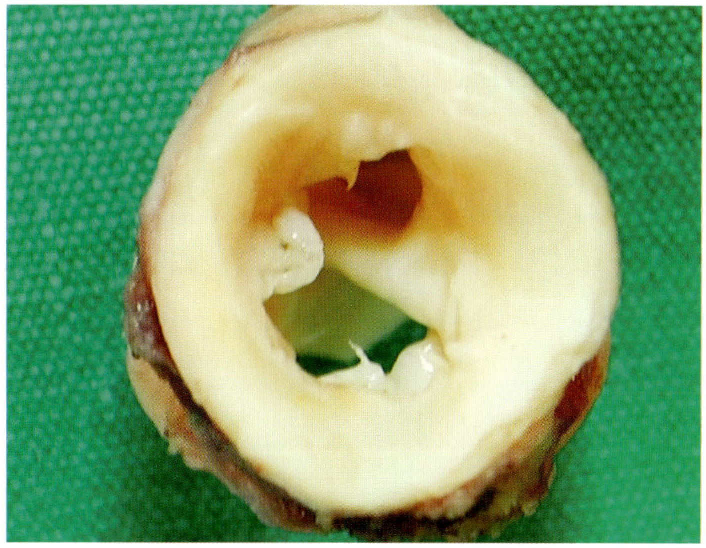

Figure 6.41 **Figure 6.42**

A surgical specimen from a 16-year-old patient with coarctation, who underwent balloon angioplasty. Note the aneurysmal dilatation denoted by the arrow. When viewed end-on (Figure 6.42), a shelf is present in the lumen.

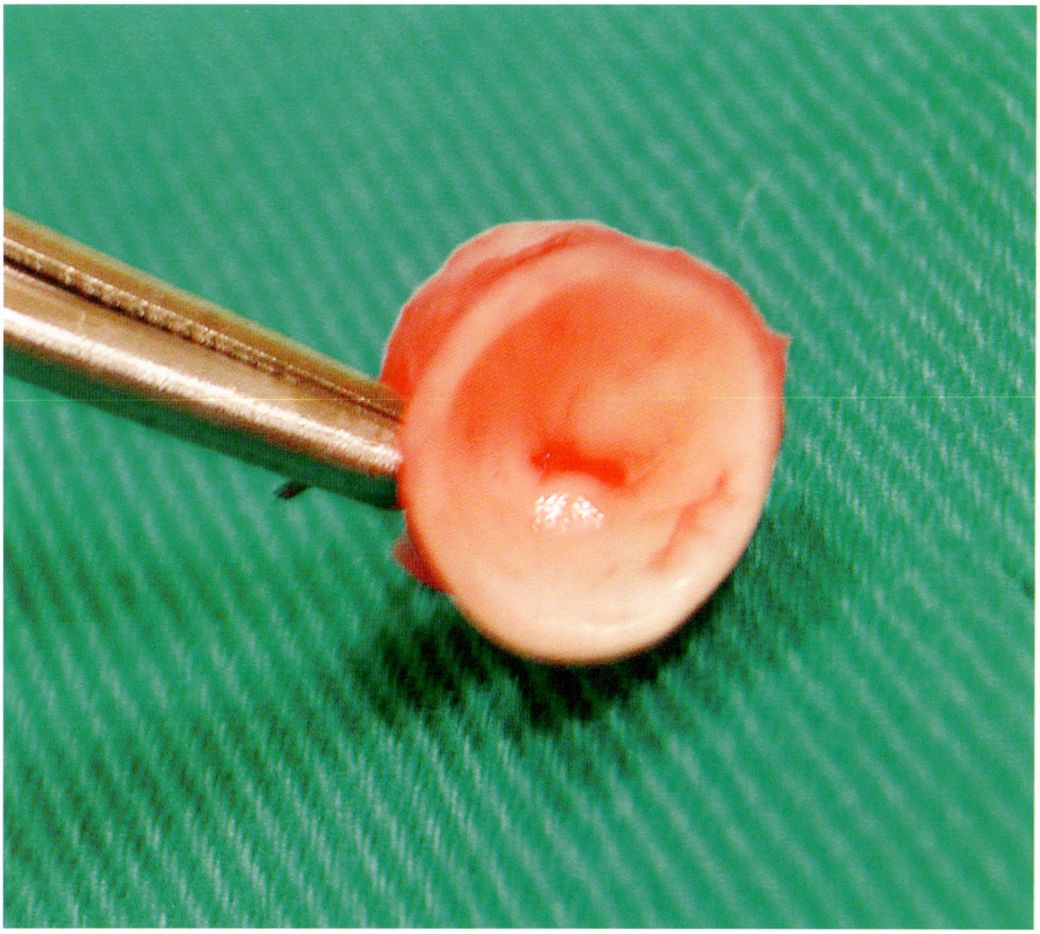

Figure 6.43. A surgical specimen from a 6-month-old infant. Note the near-complete obliteration of the lumen. The coarctation was repaired using end-to-end anastomosis.

dilatation caused by a previous balloon angioplasty is seen in Figure 6.41, and the extent of luminal narrowing is evident in Figures 6.42 and 6.43.

REFERENCES

1. Hoffman J, Kaplan S. The incidence of congenital heart disease. *J Am Coll Cardiol.* 2002;39:1890–1900.
2. Pradat P, Francannet C, Harris, JA, Robert E. The epidemiology of cardiovascular defects, Part I: a study based on data from three large registries of congenital malformations. *Pediatr Cardiol.* 2003;24:195–221.
3. Perloff JK. The variant associations of aortic isthmic coarctation. *Am J Cardiol.* 2010;106:1038–1041.
4. Celermajer DS, Greaves K. Survivors of coarctation repair: fixed but not cured. *Heart.* 2002;88:113–114.

CHAPTER 7

Interrupted Aortic Arch

Continuity of the aortic arch may be disrupted at various levels by an atretic segment or complete absence of a part of the arch. Blood supply to the aorta distal to the site of interruption is dependent on the ductus remaining widely patent. Classification is based on the location of the interruption relative to the aortic branches (Figure 7.1). The most common is type B, where the interruption is between the left common carotid and left subclavian arteries.[1] This type is also associated with chromosome 22q11 deletion.[2] Type A is when the interruption lies distal to the left subclavian artery affecting the isthmus segment of the arch, and type C is when the interruption lies between the innominate (brachiocephalic) and left common carotid arteries. Type C is very rare.

Patent ductus arteriosus (PDA) and ventricular septal defect with malalignment of the outlet septum obstructing the left ventricular outflow tract are among the commonly associated lesions.[3]

TYPE A INTERRUPTION

Figures 7.2, 7.3, and 7.7 are 2 examples of infants with type A interruption. There are several techniques to restore the continuity of the arch. We usually use the modified Blalock-Park technique, illustrated in Figure 7.4. In these 2 patients (see Figures 7.2 and 7.7), the atretic isthmus is seen as a fibrous cord. Both were repaired using the same technique, as shown in Figures 7.5 and 7.6 for the first patient and Figures 7.8 and 7.9 for the second.

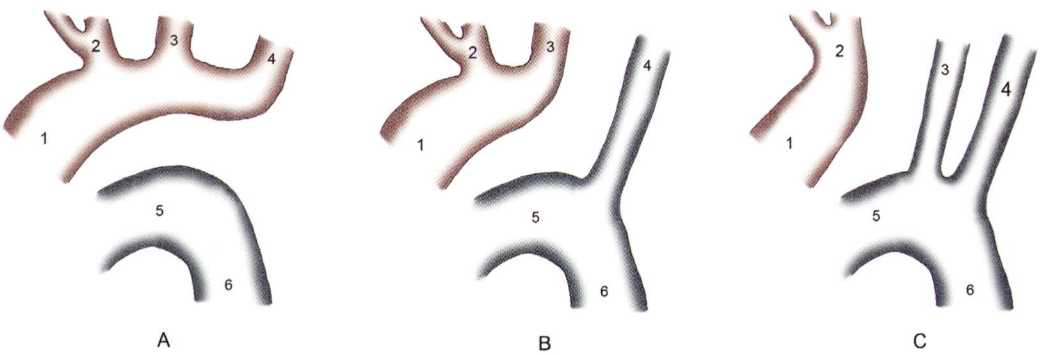

Figure 7.1. Schematic illustration of the classification of interrupted aortic arch. In type A, the interruption is distal to the origin of the subclavian artery; in type B, the interruption is between the left common carotid and left subclavian arteries; and in type C, the interruption is between the innominate and left common carotid arteries.

1. Ascending aorta
2. Innominate (brachiocephalic) artery
3. Left common carotid artery
4. Left subclavian artery
5. Ductus arteriosus
6. Descending thoracic aorta

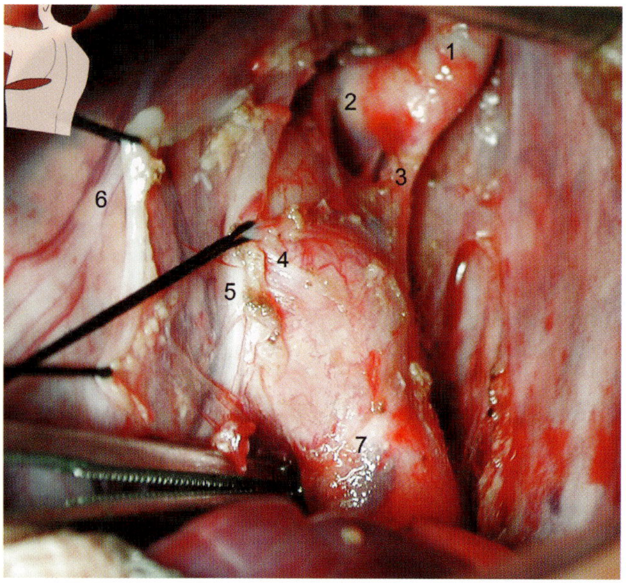

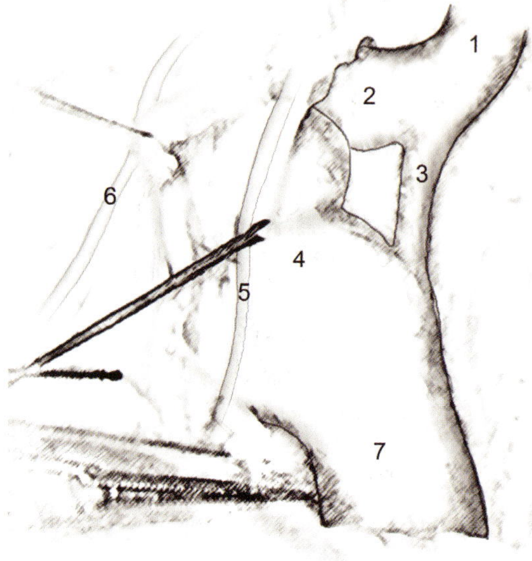

Figure 7.2 **Figure 7.3**

Type A interrupted aortic arch in a 1-month-old infant, as seen through a left lateral thoracotomy. The atretic segment (3) is merely a fibrous cord with no lumen.

1. Left subclavian artery
2. Transverse arch
3. Fibrous cord (atretic isthmus)
4. PDA
5. Left vagus nerve
6. Left phrenic nerve
7. Descending thoracic aorta

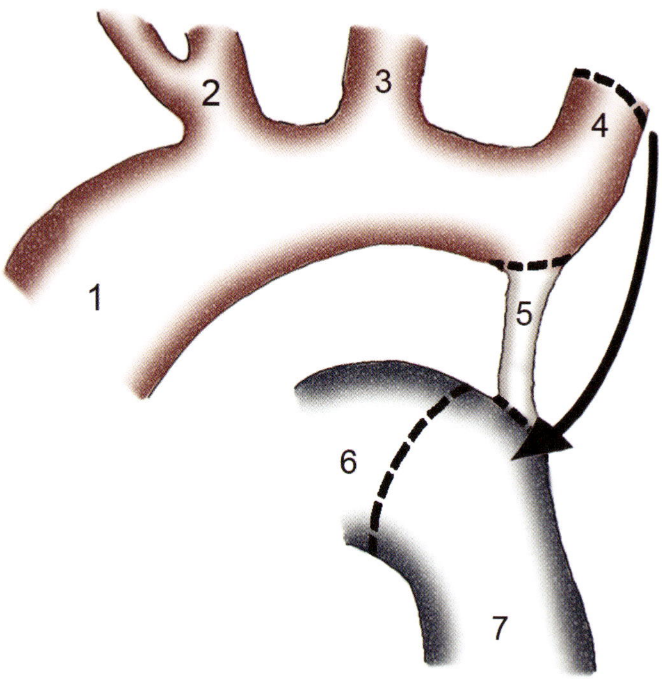

Figure 7.4. Schematic drawing of type A interrupted aortic arch with an atretic segment, similar to the patient in Figure 7.2. Surgical repair is done by excising the atretic segment, dividing the ductus, transecting the left subclavian artery, turning it down, and anastomosing it end-to-end to the descending thoracic aorta to restore continuity of the arch.

1. Ascending thoracic aorta
2. Innominate artery
3. Left common carotid artery
4. Left subclavian artery
5. Atretic segment of the arch
6. PDA
7. Descending thoracic aorta

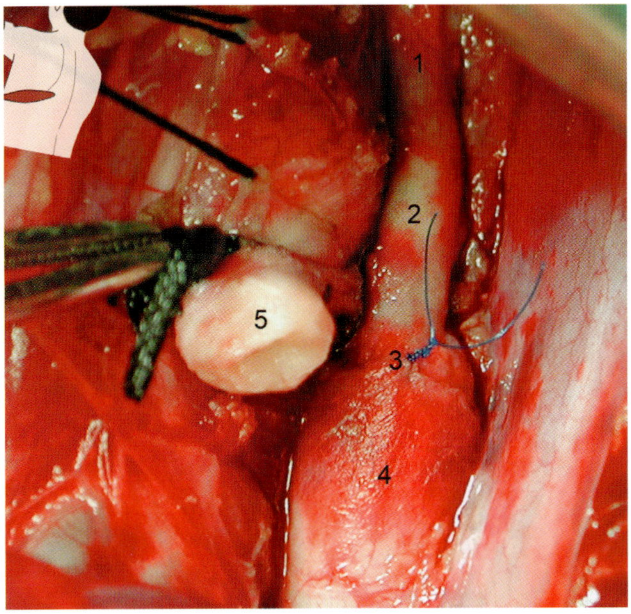

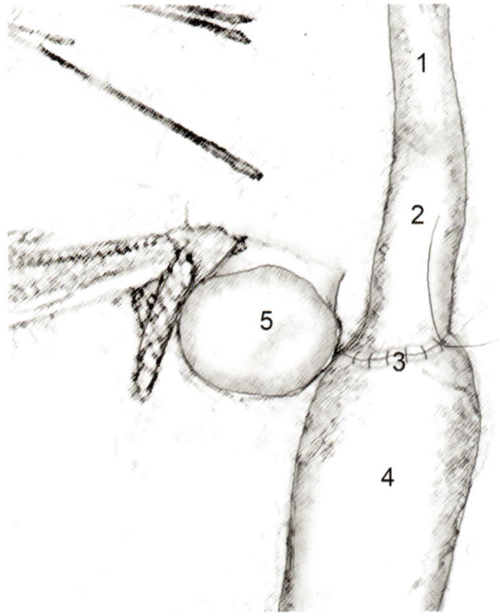

Figure 7.5 **Figure 7.6**

The same patient as in Figure 7.2 after repair using the technique illustrated in Figure 7.4.

1. Left common carotid artery
2. Left subclavian artery, now a part of the descending aorta
3. Anastomosis site
4. Descending thoracic aorta
5. Stump of ductus arteriosus

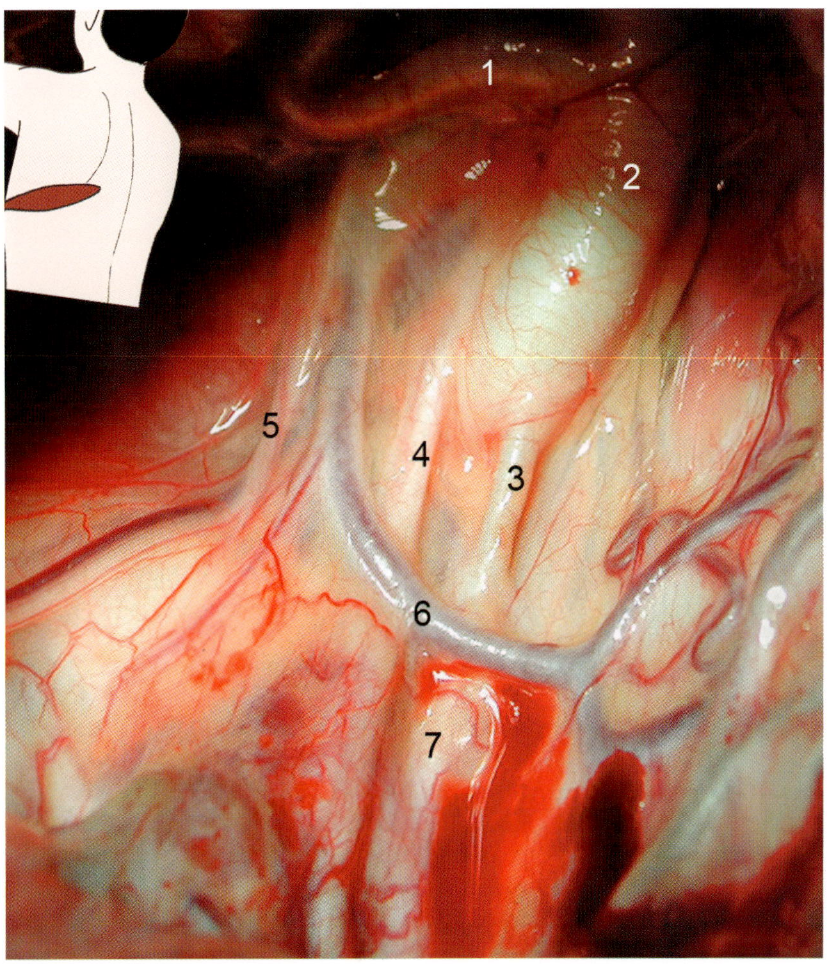

Figure 7.7. Left lateral thoracotomy view of posterior mediastinal structures before dissection, from another patient, a 3-month-old infant, with type A interruption.

1. Internal mammary artery
2. Left subclavian artery
3. Atretic segment of aortic arch
4. Left vagus nerve
5. Left phrenic nerve and pericardiophrenic vessels
6. Superior intercostal vein
7. Descending aorta

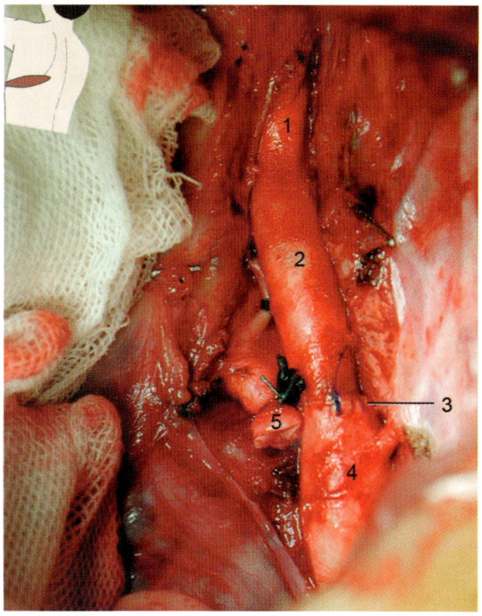

Figure 7.8

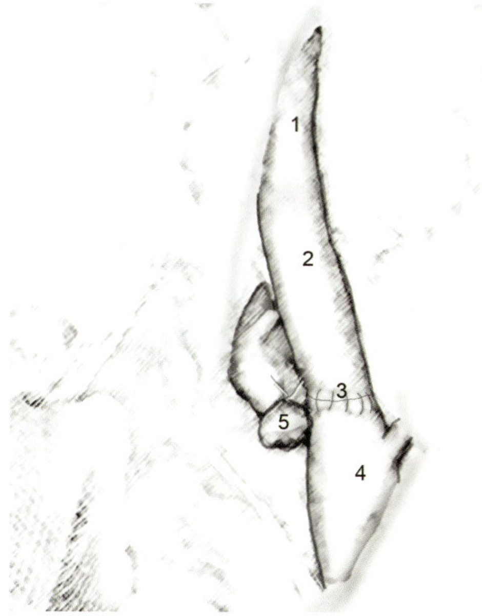

Figure 7.9

The same patient as in Figure 7.7 after repair using the technique illustrated in Figure 7.4.

1. Left common carotid artery
2. Left subclavian artery, now a part of the descending aorta
3. Anastomosis site
4. Descending thoracic aorta
5. Stump of ductus arteriosus

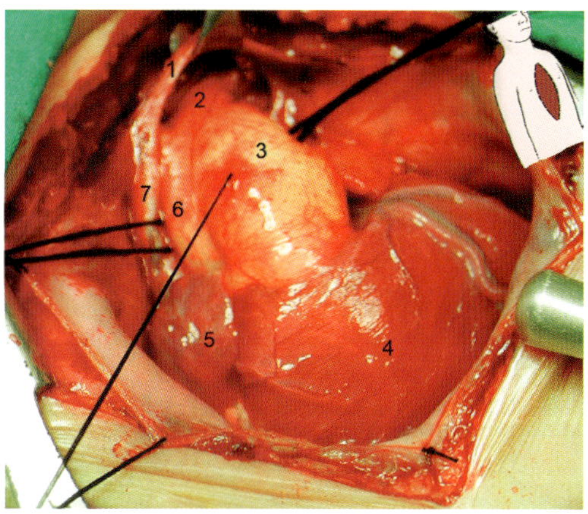

Figure 7.10

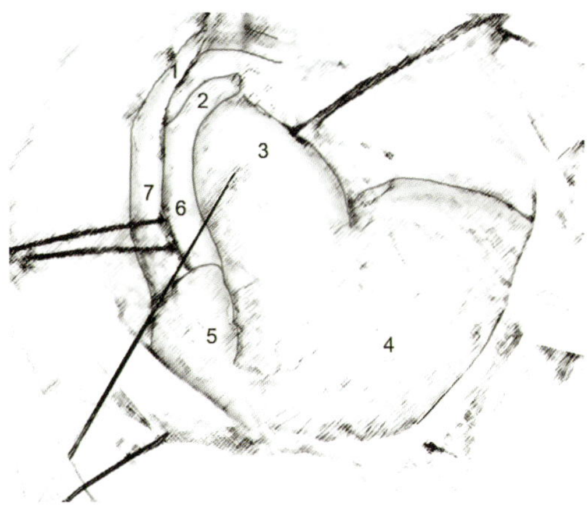

Figure 7.11

Median sternotomy view of a 3-day-old neonate with type B interruption. The descending aorta is not seen here, but becomes visible when the pulmonary artery (PA) is retracted sideways as shown in Figure 7.12.

1. Innominate vein
2. Left common carotid artery
3. Main pulmonary artery (MPA)
4. Right ventricle
5. Right atrial appendage
6. Ascending aorta
7. Superior vena cava (SVC)

TYPE B INTERRUPTION

Type B interruption may be approached from lateral thoracotomy or median sternotomy, depending on whether intracardiac repair is concomitantly performed. Figures 7.10 to 7.13 show median sternotomy views from a 3-day-old neonate. Figures 7.14 and 7.15 present a lateral thoracotomy view from a 9-month-old infant. The technique we usually use to repair type B interruption is illustrated in Figure 7.16.

Figures 7.19 to 7.26 are from a 5-month-old infant with trisomy 21, atrioventricular septal defect, and type B interruption of the aorta. This patient was thought to have type C interruption on echocardiography because 3 vessels were seen coming off the aorta proximal to the interruption. It turned out, however, that the third vessel was an anomalous vertebral artery and the left subclavian came off the aorta distal to the interruption. The repair was achieved using the technique illustrated in Figure 7.16.

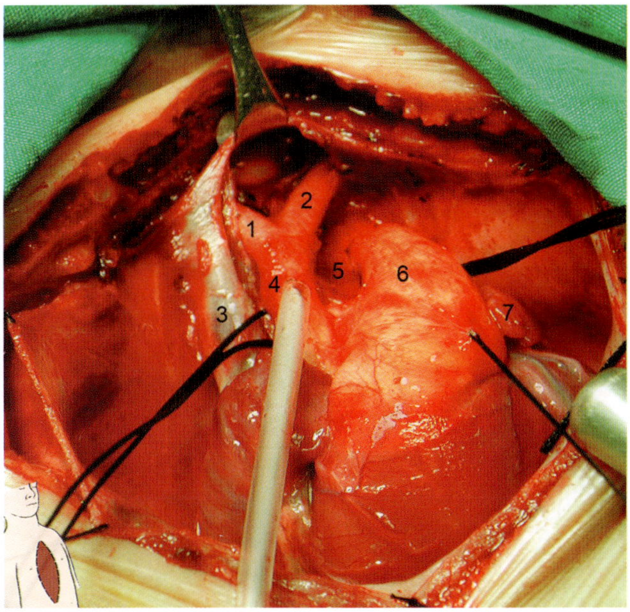

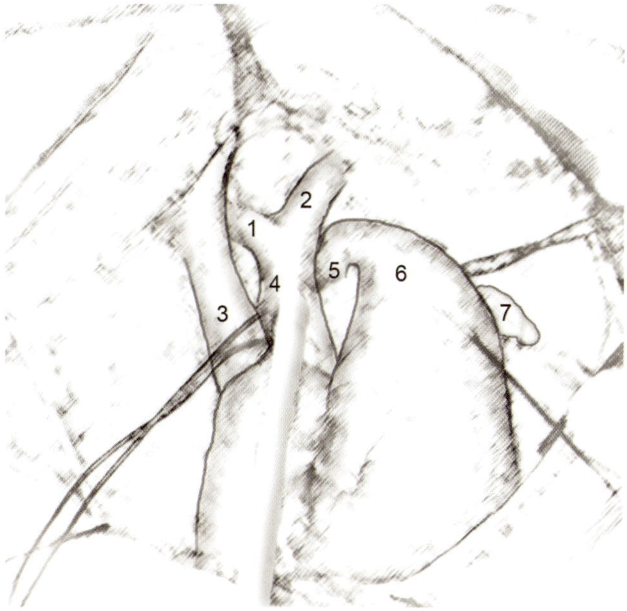

Figure 7.12 **Figure 7.13**

Same patient as in Figure 7.10 with the PA retracted to the left to show the ductus arteriosus and descending aorta. The left subclavian artery (not shown) comes off the descending aorta. Note the complete interruption of the arch after the take-off of the left common carotid artery.

1. Innominate artery
2. Left common carotid artery
3. SVC
4. Ascending aorta
5. Descending thoracic aorta
6. MPA continuing as ductus
7. Left atrial appendage

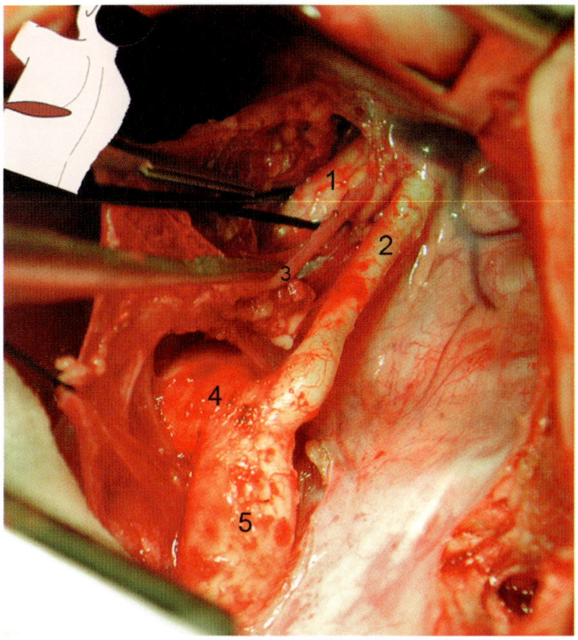

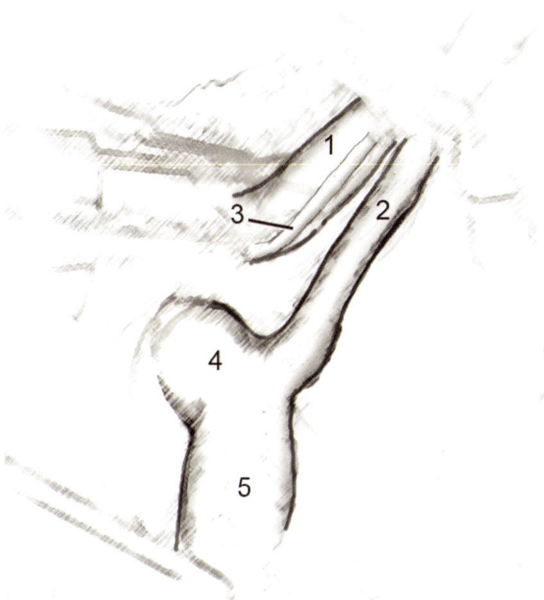

Figure 7.14 **Figure 7.15**

Left lateral thoracotomy view in a 9-month-old infant with type B interruption. A schematic illustration of this is shown in Figure 7.16, along with the operative technique used to repair this type of interruption.

1. Left common carotid artery
2. Left subclavian artery
3. Left vagus nerve
4. Ductus arteriosus
5. Descending thoracic aorta

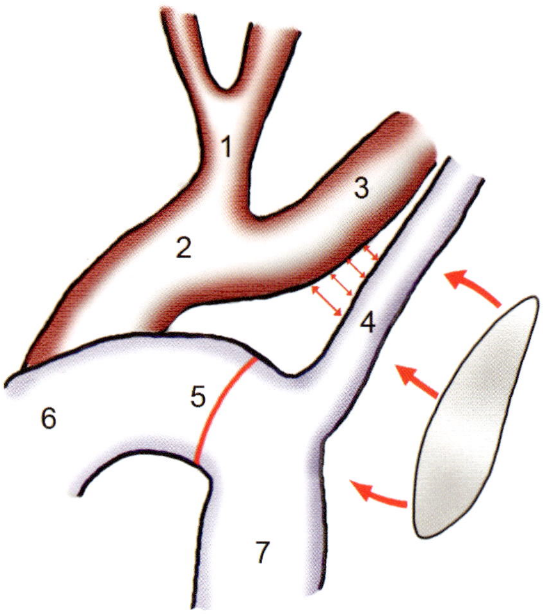

Figure 7.16. Schematic drawing of type B interruption. Continuity of the arch is restored by side-to-side anastomosis of left common carotid artery to the left subclavian artery (small arrows). The newly formed arch often needs to be enlarged by a patch. Then the ductus is divided (5) to complete the repair.

1. Innominate artery
2. Ascending aorta
3. Left common carotid artery
4. Left subclavian artery
5. Ductus arteriosus
6. MPA
7. Descending thoracic aorta

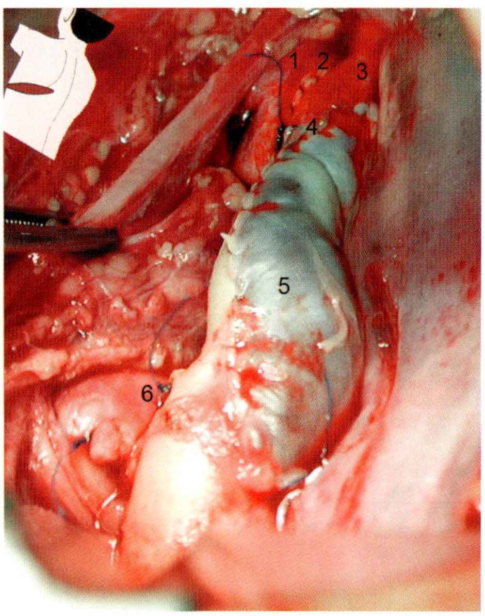

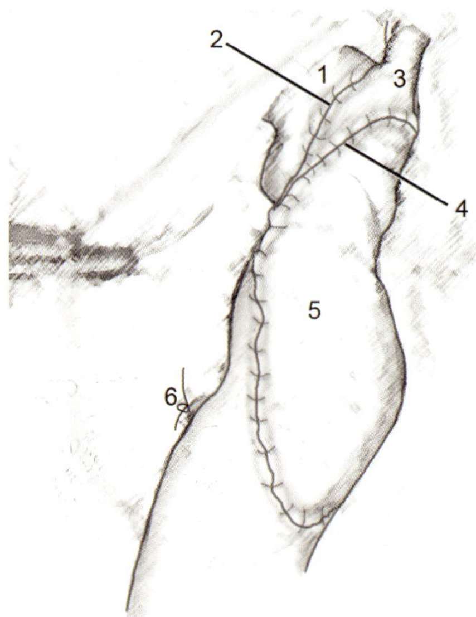

Figure 7.17 **Figure 7.18**

The same patient as in Figure 7.14 after restoration of aortic arch continuity using the technique illustrated in Figure 7.16.

1. Proximal part of left common carotid artery, now a part of surgically constructed transverse arch
2. First suture line: Side-to-side anastomosis between left common carotid and left subclavian arteries
3. Left subclavian artery
4. Second suture line: Between left subclavian artery and the patch
5. Autologous pericardial patch
6. Site of divided ductus arteriosus

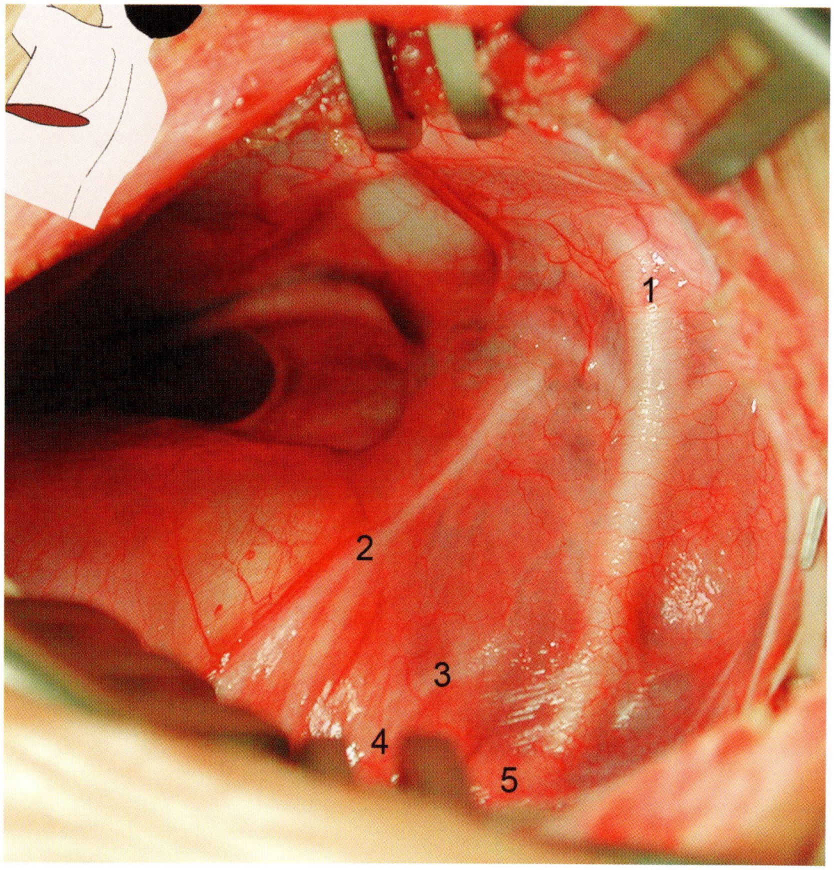

Figure 7.19. Posterior mediastinal structures as seen through a left lateral thoracotomy in a 5-month-old infant with Down syndrome and interrupted aortic arch.

1. Left subclavian artery
2. Left phrenic nerve
3. Left vagus nerve
4. Ductus arteriosus
5. Descending thoracic aorta

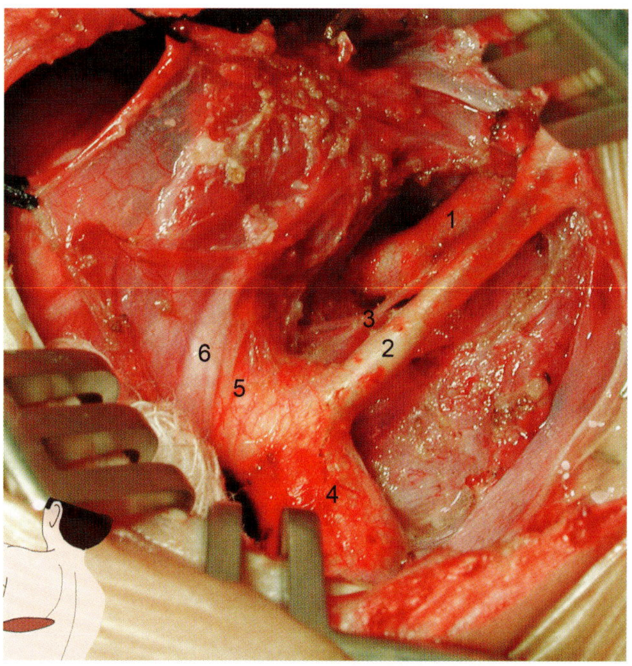

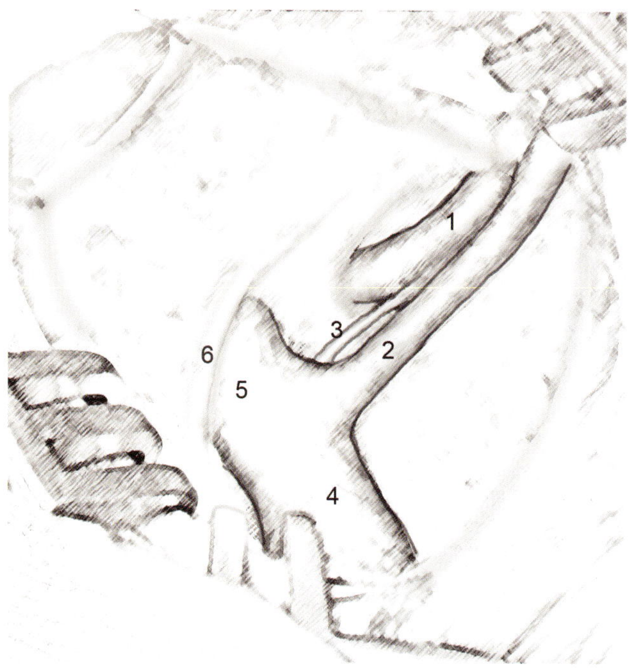

Figure 7.20 **Figure 7.21**

The same patient as in Figure 7.19 after dissection. The distal transverse arch is atretic and is present as a fibrous cord (further shown in Figure 7.22). Note that the isthmus portion of the arch is practically absent and the left subclavian artery arises directly from the junction between the ductus and the descending aorta.

1. Left common carotid artery
2. Left subclavian artery
3. Atretic distal transverse arch
4. Descending thoracic aorta
5. Ductus arteriosus
6. Left vagus nerve

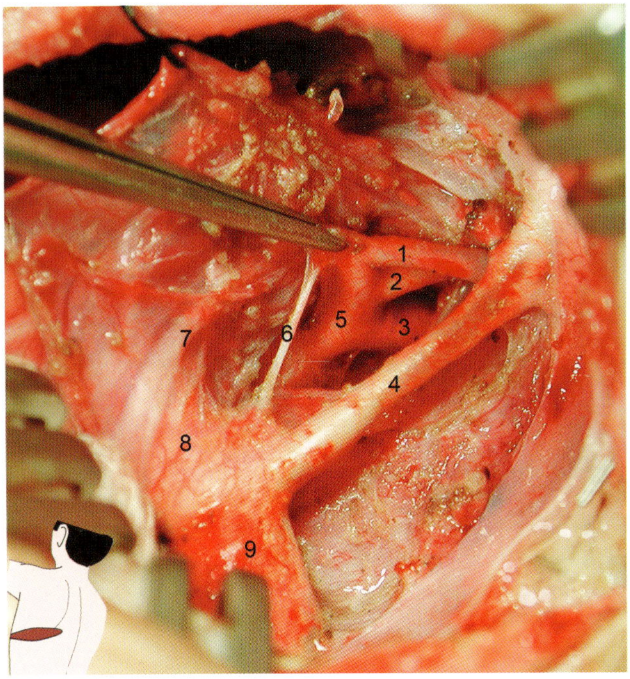

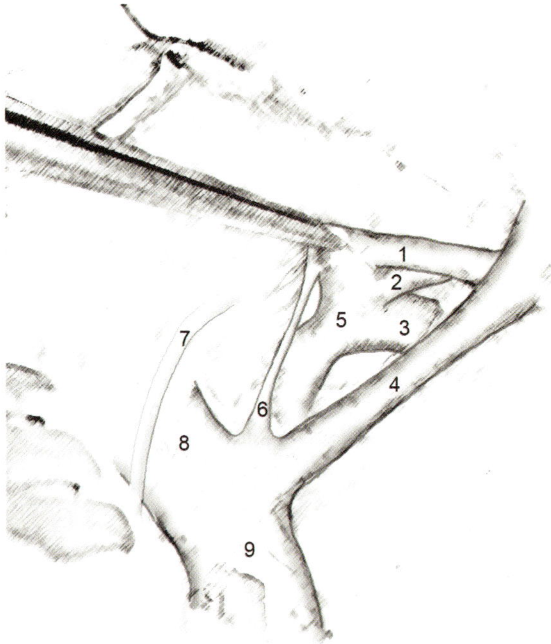

Figure 7.22 **Figure 7.23**

The same patient as in Figures 7.19 to 7.21. Note the atretic transverse arch (6) between the origin of the vertebral artery (1) and the left subclavian artery (4). See text for details.

1. Anomalous vertebral artery
2. Left common carotid artery
3. Innominate artery
4. Left subclavian artery
5. Proximal transverse arch
6. Atretic distal transverse arch
7. Left vagus nerve
8. Ductus arteriosus
9. Descending thoracic aorta

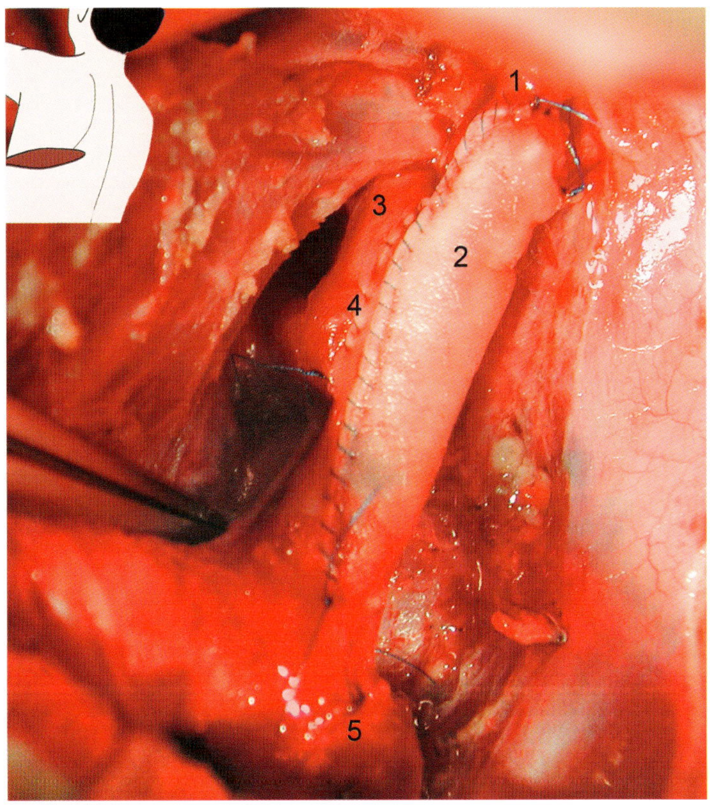

Figure 7.24. The same patient as in Figures 7.19 to 7.23 after repair using the technique illustrated in Figure 7.16. To complete the repair, the ductus arteriosus will also be divided. See Figure 7.25 for a zoomed-out view of suture lines.

1. Left subclavian artery
2. Xenograft pericardial patch
3. Left common carotid artery
4. Suture lines (see Figure 7.25)
5. Descending thoracic aorta

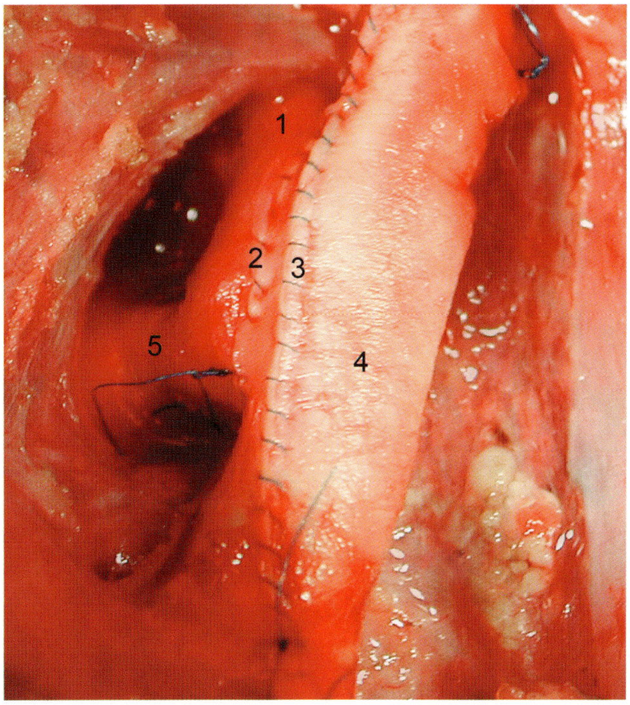

Figure 7.25

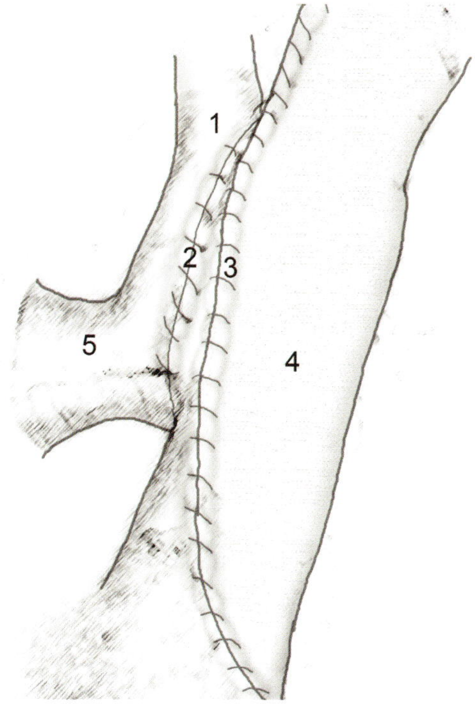

Figure 7.26

The same patient as in Figures 7.19 to 7.24 showing the anastomosis lines. Aortic arch continuity was restored using the technique illustrated in Figure 7.16.

1. Left common carotid artery
2. First suture line: Side-to-side anastomosis between left common carotid and left subclavian arteries
3. Second suture line: Between left subclavian artery and the patch
4. Xenograft pericardial patch
5. Transverse arch

REFERENCES

1. Brown J, Ruzmetov M, Okada Y, et al. Outcomes in patients with interrupted aortic arch and associated anomalies: a 20-year experience. *Eur J Cardiothoracic Surg.* 2006;29:666–674.
2. Robin N, Shprintzen R. Defining the clinical spectrum of deletion 22q11.2. *J Pediatr.* 2005;147:90–96.
3. Ho SY, Wilcox BR, Anderson RH, Lincoln JCR. Interrupted aortic arch – anatomical features of surgical significance. *Thorac Cardiovasc Surg.* 1983;31:199–205.

CHAPTER 8

Vascular Ring

VASCULAR RING

A vascular ring is formed by lack of involution of the embryonic double aortic arch or anomalous arterial branching pattern of the aorta, often in conjunction with a ductus arteriosus (or ligamentum arteriosum). The ring encircles the mediastinal structures, most importantly the trachea and esophagus. The symptoms are mainly due to mechanical compression of the trachea, the esophagus, or both.[1] Some abnormal branching patterns may also cause compression although strictly speaking do not constitute an anatomic ring.

The embryonic basis for various types of vascular ring can be simplified by analyzing a hypothetical double aortic arch, as proposed by Edwards,[2] and is illustrated in Figure 8.1.

DOUBLE AORTIC ARCH

Double aortic arch is the most common type of vascular ring.[3] It is a relatively rare anomaly that results from embryonic failure of regression of one of the primitive aortic arches. The variation in anatomy can be quite complex and is beyond the scope of this book. Symptoms usually arise from compression on the trachea and/or esophagus by the anomalous vascular structures.

Surgical correction is commonly achieved through a lateral thoracotomy. The smaller of the 2 arches is divided. A patent ductus arteriosus (PDA), when present, or ligamentum arteriosum is also divided during the repair.

The cases in this chapter present some examples of vascular rings, including a left dominant arch, a right

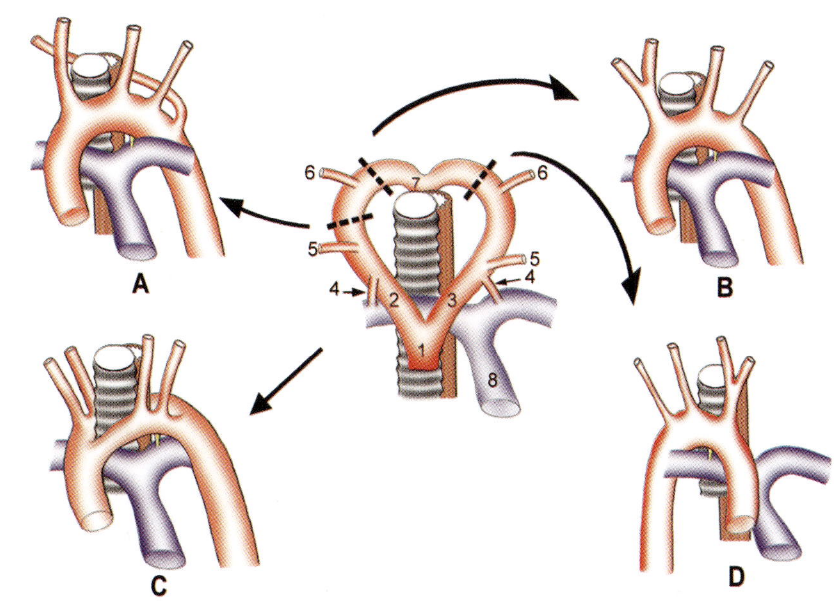

Figure 8.1. Hypothetical model of embryonic double aortic arch. The dashed lines represent where regression could take place. Some of the possible derivatives of this model are shown. **(A)** Left arch with aberrant right subclavian artery. **(B)** Normal left aortic arch. **(C)** Double aortic arch with anterior (left) arch and posterior (right) arch. **(D)** Right aortic arch with mirror-image branching pattern of the arch arteries.

1. Ventral (ascending) aorta
2. Right aortic arch
3. Left aortic arch
4. Right and left ductus arteriosus
5. Right and left common carotid arteries
6. Right and left subclavian arteries
7. Descending aorta
8. Main pulmonary artery (MPA)

Congenital Heart Disease: A Surgical Color Atlas © 2015 A. Sukru Mercan, Zakariya Hubail, S. Yen Ho.
Cardiotext Publishing, ISBN: 978-1-935395-90-4.

dominant arch, a single arch with contralateral ductus arteriosus, and an aberrant right subclavian artery.

Figures 8.2 to 8.7 are from a child with double aortic arch whose left arch was the dominant one. So the right arch was divided, thus relieving the compression on the trachea and esophagus. Upon division, the right arch self-retracts to lie to the right of the esophagus (see arrow in Figure 8.5).

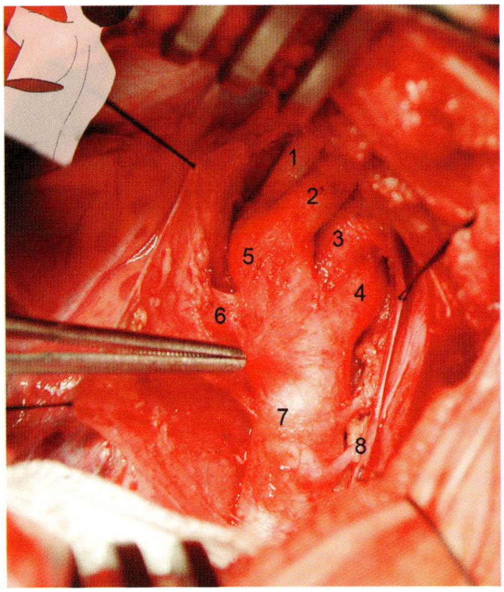

Figure 8.2

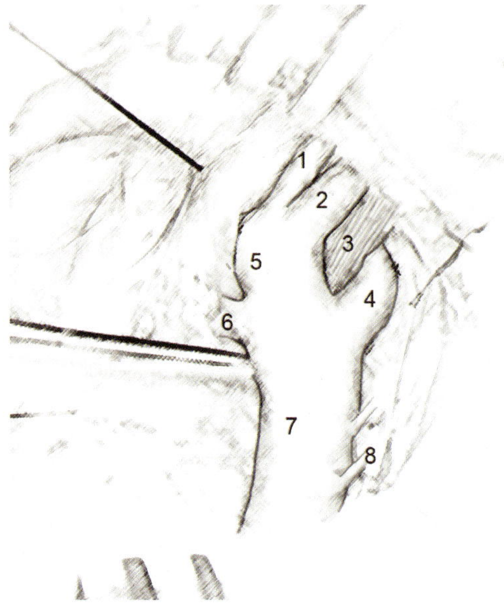

Figure 8.3

Double aortic arch as seen through a left lateral thoracotomy. The left (5) is the dominant arch. Note how the right arch (4) passes posterior to the esophagus (3).

1. Left common carotid artery
2. Left subclavian artery
3. Esophagus
4. Right aortic arch
5. Left aortic arch
6. Ligamentum arteriosum
7. Descending aorta
8. Intercostal arteries

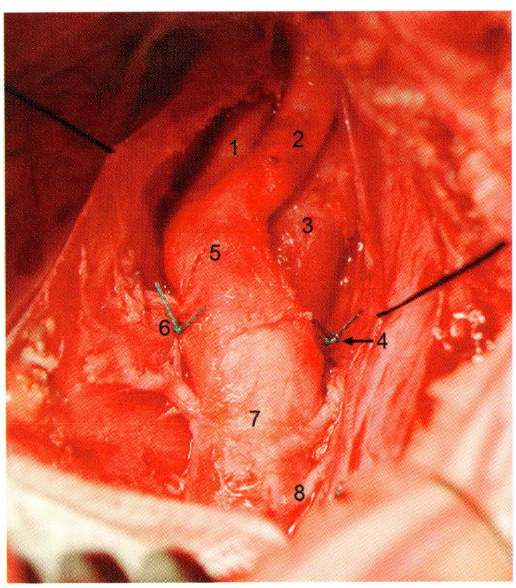

Figure 8.4

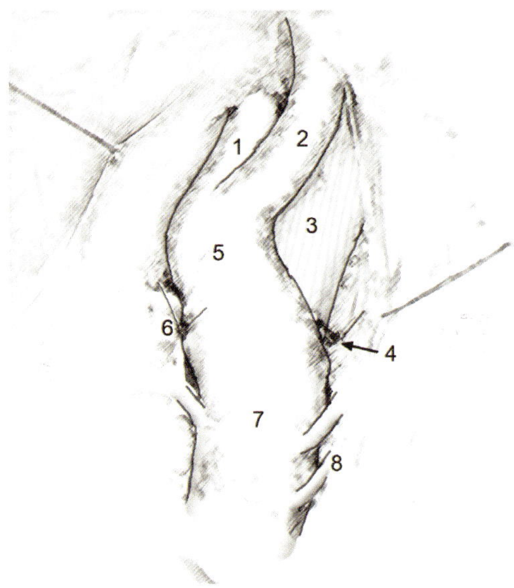

Figure 8.5

The same patient as in Figure 8.2. The right arch has been divided, and its distal stump is shown (4).

1. Left common carotid artery
2. Left subclavian artery
3. Esophagus
4. Stump of divided right arch
5. Left aortic arch
6. Ligamentum arteriosum
7. Descending aorta
8. Intercostal arteries

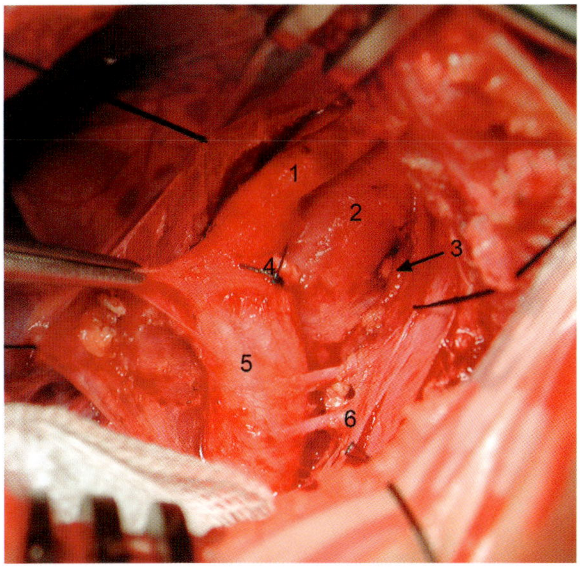

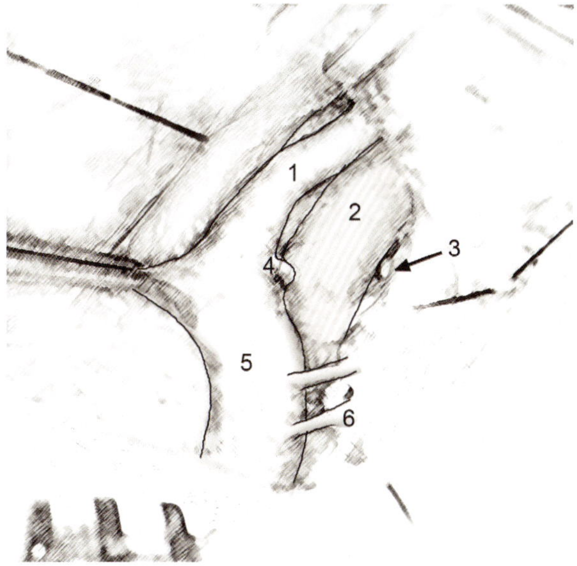

Figure 8.6 **Figure 8.7**

The same patient as in Figures 8.2 to 8.5. The left arch is retracted anteriorly to show the esophagus, now free from compression. The proximal stump of the divided right arch (3) self-retracts to a location to the right of the esophagus.

1. Left subclavian artery
2. Esophagus
3. Proximal stump of right arch
4. Distal stump of right arch
5. Descending aorta
6. Intercostal arteries

Figures 8.8 to 8.11 illustrate a double aortic arch in a 5-month-old infant. The right arch was the dominant one; therefore, the left arch and the PDA were divided.

An aortopexy is often necessary to move the right arch away from the esophagus and trachea as illustrated in Figures 8.12 to 8.18 from a 1-year-old child with right aortic arch, aberrant left subclavian artery

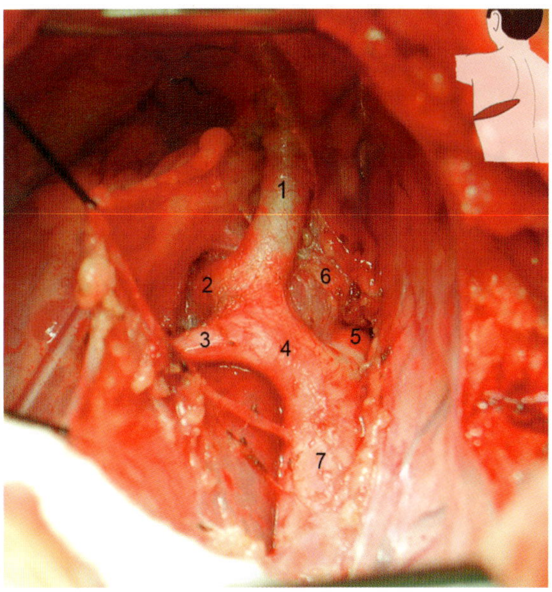

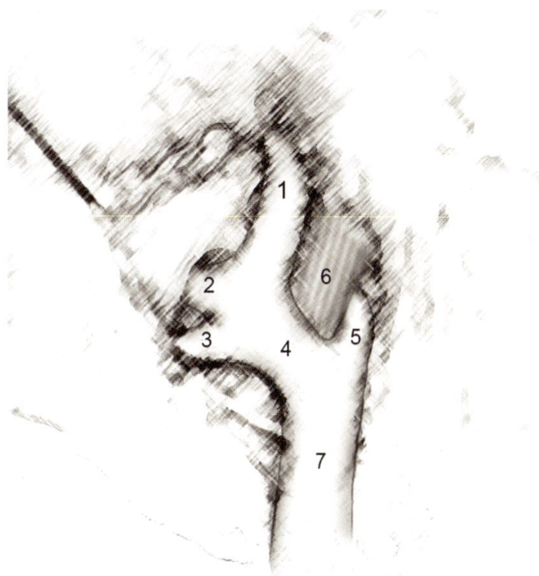

Figure 8.8 **Figure 8.9**

Left lateral thoracotomy view for a 5-month-old infant with double aortic arch. The right (5) was the dominant arch; the nondominant left arch (4) is the one that will be surgically divided to relieve the obstruction.

1. Left subclavian artery
2. Left arch
3. Ductus arteriosus
4. Part of the left arch that will be divided
5. Right arch
6. Esophagus
7. Descending aorta

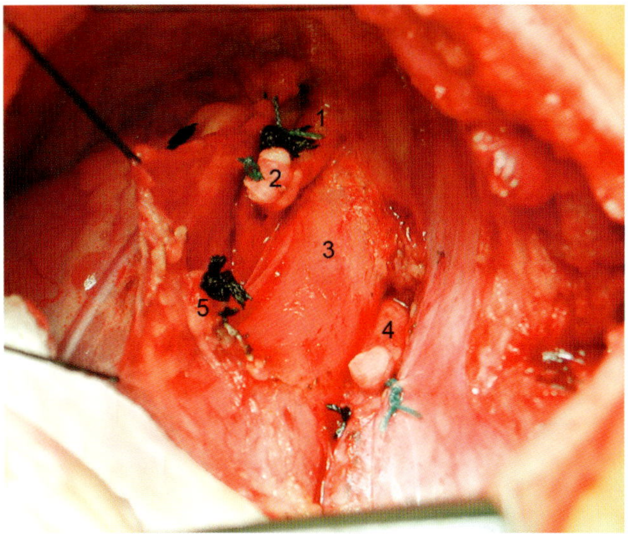

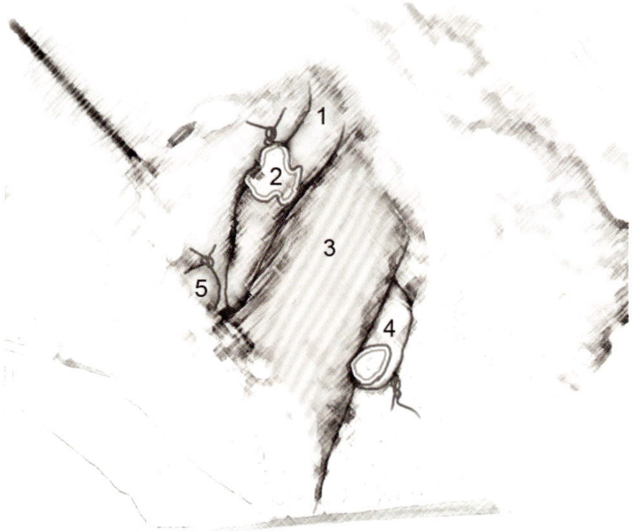

Figure 8.10 **Figure 8.11**

The same patient as in Figure 8.8. The left arch and the ductus arteriosus were divided.

1. Left subclavian artery
2. Stump of left arch
3. Esophagus
4. Right arch
5. Ductus arteriosus

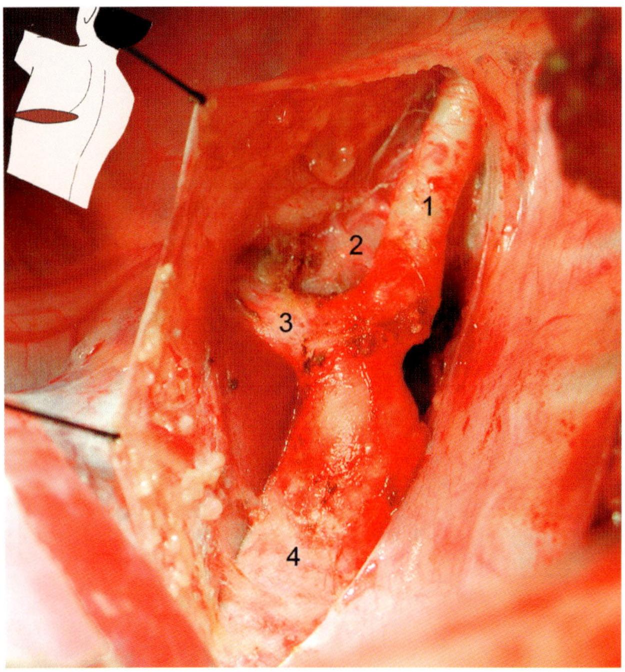

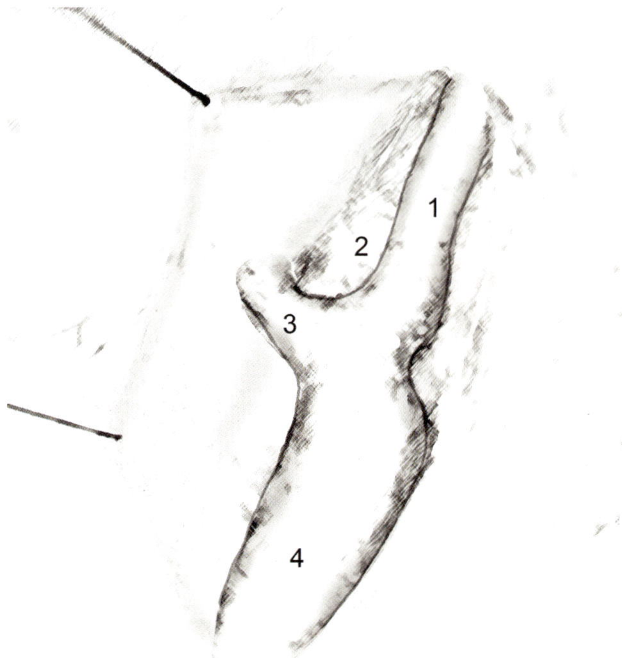

Figure 8.12 **Figure 8.13**

A 1-year-old child with a right aortic arch, an aberrant left subclavian artery, and a left ductus arteriosus as seen through a lateral thoracotomy. The right aortic arch itself is not seen here but is visible when the descending aorta is retracted anteriorly as shown in Figure 8.14.

1. Left subclavian artery
2. Esophagus
3. Ductus arteriosus
4. Descending aorta

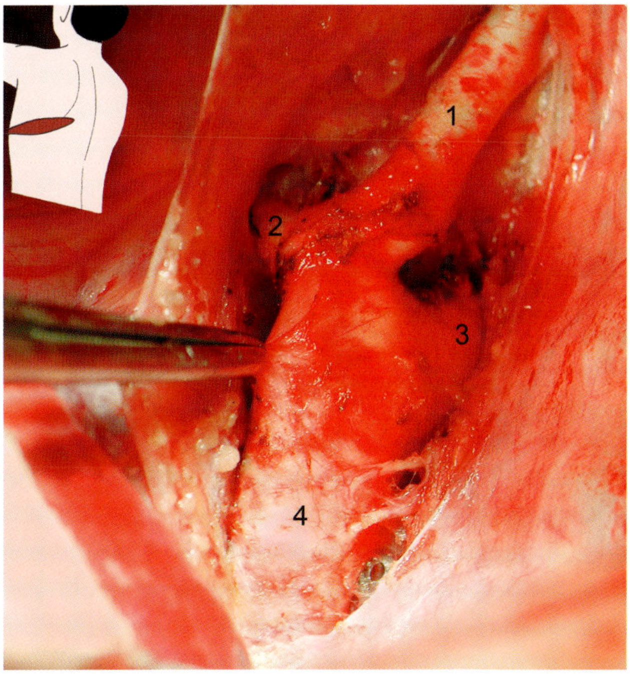

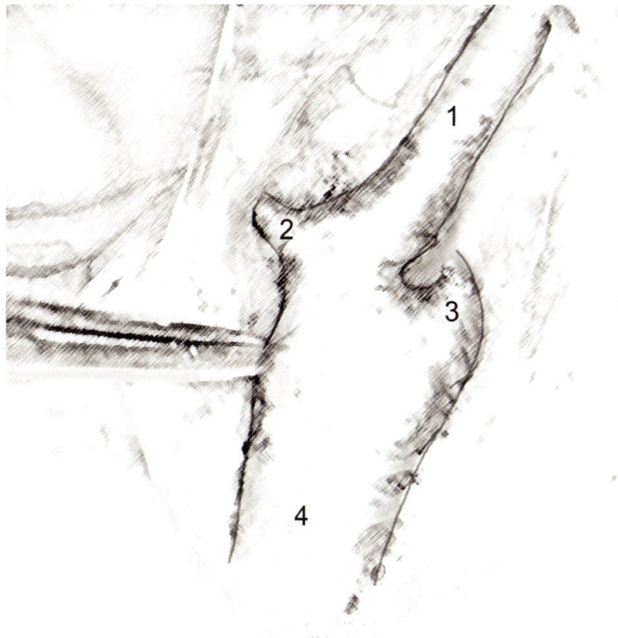

Figure 8.14 **Figure 8.15**

The same patient as in Figure 8.12. The right aortic arch is seen running posterior to the esophagus. The arch and the left ductus form a retro-eosphageal sling.

1. Left subclavian artery
2. Ductus arteriosus
3. Aortic arch
4. Descending aorta

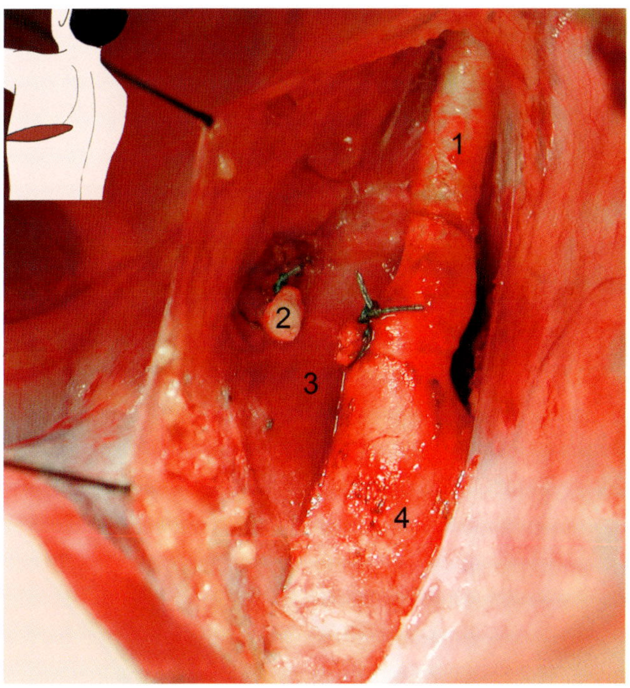

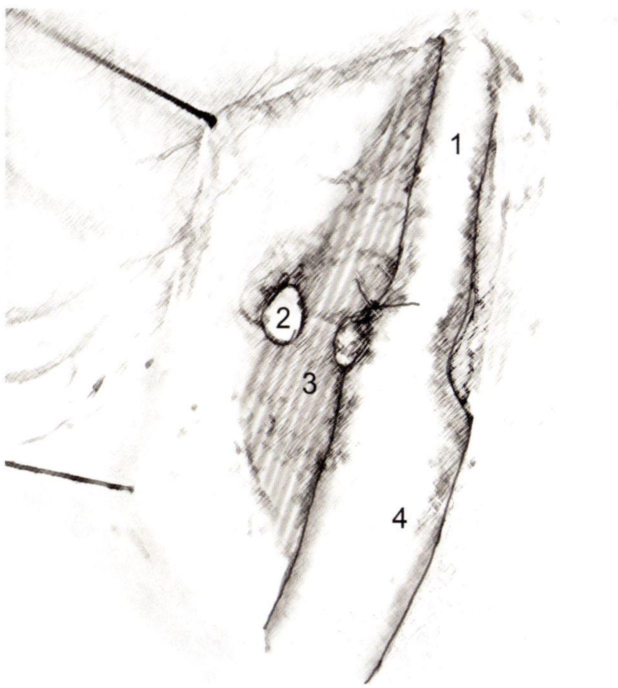

Figure 8.16 **Figure 8.17**

The same patient as in Figures 8.12 to 8.15. The ductus (2) has been divided.

1. Left subclavian artery
2. Stump of divided ductus arteriosus
3. Esophagus
4. Descending aorta

Figure 8.18. The same patient as in Figures 8.12 to 8.17. To provide more room for the mediastinal structures, an aortopexy was performed by attaching the descending thoracic aorta to the posterior thoracic wall.

1. Left subclavian artery
2. Stump of divided ductus arteriosus
3. Esophagus
4. Descending aorta
5. Posterior thoracic wall

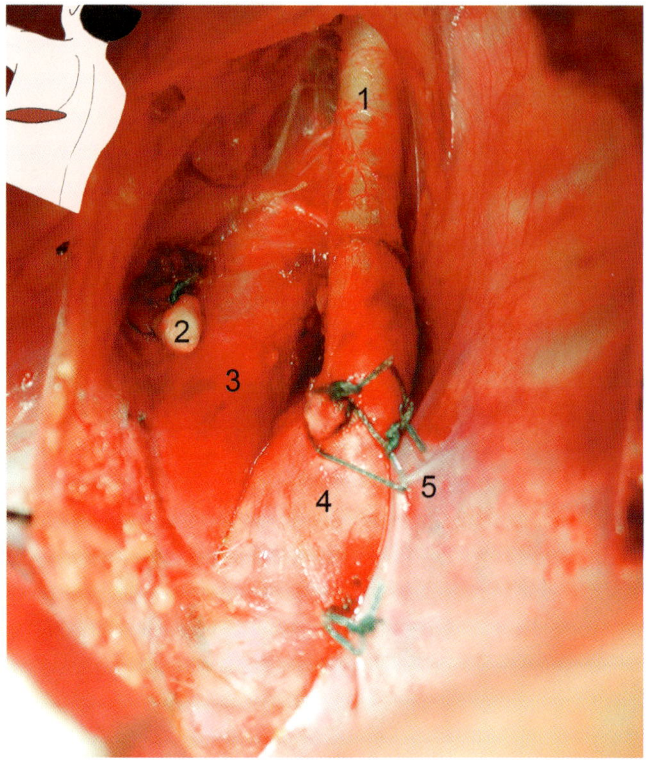

arising as the last branch of the arch, and a left ductus arteriosus.

A median sternotomy approach is chosen when concomitant intracardiac repair is also done. Figures 8.19 to 8.22 are of a 2-month-old infant with a double aortic arch. He underwent division of the right arch and closure of a concomitant ventricular septal defect (VSD). An aberrant right subclavian artery with

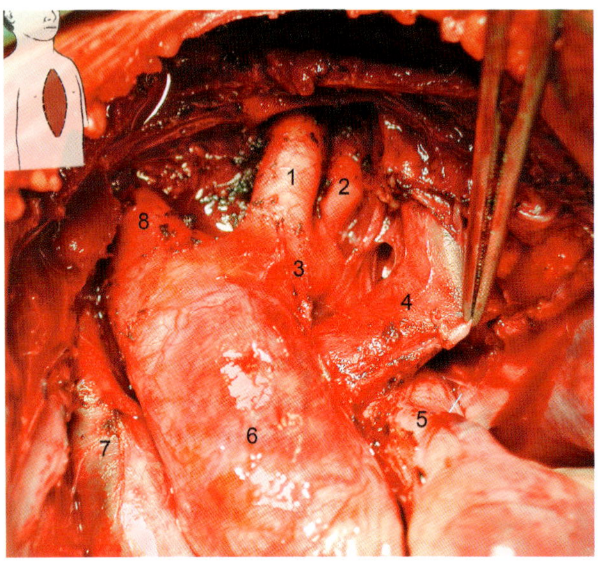

Figure 8.19

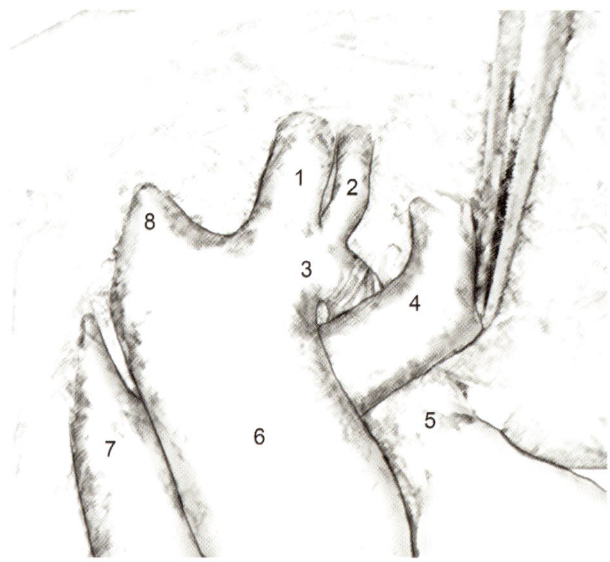

Figure 8.20

Median sternotomy view from a 2-month-old infant with double aortic arch and VSD (not shown). Note the retro-aortic innominate vein (4). The right arch is not seen in this view but becomes visible when the ascending aorta is retracted as shown in Figure 8.21.

1. Left common carotid artery
2. Left subclavian artery
3. Left aortic arch
4. Retro-aortic innominate vein
5. MPA
6. Ascending aorta
7. Superior vena cava (SVC)
8. Innominate artery

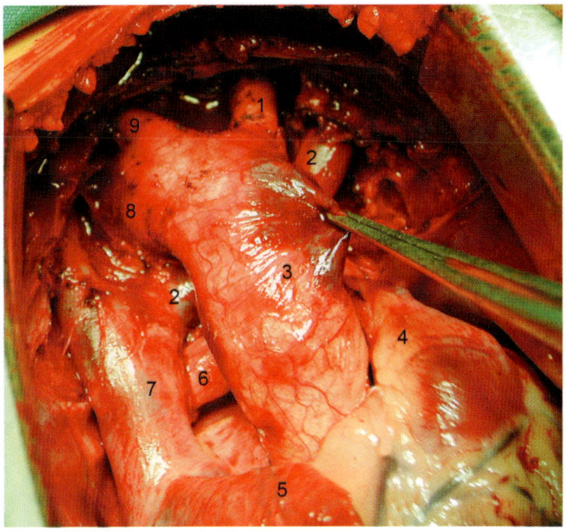

Figure 8.21

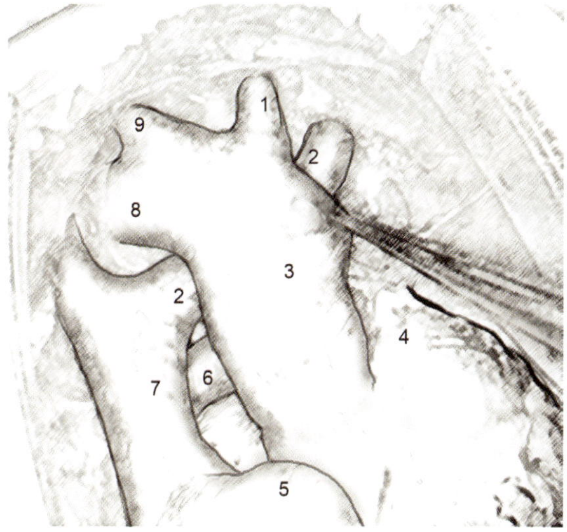

Figure 8.22

Same patient as in Figure 8.19. When the aorta is retracted, the right aortic arch becomes visible (8).

1. Left common carotid artery
2. Retro-aortic innominate vein
3. Ascending aorta
4. MPA
5. Right atrial appendage
6. Right PA
7. SVC
8. Right aortic arch
9. Innominate artery

retro-esophageal course is relatively common and is considered a normal variant. However, it may occasionally cause symptomatic compression and require treatment.[4] Figures 8.23 to 8.26 are from a 9-month-old infant with a left arch and an aberrant right subclavian artery that was treated by division. Another example is shown in Figures 8.27 to 8.32, from a 2-year-old child with failure to thrive and difficulty swallowing.

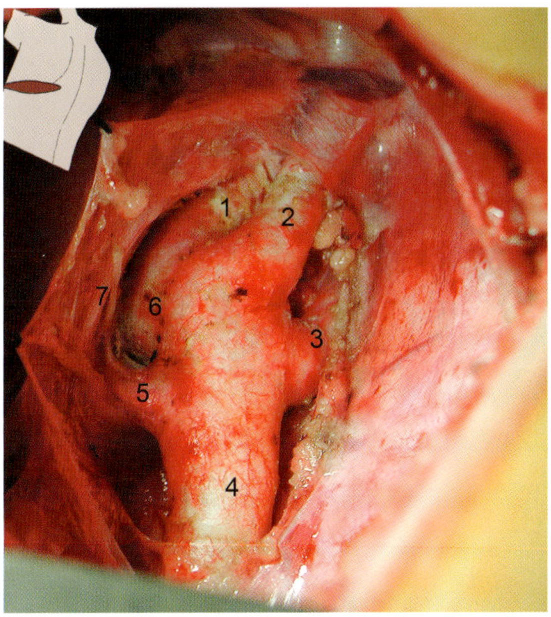

Figure 8.23

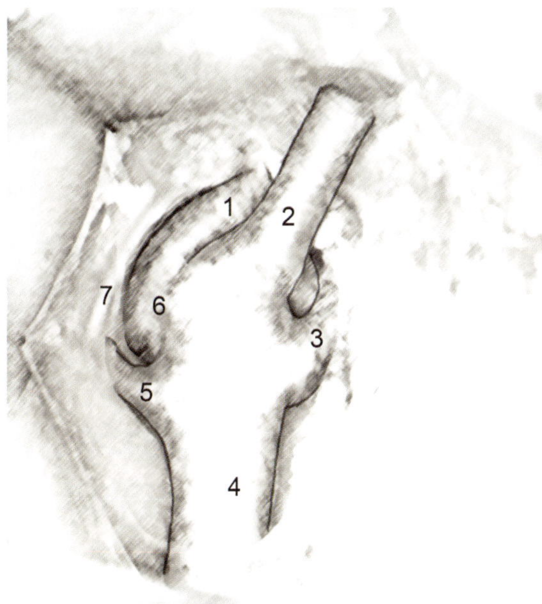

Figure 8.24

A left lateral thoracotomy view from a 9-month-old infant with aberrant right subclavian artery, running a retro-esophageal course.

1. Left common carotid artery
2. Left subclavian artery
3. Aberrant right subclavian artery
4. Descending aorta
5. Ligamentum arteriosum
6. Transverse aortic arch
7. Left vagus nerve

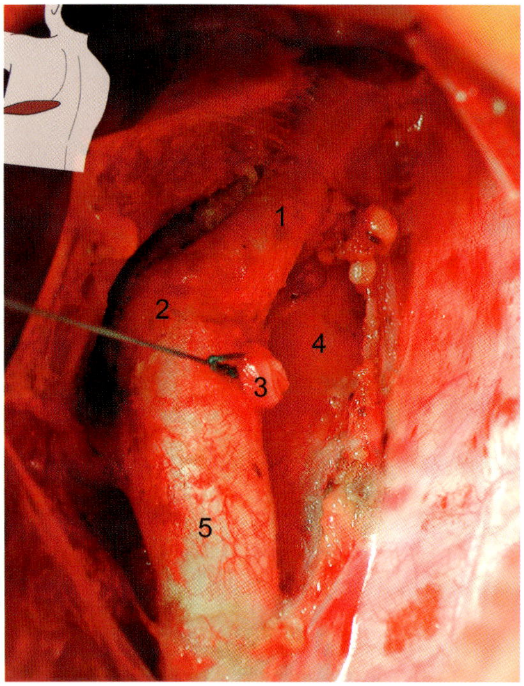

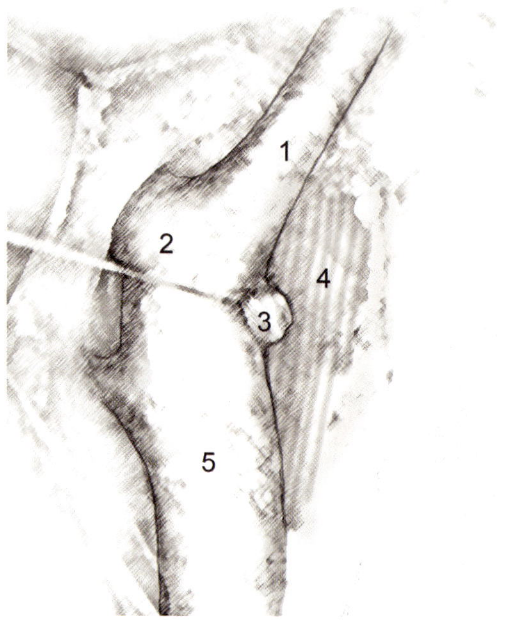

Figure 8.25 **Figure 8.26**

The same patient as in Figure 8.23. The aberrant right subclavian artery was divided at its origin (3), thus relieving the compression on the esophagus.

1. Left subclavian artery
2. Aortic arch
3. Stump of the right subclavian artery
4. Esophagus
5. Descending aorta

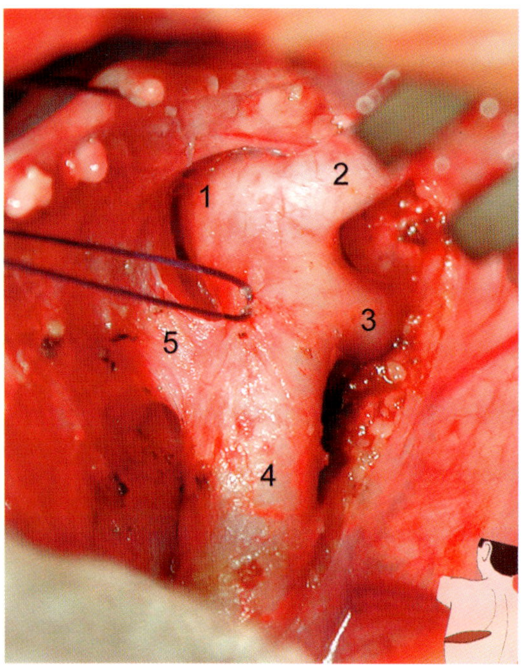

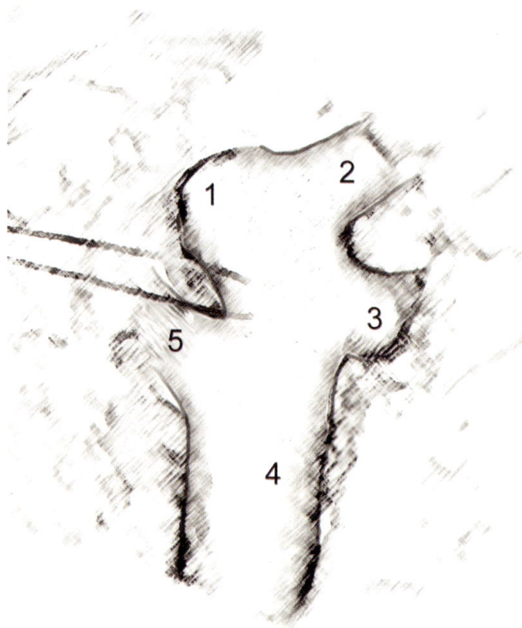

Figure 8.27 **Figure 8.28**

A left thoracotomy view of a 2-year-old child with an aberrant right subclavian artery with retro-esophageal course.

1. Aortic arch
2. Left subclavian artery
3. Right subclavian artery
4. Descending aorta
5. Ligamentum arteriosum

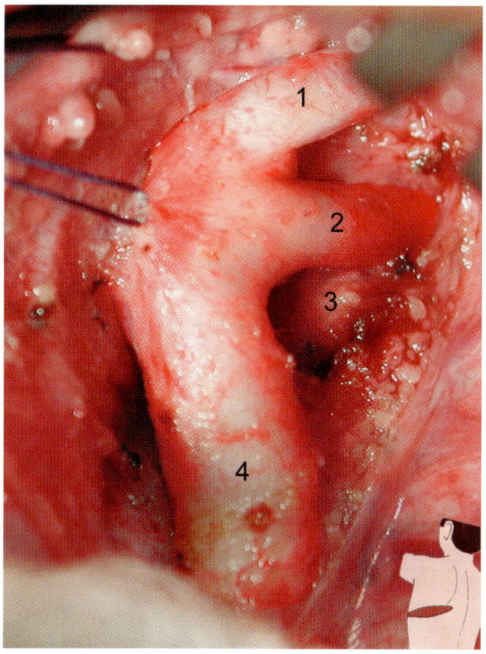

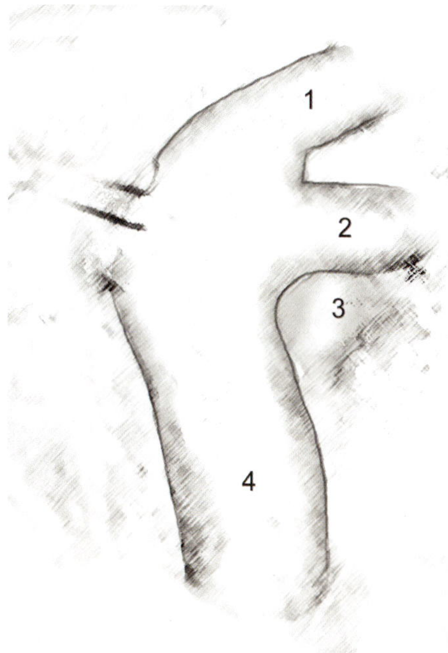

Figure 8.29 **Figure 8.30**

The same patient as in Figure 8.27, with the aortic arch retracted to reveal more of the course of the aberrant right subclavian artery.

1. Left subclavian artery
2. Right subclavian artery
3. Esophagus
4. Descending aorta

Figure 8.31. The same patient as in Figures 8.27 to 8.30. The aberrant right subclavian artery has been double-ligated at 2 points.

1. Left subclavian artery
2. Aberrant right subclavian artery
3. Esophagus
4. Descending aorta

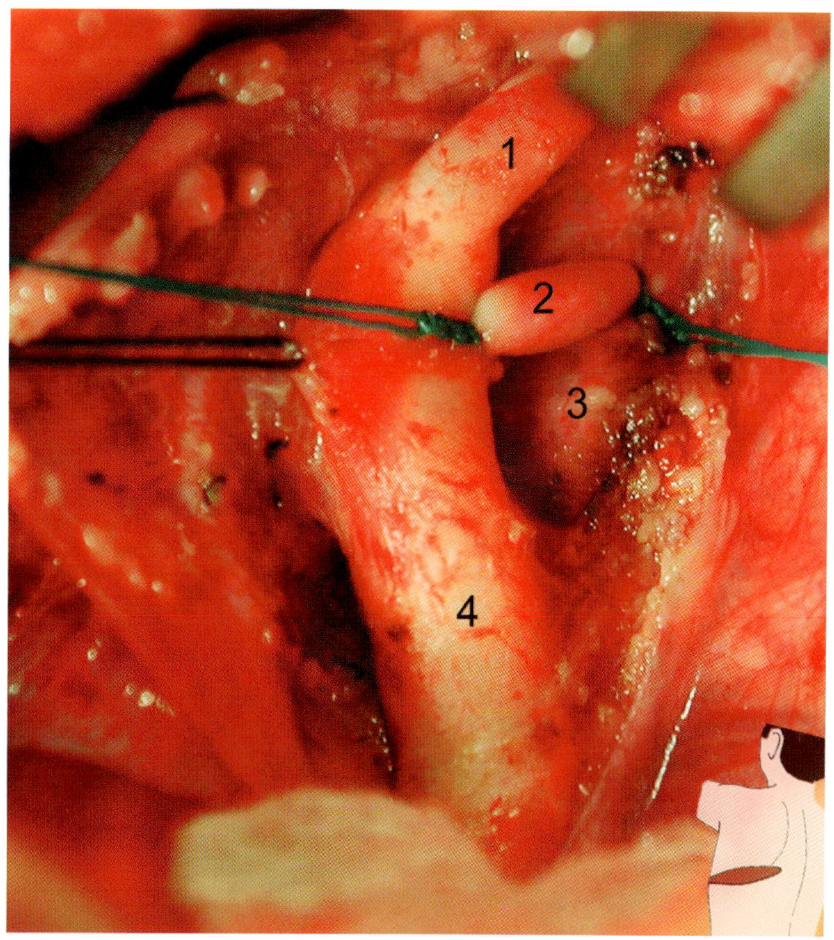

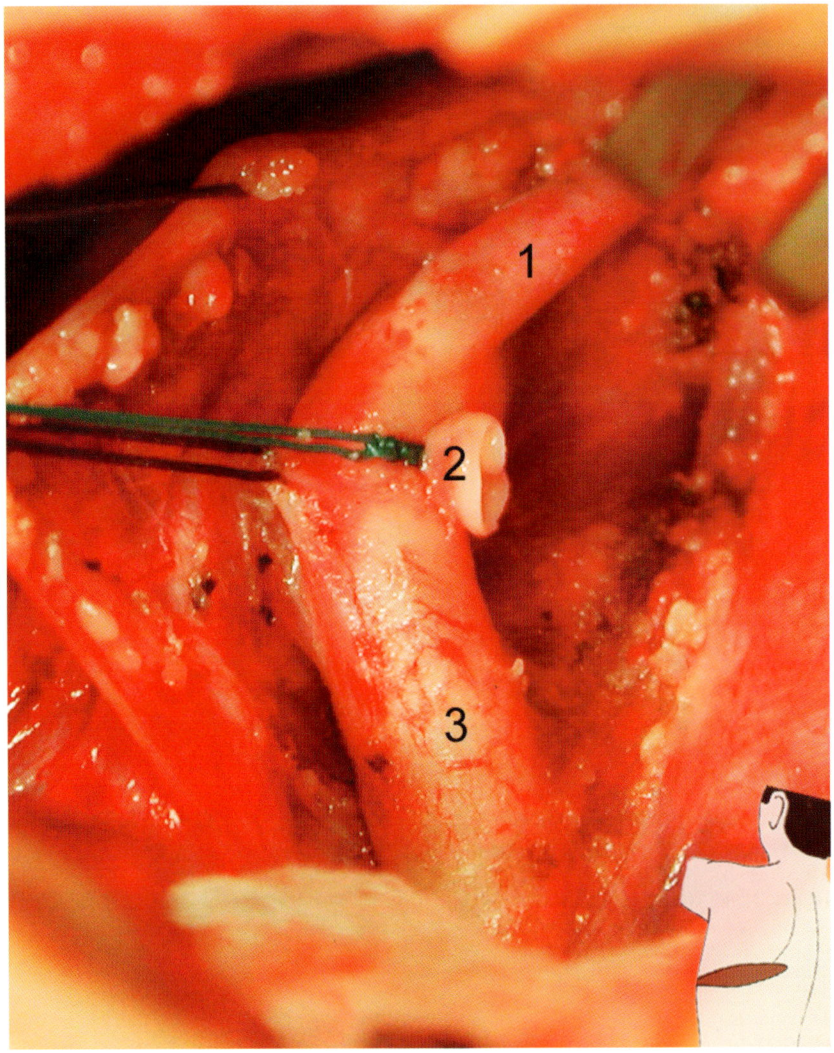

Figure 8.32. The same patient as in Figures 8.27 to 8.31. The aberrant right subclavian artery has been divided between the 2 previously placed ligatures. The proximal stump is seen, whereas the distal part has self-retracted behind the esophagus.

1. Left subclavian artery
2. Stump of aberrant right subclavian artery
3. Descending aorta

REFERENCES

1. Turner A, Gavel G, Coutts J. Vascular rings—presentation, investigation and outcome. *Eur J Pediatr.* 2005;64:266–270.
2. Edwards JE. Anomalies of the derivatives of the aortic arch system. *Med Clin N Am.* 1948;32:925–949.
3. Woods RK, Sharp RJ, Holcomb III GW, et al. Vascular anomalies and tracheoesophageal compression: a single institution's 25-year experience. *Ann Thorac Surg.* 2001;72:434–439.
4. Ramaswamy P, Lytrivi ID, Thanjan MT. Frequency of aberrant subclavian artery, arch laterality, and associated intracardiac anomalies detected by echocardiography. *Am J Cardiol.* 2008;101:677–682.

CHAPTER **9**

Aortopulmonary Window

An aortopulmonary window (APW) is a communication between the ascending aorta and the main pulmonary artery (MPA). This is a rare congenital heart disease that results from failure of complete separation between the aorta and the pulmonary artery in the embryonic truncus arteriosus. It is different from persistent truncus arteriosus because there are 2 semilunar valves (aortic and pulmonary) in APW. Rarely, the aortic valve may be atretic. A variant of APW is a communication between the ascending aorta and the right pulmonary artery.[1] Figure 9.1 shows a schematic drawing of APW.

In about half the patients, there are associated lesions such as tetralogy of Fallot (TOF), coarctation of the aorta, ventricular septal defects, interrupted aortic arch, and coronary arterial abnormalities.[2]

Clinical features are similar to those of patent ductus arteriosus (PDA). Diagnosis is made by echocardiography. Treatment is surgical and is undertaken in early infancy. The approach is through a median sternotomy.

Figures 9.2 and 9.3 are from a 5-month-old infant with a rather large APW. A vertical incision was made in the window as shown in Figures 9.4 and 9.5; the posterior wall of the window was left intact. A pericardial patch was used to close the window and separate the aorta from the pulmonary artery as illustrated in Figures 9.6 and 9.7.

Figures 9.8 to 9.10 show another example of an APW. Closure in this case was achieved through a trans-aortic approach. The communication was patch closed using autologous pericardium. Unfortunately, this patient had a residual communication and was reoperated on 3 years later (Figure 9.11). APW may be associated with type A interrupted aortic arch,[3]

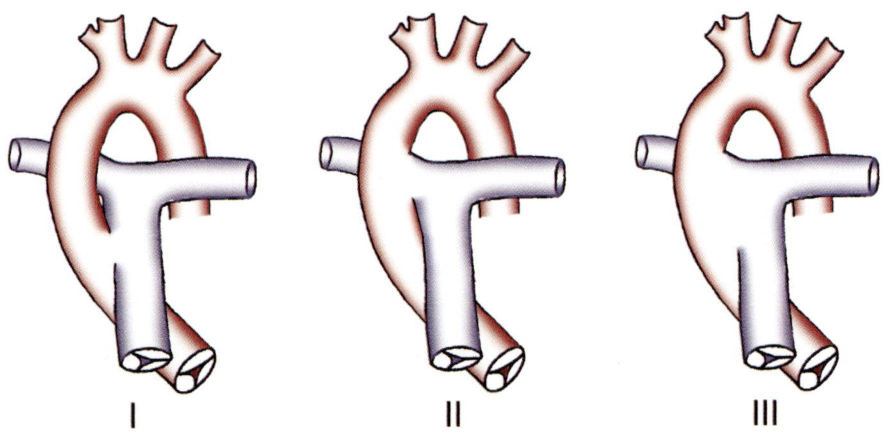

Figure 9.1. Schematic diagram of APW and its variants. In the most common form, the communication is located midway between the semilunar valves and the bifurcation of the pulmonary artery (I). More distal communications tend to be between the aorta and the right pulmonary artery (II), or the communication may be extensive (III).

Congenital Heart Disease: A Surgical Color Atlas © 2015 A. Sukru Mercan, Zakariya Hubail, S. Yen Ho.
Cardiotext Publishing, ISBN: 978-1-935395-90-4.

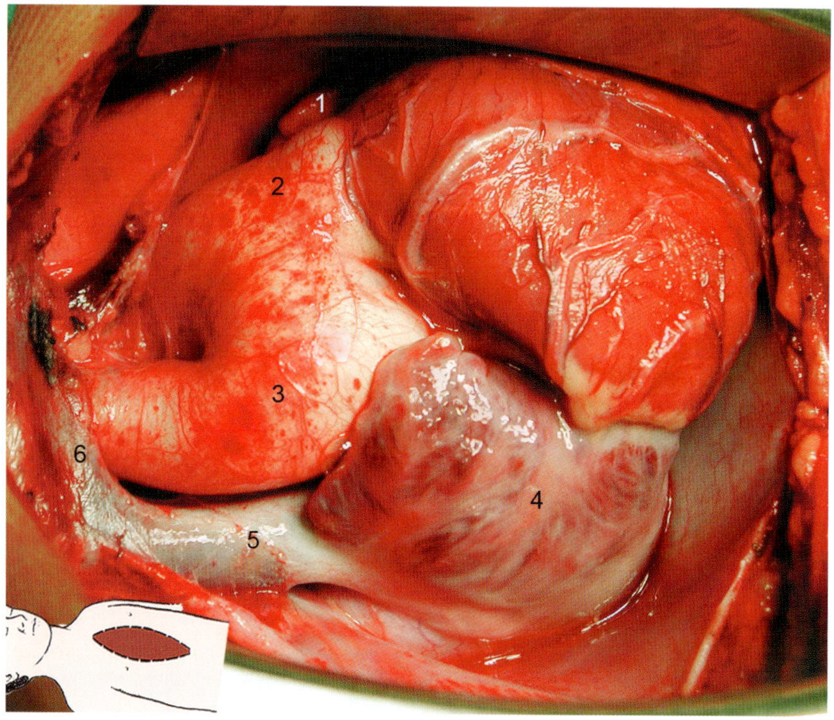

Figure 9.2. A large APW in a 5-month-old infant as seen through median sternotomy. The window is the large communication between the aorta and the MPA (between legend numbers 2 and 3).

1. Left atrial appendage (LAA)
2. MPA
3. Ascending aorta
4. Right atrial appendage (RAA)
5. Superior vena cava (SVC)
6. Innominate vein

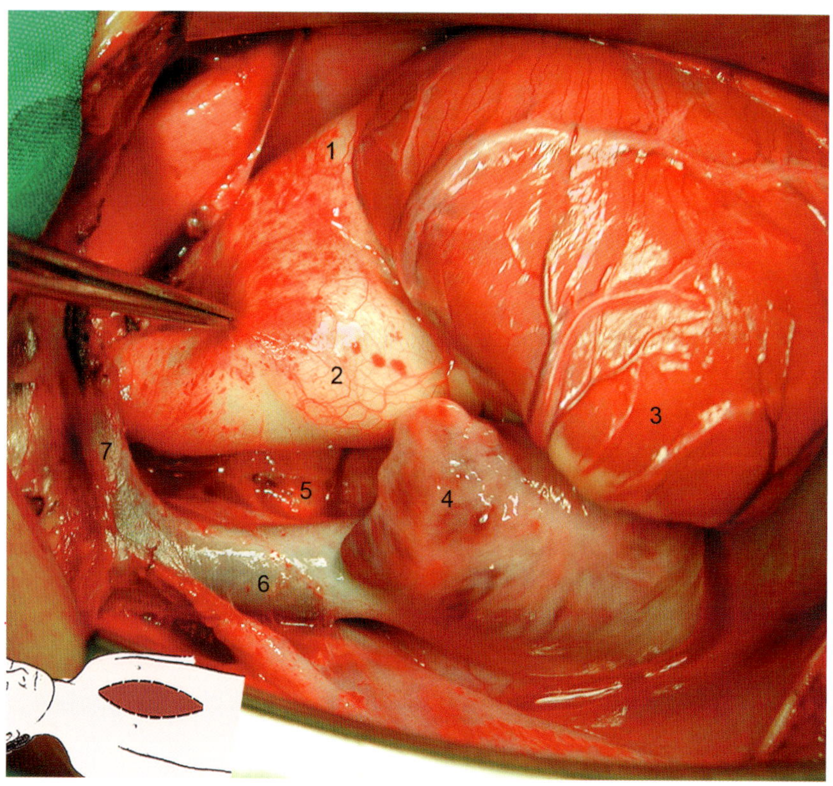

Figure 9.3. The same patient as in Figure 9.2. The aorta is retracted leftward to reveal the right pulmonary artery.

1. MPA
2. Ascending aorta
3. Right ventricle (RV)
4. RAA
5. Right pulmonary artery
6. SVC
7. Innominate vein

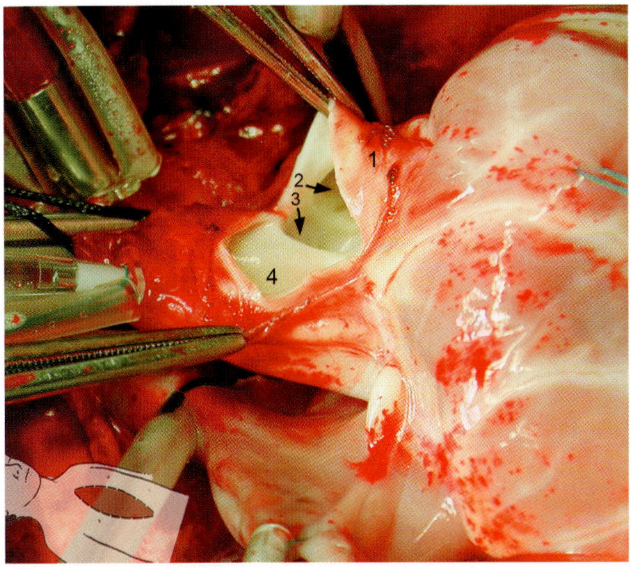

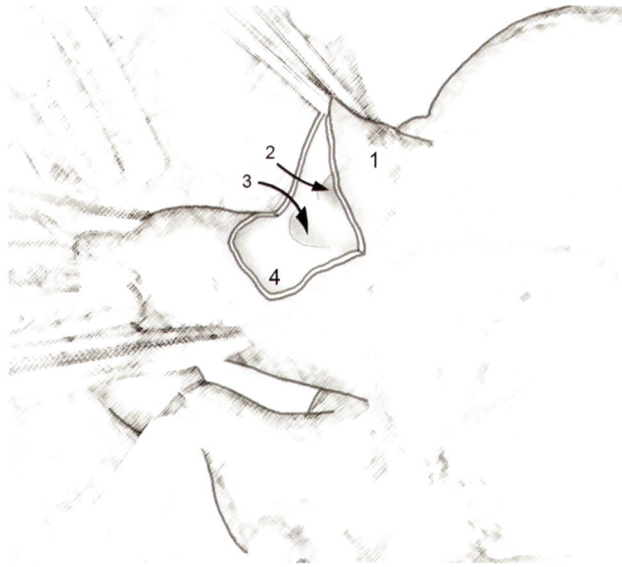

Figure 9.4 **Figure 9.5**

The same patient as in Figures 9.2 and 9.3. A vertical incision has been made in the anterior wall of the window; the posterior wall of the window was left intact. The defect was repaired using a pericardial patch, as shown in Figures 9.6 and 9.7.

1. MPA
2. Origin of left pulmonary artery
3. Origin of right pulmonary artery
4. Ascending aorta

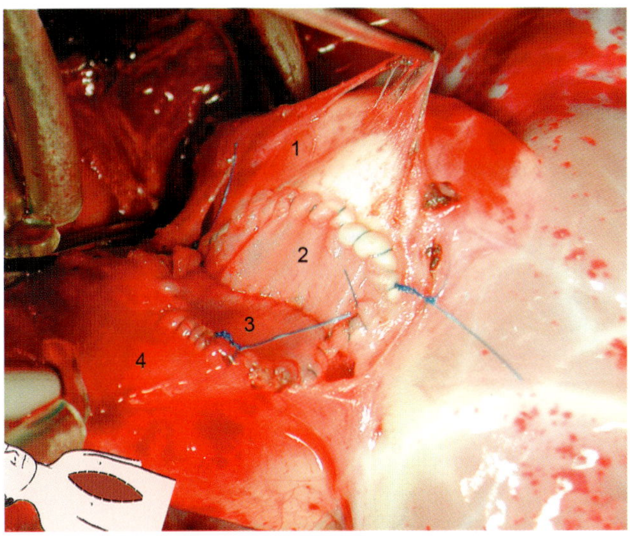

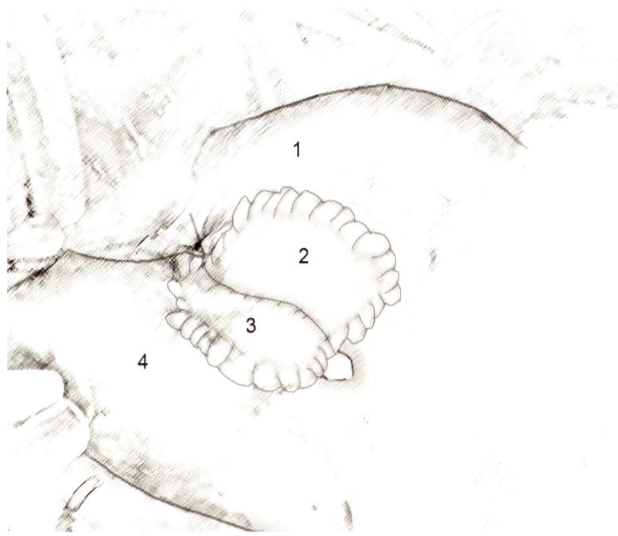

Figure 9.6 **Figure 9.7**

Same patient as in Figures 9.2 to 9.5, after repair. An autologous pericardial patch was used. The middle of the patch was sutured vertically to the posterior wall of the window, and the 2 wings of the patch were then sutured to the margin of the surgical incision, thus closing the defect and separating the 2 arteries.

1. MPA
2. Left wing of the patch closing the defect in the wall of the pulmonary artery
3. Right wing of the patch closing the defect in the wall of the aorta
4. Ascending aorta

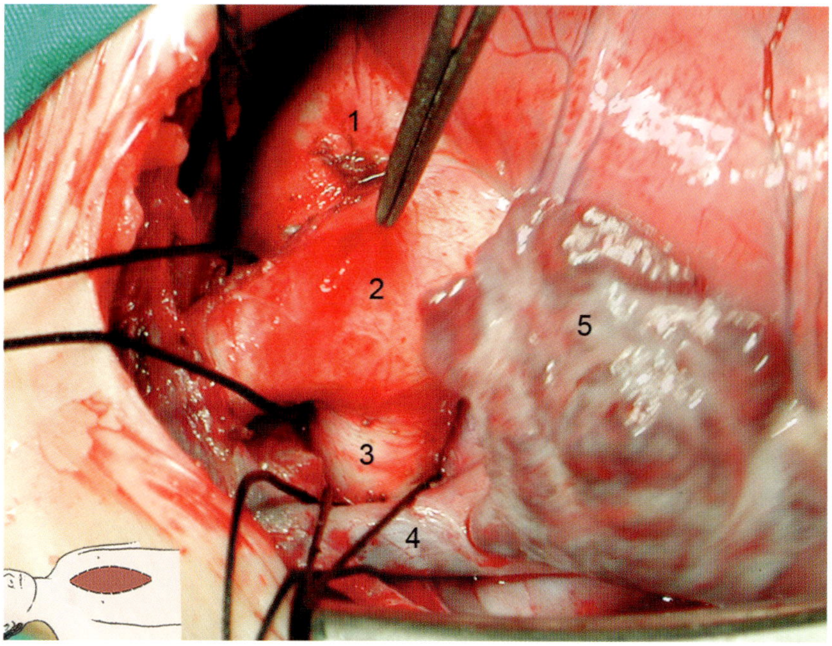

Figure 9.8. An APW in a 5-month-old infant. The communication was mostly between the ascending aorta and right pulmonary artery.

1. MPA
2. Ascending aorta
3. Right pulmonary artery
4. SVC
5. RAA

as shown in Figures 9.12 to 9.15. This is illustrated schematically in Figure 9.16.

Repair was performed through a transaortic approach. A tunnel within the lumens of the great arteries was constructed utilizing a patch and the walls of the right pulmonary artery (Figure 9.17). As a result, the deoxygenated blood is directed to the branch pulmonary arteries, whereas the oxygenated blood is directed from the ascending aorta, over the patch to the arch and through the PDA toward the

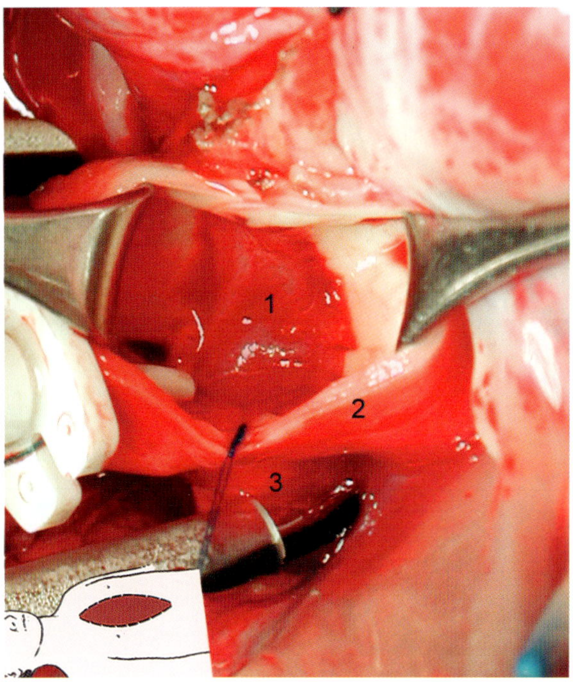

Figure 9.9

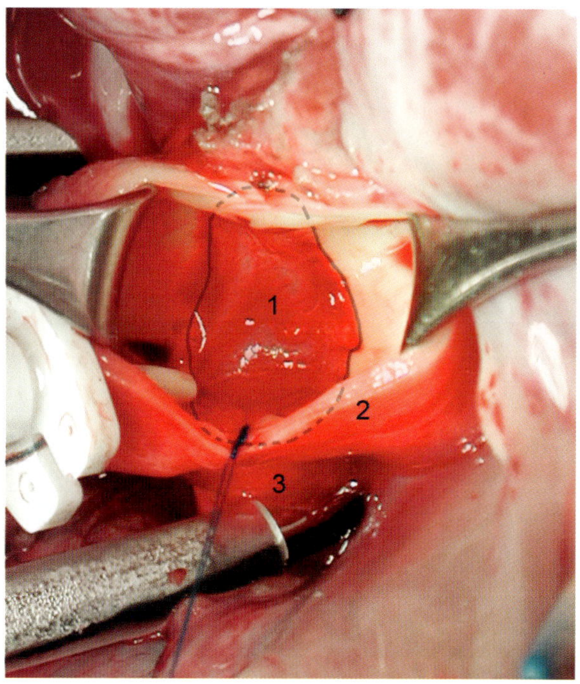

Figure 9.10

Same patient as in Figure 9.8. A transverse aortotomy has been performed. An autologous pericardial patch was used to close the window on the posterior wall of the aorta. The outline of the patch (1) is shown in Figure 9.10.

1. Autologous pericardial patch
2. Ascending aorta transversely opened
3. Right pulmonary artery

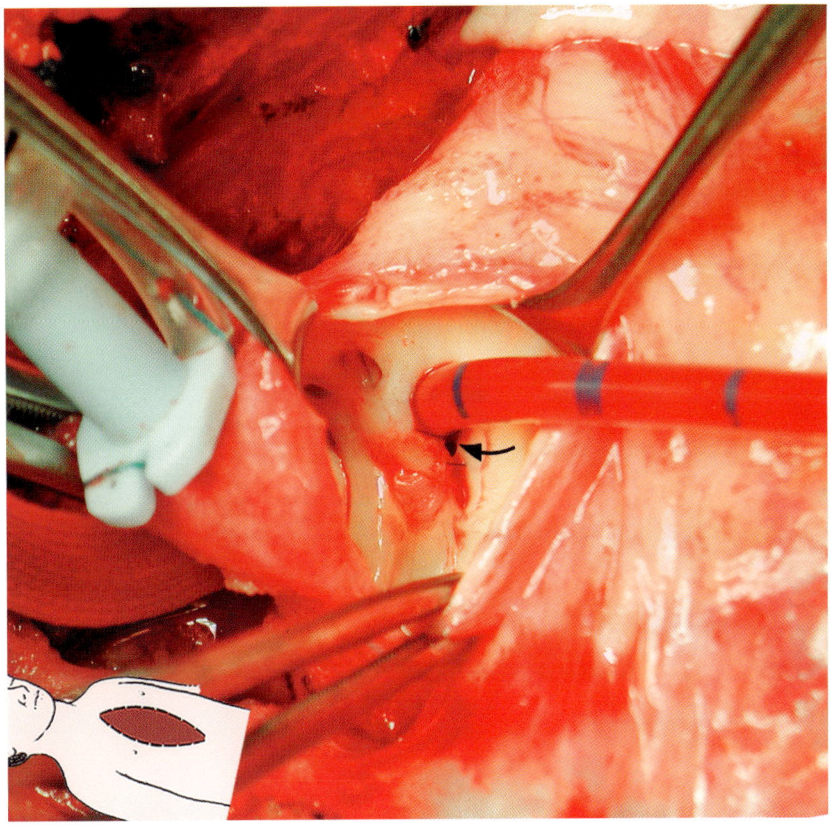

Figure 9.11. The same patient as in Figures 9.8 to 9.10, 3 years later. A residual APW is seen (arrow and catheter). The defect was in the left inferior border of the graft. It was closed by primarily suturing the edges.

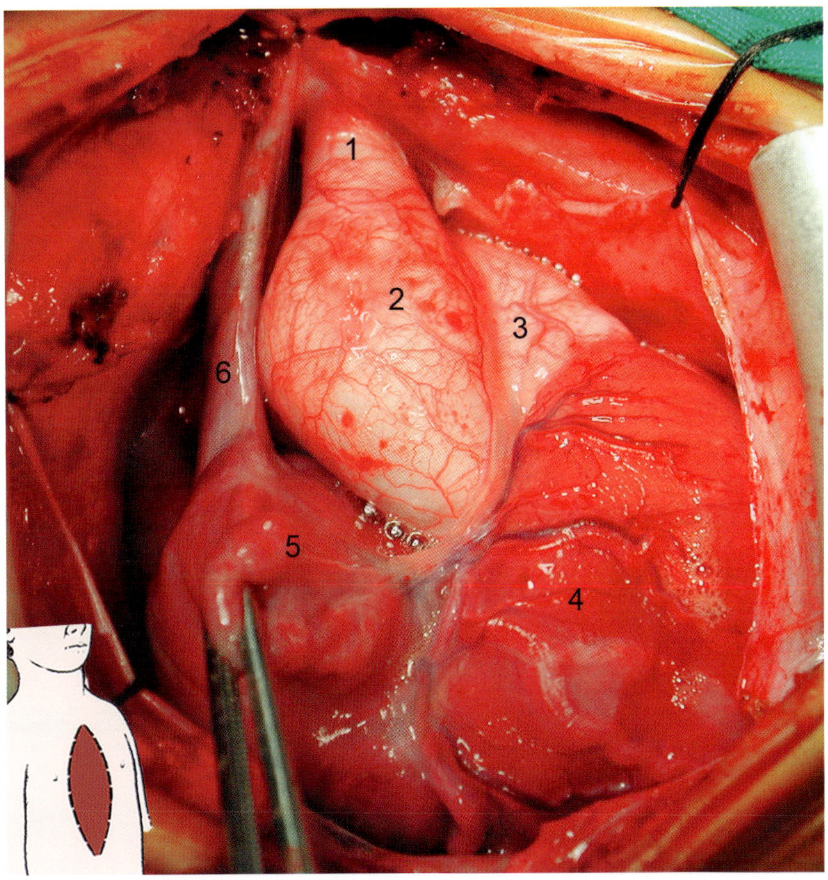

Figure 9.12. APW associated with interrupted aortic arch, type A, as seen through a median sternotomy in a 2-month-old infant.

1. Ascending aorta
2. Dilated proximal part of aorta
3. MPA
4. RV
5. RAA
6. SVC

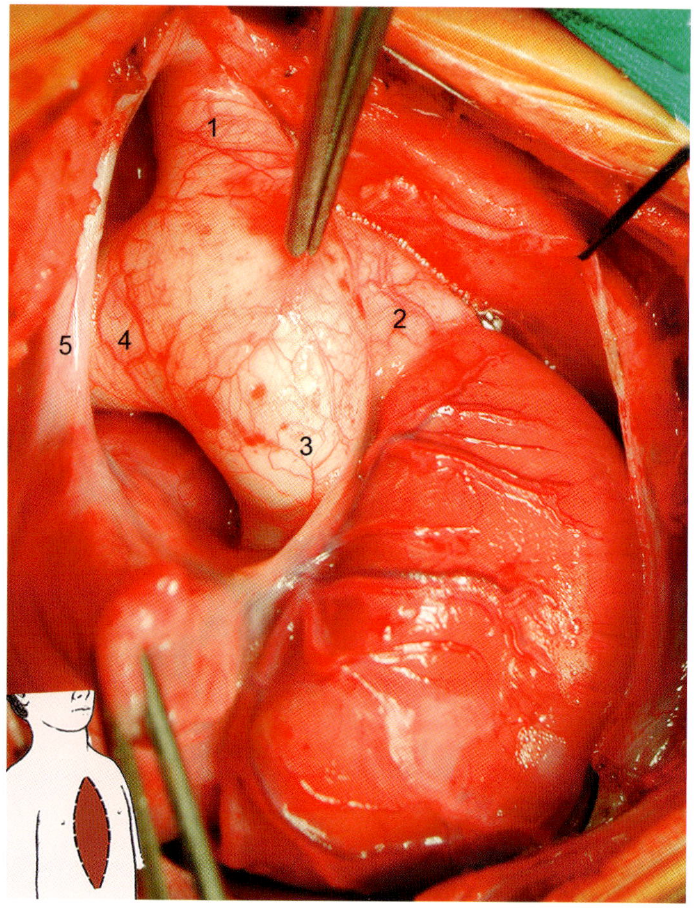

Figure 9.13. The same patient as in Figure 9.12. The aorta is retracted to the left, revealing the right pulmonary artery in direct connection with the aorta.

1. Ascending aorta
2. MPA
3. Proximal part of aorta
4. Right pulmonary artery
5. SVC

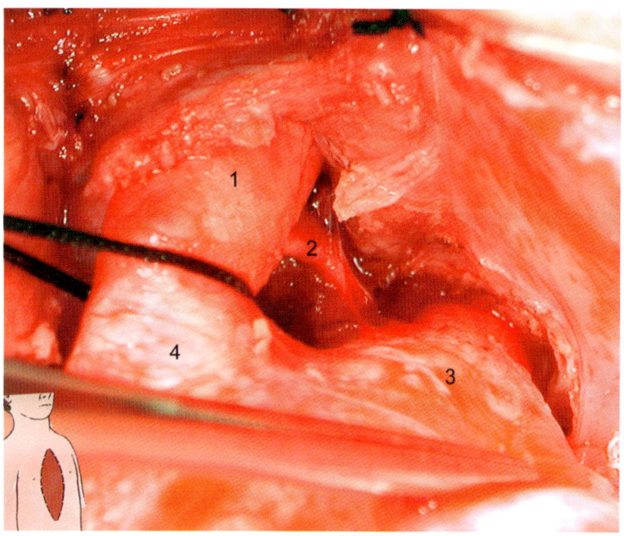

Figure 9.14

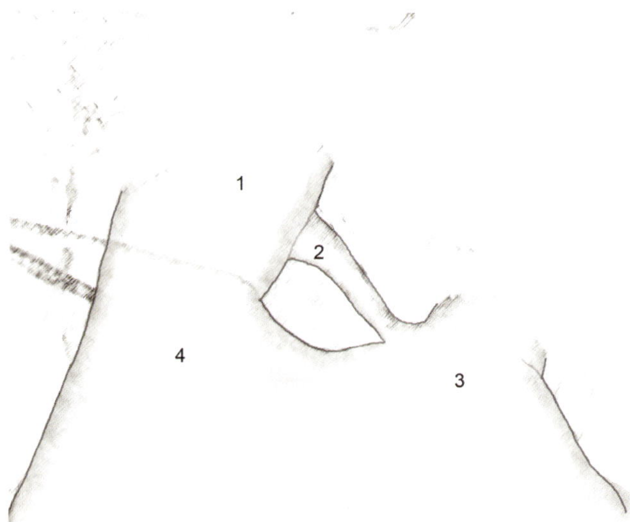

Figure 9.15

Same patient as in Figures 9.12 and 9.13, with the aorta retracted to the right to show the atretic segment of the aortic arch, present as a fibrous cord (2) that connects the transverse arch to the descending aorta. A continuation of the main pulmonary artery (3) is the PDA, which in turn feeds the descending aorta as illustrated diagrammatically in the next figure.

1. Ascending aorta and proximal transverse arch
2. Fibrous cord (atretic isthmus)
3. MPA
4. Ascending aorta

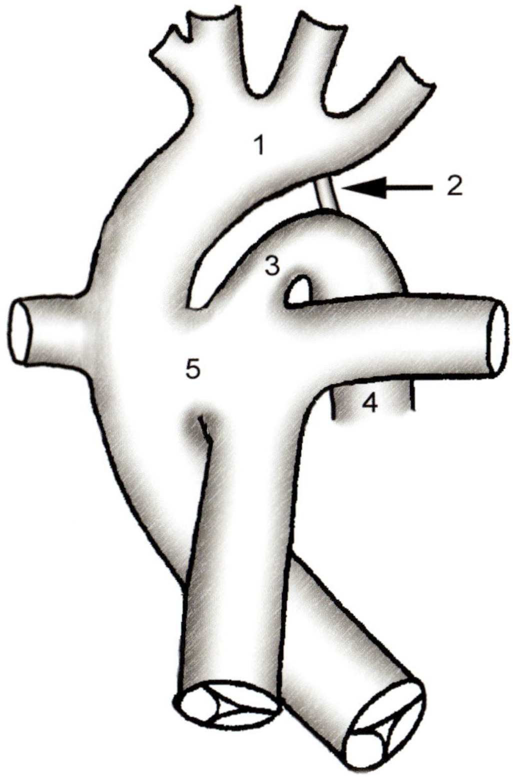

Figure 9.16. Schematic diagram of the anatomy of the lesions in the patient shown in Figures 9.13 to 9.15.

1. Transverse aortic arch
2. Fibrous cord (atretic isthmus)
3. PDA
4. Descending aorta
5. Aortopulmonary window

descending aorta. Thus the aortic and pulmonary lumens were separated and aortic arch continuity was restored. On follow-up, the ductus remained patent with no narrowing.

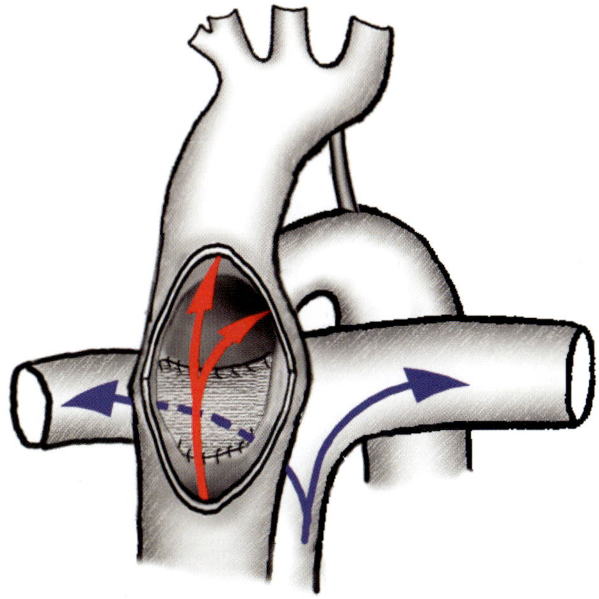

Figure 9.17. Schematic diagram illustrating the technique used to repair the patient shown in Figures 9.13 to 9.15. A tunnel within the lumens of the great arteries was constructed utilizing a patch and the walls of the pulmonary artery to direct deoxygenated blood to the branch pulmonary arteries (blue arrows). The oxygenated blood is directed from the ascending aorta, over the patch, and then through the PDA toward the descending aorta (red arrows).

REFERENCES

1. Tkebuchavaa T, von Segessera L, Vogta P, et al. Congenital aortopulmonary window: diagnosis, surgical technique and long-term results. *Europ J Cardio-thorac Surg.* 1997;11:293–297.
2. Backer C, Mavroudis C. Surgical management of aortopulmonary window: a 40-year experience. *Europ J Cardio-thorac Surg.* 2002;21:773–779.
3. Fyler DC. Report of the New England Regional Infant Cardiac Program. *Pediatrics.* 1980;65:377–461.

CHAPTER 10

Persistent Truncus Arteriosus

Persistent truncus arteriosus (or common arterial trunk) is due to failure of septation of the embryonic common arterial trunk into aorta and pulmonary artery. Thus, a single arterial vessel arises from the base of the heart and gives origin to the systemic, pulmonary, and coronary arteries. About one-third of patients have a chromosome 22q11 deletion.[1] There are 2 classification schemes commonly used to describe the different variations of this anomaly, shown together in Figure 10.1. In recent years, a simplified classification into either aortic or pulmonary dominance of the common arterial trunk has been proposed.[2]

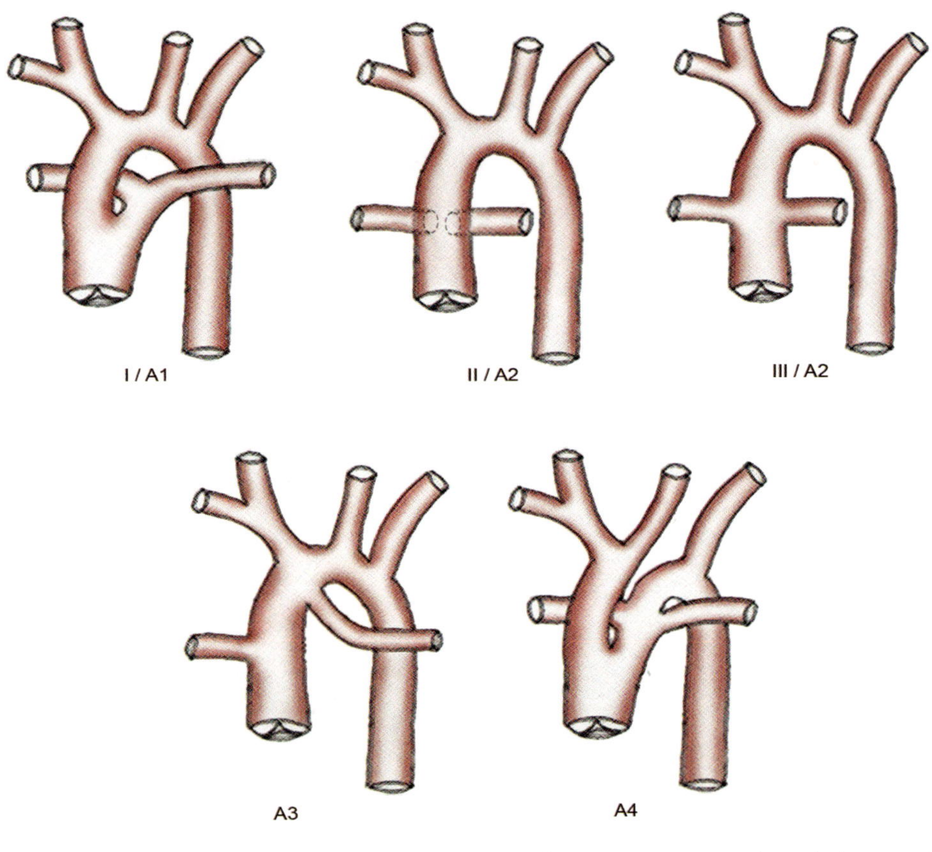

Figure 10.1. Composite diagram for the 2 classification schemes of persistent truncus arteriosus. Latin numerals refer to Collett and Edwards' classification, while alphanumeric system refers to van Praagh's classification.

Cyanosis is usually mild, and the clinical picture is dominated by pulmonary overcirculation. If left untreated, pulmonary hypertension quickly develops in these patients.[3] Surgery, therefore, is usually indicated in the neonatal period or early infancy.

Figures 10.2 and 10.3 show a surgical view through a median sternotomy of a 25-day-old neonate showing the gross anatomy of type I/A1 truncus arteriosus. Classic repair involves closing the ventricular septal defect (VSD), separating the pulmonary arteries from the common trunk, using the common trunk as the aorta, and then placing a valved conduit between the right ventricle (RV) and pulmonary arteries, as shown in Figures 10.4 to 10.8. Figures 10.9 to 10.12 are from another patient, a 1-year-old infant with type I/A1 truncus arteriosus shown before and after repair. Figures 10.13 and 10.14 show another example of type I truncus arteriosus. Note the patent ductus arteriosus (PDA), which is an uncommon finding in truncus arteriosus.[4]

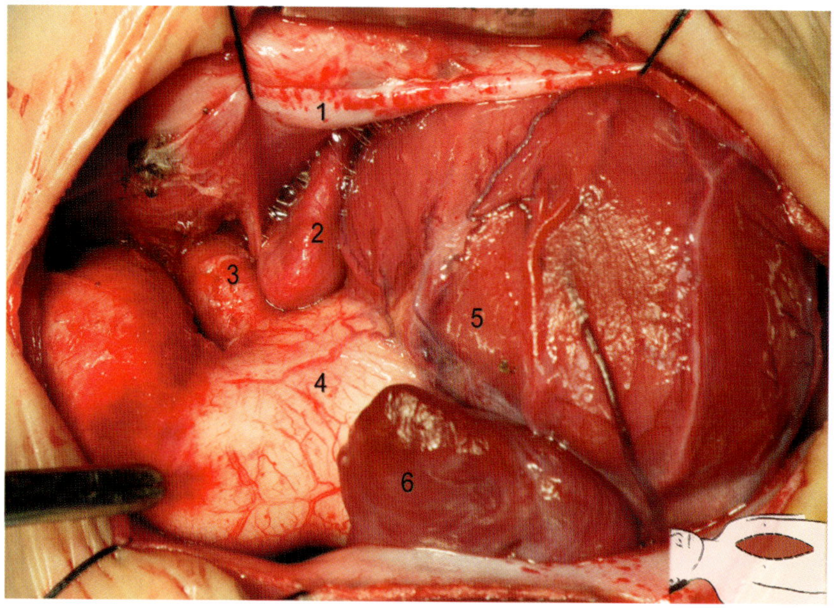

Figure 10.2. Median sternotomy view of a 25-day-old neonate with type I/A1 truncus arteriosus. The common trunk is retracted rightward to show the left pulmonary artery.

1. Pericardium
2. Left atrium
3. Left pulmonary artery
4. Common trunk
5. RV
6. Right atrial appendage (RAA)

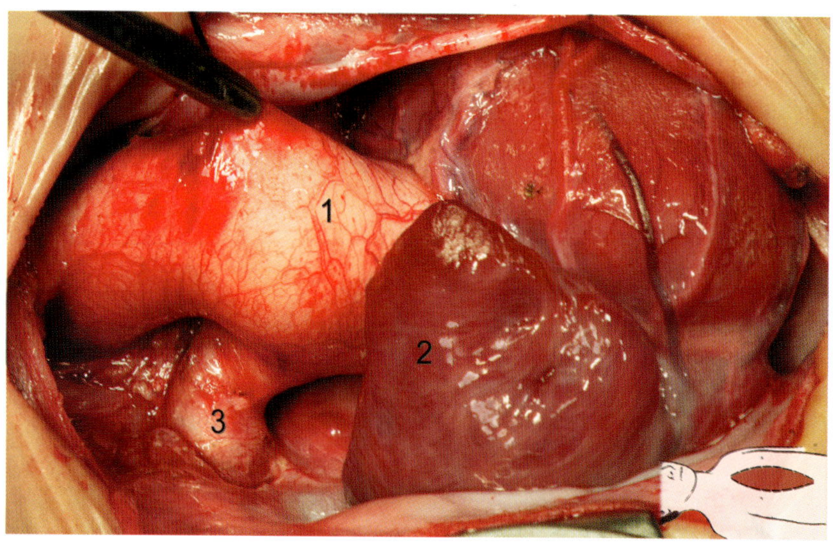

Figure 10.3. The same patient as in Figure 10.2, with truncus arteriosus retracted leftward to show the right pulmonary artery.

1. Common trunk
2. RAA
3. Right pulmonary artery

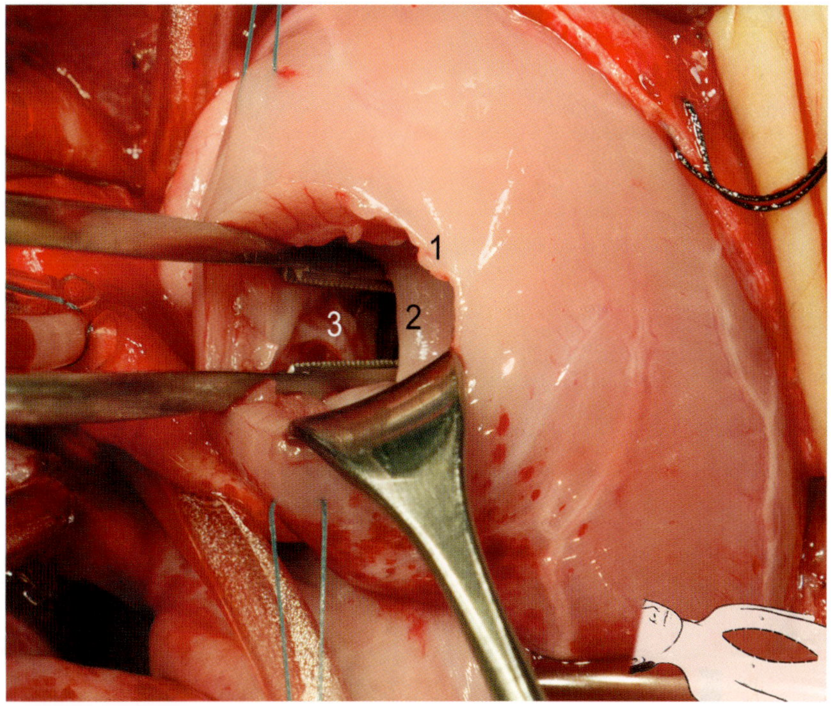

Figure 10.4. The same patient as in Figures 10.2 and 10.3. The VSD is visible through a right ventriculotomy. A pair of forceps is passed through the VSD to the left ventricle. The ventricular septum is seen forming the lower margin of the VSD.

1. Right ventriculotomy
2. Ventricular septum
3. Truncal valve

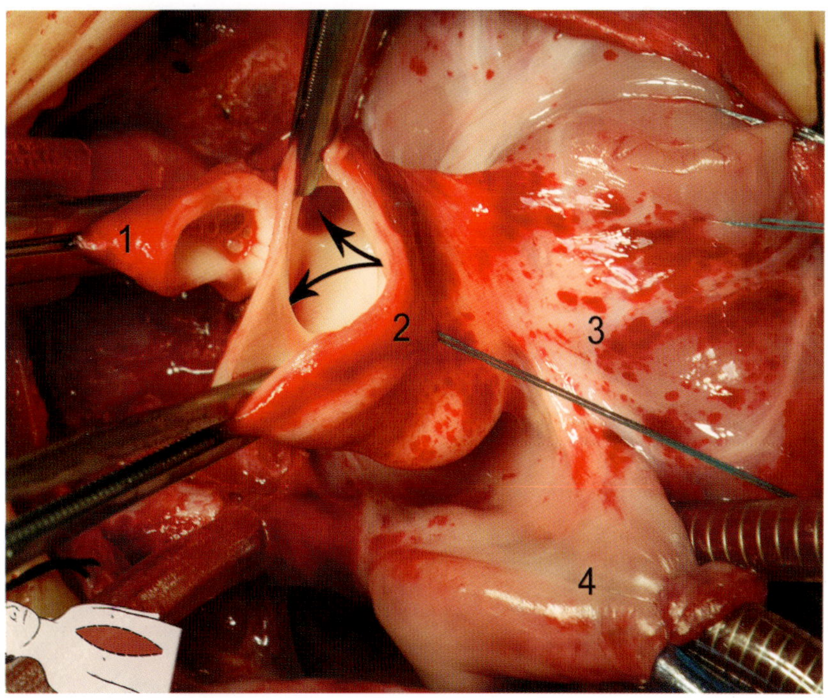

Figure 10.5. The same patient as in Figures 10.2 to 10.4 after transsection of the common trunk. A rather short main pulmonary artery gives rise to both pulmonary artery branches (indicated by the 2 arrows).

1. Ascending thoracic aorta
2. Truncus arteriosus
3. RV
4. RAA

Figure 10.6. The same patient as in Figures 10.2 to 10.5 after transsection of the common trunk. The truncal valve is bicuspid.

1. Truncal valve
2. Left pulmonary artery
3. Right pulmonary artery
4. Ascending thoracic aorta

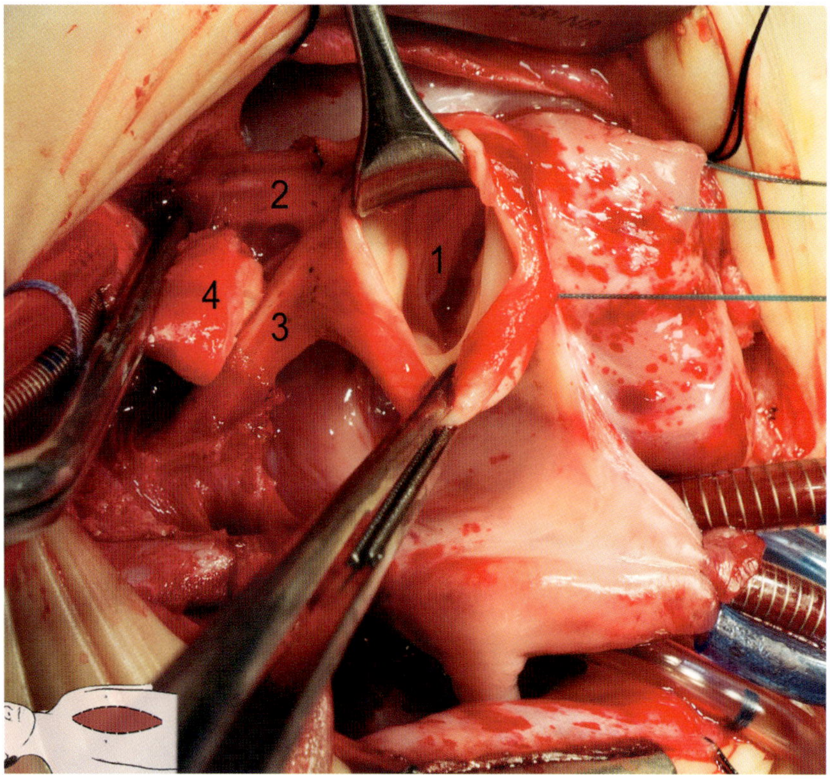

Figure 10.7. The same patient as in Figures 10.2 to 10.6. The VSD has been closed by a Dacron patch. The pulmonary arteries have been separated from the common trunk; the defect in the wall of the truncus has been repaired with a composite patch (the inner layer is a piece of Contegra graft, the outer layer is a Dacron patch).

1. Right ventriculotomy
2. Ventricular septum
3. Dacron patch closing the VSD
4. Ascending thoracic aorta
5. Composite patch (Contegra and Dacron)

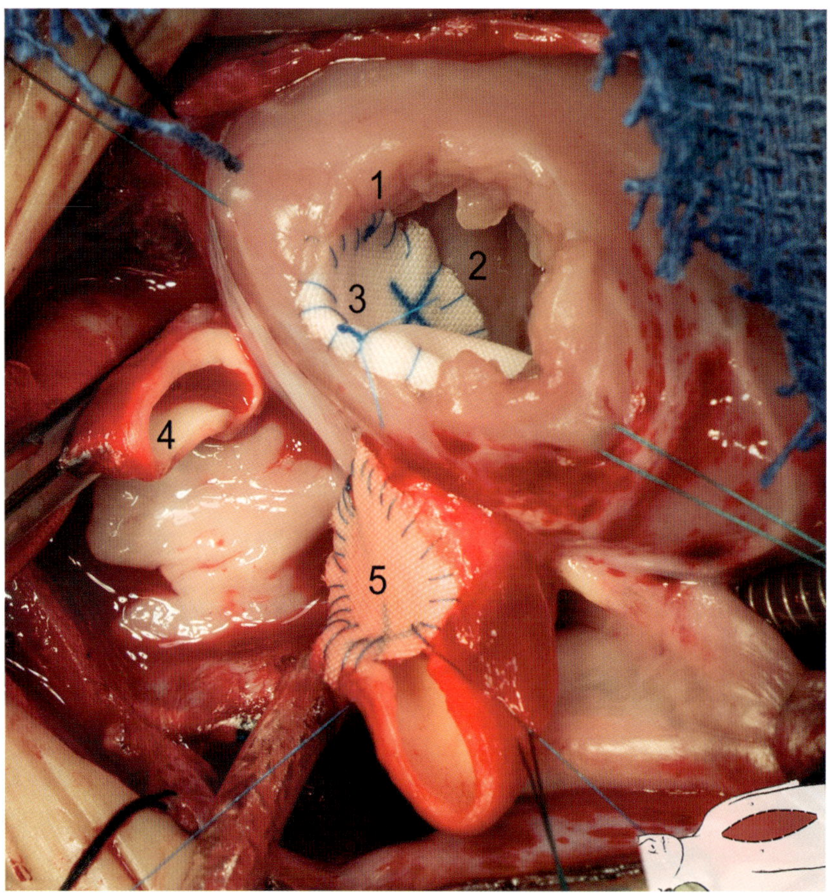

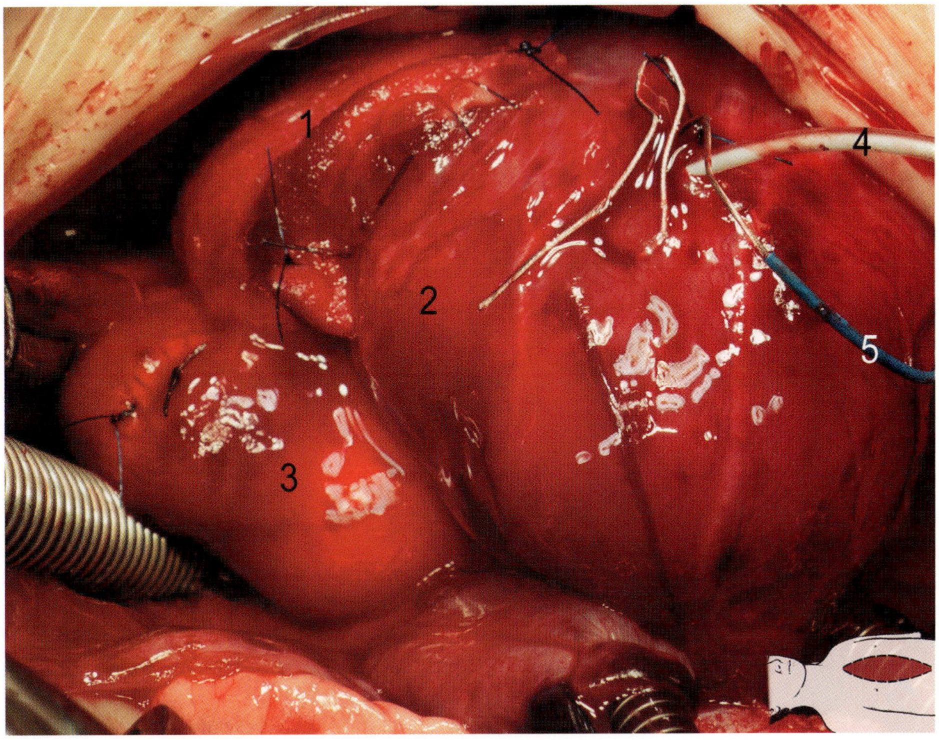

Figure 10.8. The same patient as in Figures 10.2 to 10.7 after completion of the repair. The common trunk (now aorta) has been anastomosed to the ascending thoracic aorta. A valved xenograft conduit (Contegra) has been implanted between the RV and pulmonary arteries.

1. RV-to-pulmonary artery conduit (Contegra)
2. RV
3. Ascending aorta
4. Pulmonary artery catheter
5. Temporary pacing

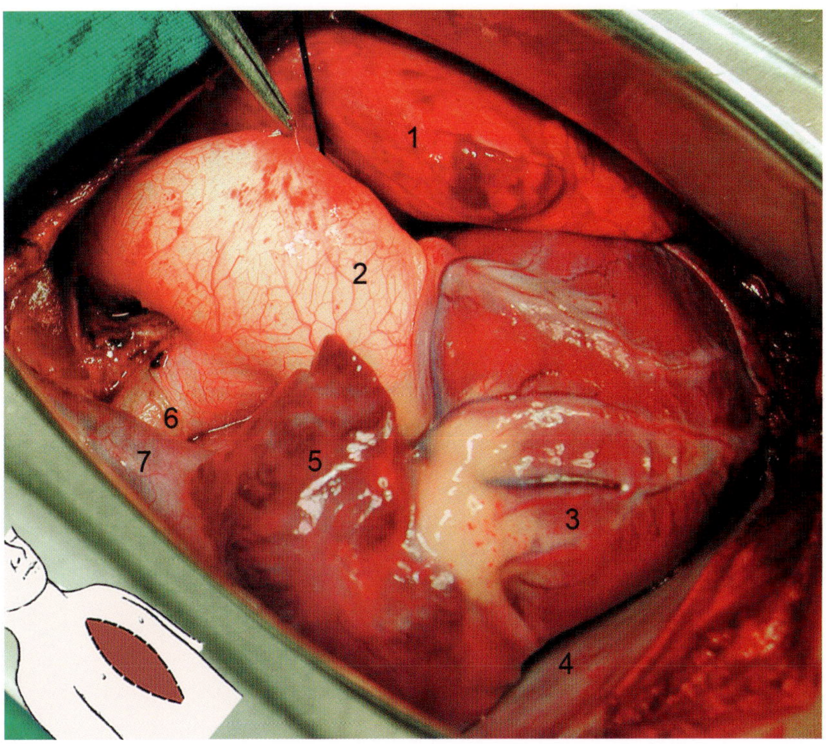

Figure 10.9. Median sternotomy view for a 1-year-old infant with type I/A1 truncus arteriosus. The truncus is retracted leftward to show the right pulmonary artery.

1. Left lung
2. Truncus arteriosus
3. RV
4. Pericardium overlying the diaphragm
5. RAA
6. Right pulmonary artery
7. Superior vena cava (SVC)

Figure 10.10. The same patient as in Figure 10.9. The common trunk is retracted rightward to show the left pulmonary artery.

1. Transverse aortic arch
2. Left pulmonary artery
3. Left atrial appendage (LAA)
4. Common trunk
5. RAA
6. RV

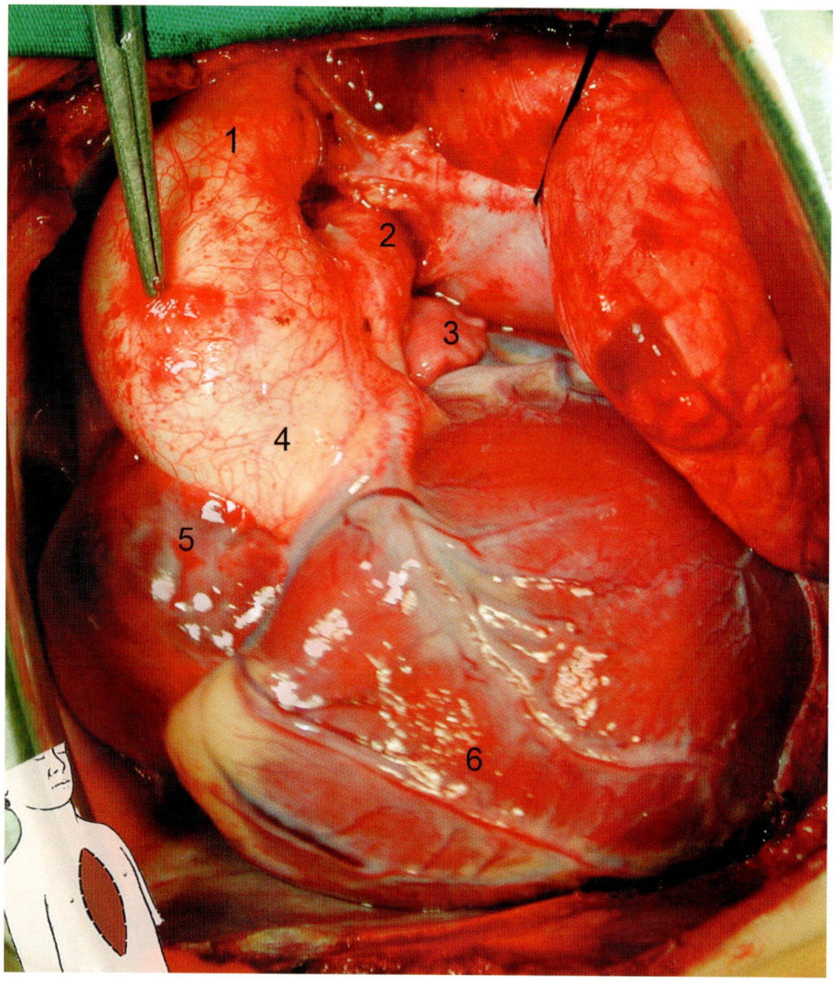

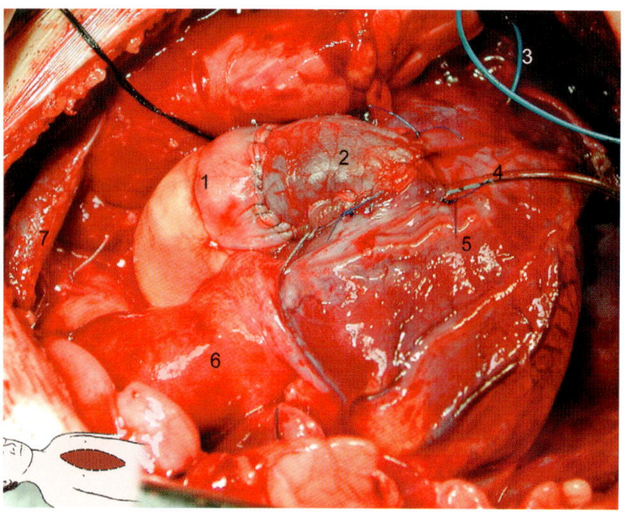

Figure 10.11

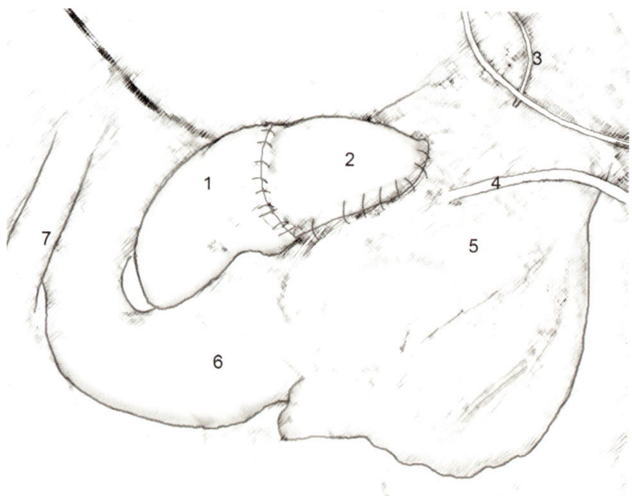

Figure 10.12

The same patient as in Figures 10.9 and 10.10 after repair using the classic technique. The common trunk has now become the aorta. A valved conduit has been placed between the pulmonary artery and the RV.

1. Valved conduit
2. Conduit hood (autologous pericardium)
3. Pacing wire
4. Pulmonary artery catheter
5. RV
6. Aorta
7. Innominate vein

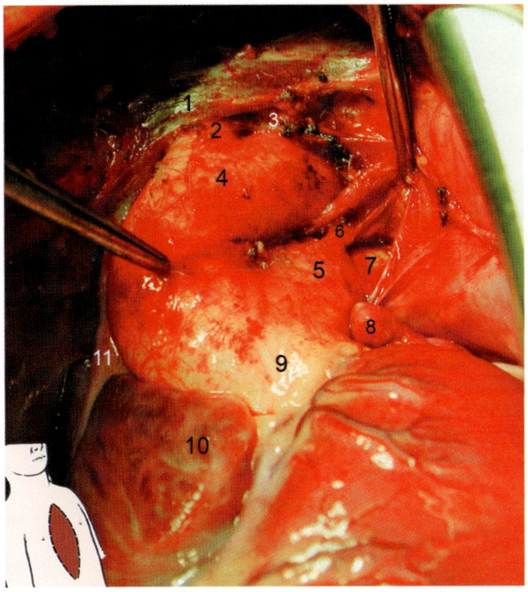

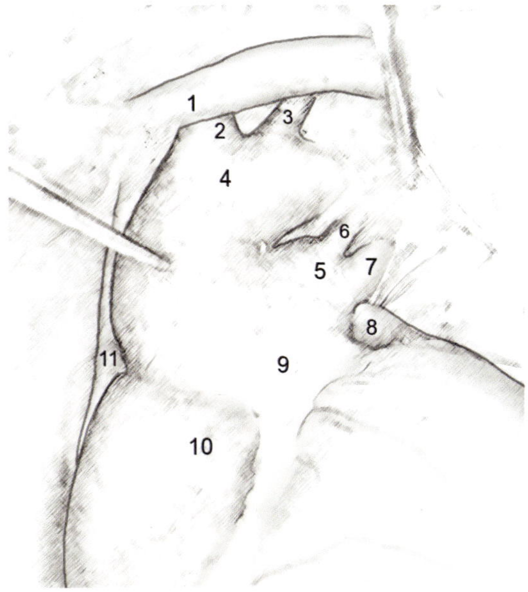

Figure 10.13 **Figure 10.14**

Truncus arteriosus type I in a 6-month-old infant. The common trunk is retracted rightward to show the left pulmonary artery and the PDA.

1. Innominate vein
2. Innominate artery
3. Left common carotid artery
4. Transverse aortic arch
5. Main pulmonary artery (MPA)
6. PDA
7. Left pulmonary artery
8. LAA
9. Common trunk
10. RAA
11. SVC

In type A4 truncus arteriosus, the aortic arch is interrupted, as shown in Figures 10.15 and 10.16. Figure 10.17 shows a 4-month-old infant with type I truncus arteriosus. Figure 10.18 shows an aortic homograft being prepared for implantation in this patient and Figure 10.19 shows the graft in place as a pulmonary artery conduit. Unfortunately, 6 months later this patient presented with aneurysmal dilatation of the homograft (Figure 10.20), which was then replaced by a xenograft valved conduit (Figure 10.21).

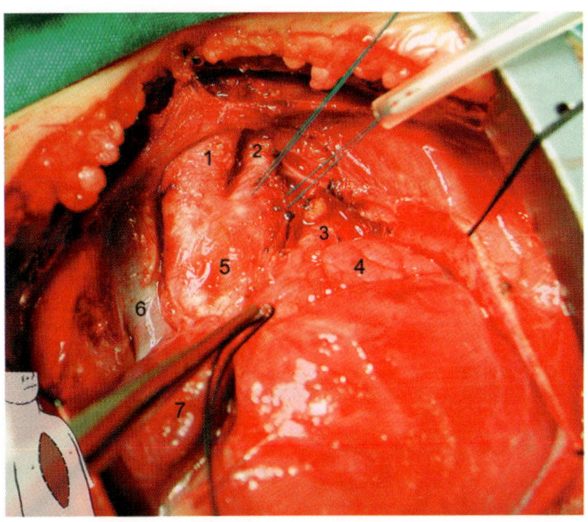

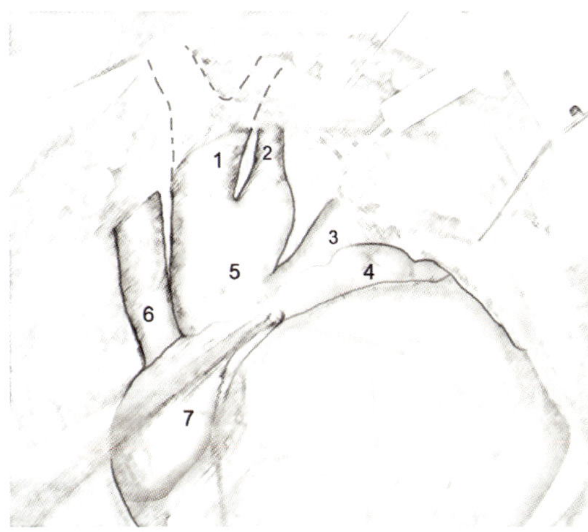

Figure 10.15 **Figure 10.16**

Truncus arteriosus type A4 in a 6-week-old infant. The aortic arch is interrupted; the descending aorta arises from the pulmonary artery.

1. Innominate artery
2. Left common carotid artery
3. MPA
4. LAA
5. Common trunk
6. SVC
7. RAA

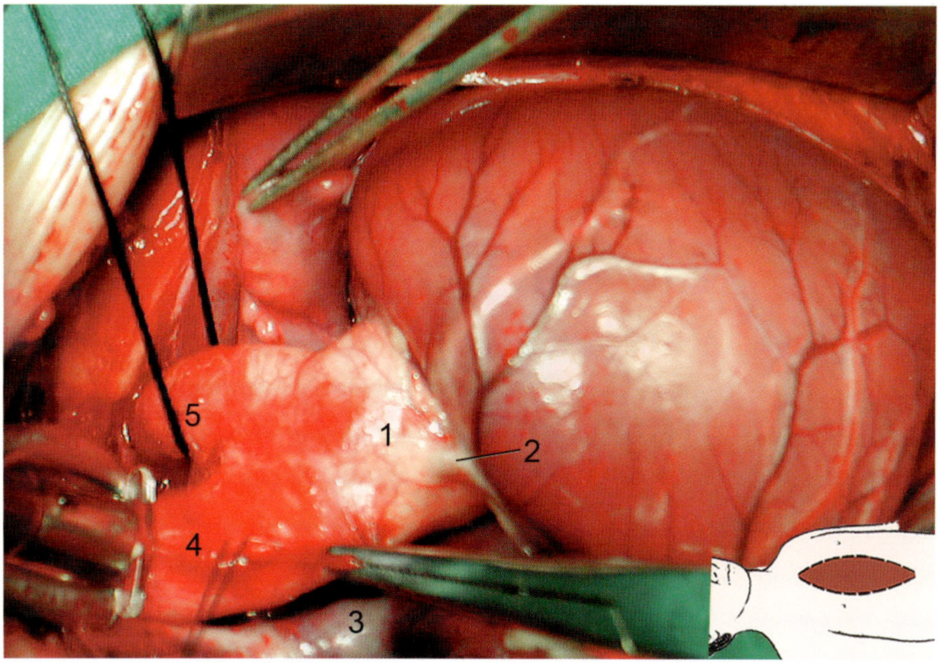

Figure 10.17. Type I truncus arteriosus in a 4-month-old infant seen through a median sternotomy.

1. Common trunk
2. Coronary artery
3. SVC
4. Ascending aorta
5. MPA

Figure 10.18. An aortic homograft is being thawed in preparation for implantation in the patient shown in Figure 10.17. Figure 10.19 shows the graft after implantation as a pulmonary artery conduit. The arrow points to the direction of blood flow.

1. Left coronary artery
2. Left ventricle outflow
3. Right coronary artery

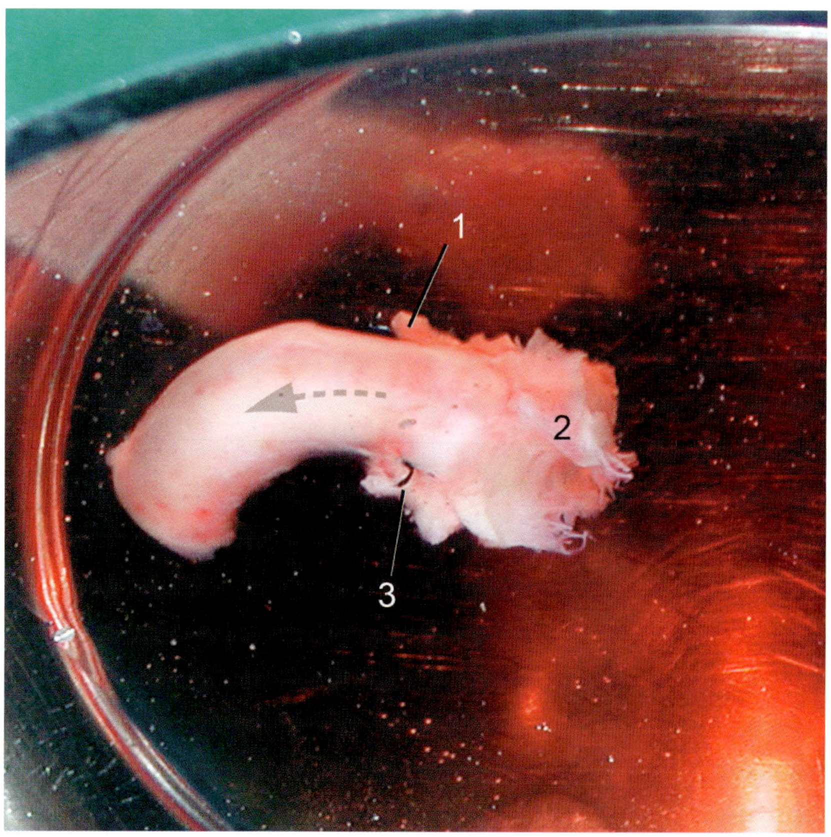

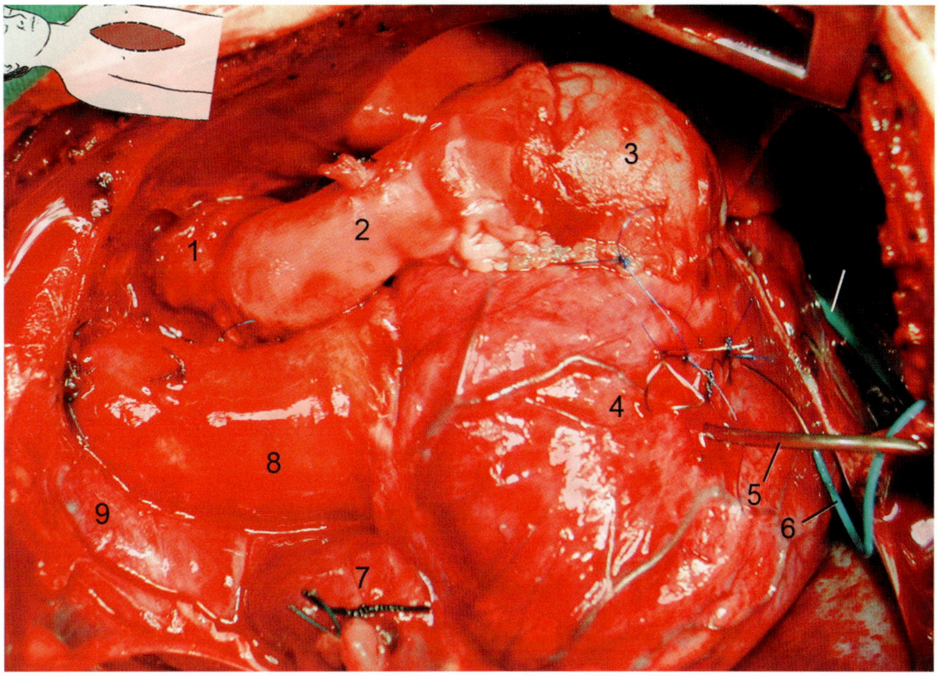

Figures 10.19. Same patient as in Figure 10.17 after repair. The aortic homograft has been implanted as a pulmonary artery conduit.

1. Distal pulmonary artery
2. Aortic homograft as pulmonary artery conduit
3. Pericardial hood
4. RV
5. Pulmonary artery catheter
6. Pacing wire
7. RAA
8. Ascending aorta
9. SVC

Figure 10.20. The same patient as in Figures 10.17 and 10.19; reoperation 6 months later for replacement of the dilated aortic homograft. The figure shows the aneurysmal homograft that was excised.

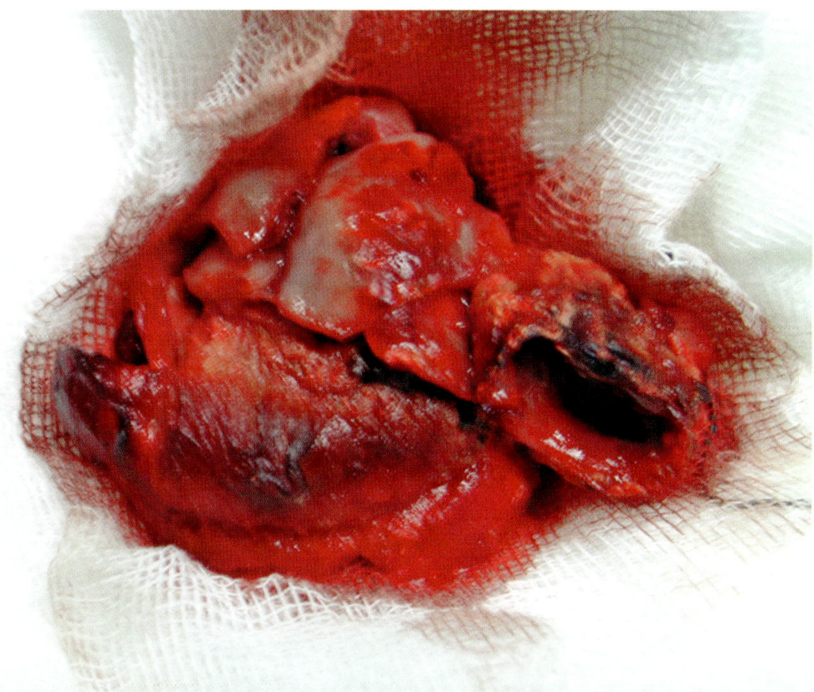

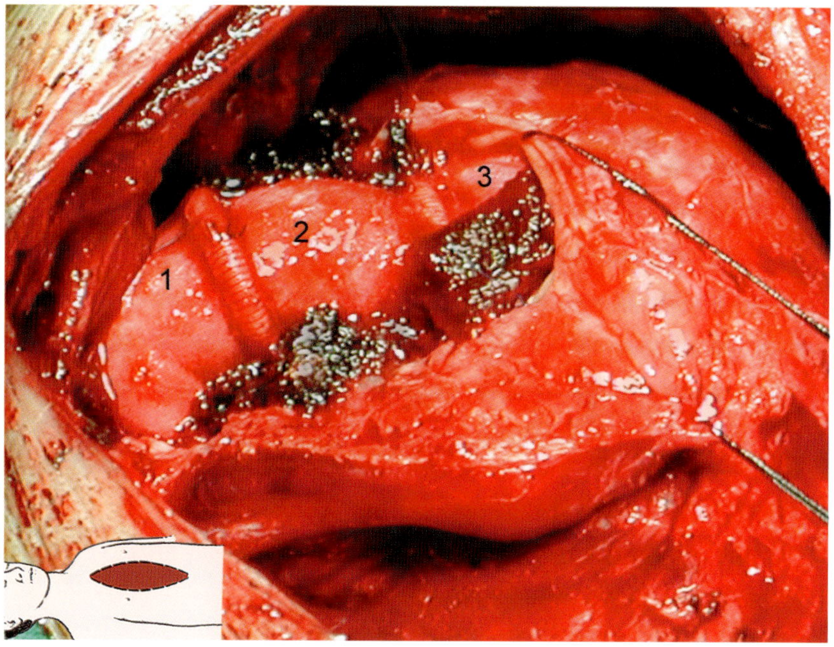

Figure 10.21. The same patient as in Figures 10.17 and 10.19, at reoperation to replace the dilated aortic homograft. A valved xenograft has been implanted as a pulmonary artery conduit.

1. Distal xenograft valved pulmonary artery conduit
2. Proximal part of xenograft
3. RV

REFERENCES

1. Momma K, Ando M, Matsuoka R. Truncus arteriosus communis associated with chromosome 22q11 deletion. *J Am Coll Cardiol.* 1997;30:1067–1071.
2. Russell HM, Marshall LJ, Anderson RH, et al. A simplified categorization for common arterial trunk. *J Thorac Cardiovasc Surg.* 2011;141:645–653.
3. Mair D, Ritter D, Davis G. Selection of patients with truncus arteriosus for surgical correction: anatomic and hemodynamic considerations. *Circulation.* 1974;49:144–151.
4. Jacobs M. Congenital Heart Surgery Nomenclature and Database Project: truncus arteriosus. *Ann Thorac Surg.* 2000;69:S50–S55.

CHAPTER 11

Cor Triatriatum

Cor triatriatum is an uncommon anomaly whereby the left atrium is partitioned into 2 chambers: a proximal chamber where the pulmonary veins (PVs) drain, and a distal chamber below the partition and above the mitral valve (Figure 11.1). The pulmonary venous chamber thus created may communicate with the distal left atrium, the right atrium, or both. This condition differs from supravalvar stenosing mitral ring (or membrane) in that the mouth of the left atrial appendage (LAA) lies below the level of the partition, whereas in supravalvar ring the appendage orifice lies above the membrane.[1]

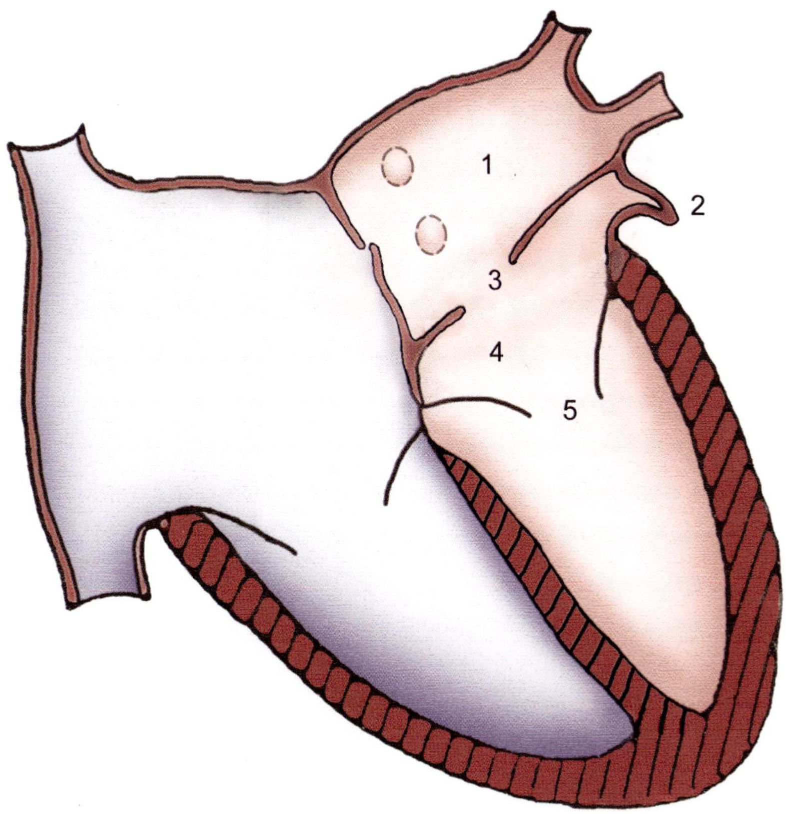

Figure 11.1. A schematic diagram of cor triatriatum. A membrane divides the left atrial cavity into 2 chambers. Many varieties can exist; the one illustrated here has a proximal chamber that receives the PVs and communicates with the right atrium via an interatrial communication and communicates with the distal chamber below the membrane, which in turn drains into the LV. Note the location of the LAA in the distal chamber below the membrane.

1. Proximal chamber
2. LAA
3. The dividing membrane
4. Distal chamber
5. Mitral valve

Congenital Heart Disease: A Surgical Color Atlas © 2015 A. Sukru Mercan, Zakariya Hubail, S. Yen Ho.
Cardiotext Publishing, ISBN: 978-1-935395-90-4.

Figure 11.2. Right atriotomy view of a 3-month-old infant with cor triatriatum. A suction catheter is passed through the foramen ovale. The arrow points to the direction of the tricuspid valve.

1. Right ventricle (RV)
2. Catheter in foramen ovale
3. Right atrial wall
4. Ascending aorta

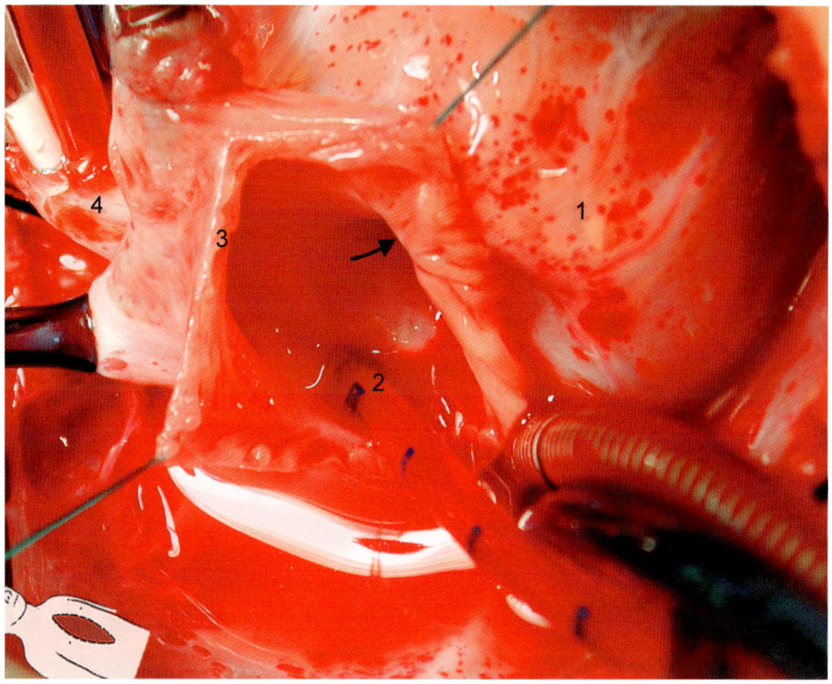

Anomalies of pulmonary venous connections are a common association[2] and along with site of atrial septal defect (ASD), give rise to many subtypes of cor triatriatum. Symptoms are usually caused by pulmonary venous hypertension, simulating mitral stenosis.[3] This anomaly is usually diagnosed noninvasively by echocardiography. Treatment is surgical resection of the partition, which may comprise a muscular shelf or a deep infolding of the atrial wall, through a median sternotomy approach, on cardiopulmonary bypass. Figures 11.2 to 11.5 are from a 3-month-old infant with cor triatriatum. Accessed through a transseptal approach from the right atrium, the dividing shelf is visible in Figure 11.3. A small orifice is the only

Figure 11.3. The same patient as in Figure 11.2. The left atrium is accessed through an atrial septostomy. The membrane dividing the left atrium is seen (2). The arrow points to the direction of the tricuspid valve.

1. Right atrial wall
2. Dividing membrane
3. Atrial septum (cut edge)

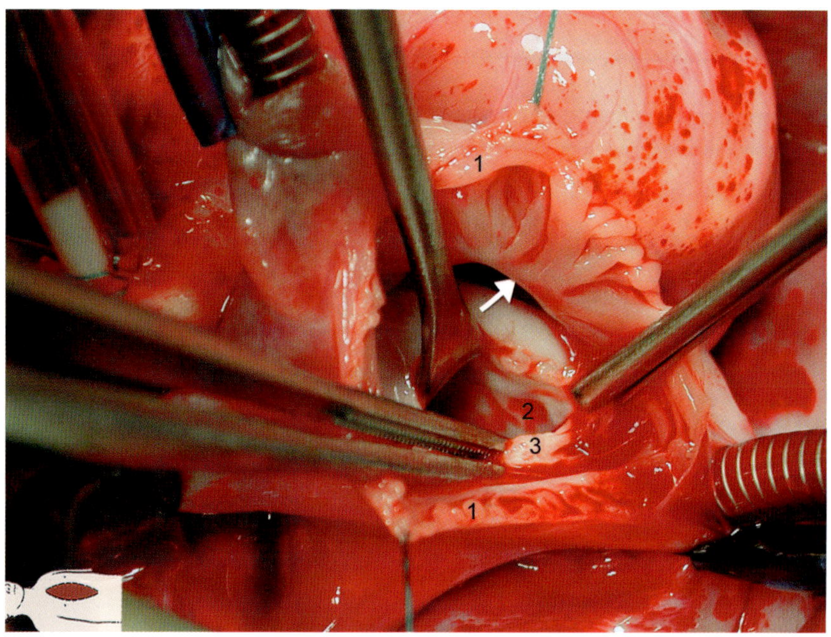

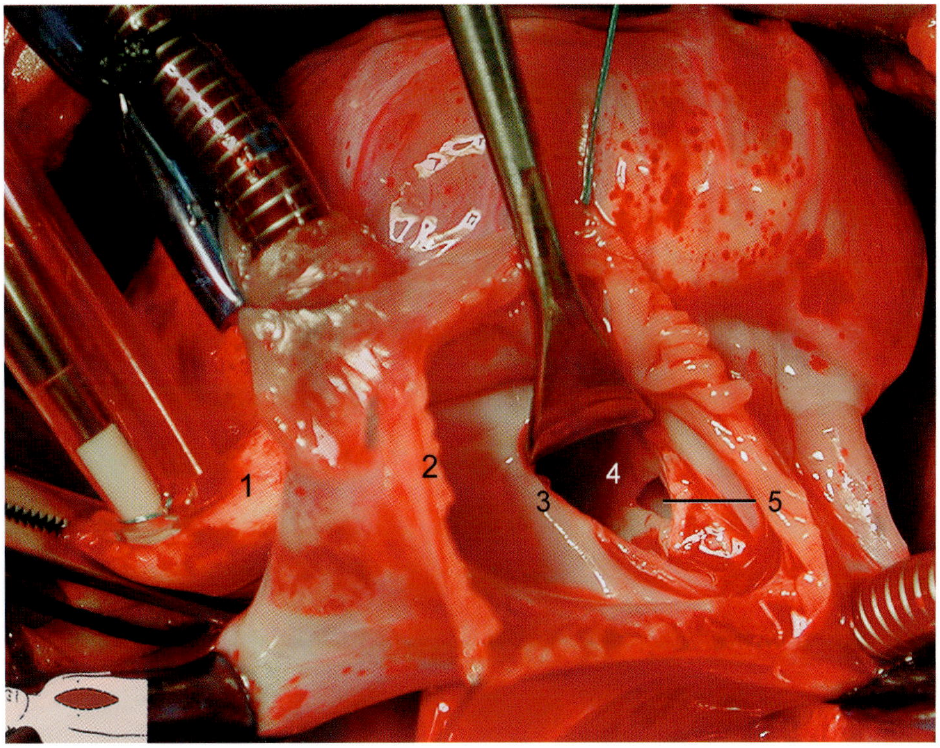

Figure 11.4. The same patient as in Figures 11.2 and 11.3. A small orifice is seen in the membrane. It is the only communication between the proximal chamber of the left atrium, where PVs drain, and the distal chamber, which opens to the mitral valve.

1. Ascending aorta
2. Right atrial wall
3. Atrial septum (cut edge)
4. Dividing membrane
5. Orifice in dividing membrane

Figure 11.5. The same patient as in Figures 11.2 to 11.4 after resection of most of the membrane. In this picture, the remnant of the dividing membrane is pulled out through the atrial septostomy site.

1. Right atrial wall
2. Left atrial cavity
3. Dividing membrane
4. Interatrial septum

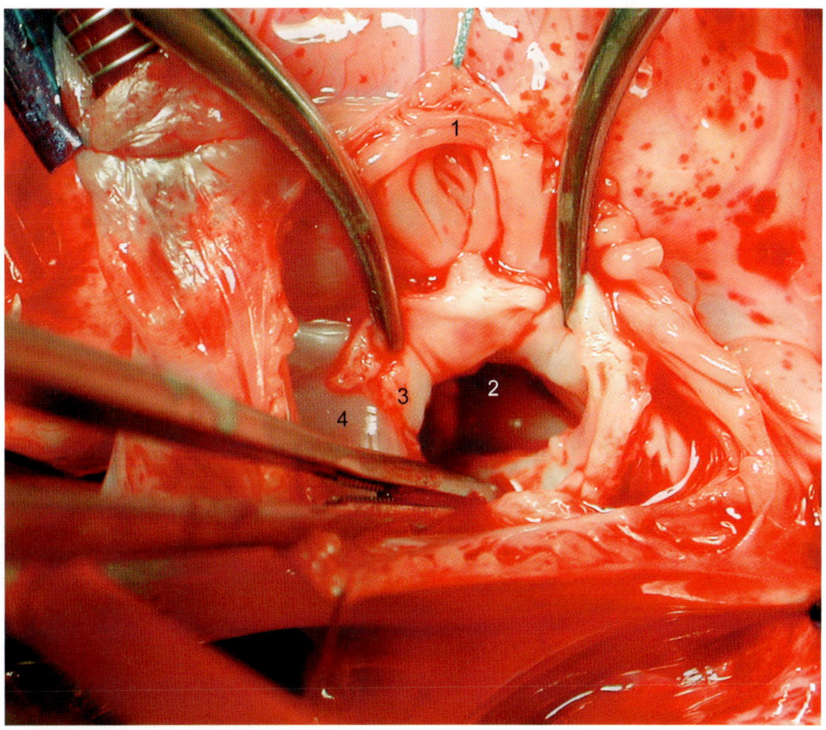

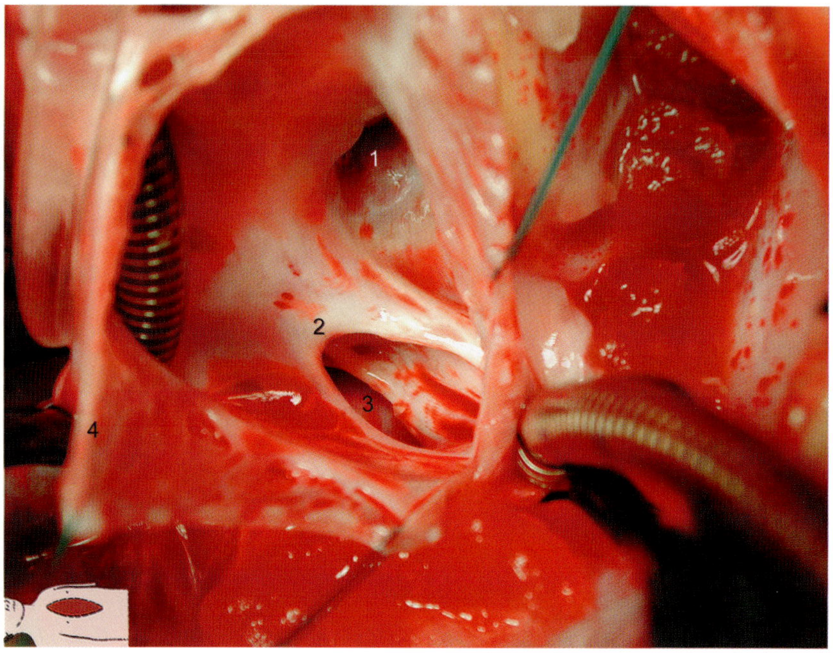

Figure 11.6. Right atriotomy view of an 18-month-old child with cor triatriatum and ASD.

1. Tricuspid valve
2. Interatrial septum
3. Left atrial cavity seen through ASD
4. Right atrial wall

communication between the 2 chambers of the divided left atrium. This was treated by resecting the shelf. Another example of cor triatriatum with an ASD is shown in Figures 11.6 to 11.10.

Figures 11.11 to 11.21 are from a 7-month-old infant with cor triatriatum, large ASD, and abnormal pulmonary venous drainage. There is infolding of the left atrial wall, resulting in a funnel-shaped left atrium. The PVs connect normally to the left atrium, which has no clear septation from the right atrium. The distal chamber, and thence the left ventricle (LV), receives blood from the right atrium through a small orifice. This is an example of a normal pulmonary venous connection, but abnormal drainage.

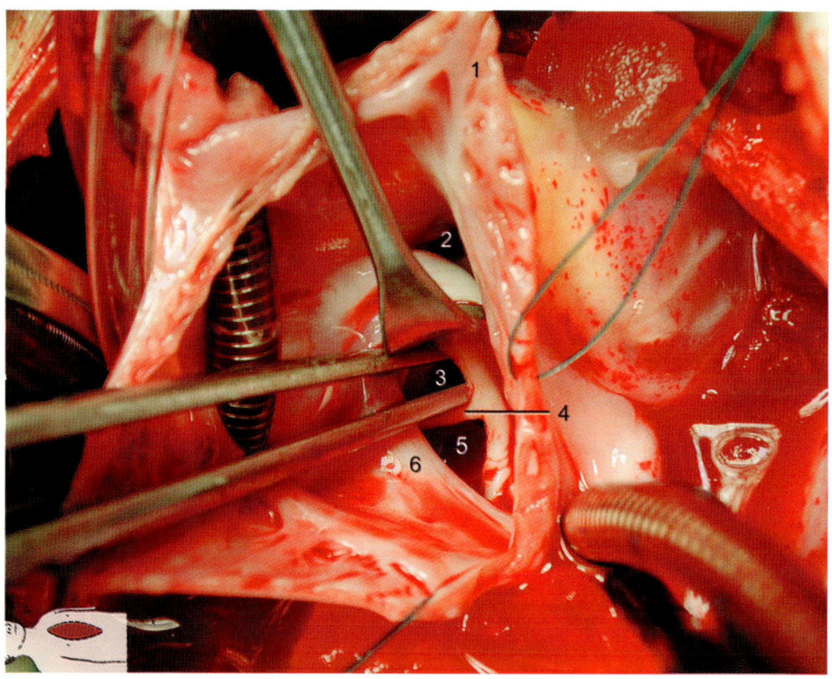

Figure 11.7. The same patient as in Figure 11.6. The edge of the ASD is retracted to better show the left atrial cavity. The cor triatiatum membrane is seen dividing the left atrium into 2 chambers.

1. Right atrial wall
2. Tricuspid valve
3. Distal chamber
4. Dividing membrane
5. Proximal (pulmonary venous) chamber
6. Interatrial septum

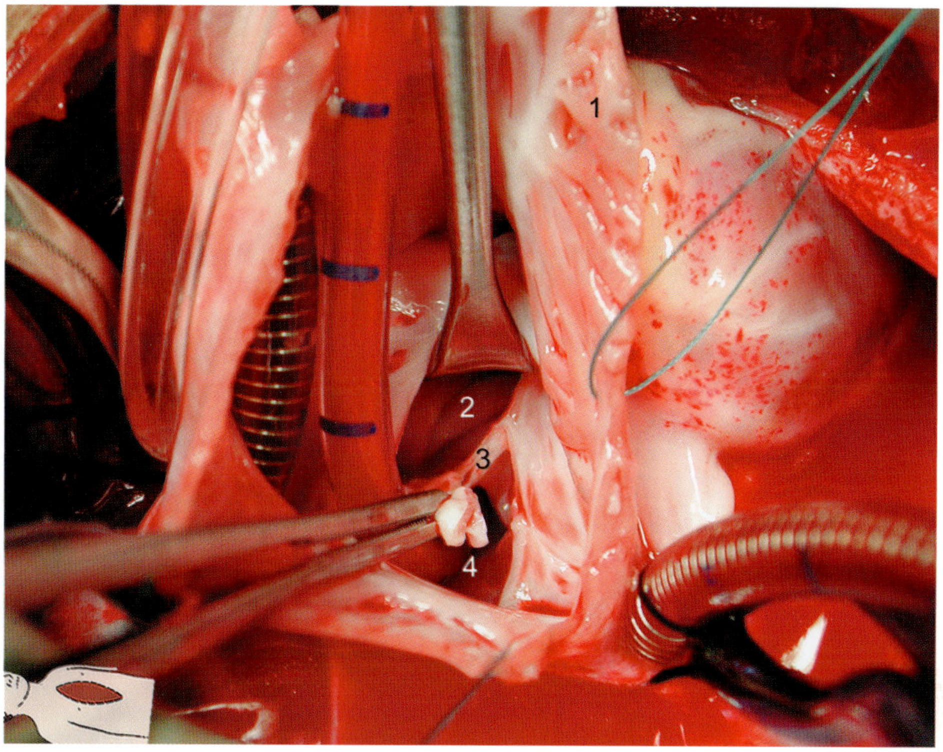

Figure 11.8. The same patient as in Figures 11.6 and 11.7 during resection of the membrane.

1. Right atrial wall
2. Distal chamber
3. Dividing membrane
4. Proximal (pulmonary venous) chamber

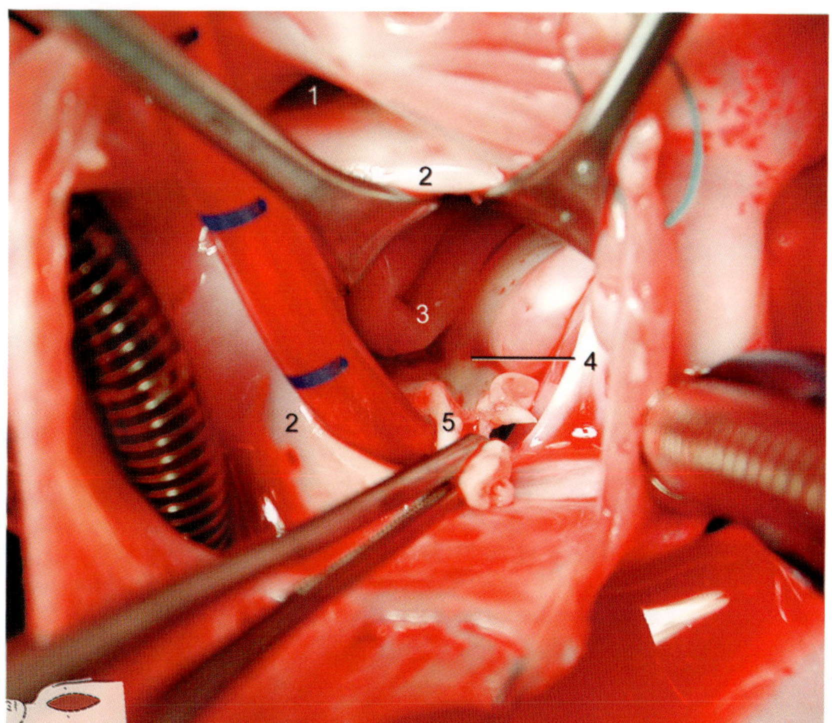

Figure 11.9. The same patient as in Figures 11.6 to 11.8. The remnant of the dividing membrane is retracted down, showing the distal chamber of the divided left atrium. Note that the LAA opens into the distal (supramitral) chamber.

1. Site of tricuspid valve
2. Interatrial septum
3. Base of LAA
4. Junction of the dividing membrane and the left atrial posterior free wall
5. Dividing membrane

Figure 11.10. The same patient as in Figures 11.6 to 11.9. The remnant of the dividing membrane is retracted up, showing the proximal chamber (pulmonary venous chamber) of the divided left atrium.

1. Right atrial wall
2. Site of tricuspid valve
3. Distal left atrial chamber
4. Dividing membrane
5. Proximal left atrial chamber
6. Interatrial septum

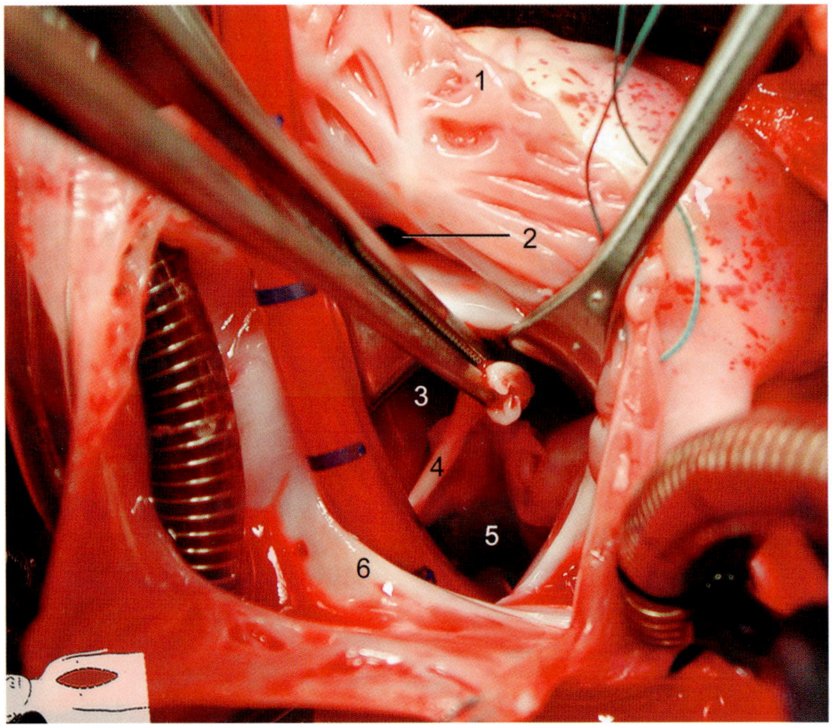

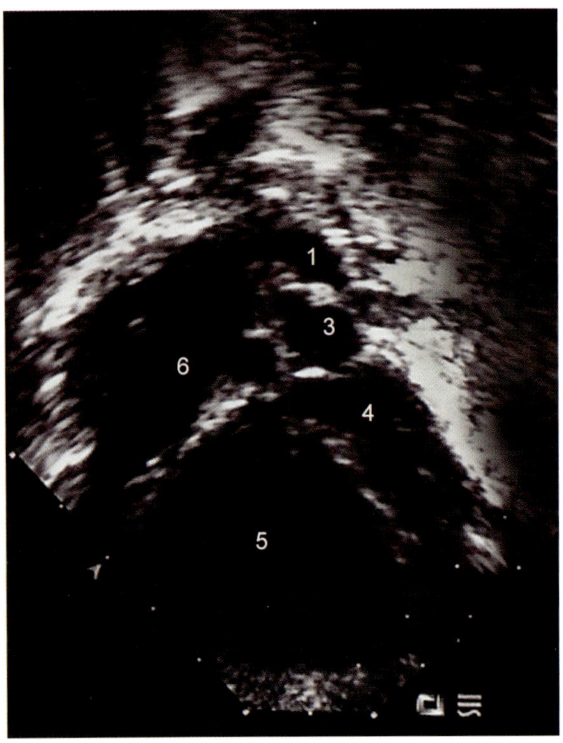

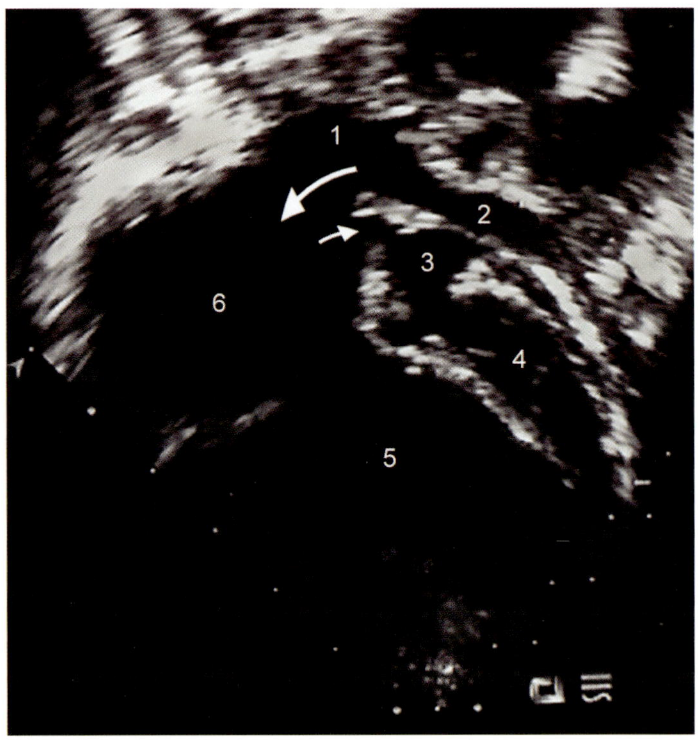

Figure 11.11 **Figure 11.12**

An echocardiogram from a 7-month-old infant with cor triatriatum. The 4-chamber views show division of the left atrium into 2 chambers: a proximal chamber that receives the PVs and communicates with the right atrium (large arrow), and a distal chamber connected to the mitral valve. The distal left atrial chamber receives blood from the right atrium (small arrow).

1. Proximal left atrial chamber
2. Pulmonary vein (PV)
3. Distal left atrial chamber
4. LV
5. RV
6. Right atrium

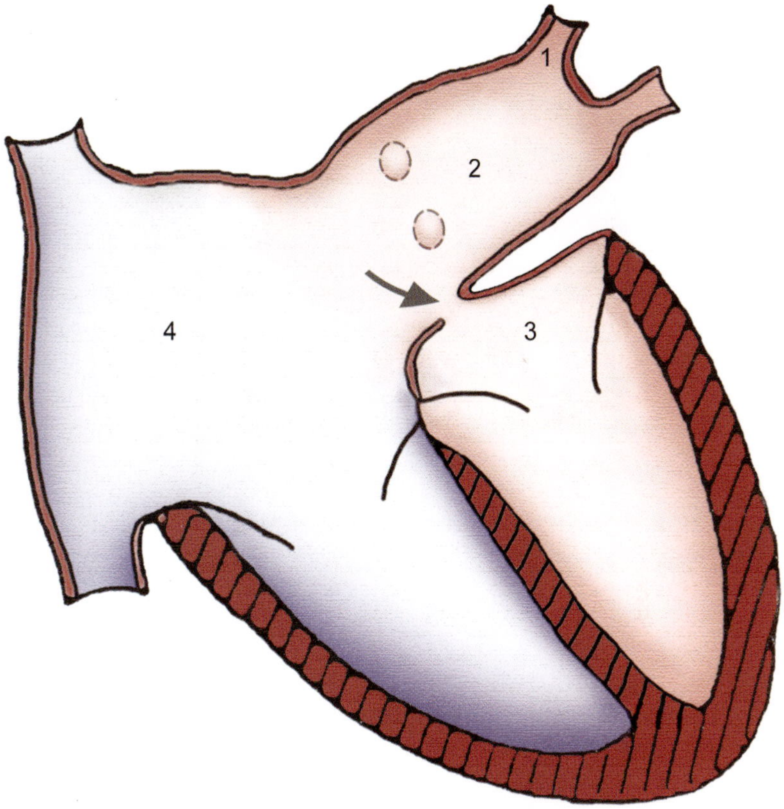

Figure 11.13. Diagrammatic illustration of the patient shown in Figures 11.11 and 11.12. The arrow points to the orifice that leads to the distal left atrium.

1. PV
2. Proximal chamber of left atrium
3. Distal chamber of left atrium
4. Right atrium

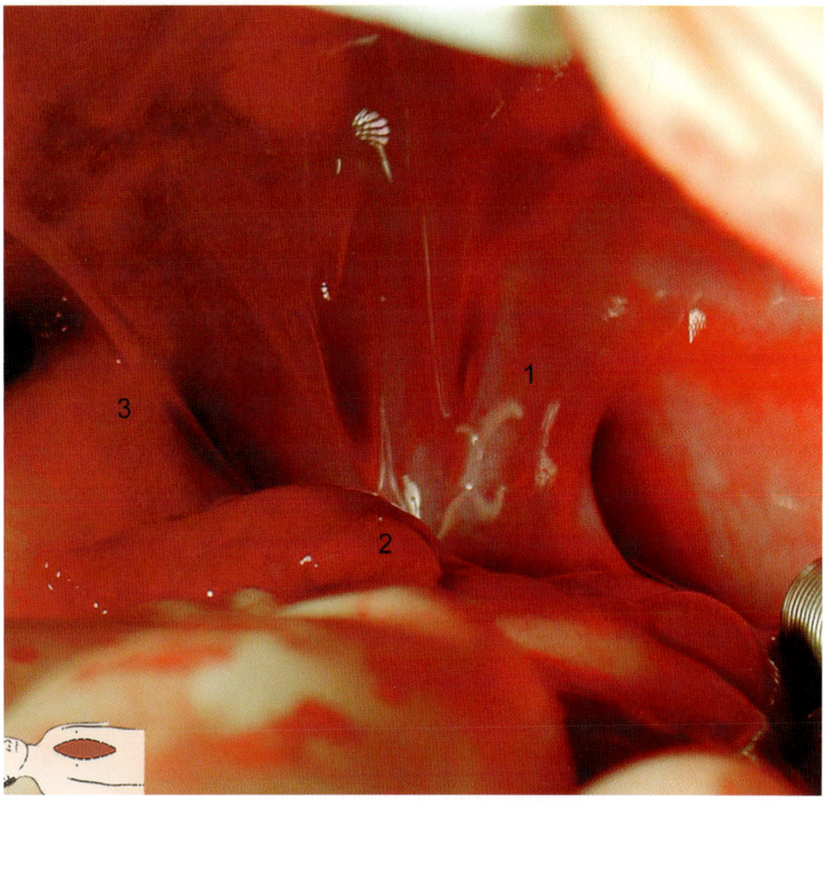

Figure 11.14. Intraoperative view via median sternotomy of the same patient whose echocardiogram is shown in Figures 11.11 and 11.12. The heart base is retracted rightward to show the left PVs, which connect normally to the left atrium. The 2 veins join each other before entering the atrium.

1. Left lower PV
2. LAA
3. Left pulmonary artery

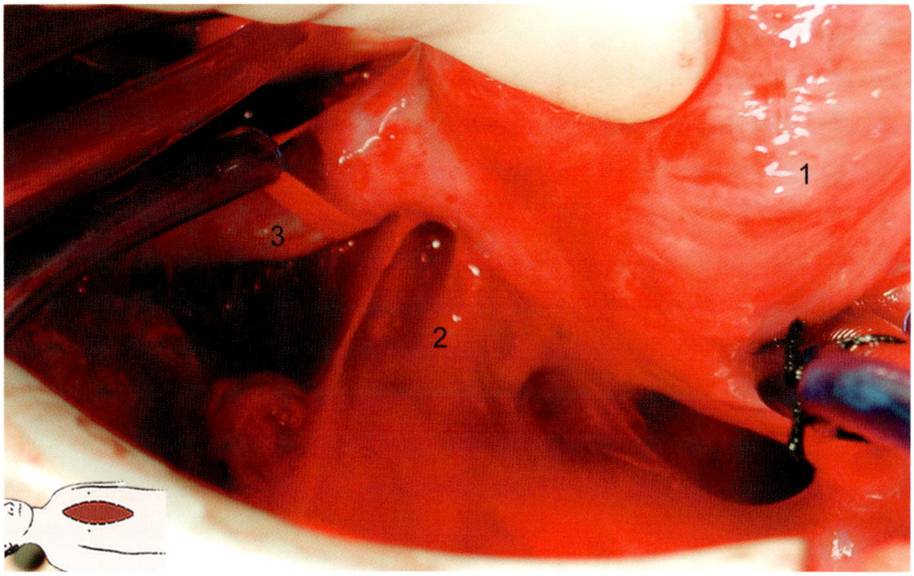

Figure 11.15. The same patient as in Figure 11.14 with the base of the heart retracted leftward to show the right PVs, which connect normally to the left atrium.

1. Right atrium
2. Right PV
3. Superior vena cava (SVC)

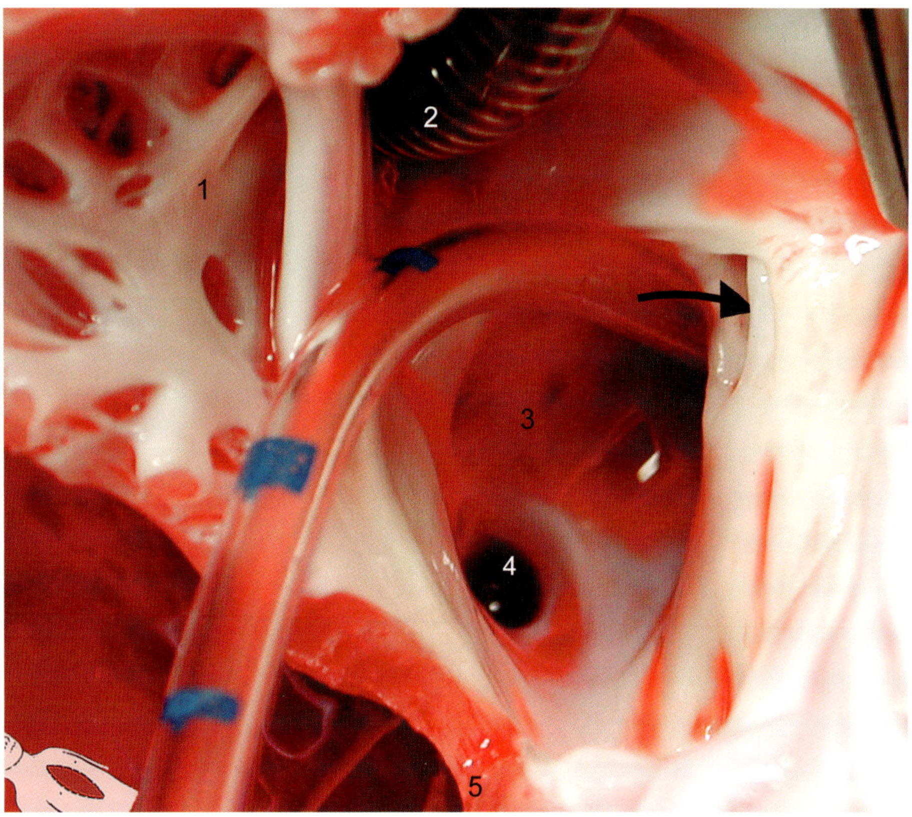

Figure 11.16. Right atriotomy view of the same patient shown in Figures 11.14 and 11.15. No discernible interatrial septum is seen. The PVs, which connect to the left atrium, freely communicate with the right atrium, in effect resulting in anomalous pulmonary venous drainage (see text). The arrow points to the orifice that leads to the distal left atrial chamber.

1. Right atrial free wall
2. Venous cannula draining SVC
3. Proximal left atrial chamber
4. PV
5. Right atriotomy incision

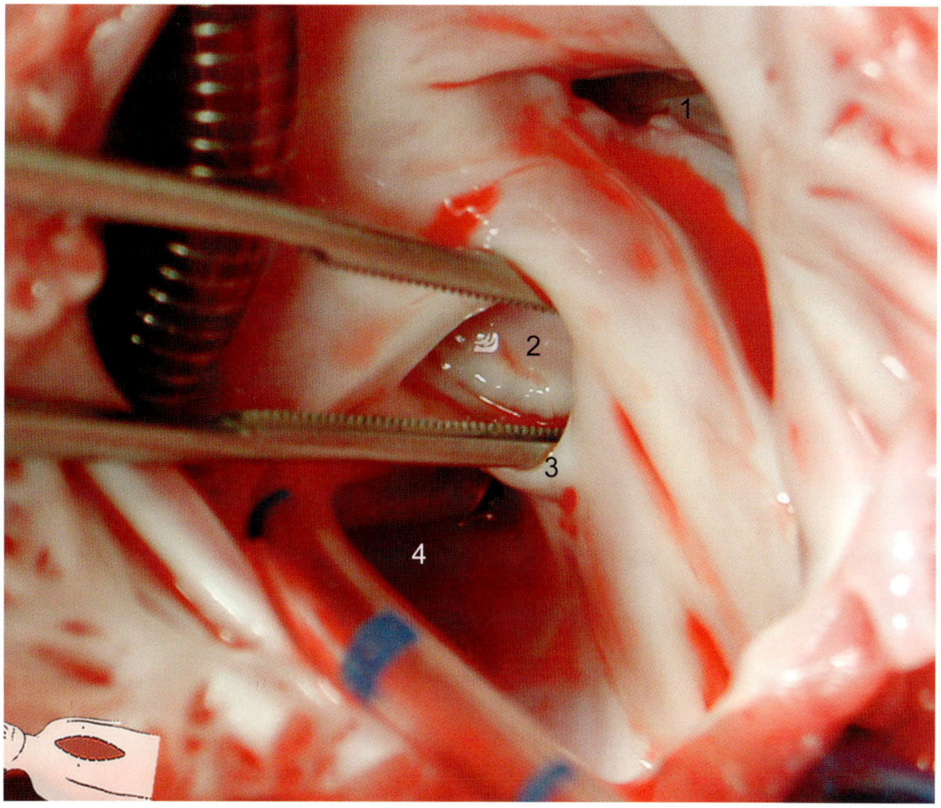

Figure 11.17. The same patient as in Figures 11.14 to 11.16. The orifice leading to the distal left atrial chamber is probed open with forceps.

1. Tricuspid valve
2. Distal left atrial chamber
3. Edge of orifice
4. Proximal left atrial chamber

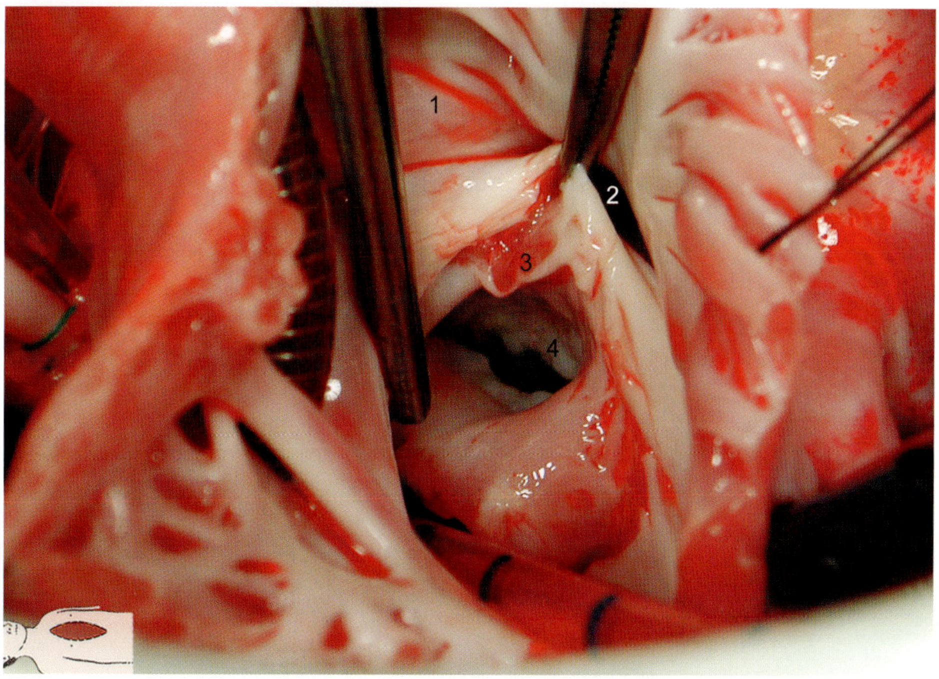

Figure 11.18. The same patient as in Figures 11.14 to 11.17. The orifice is enlarged by cutting its edges. The inside of the distal left atrial chamber is visible.

1. Right atrium
2. Site of tricuspid valve
3. Edge of orifice
4. Mitral valve

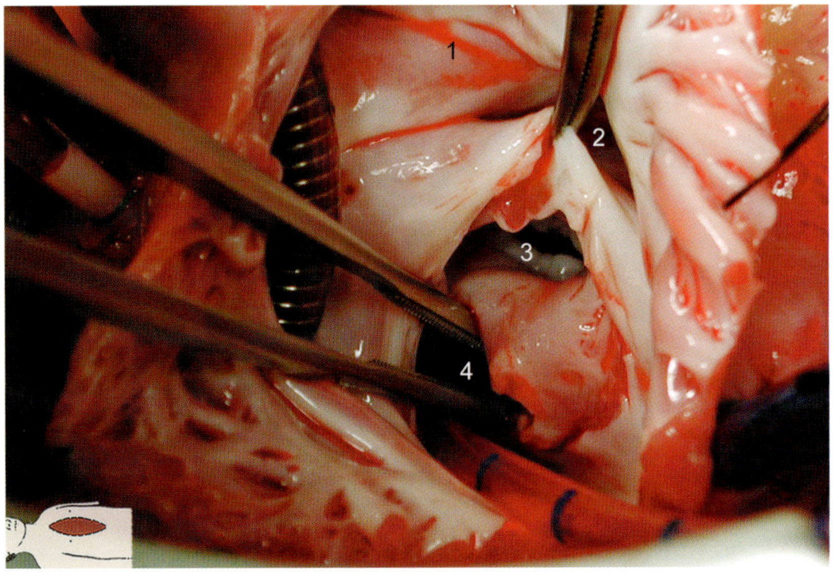

Figure 11.19. The same patient as in Figures 11.14 to 11.18. The left atrial posterolateral wall has been incised in order to enlarge the left atrial cavity. The forceps pass to the outside of the heart.

1. Right atrium
2. Site of tricuspid valve
3. Mitral valve
4. Forceps passing through atrial incision to outside the heart

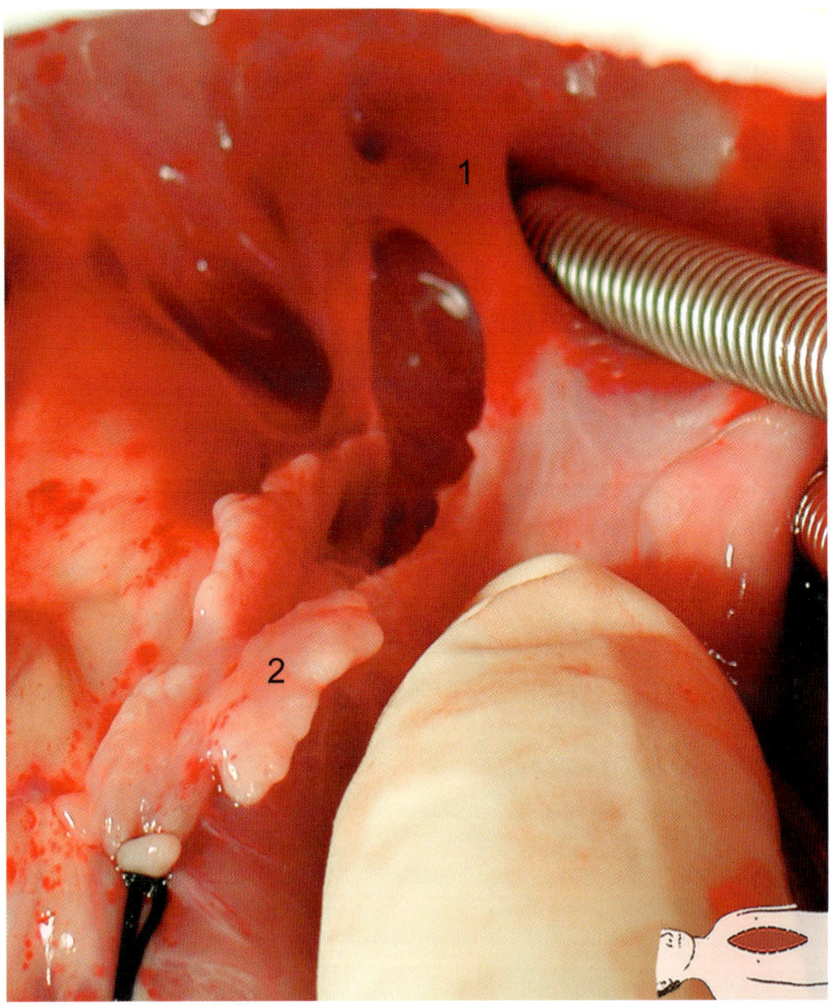

Figure 11.20. The same patient as in Figures 11.14 to 11.19, showing the incision in the left atrial wall from outside the heart. The incision has been extended to the PVs. A patch (not shown) was then sutured to enlarge the left atrium and PVs.

1. Left lower PV
2. LAA

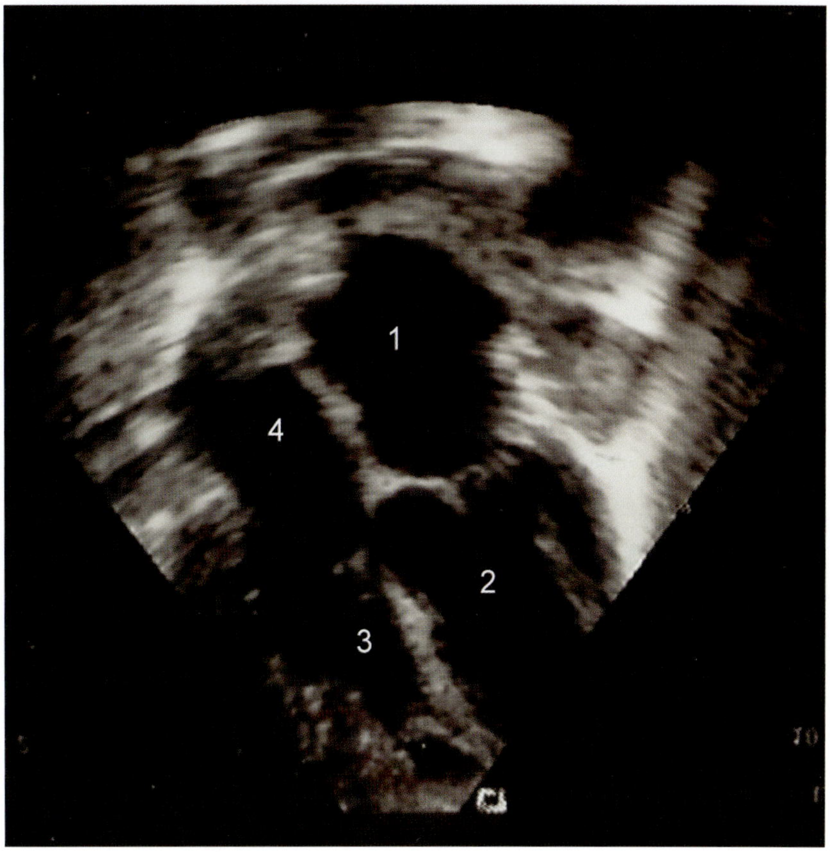

Figure 11.21. A postoperative echocardiogram of the same patient shown in Figures 11.14 to 11.20. It shows a fairly normal-looking heart after repair of the anomalous pulmonary venous drainage and septation of the atria.

1. Left atrium
2. LV
3. RV
4. Right atrium

REFERENCES

1. Jacobstein MD, Hirschfield SS. Concealed left atrial membrane: pitfalls in the diagnosis of cor triatriatum and supravalvar mitral ring. *Am J Cardiol.* 1982;49:780–786.
2. Alphonso N, Nørgaard M, Newcomb A, et al. Cor triatriatum: presentation, diagnosis and long-term surgical results. *Ann Thorac Surg.* 2005;80:1666–1671.
3. Gheissari A, Malm JR, Bowman FO Jr, Bierman FZ. Cor triatriatum sinistrum: one institution's 28-year experience. *Pediatr Cardiol.* 1992;13:85–88.

CHAPTER 12

Anomalous Pulmonary Venous Connections

PARTIALLY ANOMALOUS PULMONARY VENOUS CONNECTION

In this condition, one or more, but not all, pulmonary veins (PVs) connect to the right atrium, directly or by means of another vein. It is most commonly associated with a sinus venosus interatrial communication (so-called sinus venosus atrial septal defect [ASD]).[1]

On gross inspection, the anomalous veins can usually be seen connecting to the superior vena cava (SVC) as in the patients shown in Figures 12.1 to 12.5 from a 7-year-old child and Figures 12.6 to 12.9 from

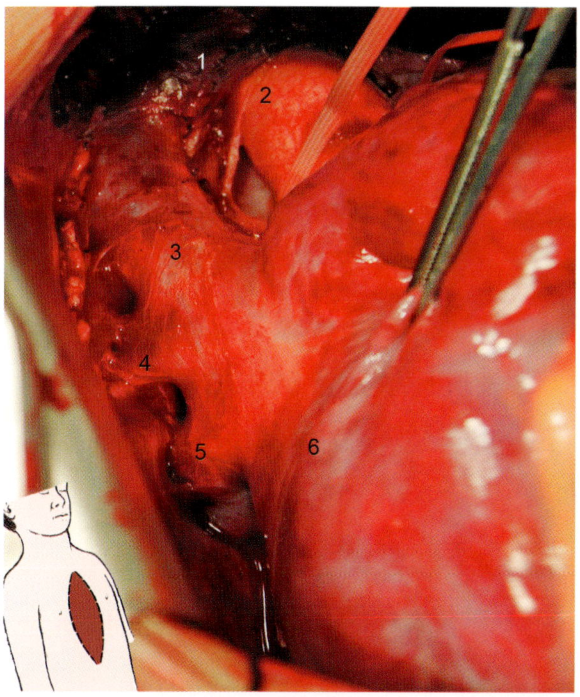

Figure 12.1

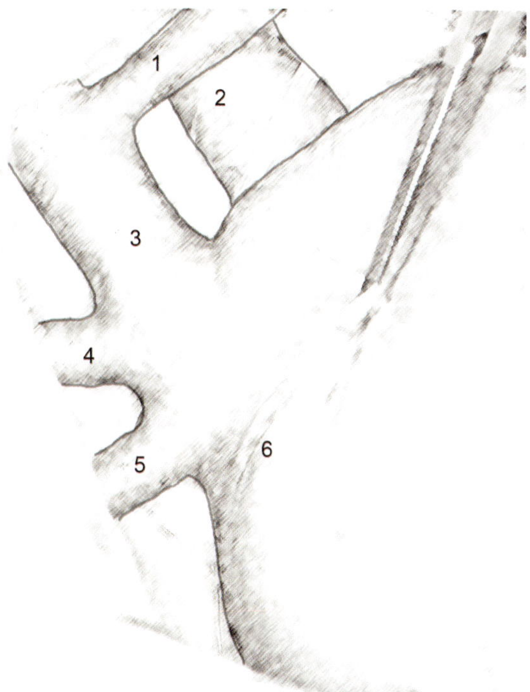

Figure 12.2

Partially anomalous pulmonary venous connection to the SVC as seen through a median sternotomy in a 7-year-old child.

1. Innominate vein
2. Ascending aorta
3. SVC
4. Right upper PV
5. Right lower PV
6. Right atrium

Figure 12.3. The same patient as in Figure 12.1, now on cardiopulmonary bypass. A right atriotomy has been performed. A superior sinus venosus ASD is seen. See Figure 12.4 for a close-up view.

1. SVC venous catheter
2. Margin of sinus venosus ASD
3. Limbus of fossa ovalis
4. Fossa ovalis

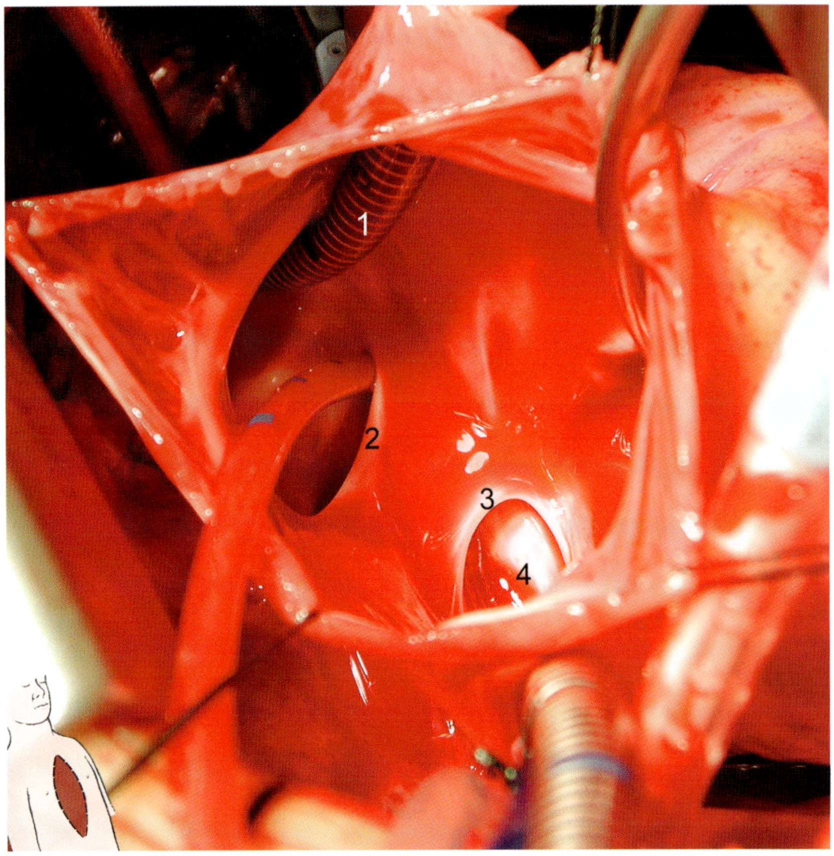

Figure 12.4. A close-up view of the same patient as in Figure 12.3. The arrow points to the opening of the anomalously connected right upper PV.

1. SVC venous cannula
2. Margin of sinus venosus ASD
3. Suction catheter draining left atrium
4. Opening of right upper PV

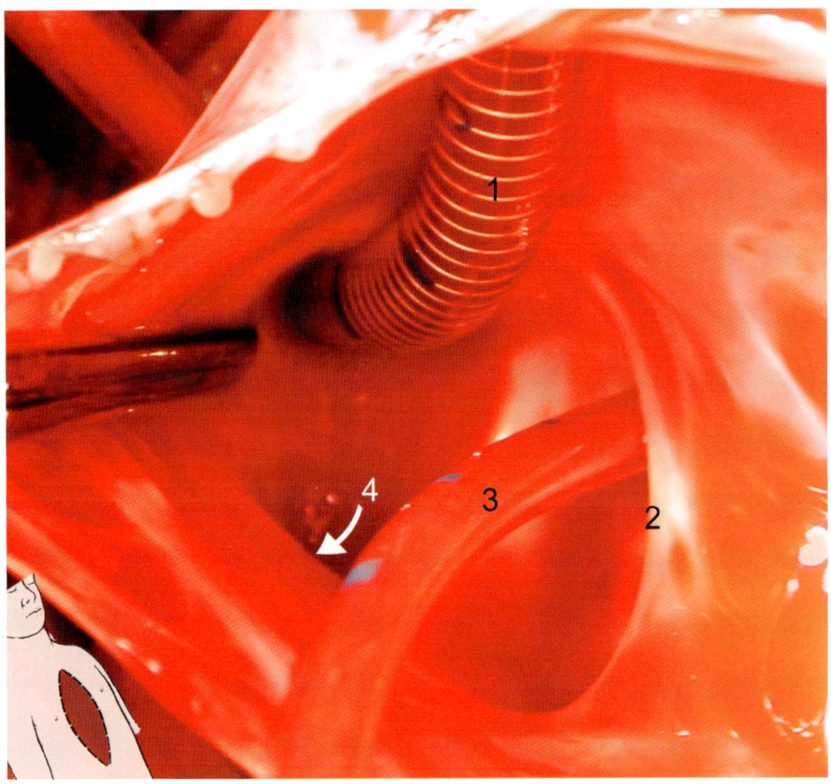

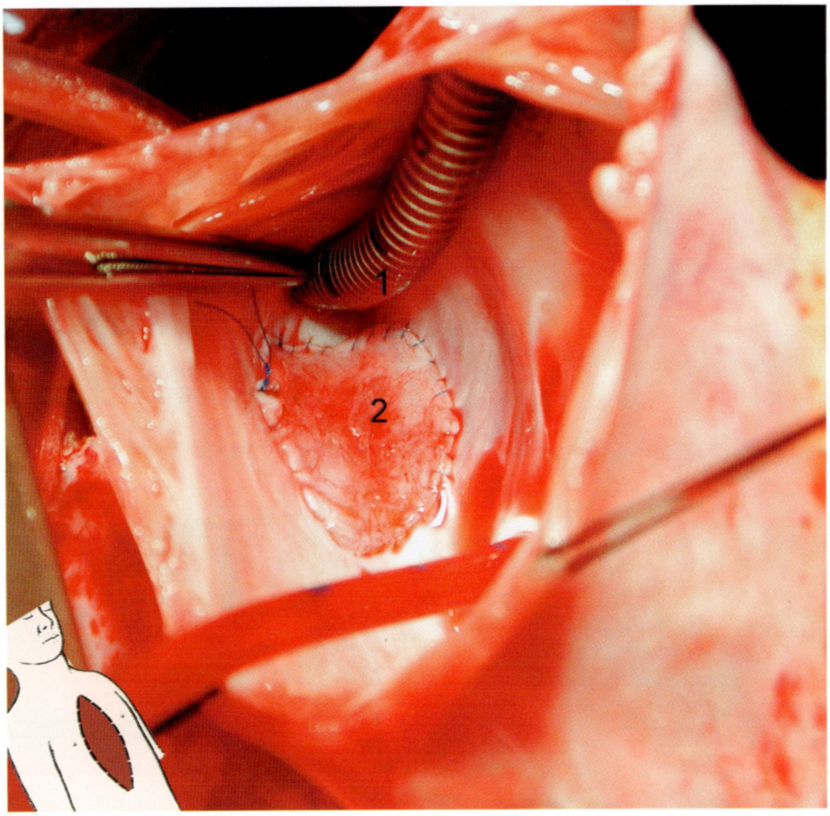

Figure 12.5. The same patient as in Figures 12.1 to 12.4. The ASD has been closed with an autologous pericardial patch, redirecting the drainage of the anomalous veins to the left atrium. The SVC was left to open directly into the right atrium.

1. SVC venous cannula
2. Autologous pericardial patch

a 6-year-old child. Both were treated using the same technique; that is, an autologous pericardial patch was used to close the sinus venosus ASD in a way that directs the pulmonary venous blood to the left atrium. The SVC is left to drain directly to the right atrium (Figures 12.5 and 12.9).

Occasionally, 3 veins are seen draining the right lung, which is a normal anatomic variant, because

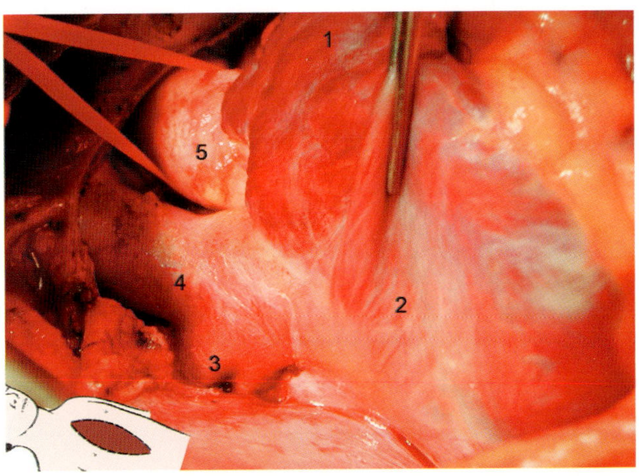

Figure 12.6

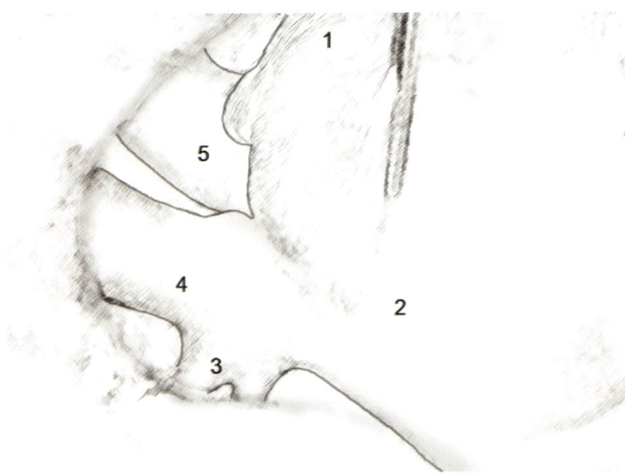

Figure 12.7

Partially anomalous pulmonary venous connection to the SVC as seen through a median sternotomy in a 6-year-old child. Both right PVs connect to the right atrium–SVC junction.

1. Right atrial appendage (RAA)
2. Right atrium
3. Right PVs
4. SVC
5. Ascending aorta

Figure 12.8. Same patient as in Figures 12.6 and 12.7. The sinus venosus ASD and anomalous PVs are viewed from within the right atrium.

1. SVC venous cannula
2. Margin of sinus venous ASD
3. Catheter draining left atrium
4. Opening of right PV

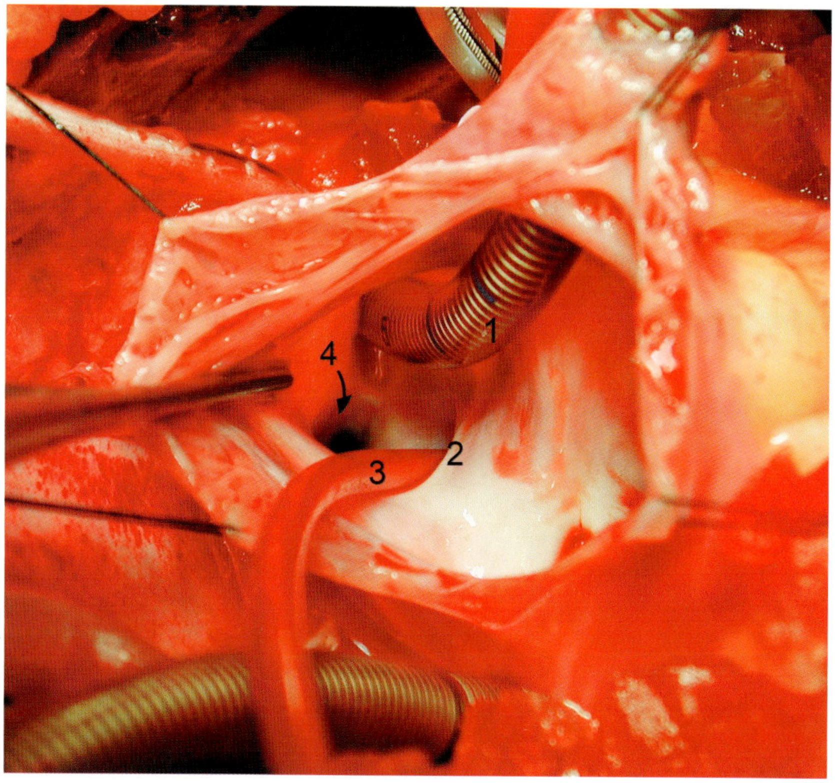

Figure 12.9. The same patient as in Figures 12.6 to 12.8. The ASD has been closed with an autologous pericardial patch, redirecting the drainage of the anomalous veins to the left atrium.

1. SVC venous cannula
2. Autologous pericardial patch closing the ASD
3. Limbus of fossa ovalis
4. Blood pooled at fossa ovalis

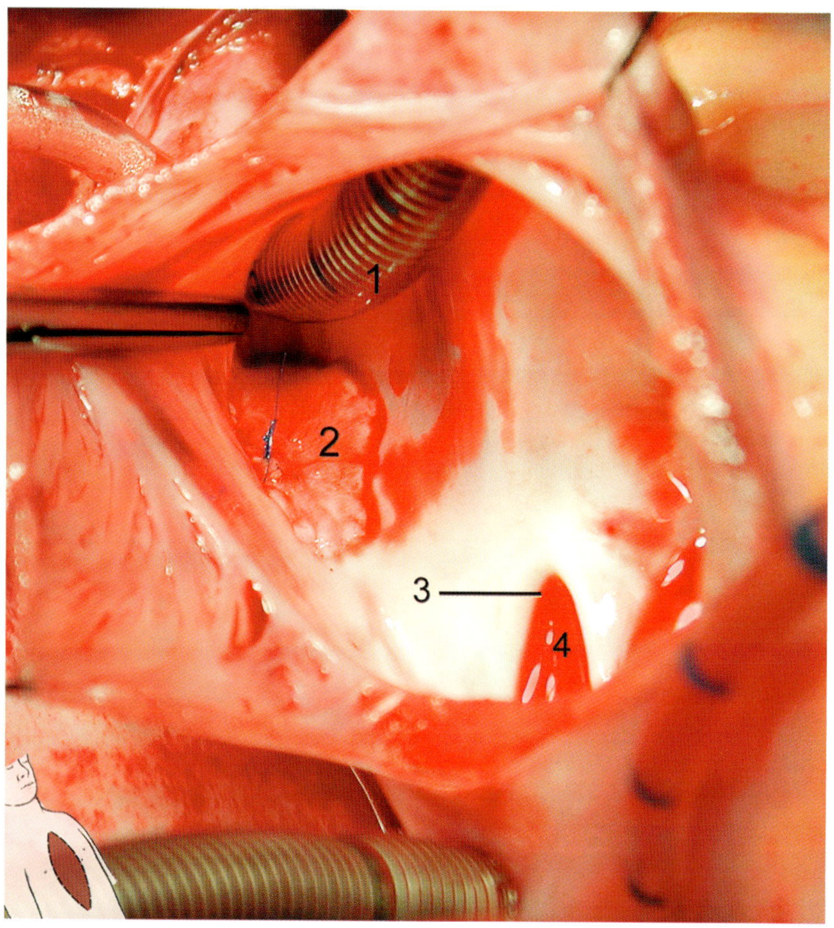

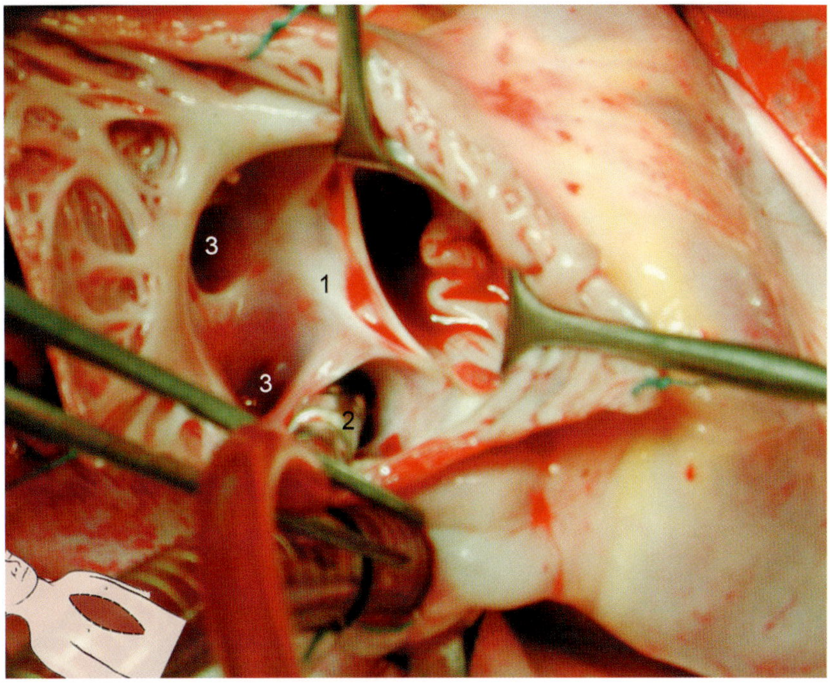

Figure 12.10. Partially anomalous pulmonary venous connection in a 6-year-old child. Three veins are seen draining anomalously to the right atrium.

1. Atrial septum
2. Metallic sump in a PV
3. Anomalous PVs

the right lung has 3 lobes. However, a third vein could as well be coming from the left lung and anomalously connecting to the right side of the heart. Figures 12.10 and 12.11 show a sinus venosus defect with 3 PVs draining anomalously to the right atrium. In this patient, the true atrial septum was intact, so an ASD was created to redirect pulmonary venous flow to the left atrium.

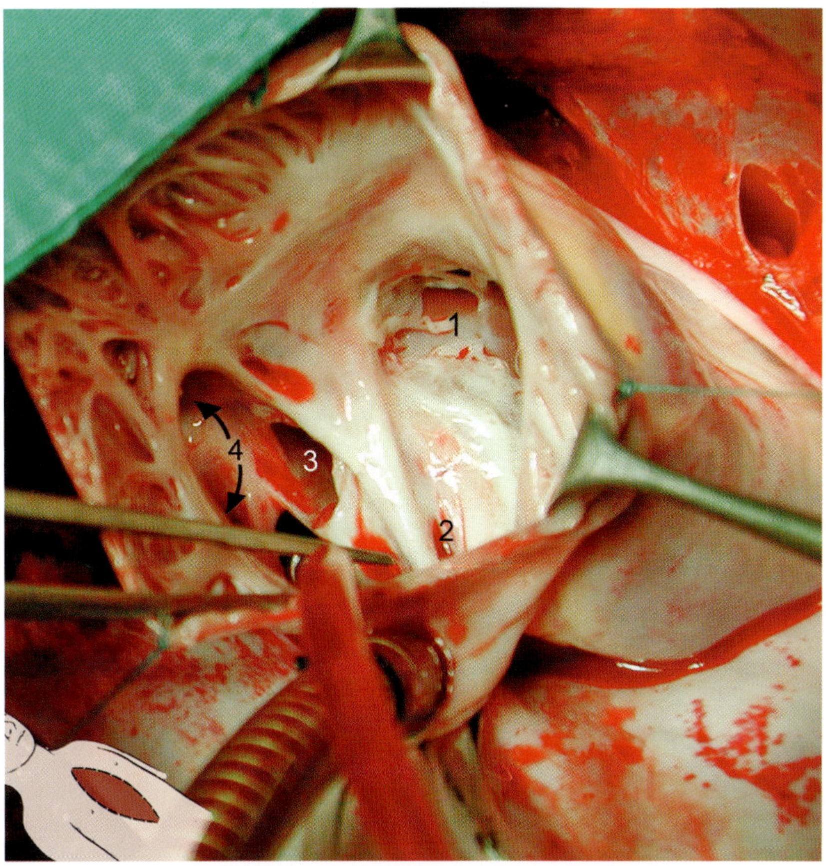

Figure 12.11. The same patient as in Figure 12.10. An ASD (3) has been created in order to redirect the anomalous venous blood so that it drains into the left atrium.

1. Tricuspid valve
2. Coronary sinus opening
3. Surgically created ASD
4. Anomalous PVs

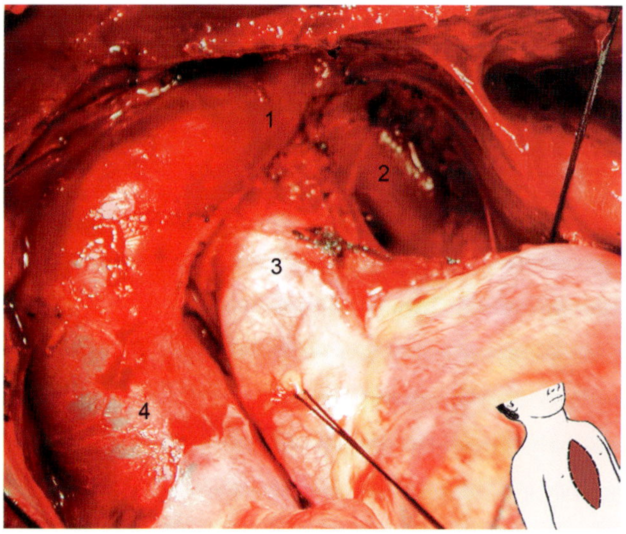

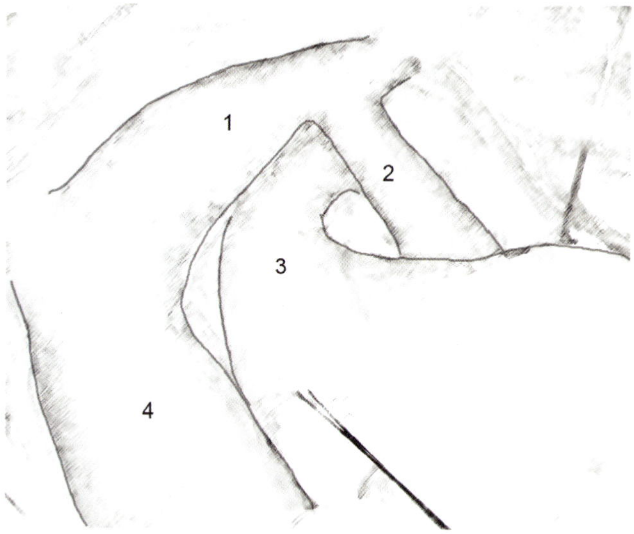

Figure 12.12 **Figure 12.13**

Partially anomalous pulmonary venous connection in an 18-year-old patient. The left-sided PVs drain to the innominate vein via a vertical vein. The right upper PV connects to the SVC (4), whereas the right lower vein drains normally to the left atrium (not shown).

1. Innominate vein
2. Vertical vein
3. Ascending aorta
4. SVC

Figures 12.12 to 12.16 show a mixed-type partially anomalous pulmonary venous connection in an 18-year-old patient. The left-sided PVs drain to the innominate vein via a vertical vein, the right upper PV connects to the SVC, and the right lower vein drains normally to the left atrium. Another example is shown in Figures 12.17 and 12.18, from a 27-year-old patient.

Figure 12.14. A close-up view of the vertical vein.

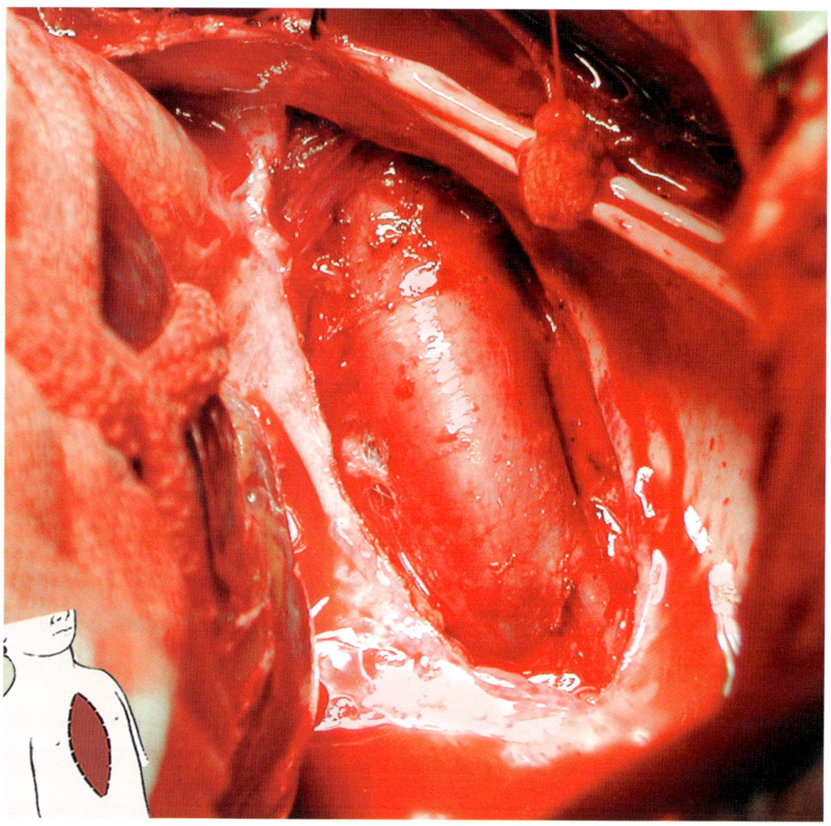

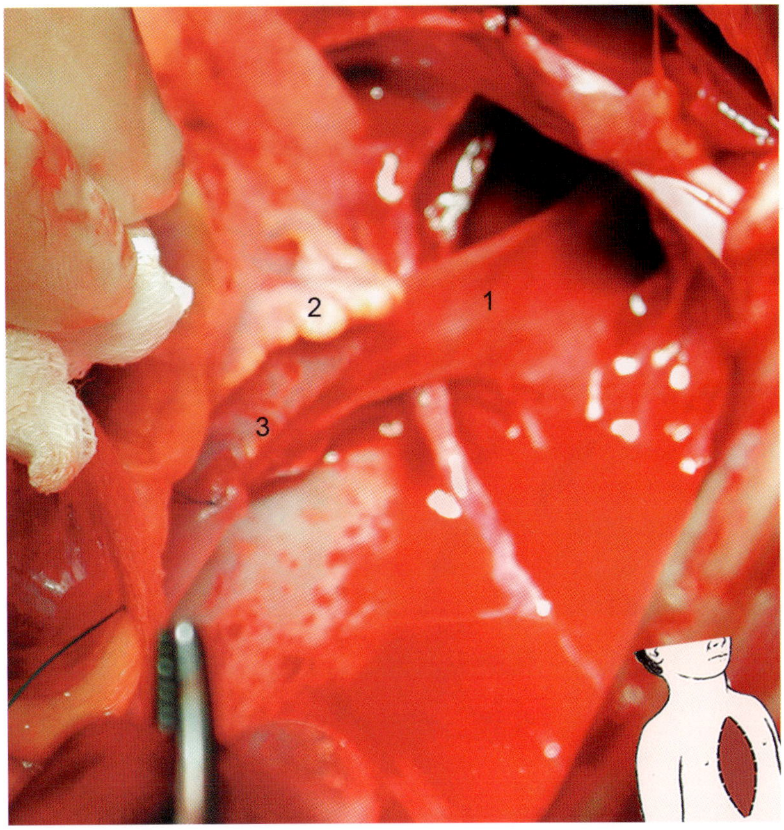

Figure 12.15. The same patient as in Figures 12.12 to 12.14. The vertical vein was divided, turned down, and anastomosed directly to the left atrium.

1. Vertical vein
2. Left atrial appendage (LAA)
3. Anastomosis of vertical vein to left atrium

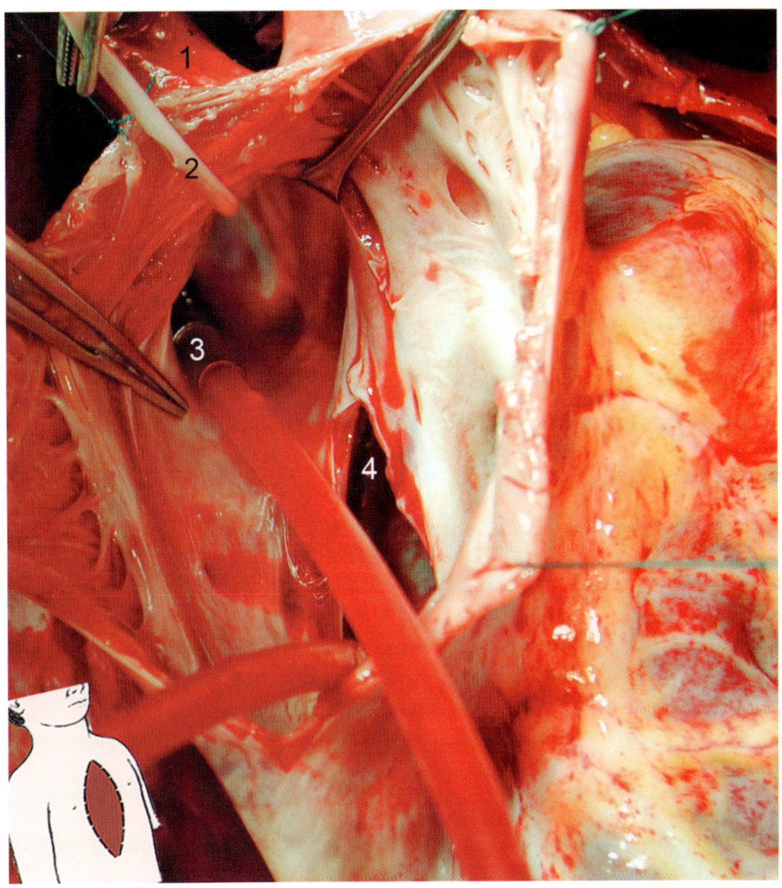

Figures 12.16. The same patient as in Figures 12.12 to 12.15. The right upper PV connects to the right atrium. The ASD (4) was enlarged, then an autologous pericardial patch (not shown) was used to reroute anomalous venous flow and close the ASD.

1. SVC
2. Central venous catheter
3. Suction catheter in right upper PV
4. ASD—surgically enlarged

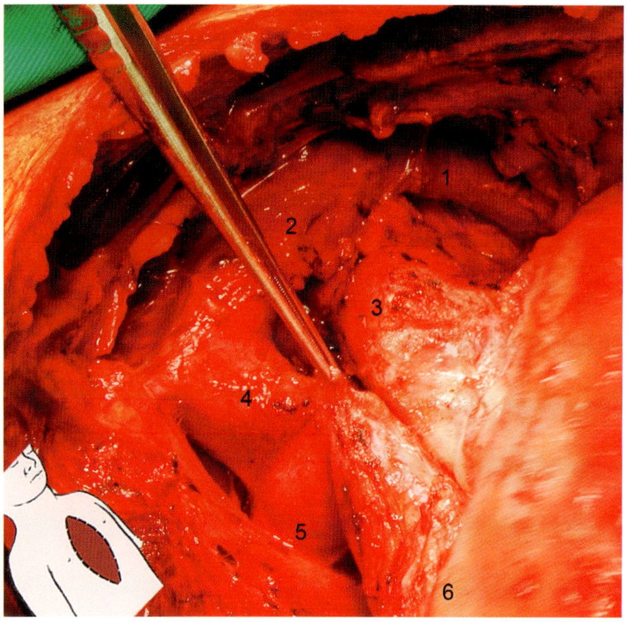

Figure 12.17

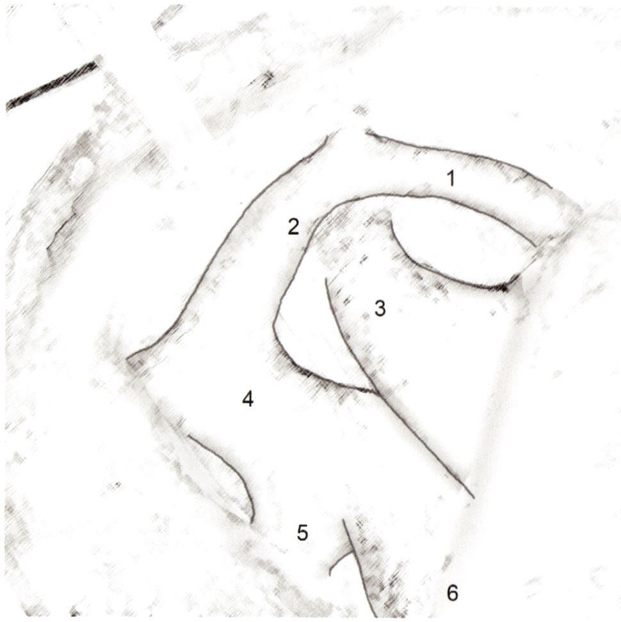

Figure 12.18

Mixed-type partially anomalous pulmonary venous connection in a 27-year-old patient. Left upper PV drains to the innominate vein through a vertical vein, and the right upper PV drains directly to the SVC.

1. Vertical vein
2. Innominate vein
3. Ascending aorta
4. SVC
5. Right upper PV
6. Right atrium

TOTALLY ANOMALOUS PULMONARY VENOUS CONNECTION

The PVs do not connect to the left atrium at all in this condition. Totally anomalous pulmonary venous connection (TAPVC) should be distinguished from totally anomalous pulmonary venous drainage (TAPVD). In the latter condition, the PVs connect to the left atrium but, because of the lack of egress through the atrioventricular valve or an interatrial communication, left atrial blood is diverted via a pulmonary-to-systemic collateral vein (usually a levoatrial cardinal vein) to drain directly or indirectly to the right atrium.

In TAPVC, there are 3 levels at which the anomalous venous connection can be made: supracardiac, cardiac, and infracardiac. The most common type is supracardiac connection to the innominate vein[2] or directly to the SVC. The cardiac type connects to the coronary sinus or directly to the right atrium, whereas the infracardiac type connects subdiaphragmatically, for example, to the portal vein, inferior caval vein, or gastric veins. A mixed-type connection takes place when the PVs drain to more than one site. Figures 12.19 and 12.20 illustrate a patient with typical supracardiac TAPVC to the innominate vein. The vertical vein may become obstructed along its course, as shown in Figures 12.21 to 12.23. The pulmonary venous confluence is usually located behind the atria, inferior to the branch pulmonary arteries (PAs), as shown in Figures 12.24 and 12.25. Surgical repair is achieved by ligating the vertical vein, anastomosing the pulmonary venous confluence to the left atrium (Figures 12.26–12.32), and closing the ASD. Rarely, the individual veins may open directly to the right atrium as in the 8-month-old infant shown in Figures 12.33 to 12.35. This patient also had 2 (outlet and inlet) ventricular septal defects (VSDs).

Infracardiac anomalous pulmonary venous connection is the type most likely to get obstructed and can present as a surgical emergency.[3] Figures 12.36 to 12.38 are 2 examples of infracardiac connections. Figures 12.38 and 12.39 are from patients with mixed-type anomalous connection.

Anomalous pulmonary venous connection is also seen as a part of more complex heart disease and in heterotaxy syndromes.[4] Figures 12.40 and 12.41 are from a 6-year-old child with univentricular physiology (unbalanced complete atrioventricular septal defect [AVSD], hypoplastic right ventricle (RV), and severe pulmonary stenosis). He underwent a Glenn shunt, but could not be weaned from cardiopulmonary bypass, and further intraoperative inspection

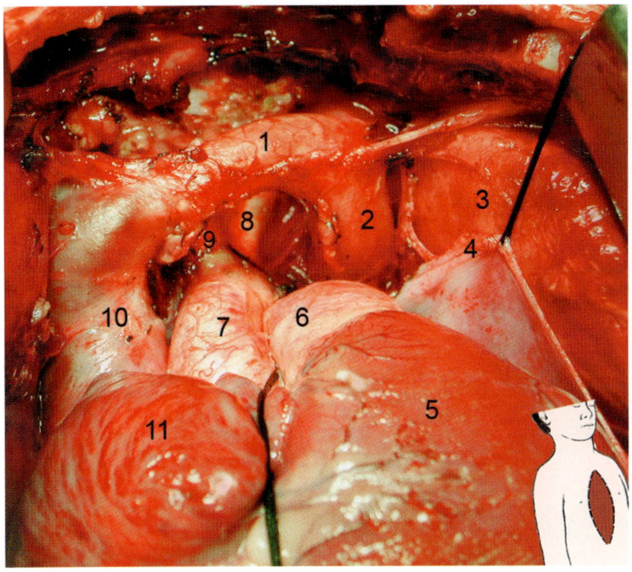

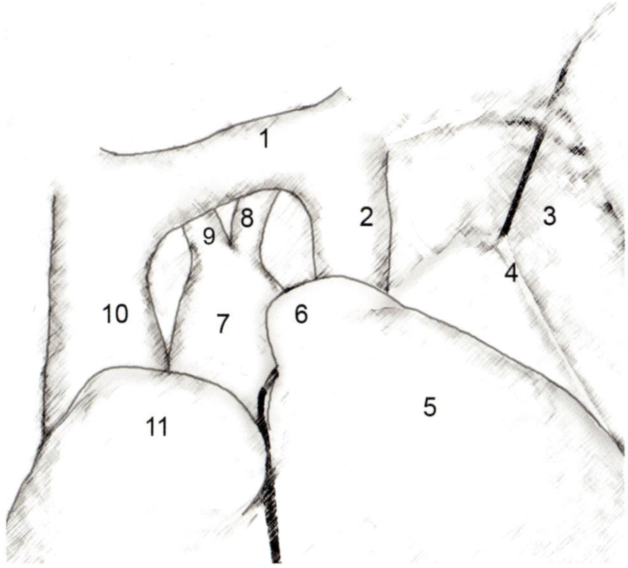

Figure 12.19 **Figure 12.20**

TAPVC to the SVC via a vertical vein as seen through a median sternotomy in a 6-month-old infant.

1. Innominate vein
2. Vertical vein
3. Left lung
4. Pericardium
5. RV
6. Main pulmonary artery (MPA)
7. Ascending aorta
8. Left common carotid artery
9. Innominate artery
10. SVC
11. RAA

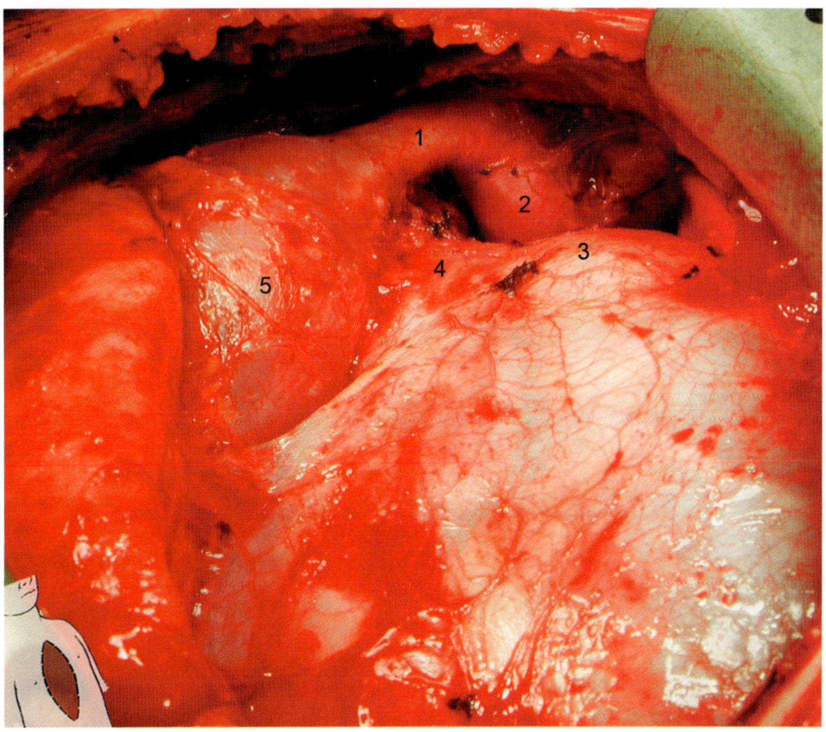

Figure 12.21. Supracardiac TAPVC to SVC in an 18-month-old child. The veins are stenosed at 2 levels shown here (1) and in Figure 12.22. Note the aneurysmal dilatation of the innominate vein.

1. Innominate vein
2. Vertical vein
3. MPA
4. Ascending aorta
5. Innominate vein with aneurysmal dilatation

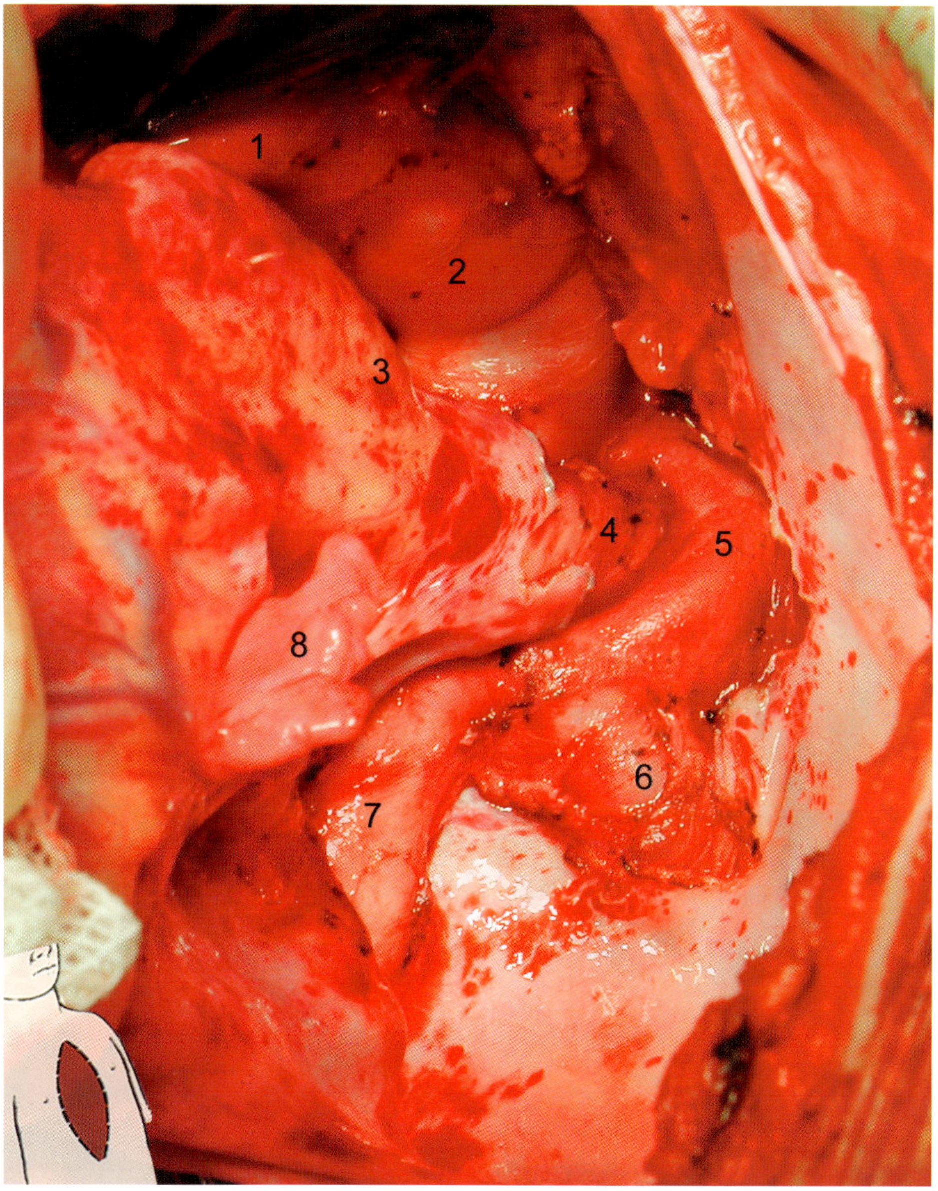

Figure 12.22. Same patient as in Figure 12.21. The heart is retracted rightward for a better view of the vertical vein. There is stenosis of the vertical vein where it passes anterior to the left PA. Note the dilated segment (2) distal to the stenosis. See Figure 12.23 for a diagrammatic illustration.

1. Innominate vein
2. Dilated segment of vertical vein
3. MPA
4. Left PA
5. Vertical vein
6. Confluence of left PVs
7. Confluence of right PVs
8. LAA

revealed TAPVC to the innominate vein, not diagnosed preoperatively. This was repaired in the same session.

One of the important long-term complications of anomalous pulmonary venous connections is the development of PV stenosis. The so-called "sutureless technique" has been devised to tackle this issue.[5] A pedicle of pericardium is sutured *in situ* to the left atrial wall around the veins (Figure 12.42), a technique that has some resemblance to the reconstruction of the neo-left atrium in the Senning atrial switch.

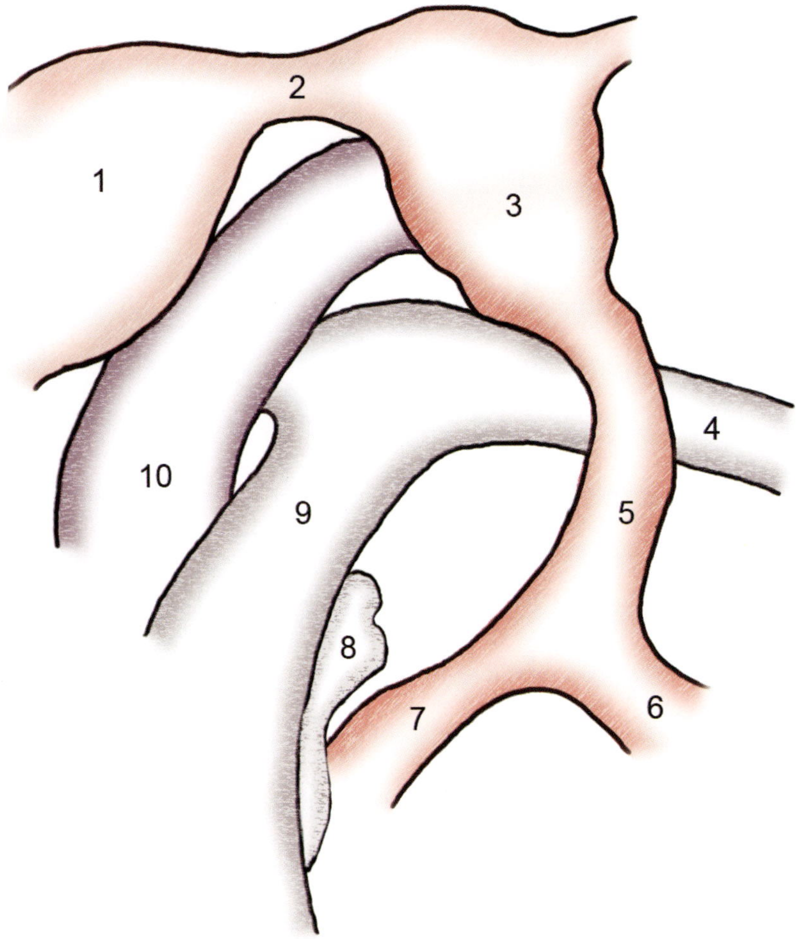

Figure 12.23. Schematic illustration of the anatomy shown in Figures 12.21 and 12.22. There is narrowing at 2 levels: where the vertical vein passes anterior to the left PA and in the innominate vein.

1. Innominate vein with aneurysmal dilatation
2. Narrow segment of innominate vein
3. Dilated segment of vertical vein
4. Left PA
5. Vertical vein
6. Confluence of left PVs
7. Confluence of right PVs
8. LAA
9. MPA
10. Ascending aorta

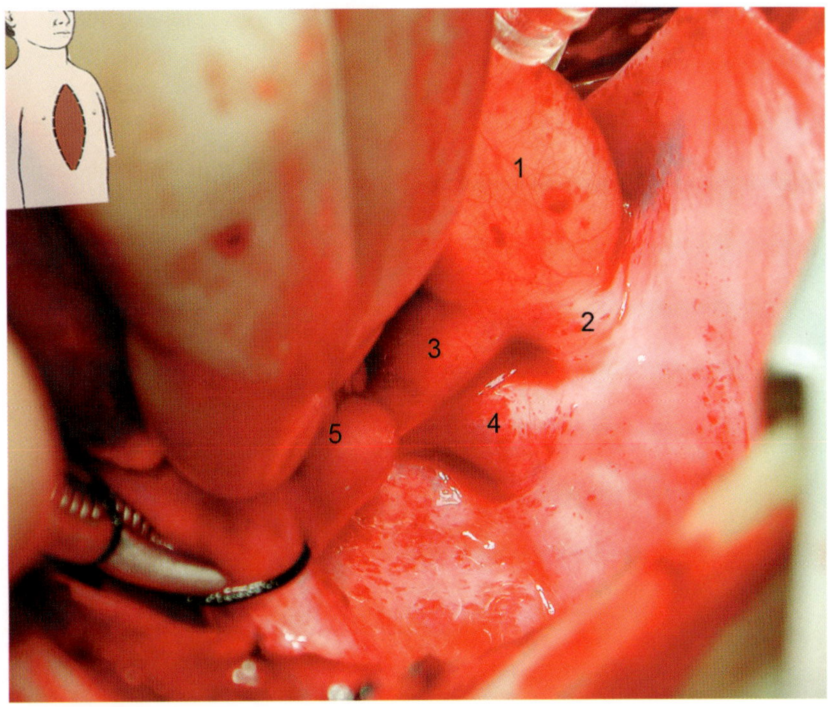

Figure 12.24. Supracardiac TAPVC to the SVC seen through a median sternotomy in a 5-month-old infant. The pulmonary venous confluence (4) is seen behind the heart just inferior to the bifurcation of PA.

1. MPA
2. Left PA
3. Right PA
4. Pulmonary venous confluence
5. Left atrium

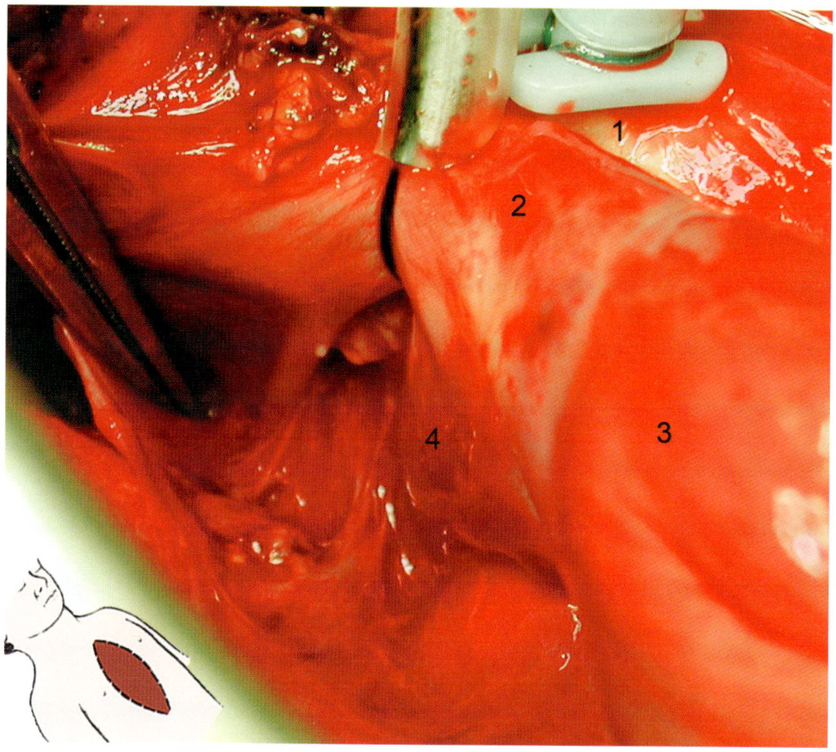

Figure 12.25. The same patient as in Figure 12.24. The SVC is retracted upward and leftward. The pulmonary venous confluence drains directly to the SVC immediately above its junction with the right atrium.

1. Ascending aorta
2. SVC
3. Right atrium
4. Connection of the pulmonary venous confluence to the right atrium

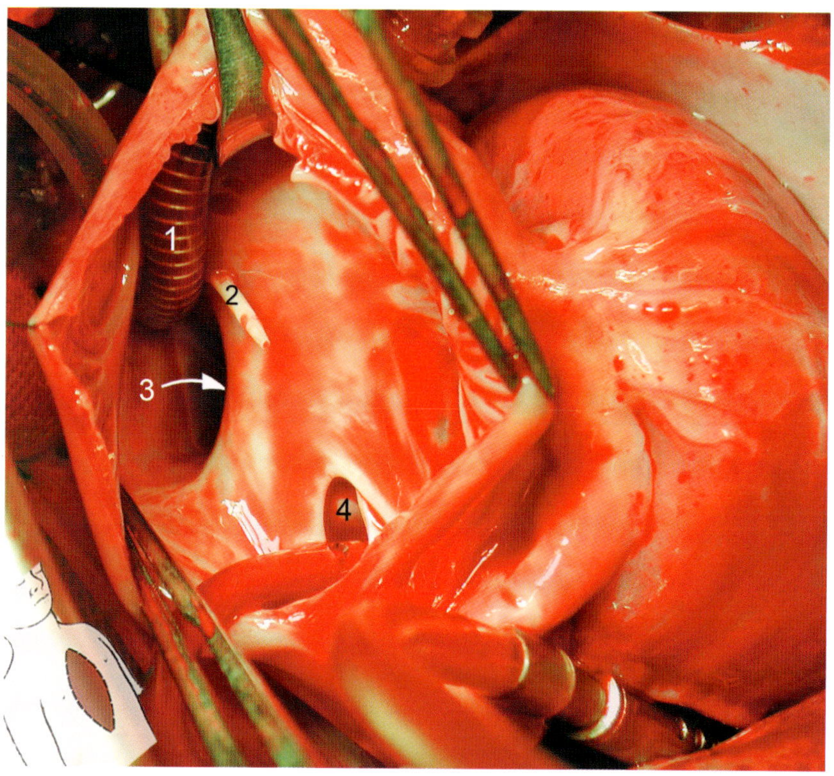

Figure 12.26. The same patient as in Figures 12.24 and 12.25 viewed from within the right atrium. The pulmonary venous confluence drains directly to the SVC immediately above its junction with the right atrium.

1. SVC venous cannula
2. Central venous catheter
3. Opening of pulmonary venous confluence
4. Foramen ovale

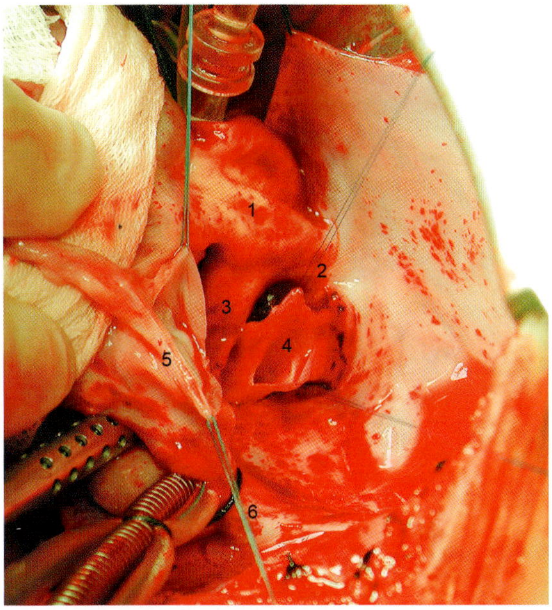

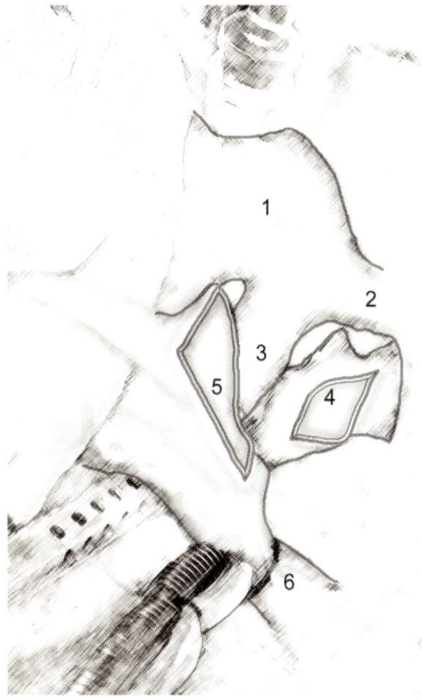

Figure 12.27 **Figure 12.28**

The same patient as in Figures 12.24 to 12.26. The heart is retracted rightward. On cardiopulmonary bypass, incisions are made in adjacent areas of the pulmonary venous confluence and left atrium.

1. MPA
2. Left PA
3. Right PA
4. Pulmonary venous confluence
5. Left atrium
6. Inferior vena cava (IVC)

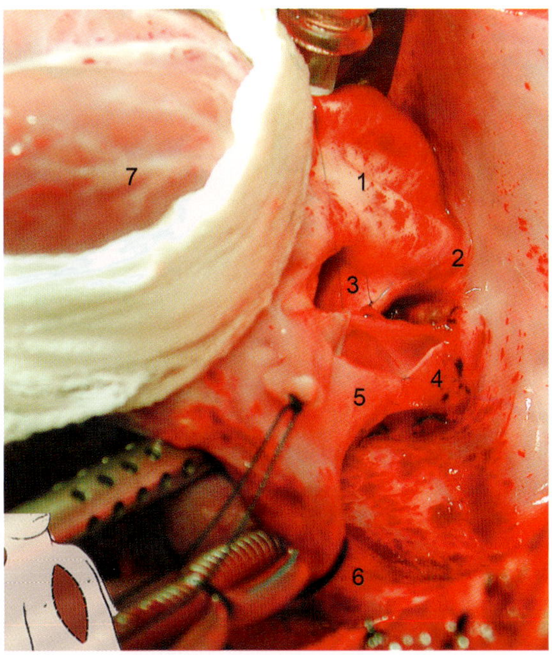

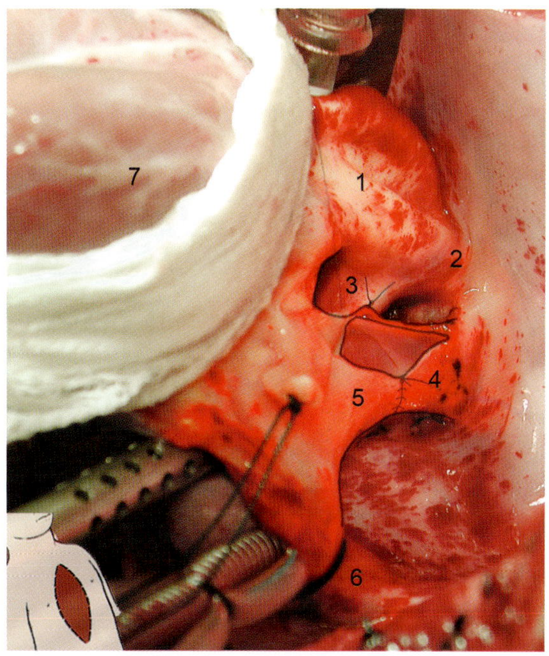

Figure 12.29 **Figure 12.30**

The same patient as in Figures 12.24 to 12.28. The pulmonary venous confluence is being anastomosed to the left atrium. In Figure 12.30, the area of anastomosis and the sutures are outlined in ink.

1. MPA
2. Left PA
3. Right PA
4. Pulmonary venous confluence
5. Left atrium
6. IVC
7. The heart retracted rightward

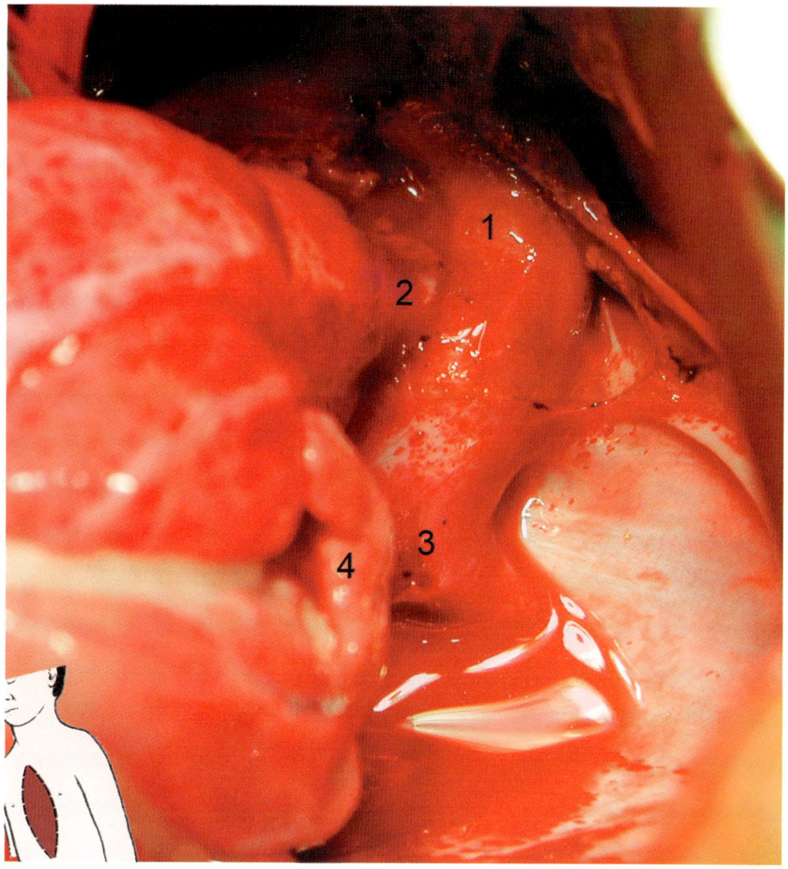

Figure 12.31. Supracardiac TAPVC in a 4-month-old infant as seen through a median sternotomy. The PVs join to form a confluence behind the left atrium and then drain via the vertical vein to the innominate vein.

1. Vertical vein
2. Left PA
3. Pulmonary venous confluence
4. LAA

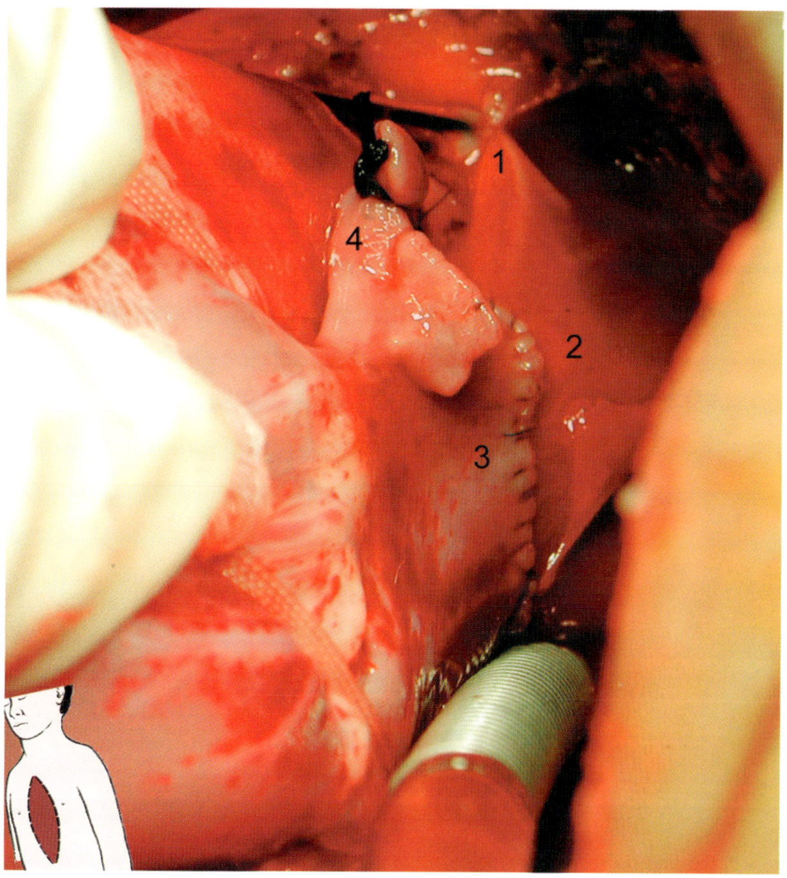

Figure 12.32. The same patient as in Figure 12.31 after repair. The venous confluence was anastomosed to the left atrium and the vertical vein was ligated.

1. Vertical vein
2. Pulmonary venous confluence
3. Left atrium
4. LAA

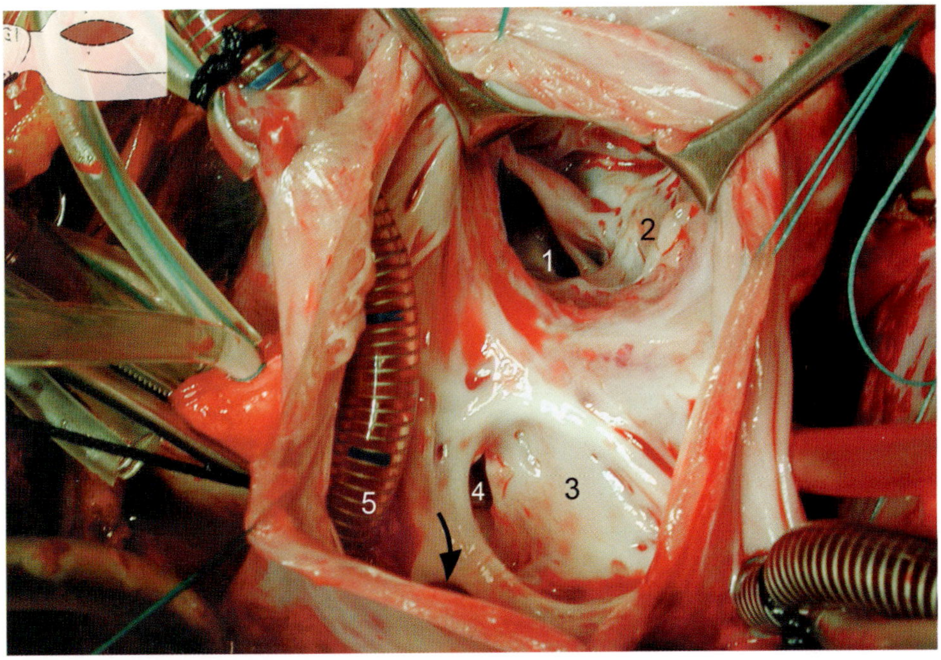

Figure 12.33. Right atriotomy view of an 8-month-old infant with cardiac anomalous pulmonary venous connection and 2 VSDs (outlet and inlet defects). The right atrium is markedly dilated. The arrow points to the entrance of one of the anomalous PVs (further shown in Figures 12.34 and 12.35).

1. Inlet VSD
2. Tricuspid valve
3. Fossa ovalis
4. Patent foramen ovale
5. Venous cannula draining the SVC

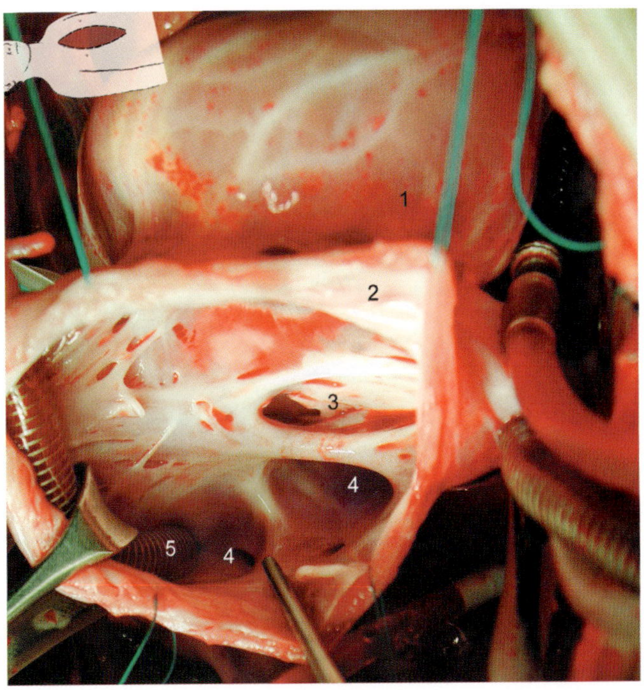

Figure 12.34

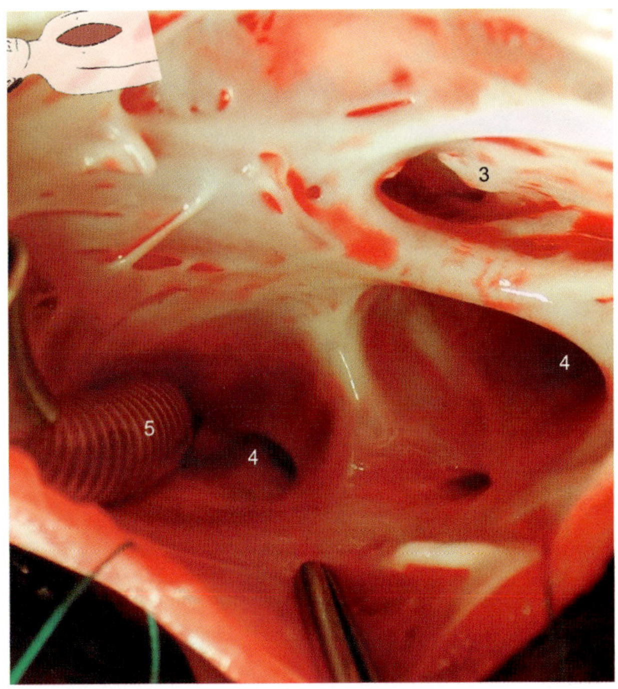

Figure 12.35

The same patient as in Figure 12.33. The right atrial wall is retracted to show the openings of the PVs. Figure 12.35 is a close-up view of the openings of the PVs.

1. RV
2. Right atrial wall
3. Fossa ovalis
4. Openings of anomalous PVs
5. SVC cannula

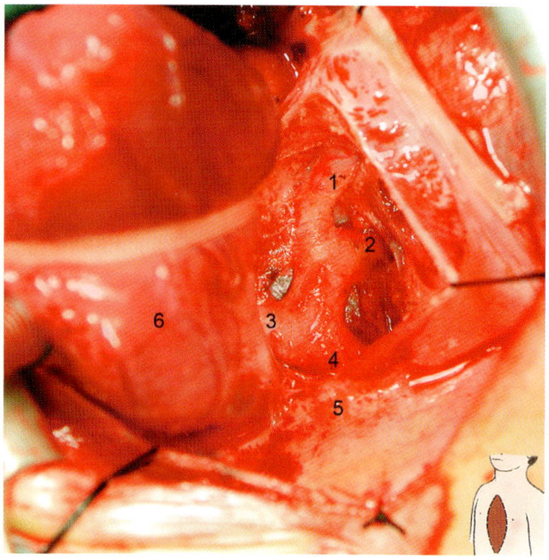

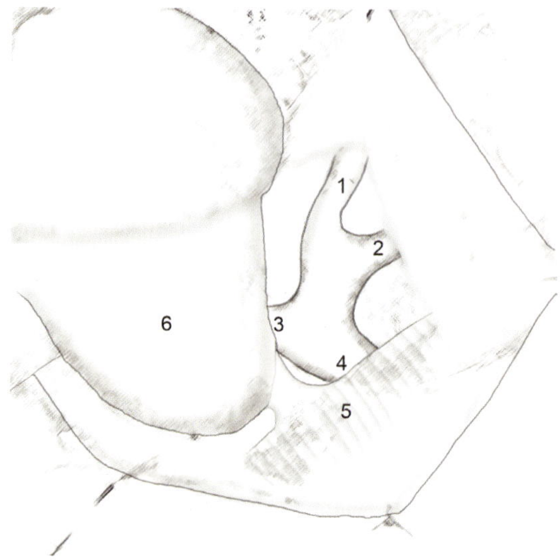

Figure 12.36 **Figure 12.37**

Infracardiac TAPVC in a 3-day-old neonate. The vertical vein descends downward to the abdomen through the diaphragm. It drains into the portal vein (not shown).

1. Left upper PV
2. Left lower PV
3. Confluence of right PVs
4. Vertical vein
5. Pericardium overlying the diaphragm
6. The heart retracted rightward

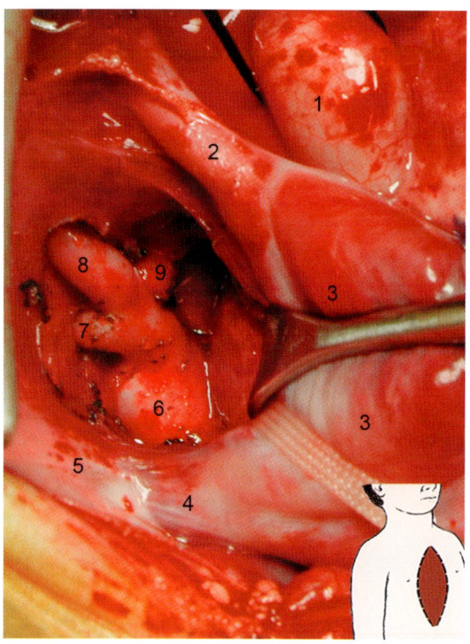

Figure 12.38. TAPVC in a 19-day-old neonate, median sternotomy view with the heart retracted leftward. This was a mixed type; 3 veins were draining infradiaphragmatically, whereas the left lower PV (not shown) was draining to the coronary sinus.

1. Ascending aorta
2. SVC
3. Right atrium
4. IVC
5. Diaphragmatic surface
6. Vertical vein
7. Right lower PV
8. Right upper PV
9. Left upper PV

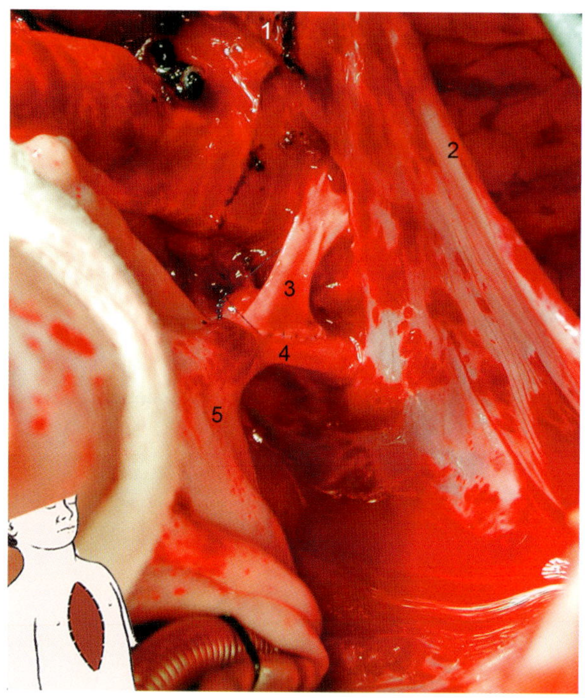

Figure 12.39. Mixed-type supracardiac TAPVC in a 4-month-old infant. The left upper PV was connected to the innominate vein via a vertical vein, whereas the other 3 veins joined to form a confluence that connected to the coronary sinus. The vertical vein was divided, turned down, and anastomosed to the pulmonary venous confluence.

1. Innominate vein
2. Pericardium
3. Vertical vein—divided, turned down, and anastomosed to the confluence
4. Pulmonary venous confluence
5. Left atrium

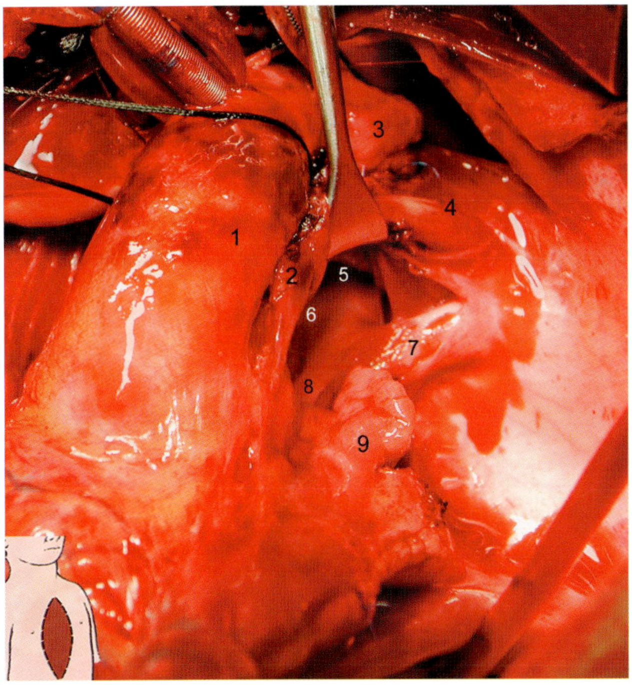

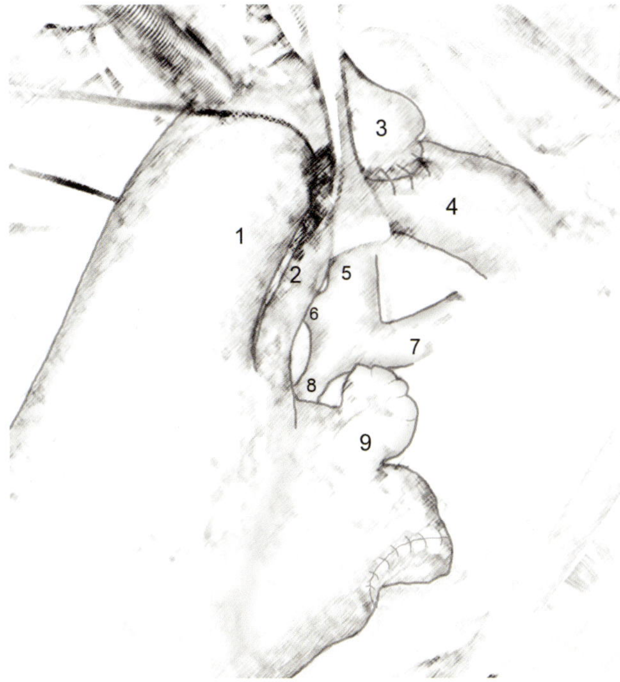

Figure 12.40 **Figure 12.41**

Supracardiac TAPVC to innominate vein in a 6-year-old child with unbalanced AVSD and severe pulmonary stenosis. A Glenn shunt has already been performed (see text).

1. Ascending aorta
2. MPA
3. SVC (left sided)
4. Left PA
5. Vertical vein
6. Right upper PV
7. Left upper PV
8. Right lower PV
9. LAA

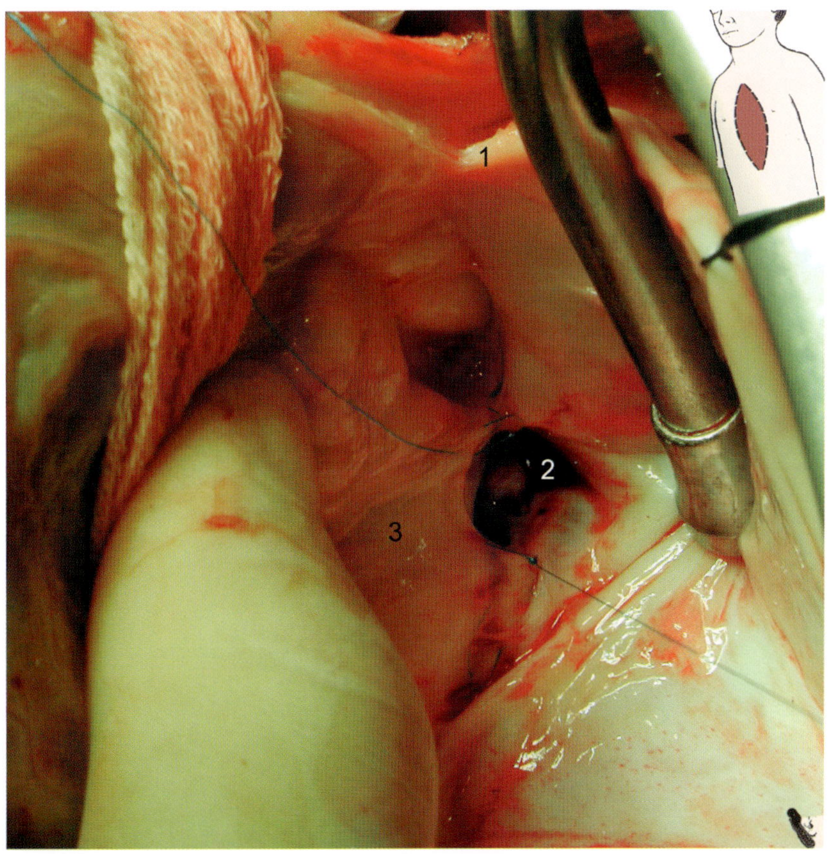

Figure 12.42. Intraoperative view of a child with TAPVC who developed PV stenosis a few months after repair. The vein has been split open and a pedicle of *in situ* pericardium is being sutured to the left atrial wall around the vein, affecting the so-called "sutureless anastomosis."

1. Pericardium
2. PV
3. Left atrium

REFERENCES

1. Van Praagh S, Carrera ME, Sanders SP, et al. Sinus venosus defects: unroofing of the right pulmonary veins anatomic and echocardiographic findings and surgical treatment. *Am Heart J.* 1994;128:365–379.
2. Burroughs JT, Edwards JE. Total anomalous pulmonary venous connection. *Am Heart J.* 1960;59:913–931.
3. McCrindle BW, Parikh A, Gow RM, Williams WG, Freedom RM. Outcomes of total anomalous pulmonary venous drainage—340 cases. Annual meeting of the AEPC. *Cardiol Young.* 2000;10(Suppl 2):43–44.
4. Heineman MK, Hanley FL, Van Praagh S, et al. Total anomalous pulmonary venous drainage in newborns with visceral heterotaxy. *Ann Thorac Surg.* 1994;57:88–91.
5. Najm H, Caldarone CA, Smallhorn JF, Coles JG. A sutureless technique for the relief of pulmonary vein stenosis with the use of *in situ* pericardium. *J Thorac Cardiovasc Surg.* 1998;115:468–470.

CHAPTER 13

Tetralogy of Fallot

Tetralogy of Fallot (TOF) is the most common cyanotic congenital heart disease.[1] The classic 4 lesions that constitute the tetralogy are right ventricular outflow tract (RVOT) obstruction, ventricular septal defect (VSD), overriding of the aorta, and right ventricle (RV) hypertrophy. The classical substrate of muscular subpulmonary obstruction is antero-cephalad deviation of the outlet septum. Hypertrophy of septo-parietal trabeculations exacerbates the obstruction. Most commonly, the VSD is perimembranous and the atrioventricular (AV) conduction bundle is in the immediate vicinity of its postero-inferior margin. The spectrum of the disease ranges from "pink tetralogy," in which there is minimal pulmonic stenosis, to pulmonary atresia with VSD. Absent pulmonary valve syndrome shares some of the above features and is considered a variant of TOF. TOF with pulmonary atresia will be discussed along with pulmonary atresia in chapter 14.

The disease may not be manifest at birth, but as the degree of RV outflow obstruction increases, the clinical features become apparent. There is controversy over the choice of surgical intervention when a patient becomes cyanosed in the neonatal period or early infancy. Classically, a two-stage approach was employed with an initial systemic-to-pulmonary arterial shunt, to be followed later by complete repair. This approach is still popular among many surgeons, but many centers prefer a single-stage complete repair, even in small infants.[2]

SYSTEMIC-TO-PULMONARY ARTERIAL SHUNT

The most popular type of systemic-to-pulmonary arterial shunt is a modified Blalock-Taussig (BT) shunt. The shunt is usually placed between the subclavian artery and the ipsilateral pulmonary artery (PA) through a lateral thoracotomy approach. Figures 13.1 to 13.8 are from a 5-day-old neonate with TOF and severe pulmonary stenosis. The aortic arch was right sided. An atypically long and narrow left-sided ductus supplied blood to the pulmonary tree (Figure 13.1). A right-modified BT shunt was placed between the right subclavian artery and the right PA (Figures 13.2–13.8). Figures 13.9 to 13.11 are from a 5-month-old infant with TOF, a right aortic arch, and a retro-aortic innominate vein. A left-modified BT shunt was placed between the left subclavian artery and the left PA. Further examples of BT shunts are shown in chapter 14.

COMPLETE REPAIR

Complete repair is performed via a standard median sternotomy and right atriotomy or right ventriculotomy according to the surgeon's preference and details of the anatomy. The VSD is closed and the RV outflow obstruction is relieved. The pulmonary valvar stenosis may be relieved by valvotomy, transannular patch, or valve replacement according to the severity of the stenosis. The main and branch PAs may need to be augmented.

Figure 13.12 shows the gross outside anatomy of TOF as seen through a median sternotomy before cardiopulmonary bypass in a 5-month-old infant. Ventriculotomy through the RVOT (infundibulotomy) will expose the subpulmonary obstruction, examples of which are shown in Figures 13.13 to 13.15. The area of stenosis can also be exposed through a right atriotomy as shown in Figure 13.16. After relief of the outflow obstruction, the VSD is closed, as shown in Figures 13.17 to 13.19.

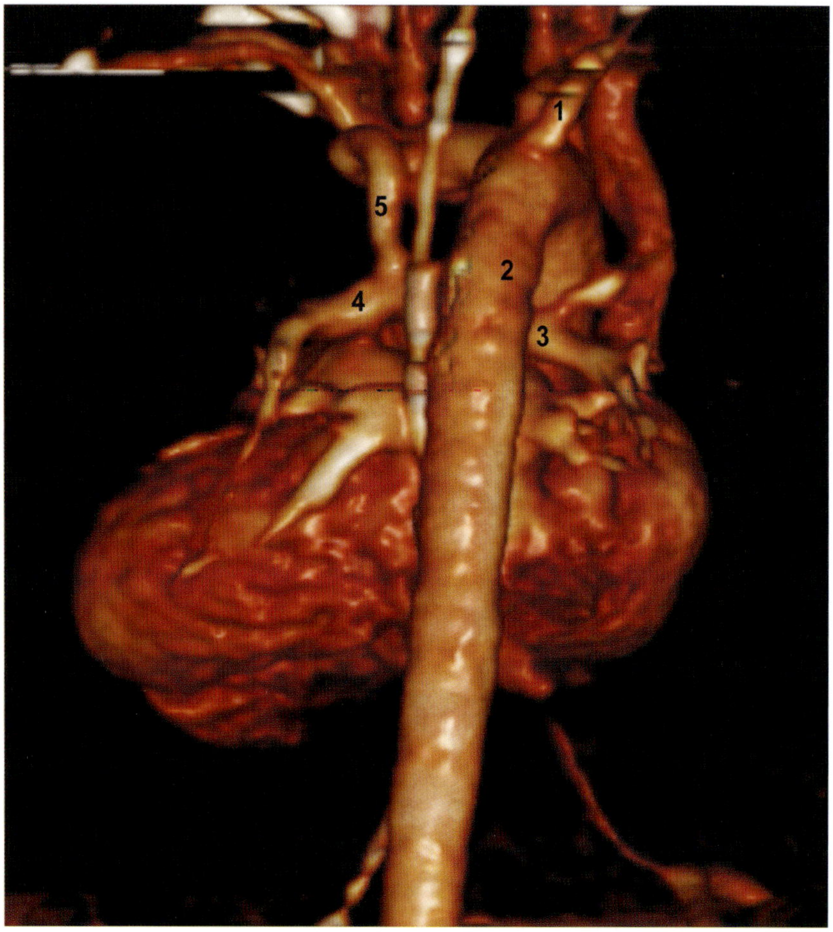

Figure 13.1. A reconstructed computed tomography (CT) image from a 5-day-old neonate with TOF and severe pulmonary stenosis. A posterior view is shown. The aortic arch is right sided, and a long and narrow ductus (5) connects the left subclavian artery to the left PA.

1. Right subclavian artery
2. Descending thoracic aorta
3. Right PA
4. Left PA
5. Ductus

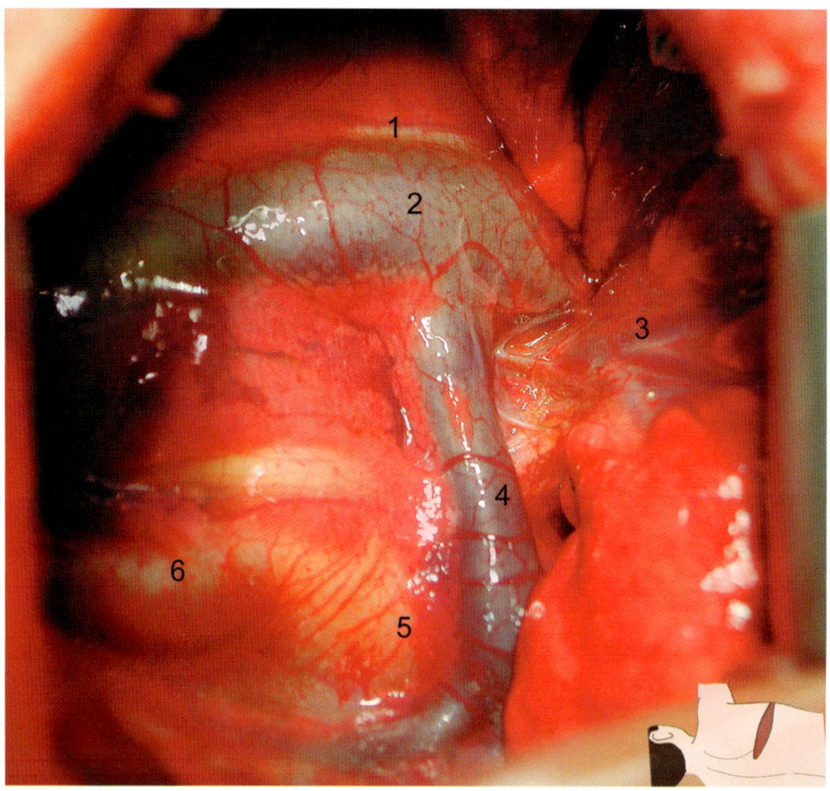

Figure 13.2. Right lateral thoracotomy view of the same patient whose CT image is shown in Figure 13.1. The right lung is retracted downward. The mediastinal structures and right aortic arch are covered by pleura.

1. Right phrenic nerve
2. Superior vena cava (SVC)
3. Hilum of right lung
4. Azygos vein
5. Descending thoracic aorta
6. Right subclavian artery

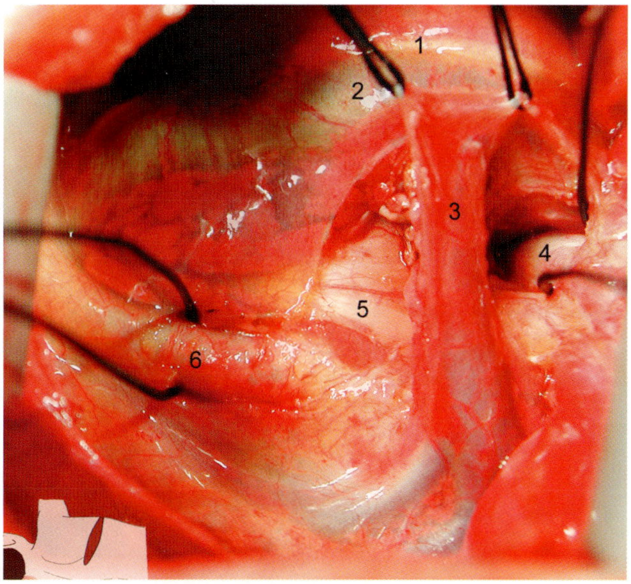

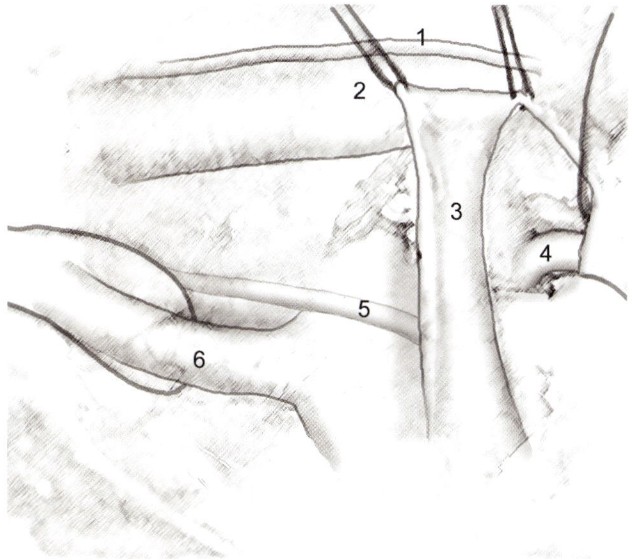

Figure 13.3 **Figure 13.4**

The same patient as in Figures 13.1 and 13.2. The mediastinal pleura have been opened. The azygos vein and right PA have been dissected and mobilized. Note the small size of the right PA.

1. Right phrenic nerve
2. SVC
3. Azygos vein
4. Right PA
5. Right vagus nerve
6. Right subclavian artery

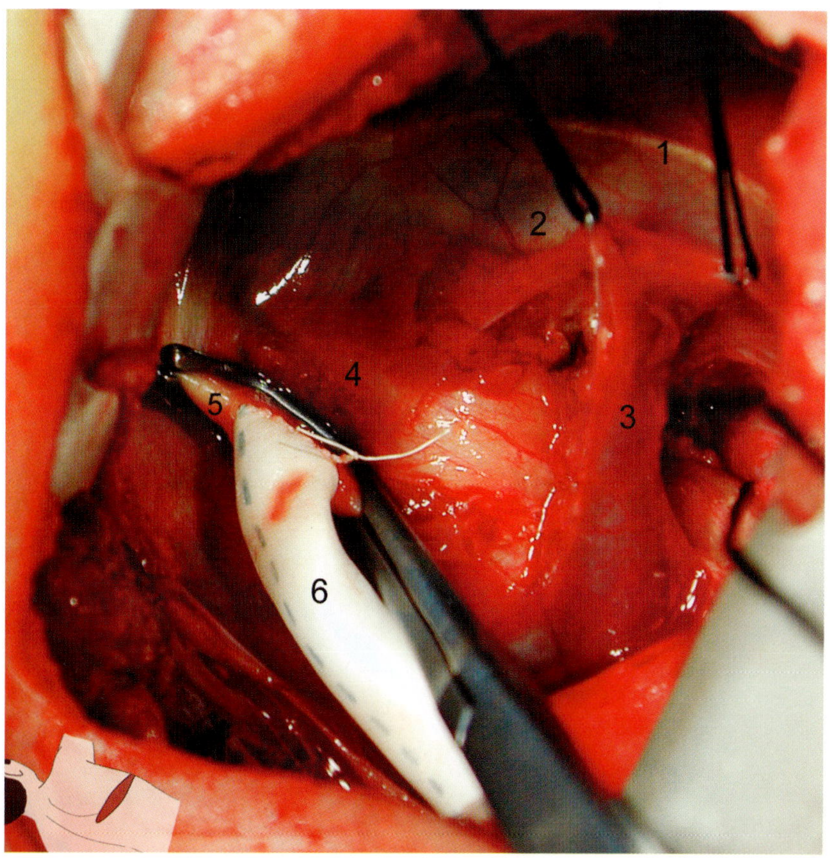

Figure 13.5. The same patient as in Figures 13.1 to 13.4. A 4 mm ePTFE (Gore-Tex) tube graft is used to construct the shunt. The systemic end of the shunt has already been anastomosed to the right subclavian artery using continuous sutures.

1. Right phrenic nerve
2. SVC
3. Azygos vein
4. Right vagus nerve
5. Right subclavian artery (clamped)
6. Tube graft (4 mm ePTFE)

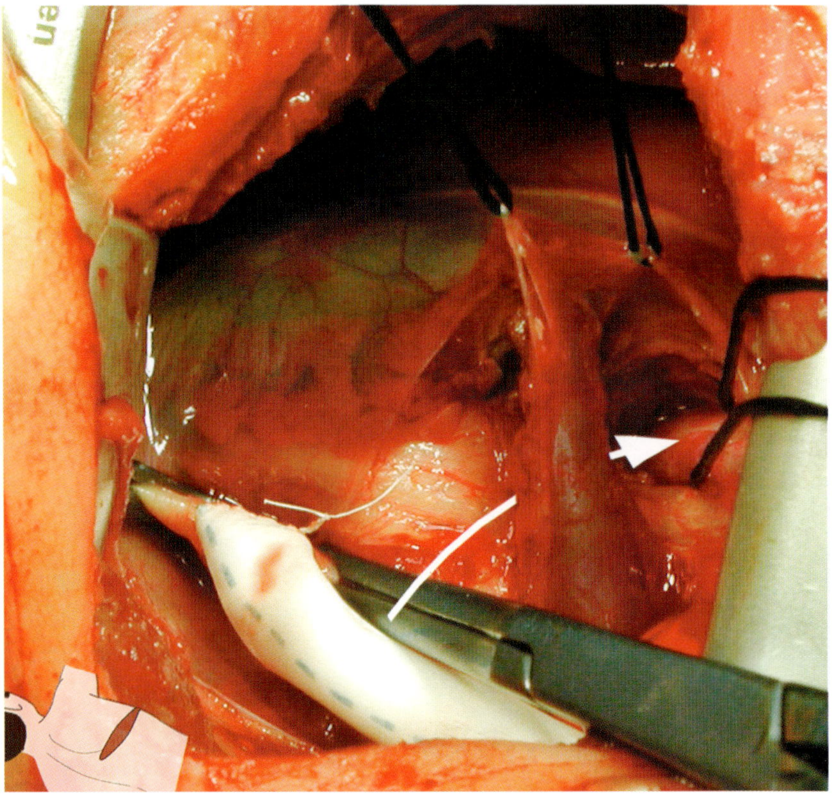

Figure 13.6. The same patient as in Figures 13.1 to 13.5. The systemic end of the shunt has already been anastomosed to the right subclavian artery. The pulmonary end will be passed medial to the azygos (arrow) to the right lung hilum, where it will be anastomosed to the right PA.

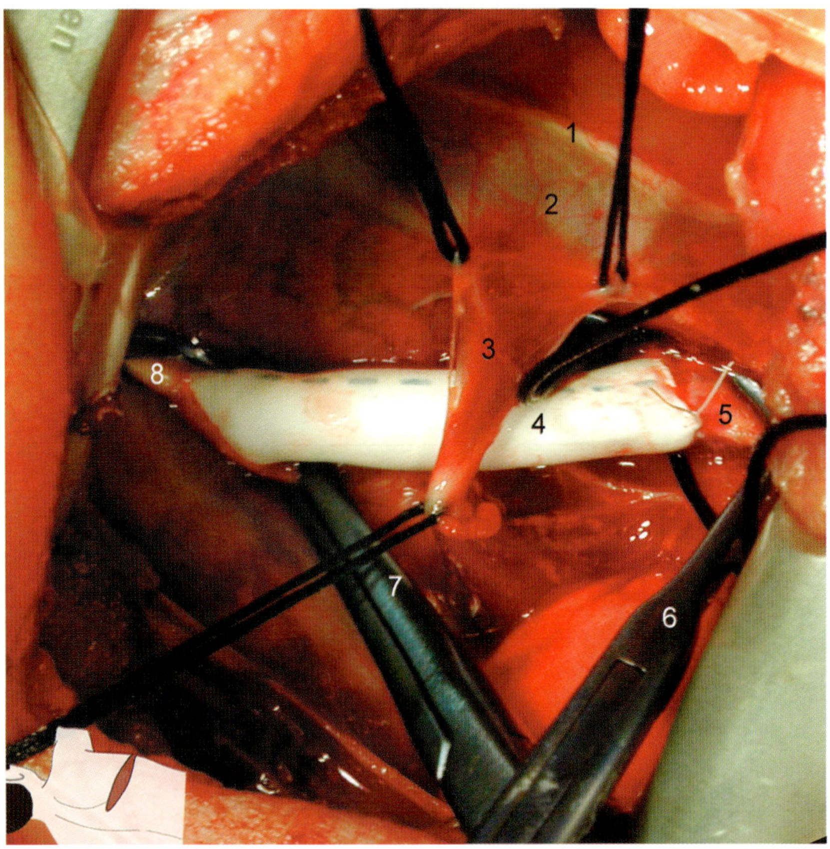

Figure 13.7. The same patient as in Figures 13.1 to 13.6. A C-shaped clamp was placed around the right PA. The graft is cut to adjust its length so that it lies straight. The pulmonary end of the shunt is then anastomosed to the right PA.

1. Right phrenic nerve
2. SVC
3. Azygos vein
4. Tube graft (4 mm ePTFE)
5. Right PA
6. Right PA clamp
7. Right subclavian artery clamp
8. Right subclavian artery

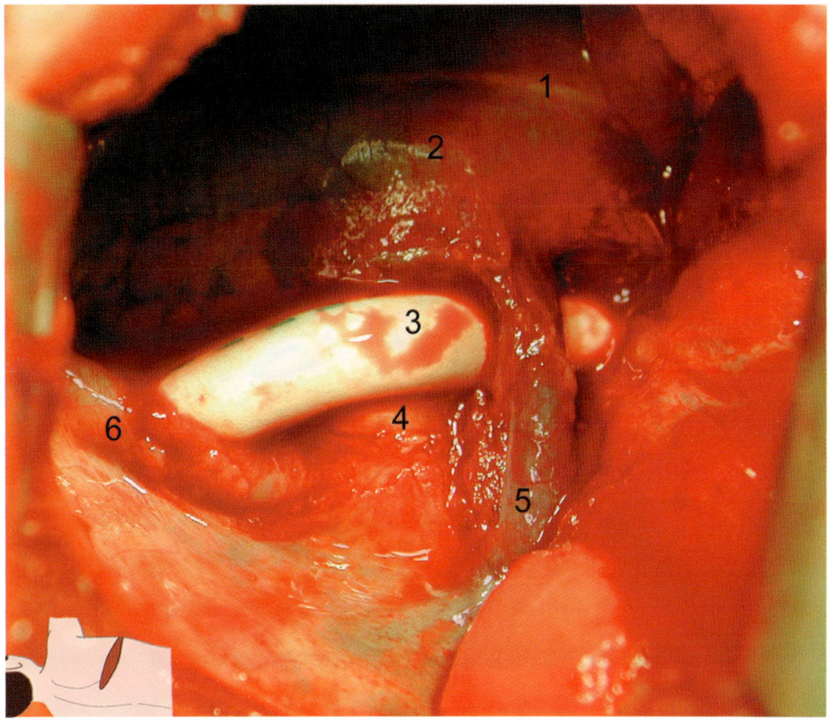

Figure 13.8. The same patient as in Figures 13.1 to 13.7. Both vascular clamps have been released. Blood is now shunted from the systemic circulation to the pulmonary circulation, circumventing the pulmonary valve stenosis.

1. Right phrenic nerve
2. SVC
3. BT shunt (4 mm ePTFE)
4. Aortic arch
5. Azygos vein
6. Right subclavian artery

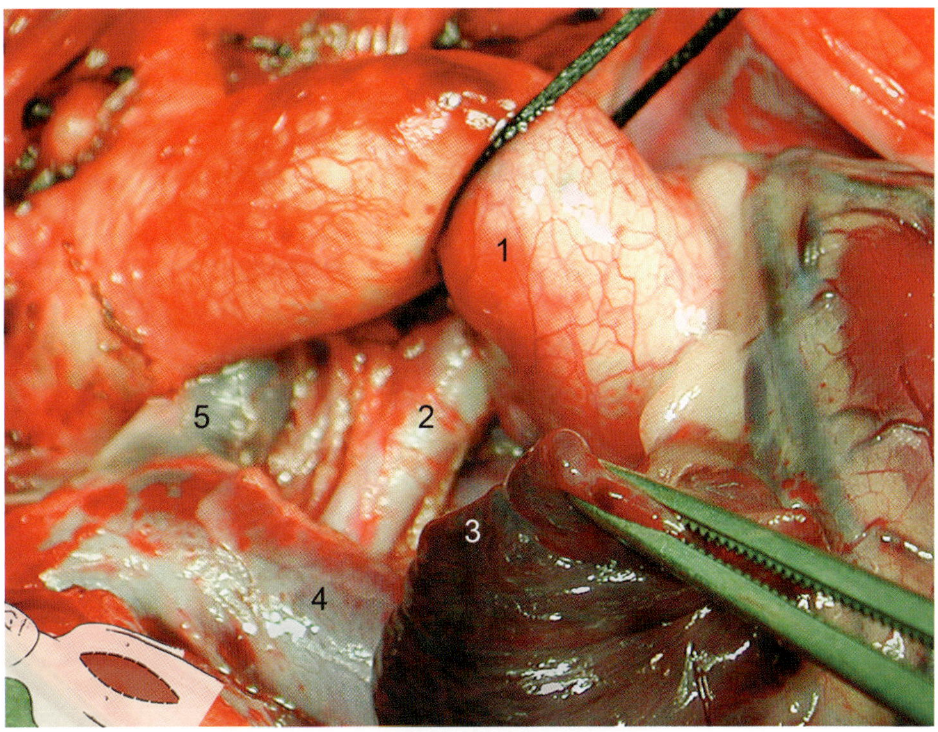

Figure 13.9. Median sternotomy view of a 5-month-old infant with TOF. The hypoplastic right PA is shown. The aortic arch is right sided. Note the retro-aortic innominate vein.

1. Ascending aorta
2. Right PA
3. Right atrial appendage (RAA)
4. SVC
5. Retro-aortic innominate vein

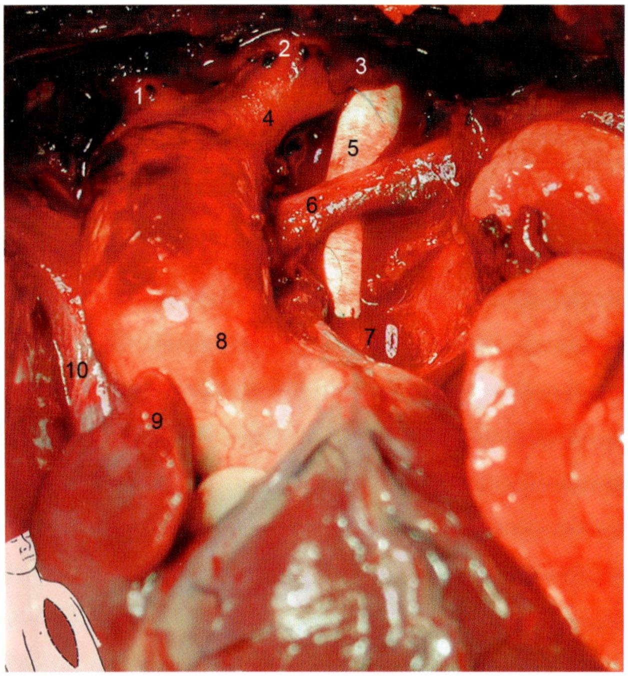

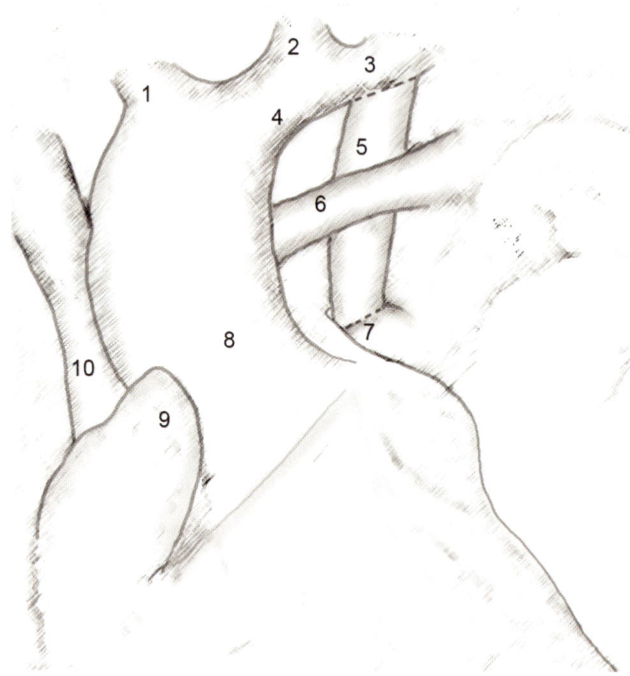

Figure 13.10 **Figure 13.11**

The same patient as in Figure 13.9. The size of the PAs was deemed too small for complete repair, so a left-modified BT shunt was placed between the left subclavian artery and the left PA. A 5 mm ePTFE tube graft was used. Note the mirror-image branching of the right aortic arch.

1. Right common carotid artery
2. Left common carotid artery
3. Left subclavian artery
4. Innominate (brachiocephalic) artery
5. Modified BT shunt (5 mm ePTFE)
6. Retro-aortic innominate vein
7. Left PA
8. Ascending aorta
9. RAA
10. SVC

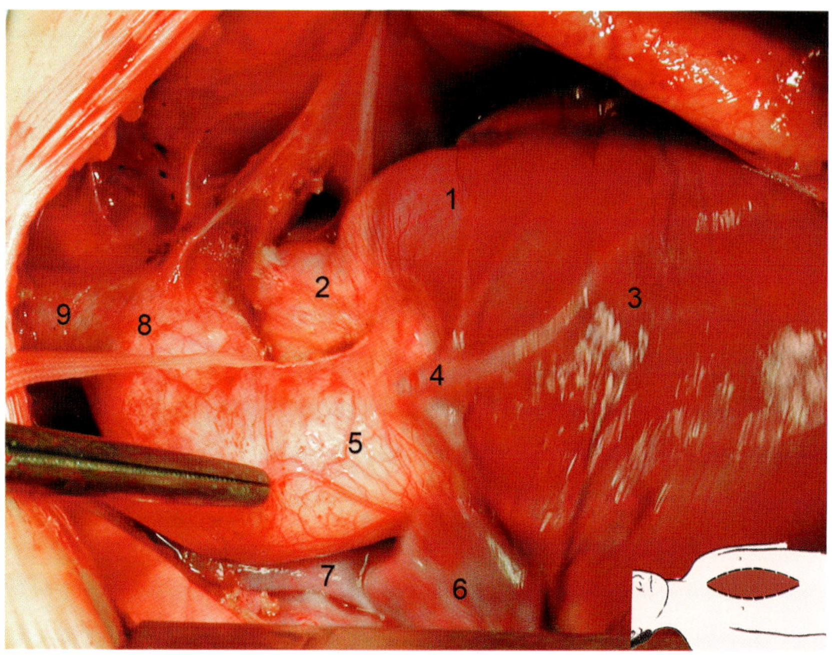

Figure 13.12. Median sternotomy view of a 5-month-old infant with TOF. The gross outside anatomy is shown.

1. Outflow part of RV
2. Main pulmonary artery (MPA)
3. RV
4. Right coronary artery and its branches
5. Ascending aorta
6. Right atrium
7. SVC
8. Transverse aortic arch
9. Innominate artery

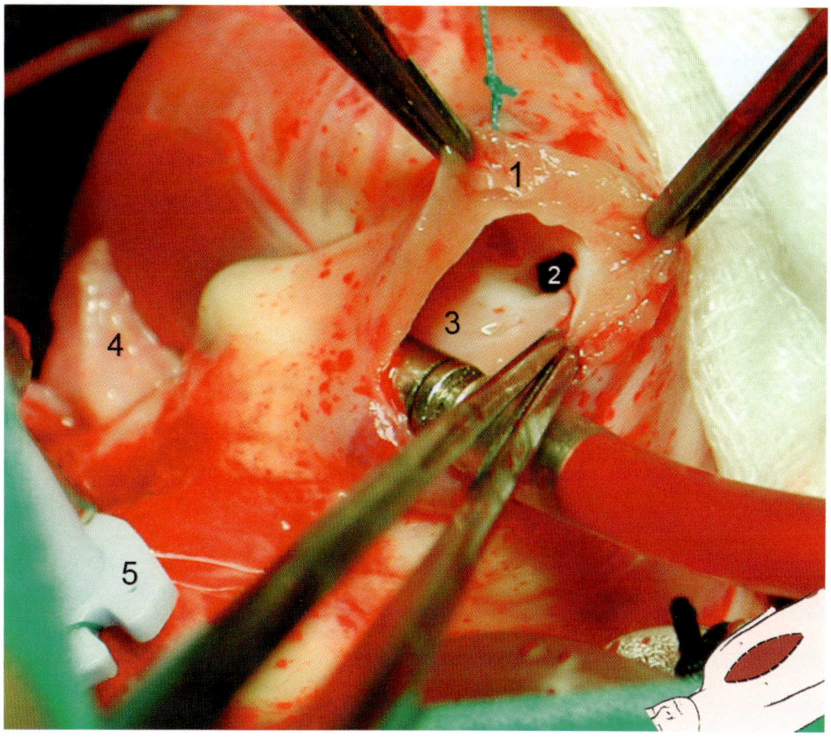

Figure 13.13. Right ventriculotomy through the RVOT in a 10-month-old infant with TOF. Note the tight infundibular stenosis.

1. Right ventriculotomy incision
2. Os infundibulum
3. Outlet septum
4. Left atrial appendage (LAA)
5. Cardioplegia catheter in ascending aorta

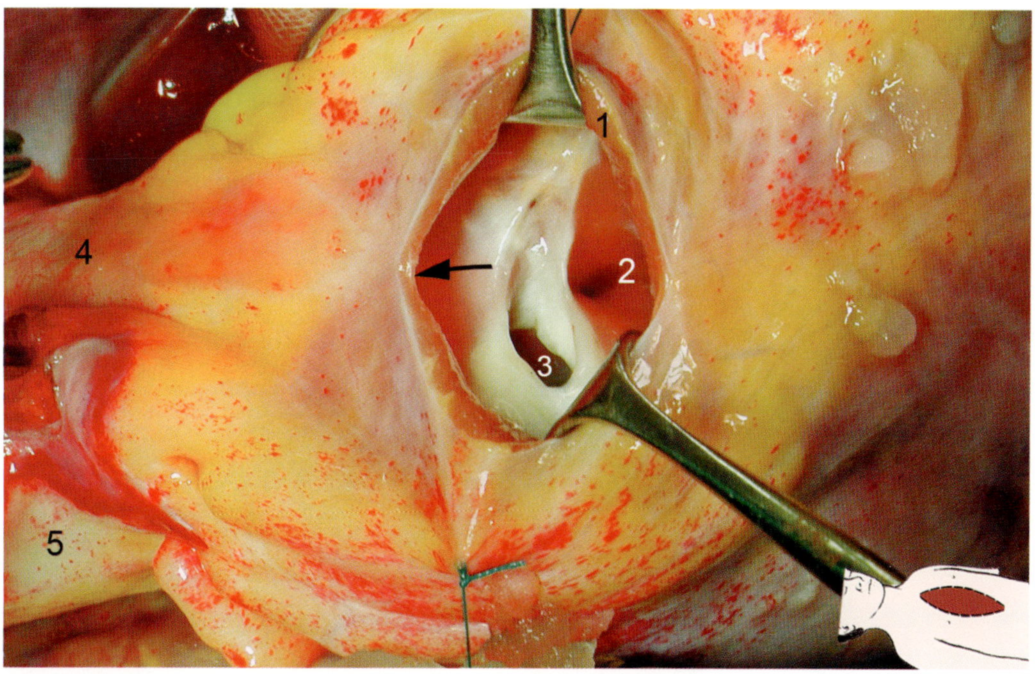

Figure 13.14. Right ventriculotomy revealing the RVOT in a 12-year-old child with TOF. In this patient, the obstruction was at the subpulmonary level and there was no pulmonary valvar stenosis. The arrow points to direction of the pulmonary valve.

1. Right ventriculotomy incision
2. Outlet part of RV
3. Os infundibulum
4. MPA
5. Ascending aorta

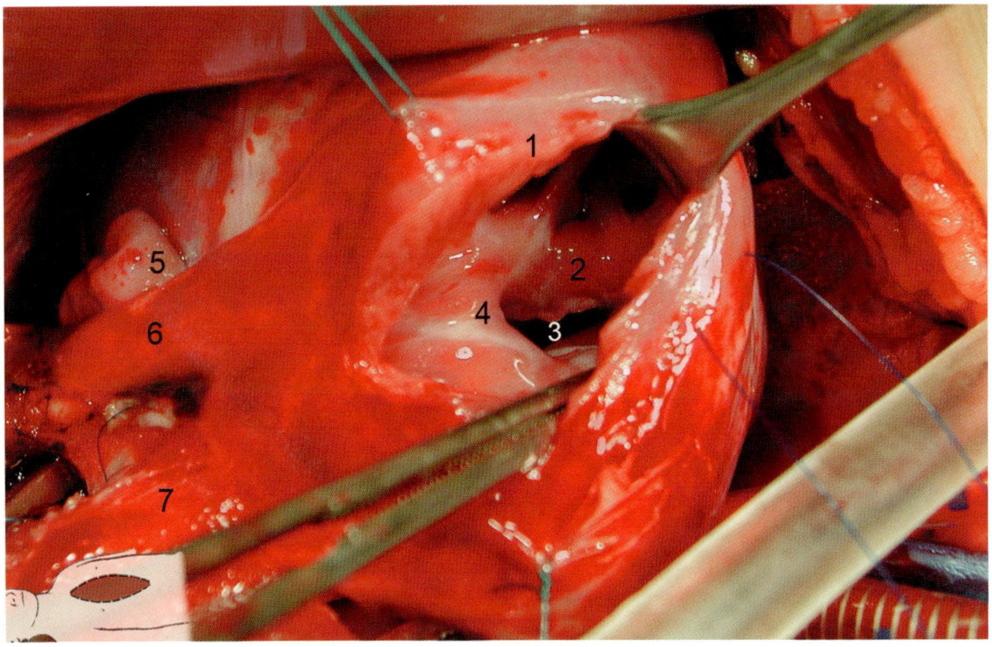

Figure 13.15. Right ventriculotomy view in a 6-month-old infant with TOF. In this patient, the obstruction was due to muscular hypertrophy at the subvalvar level. Note the hypoplastic MPA.

1. Right ventriculotomy incision
2. Septomarginal trabeculation
3. Os infundibulum
4. Outlet septum
5. LAA
6. MPA
7. Ascending aorta

Figure 13.16. Severe RV outflow stenosis as seen through a right atriotomy in a 2-year-old child with TOF. The arrow points to the VSD (not visible) behind the tricuspid valve.

1. SVC cannula passing through the RAA
2. Right atriotomy incision
3. RV outflow stenosis
4. Tricuspid valve annulus

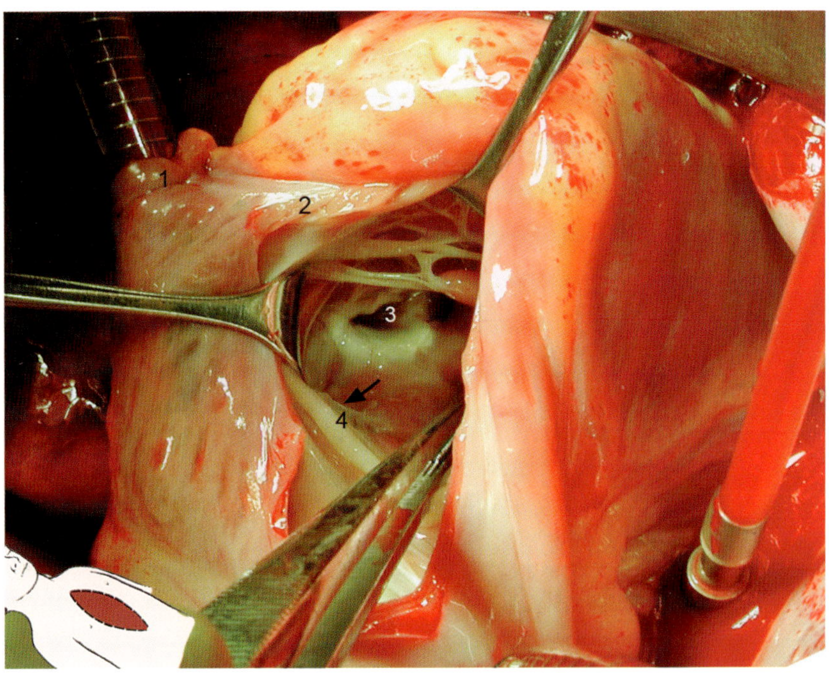

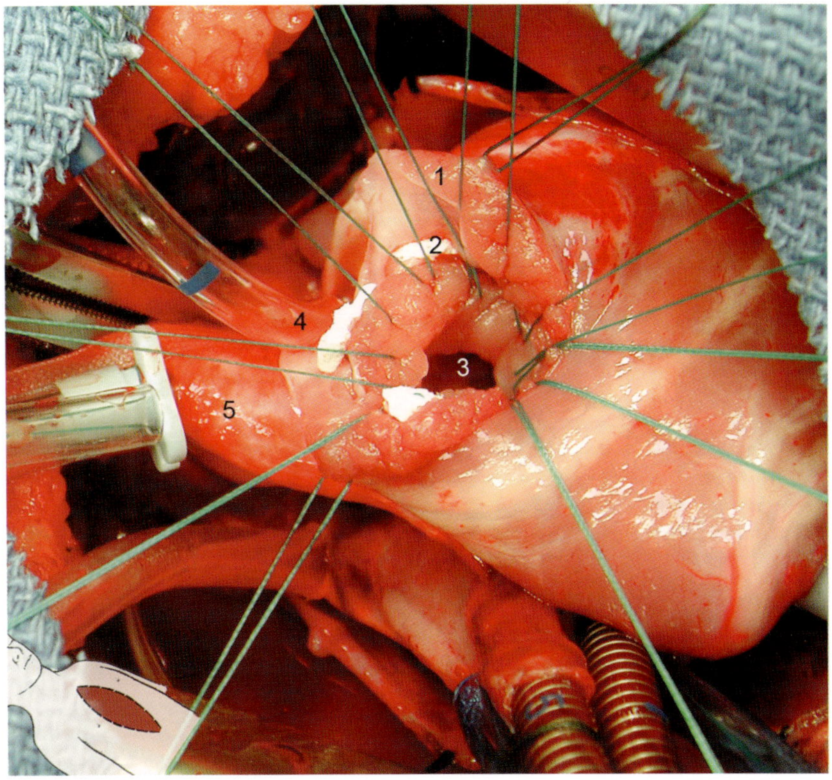

Figure 13.17. Right ventriculotomy view in a 5-month-old infant with TOF. The obstructing muscle bundles have been excised to reveal the RV outflow obstruction. Pledgets have been placed around the VSD in preparation for closure by interrupted mattress sutures and a Dacron patch.

1. Right ventriculotomy incision
2. Teflon pledgets
3. VSD
4. Suction catheter in MPA
5. Ascending aorta

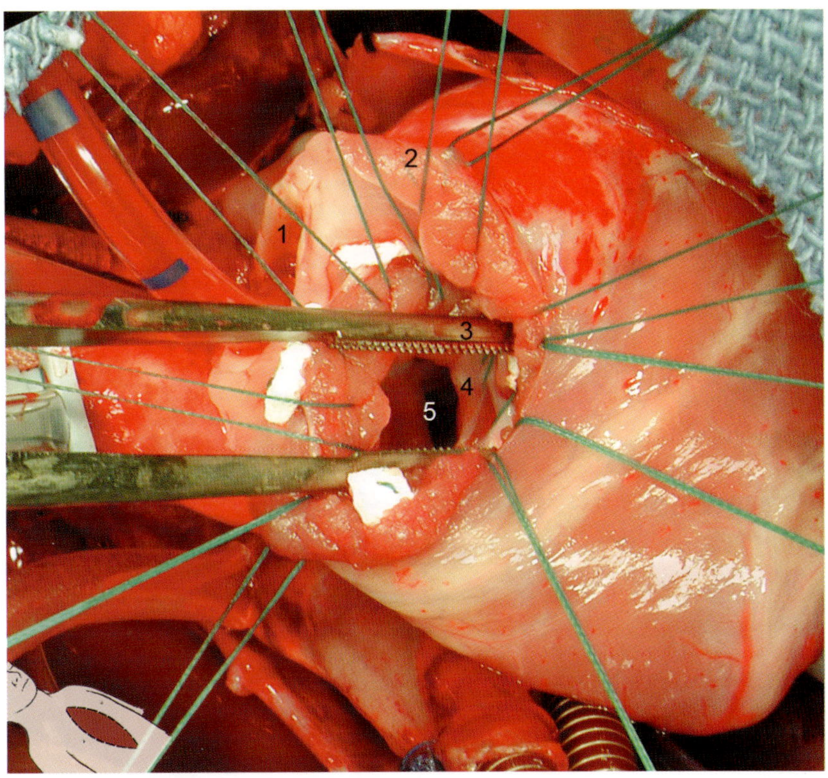

Figure 13.18. The same patient as in Figure 13.17 with forceps retracting the RVOT to reveal the lower margin of the VSD. Note the inferior pledgets of the VSD.

1. MPA
2. Right ventriculotomy incision
3. Forceps passing to RV
4. Ventricular septum and inferior margin of VSD
5. VSD

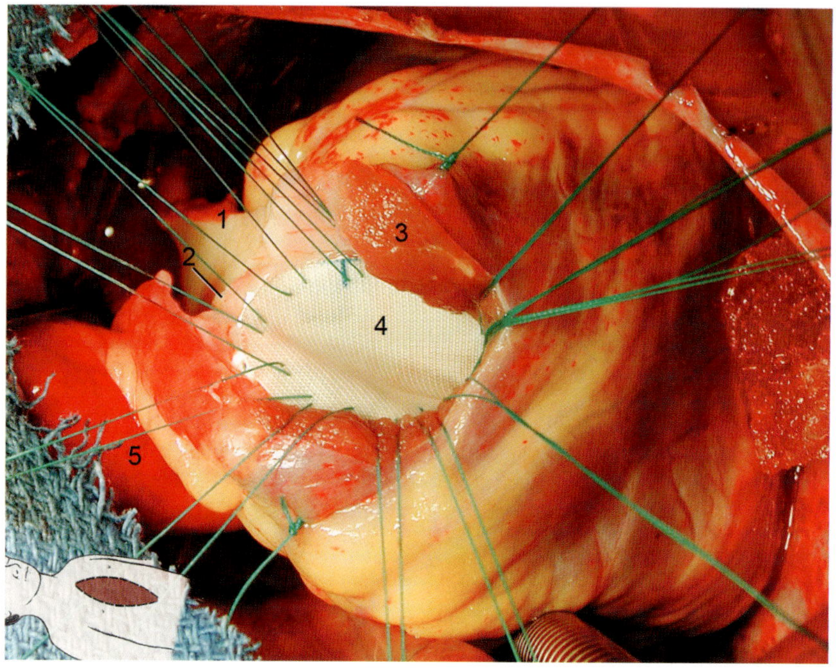

Figure 13.19. Right ventriculotomy view in a 9-year-old child with TOF during closure of the VSD using a Dacron patch and pledget-supported interrupted mattress sutures.

1. MPA
2. Pulmonary valve
3. Right ventriculotomy incision
4. Dacron patch
5. Ascending aorta

An outlet doubly committed juxtaarterial VSD is occasionally seen (Figures 13.20–13.21) and is particularly common in Asian populations.[3] Strictly speaking, this variant does not satisfy the anatomical criterion for TOF, namely, antero-cephalad deviation of the outlet septum, because this type of VSD lacks an outlet septum in its cephalad margin. Nevertheless, the obstruction to flow at the pulmonary ventriculo-arterial junction and overriding aorta confers similar physiology as TOF.

Figure 13.22 shows a transannular pericardial patch placed in a 3-year-old child with TOF to relieve

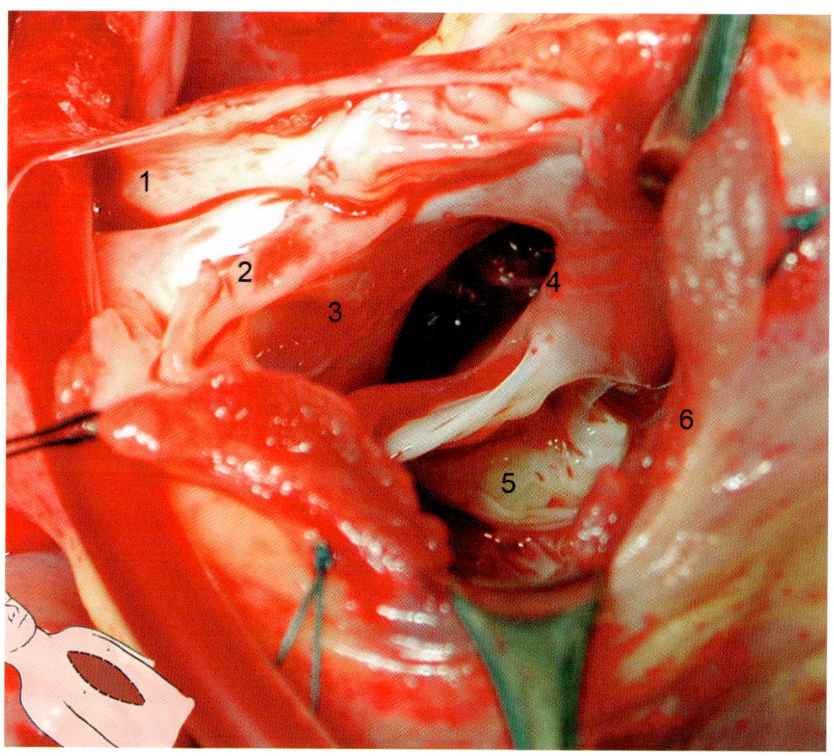

Figure 13.20. A 4-year-old child with outlet doubly committed juxtaarterial VSD as seen through a right ventriculotomy. Note that the inferior margin of the VSD is muscular, whereas the superior margin is bordered by semilunar valves.

1. Pulmonary trunk
2. Pulmonary valve
3. Aortic valve
4. Muscular inferior margin of the VSD
5. Tricuspid valve
6. Right ventriculotomy incision

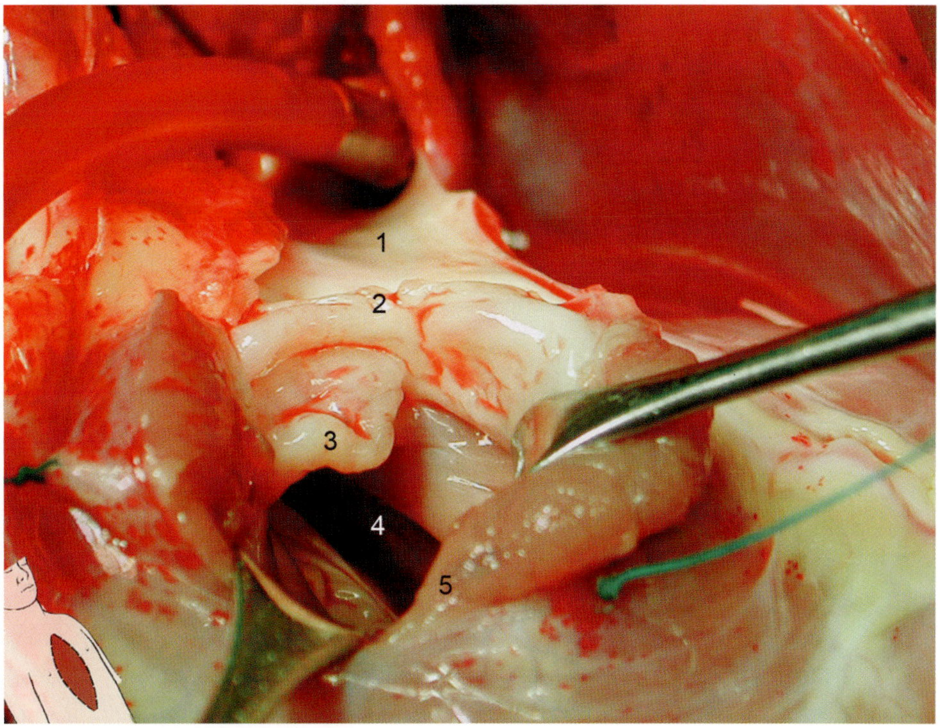

Figure 13.21. Another example of an outlet doubly committed juxtaarterial VSD in a 2-year-old child. Note the prolapsed pulmonary valve leaflet into the VSD toward the left ventricle.

1. Pulmonary trunk
2. Pulmonary valve
3. Prolapsed pulmonary valve leaflet
4. VSD
5. Right ventriculotomy incision

Figure 13.22. Median sternotomy view in a 3-year-old child after repair of TOF. Pulmonary valve stenosis has been relieved by placing a transannular pericardial patch.

1. Transannular pericardial patch
2. Pacing wire
3. RV
4. Ascending aorta

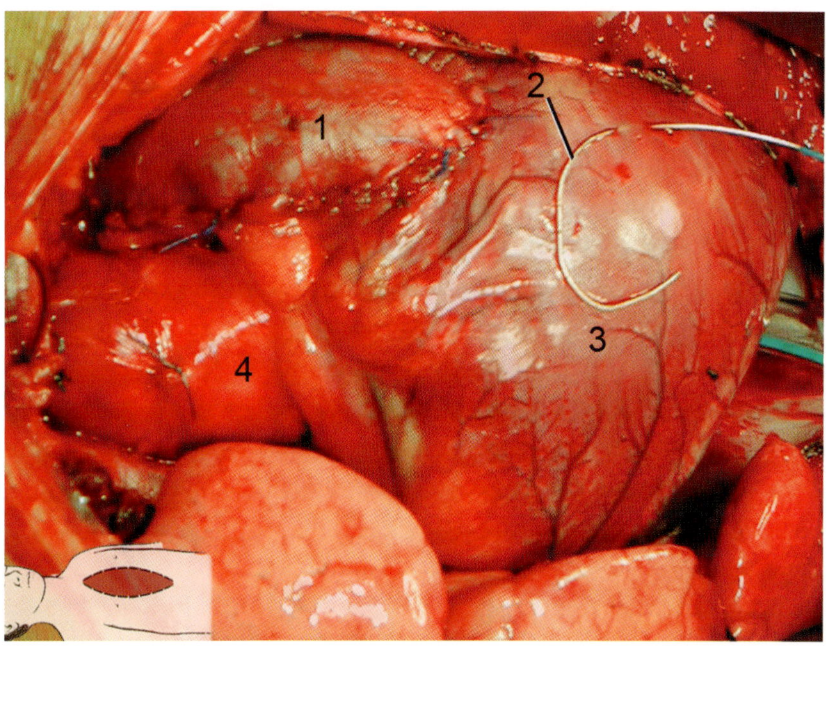

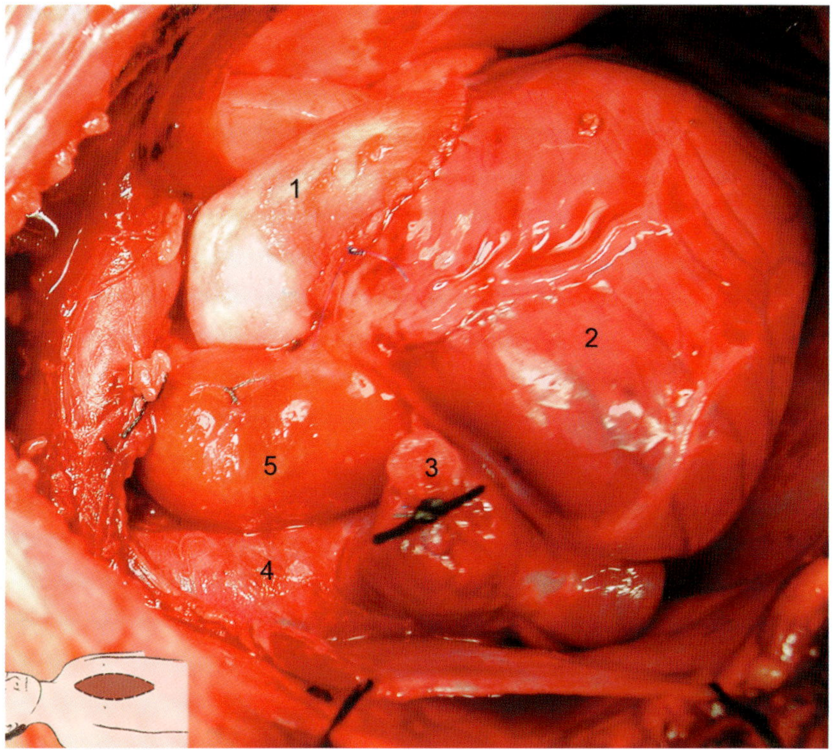

Figure 13.23. Median sternotomy view in an 8-month-old child after repair of TOF. A bovine jugular vein valved conduit (Contegra) has been placed between the RV and the pulmonary arteries (PAs).

1. Contegra conduit
2. RV
3. RAA
4. SVC
5. Ascending aorta

pulmonary stenosis. An RV-to-PA conduit may need to be implanted in cases of TOF with hypoplastic pulmonary valve. Figure 13.23 is from an 8-month-old infant with TOF. A bovine jugular vein valved conduit (Contegra) has been placed between the RV and the PA. In some patients, an abnormal coronary artery pattern may preclude cutting through the pulmonary valve or subvalvar area, and may necessitate placing a conduit to bypass the obstruction, as in the patient shown in Figures 13.24 and 13.25. Figure 13.26 shows an unusual coronary artery pattern. When a nonvalved conduit is used, free pulmonary regurgitation develops (Figure 13.27). Occasionally, one of the PAs may arise directly from the aorta, as shown in Figures 13.28 to 13.30.

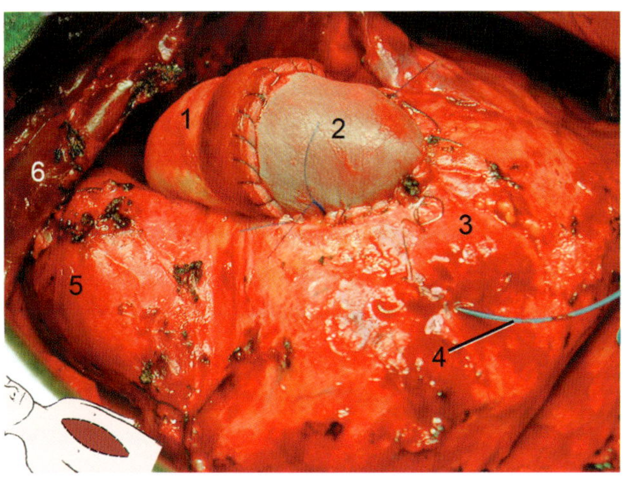

Figure 13.24

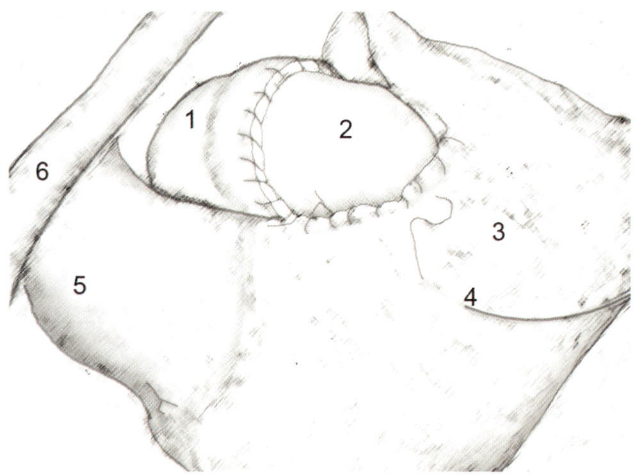

Figure 13.25

Median sternotomy view in a 5-year-old child with TOF after repair. The right coronary artery was arising from the left coronary artery, and thus a transannular patch could not be placed. A Cryolife Ross xenograft conduit (15 mm) was used to bypass the RVOT and relieve the pulmonary stenosis.

1. Cryolife Ross conduit (15 mm)
2. Pericardial hood
3. RV
4. Temporary pacing wire
5. Ascending aorta
6. Innominate vein

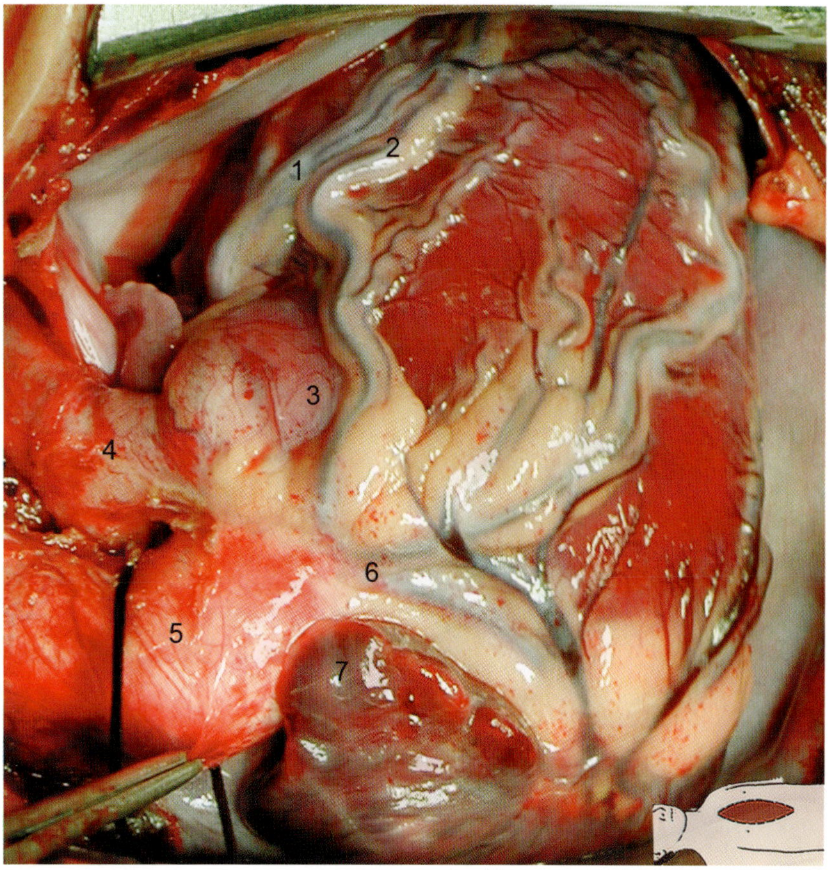

Figure 13.26. An unusual coronary artery pattern in a 2-year-old child with TOF. Two anterior descending coronary arteries are seen.

1. "Left" anterior descending coronary artery
2. "Right" anterior descending coronary artery
3. Outflow part of RV
4. MPA
5. Ascending aorta
6. Right coronary artery
7. RAA

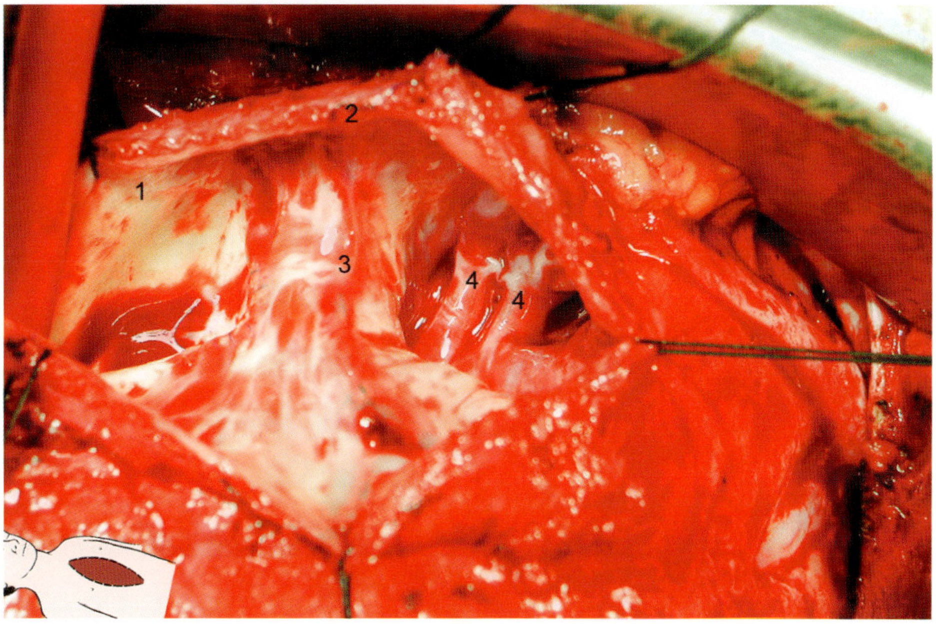

Figure 13.27. A reoperation view in a 6-year-old child who had TOF repaired with a conduit. There is no pulmonary valve, so severe regurgitation developed. Note the residual muscle bundles (4) in the RVOT. A new xenograft conduit was implanted (not shown) after removal of the old conduit and resection of all muscle bundles.

1. PA
2. Old conduit, split open
3. Pulmonary annulus, no valve
4. Obstructing residual muscle bundles

Figure 13.28. A cross-sectional CT cut through the chest in an 18-month-old child with TOF. The MPA does not branch; it gives rise to the left PA only. The right PA arises directly from the ascending aorta.

1. Ascending aorta
2. MPA continuing as left PA
3. Left lung
4. Descending thoracic aorta
5. Right lung

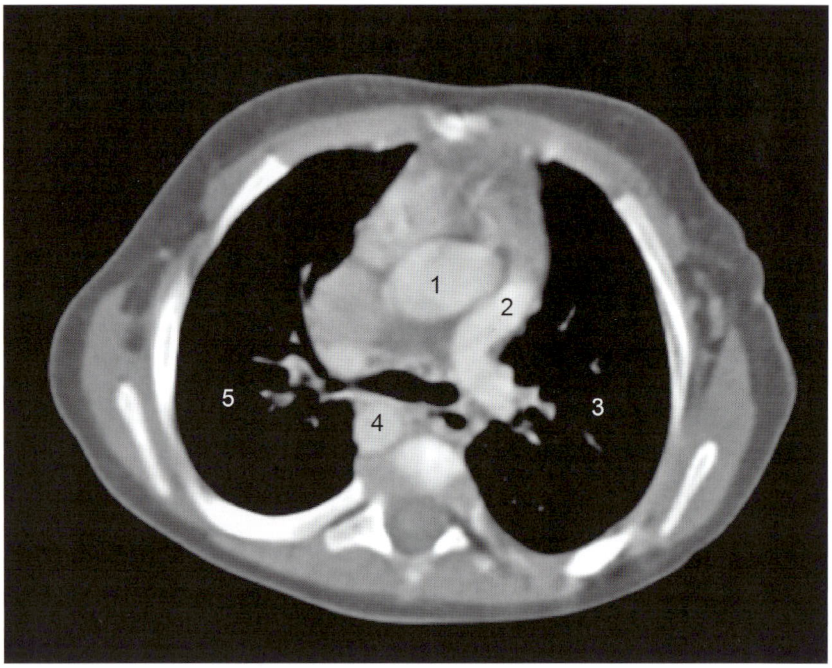

Figure 13.29. The same patient as in Figure 13.28, during surgery. The MPA continues as the left PA. The right PA arises directly from the ascending aorta, as shown in Figure 13.30.

1. Innominate vein
2. Aorta
3. Left PA
4. MPA
5. RV
6. RAA
7. SVC

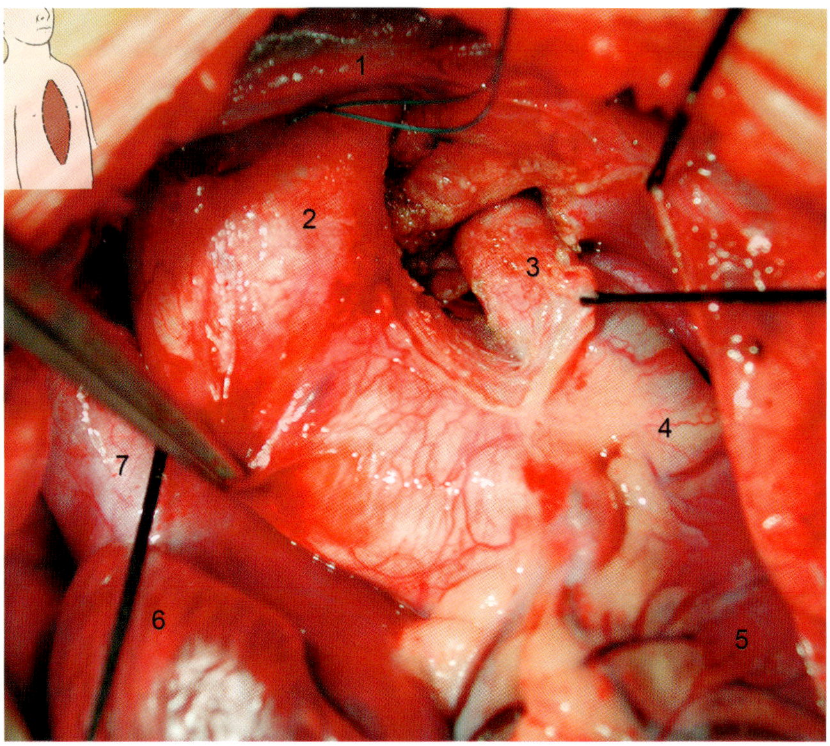

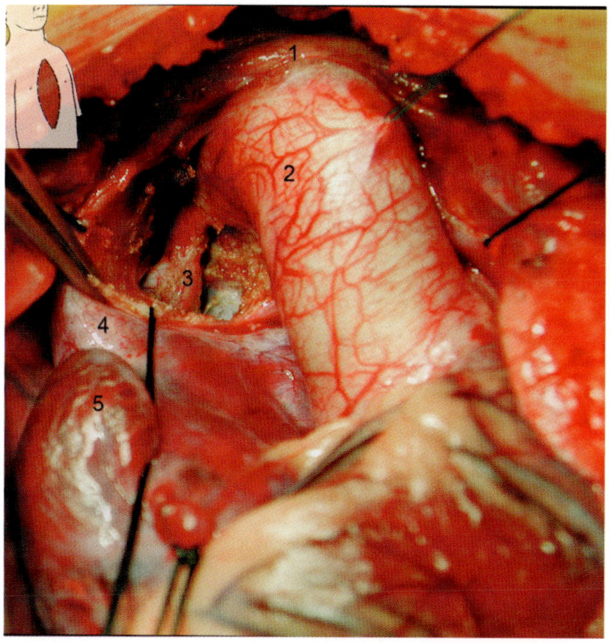

Figure 13.30. The same patient as in Figures 13.28 and 13.29 with the aorta retracted leftward. The right PA is seen arising directly from the aorta.

1. Innominate vein
2. Ascending aorta
3. Right PA
4. SVC
5. RAA

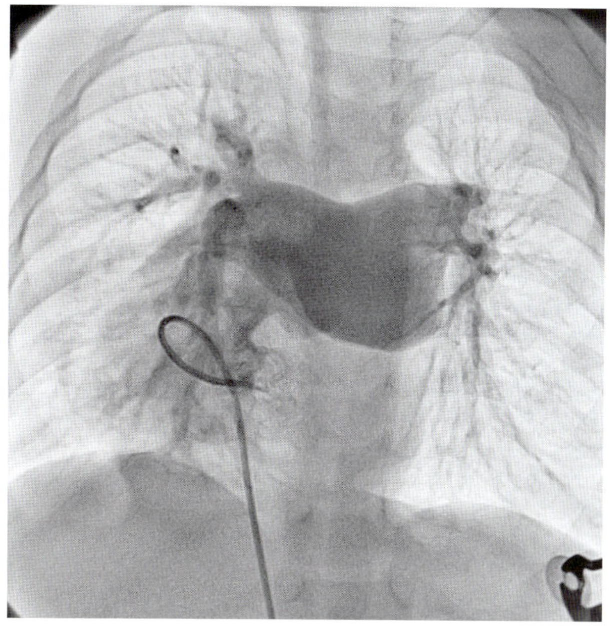

Figure 13.31. Pulmonary angiogram of a 1-year-old child with absent pulmonary valve syndrome. Note the massive dilatation of the PAs.

TETRALOGY OF FALLOT WITH ABSENT PULMONARY VALVE

Also called absent pulmonary valve syndrome, this variant of TOF is characterized, in addition to the features of TOF, by absent or rudimentary pulmonary valve leaflets, dilatation of main and branch PAs, and congenital absence of the ductus arteriosus in most cases. There is often compression of the airways by the enlarged PAs, which may cause significant respiratory distress.[4] Many palliative and corrective procedures have been devised to relieve compression and restore normal physiology.[5]

Figure 13.31 shows a preoperative angiogram of a 1-year-old child with absent pulmonary valve syndrome, showing the massively dilated PAs. Figures 13.32 and 13.33 are intraoperative views of the same patient. Another example is shown in Figures 13.34 to 13.36. Repair was achieved by plicating both branch PAs to reduce their size. Then a xenograft conduit (12 mm Cryolife Ross) was implanted between the RV and the PAs.

The rudimentary pulmonary valve of a 1-week-old neonate with absent pulmonary valve syndrome is shown in Figures 13.37 to 13.39. The normally semilunar-shaped valve leaflets are almost absent. The branch PAs may not be confluent; one of the PAs may originate from the ductus or aorta. Two examples are shown in Figures 13.40 to 13.46.

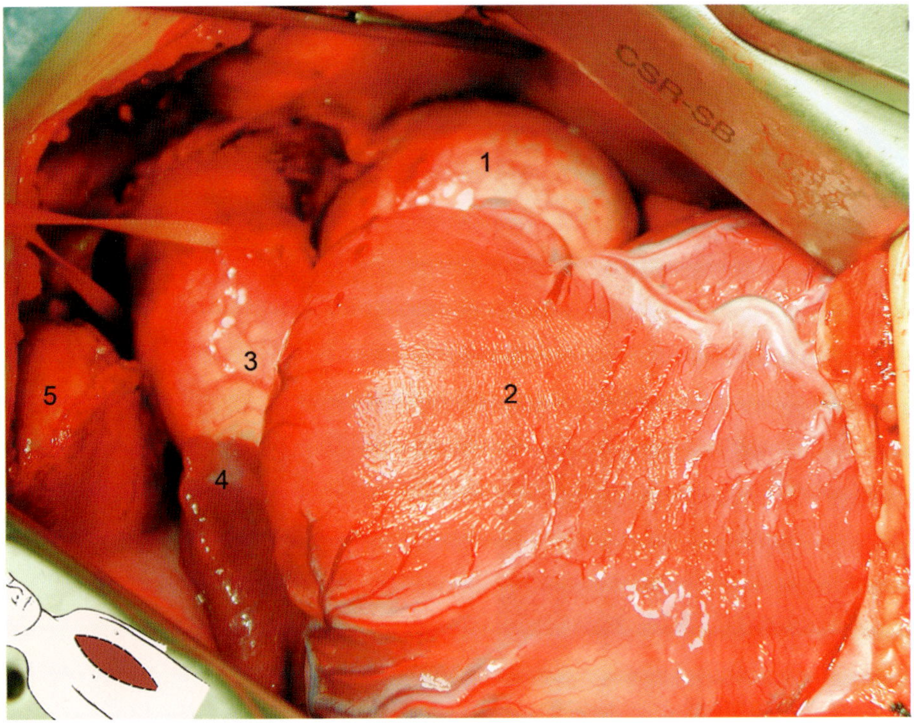

Figure 13.32. An operative view of the same patient as in Figure 13.31. The MPA is hugely dilated.

1. MPA
2. RV
3. Ascending aorta
4. RAA
5. Right lung

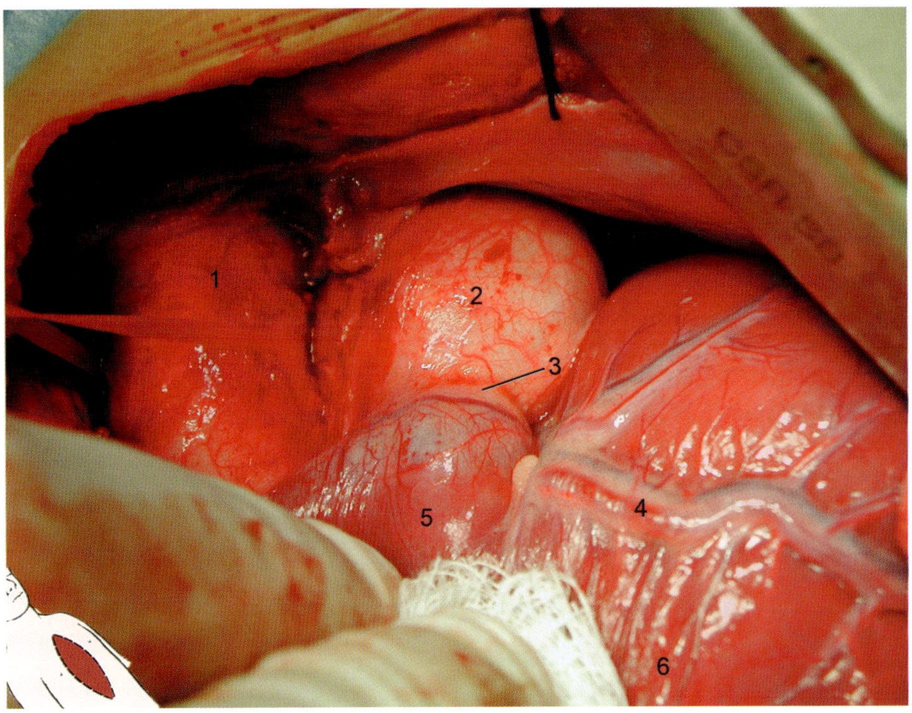

Figure 13.33. The same patient as in Figures 13.31 and 13.32. Note the tight pulmonary valve annulus (3) at the ventriculo-arterial junction and the dilated MPA.

1. Ascending aorta
2. MPA
3. Region of pulmonary valve
4. Left anterior descending coronary artery
5. RV outflow
6. RV

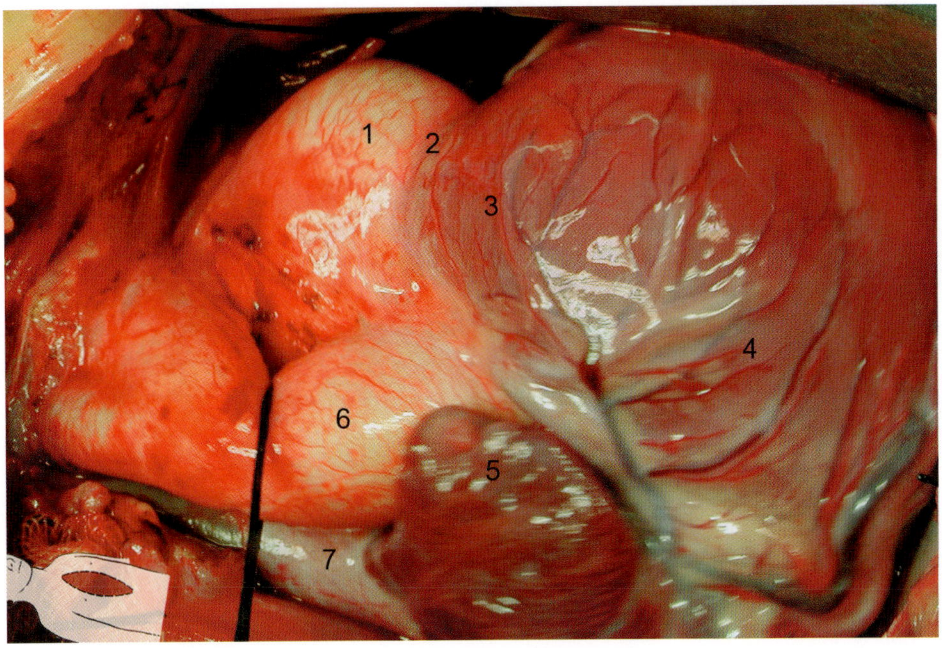

Figure 13.34. Median sternotomy view of 4-month-old infant with absent pulmonary valve syndrome. The MPA is dilated.

1. MPA
2. Pulmonary valve annulus
3. RV outflow
4. RV
5. RAA
6. Ascending aorta
7. SVC

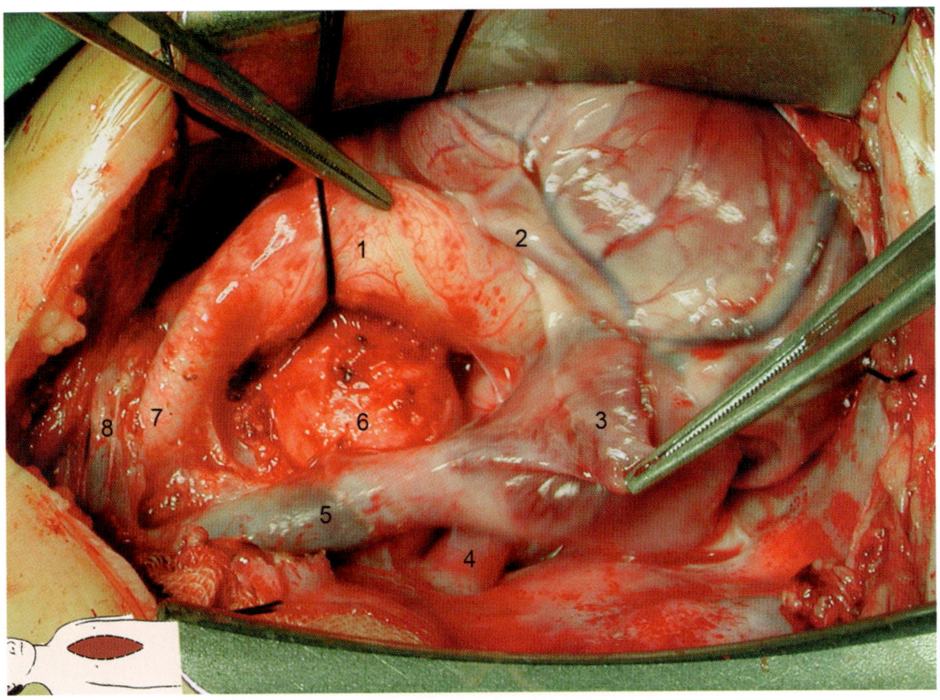

Figure 13.35. The same patient as in Figure 13.34. The aorta is retracted leftward to reveal the massively dilated right PA.

1. Ascending aorta
2. Right coronary artery
3. RAA
4. Right upper pulmonary vein
5. SVC
6. Right PA
7. Innominate artery
8. Innominate vein

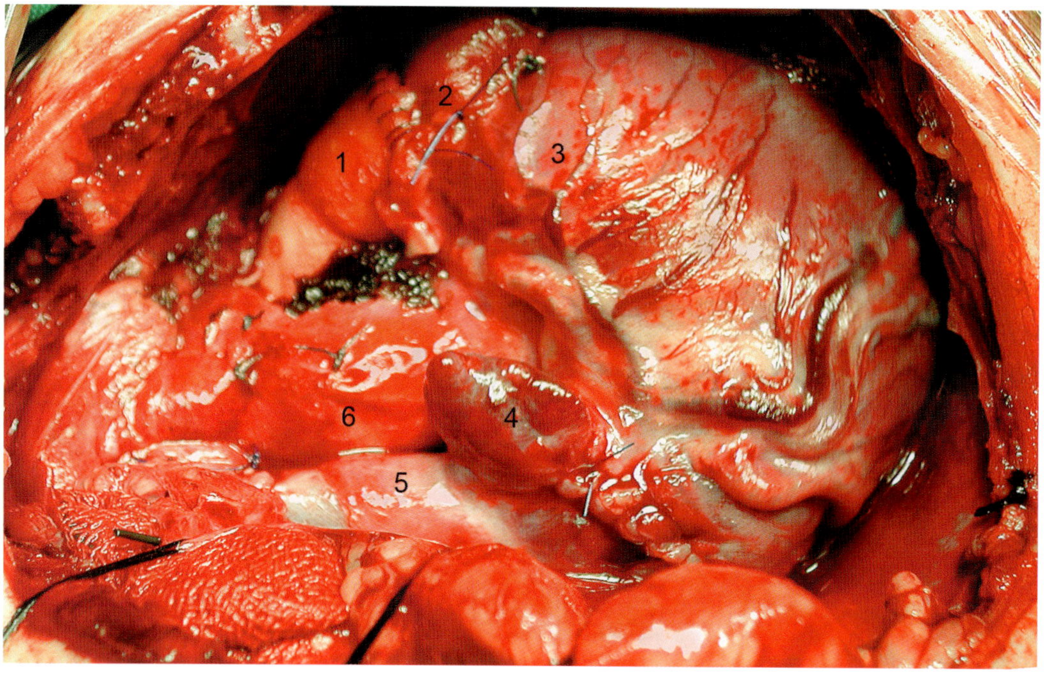

Figure 13.36. The same patient as in Figures 13.34 and 13.35, after repair. Reduction angioplasty was done by plicating both branch PAs. The VSD was closed in the usual manner, and a xenograft conduit (12 mm Cryolife Ross) was implanted between the RV and the PA.

1. Conduit (12 mm Cryolife Ross)
2. Conduit hood
3. RV
4. RAA
5. SVC
6. Ascending aorta

Figure 13.37. Intraoperative view of the pulmonary valve in a 1-week-old neonate with absent pulmonary valve syndrome. Note the rudimentary ridge representing almost absent pulmonary valve leaflets (2).

1. Opened MPA
2. Pulmonary valve "leaflet"
3. RV outflow
4. IVC venous cannula
5. SVC venous cannula going through RAA
6. Ascending aorta
7. LAA

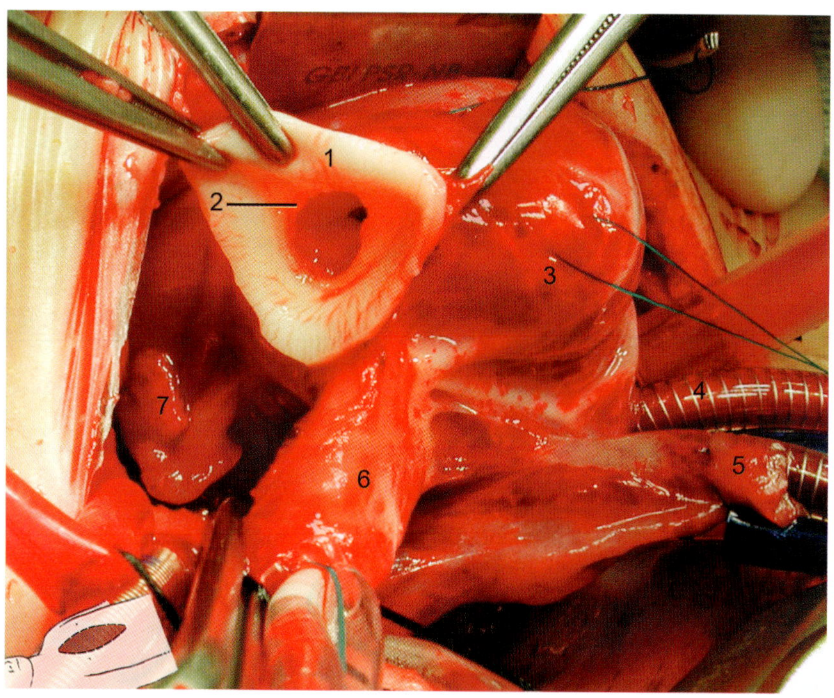

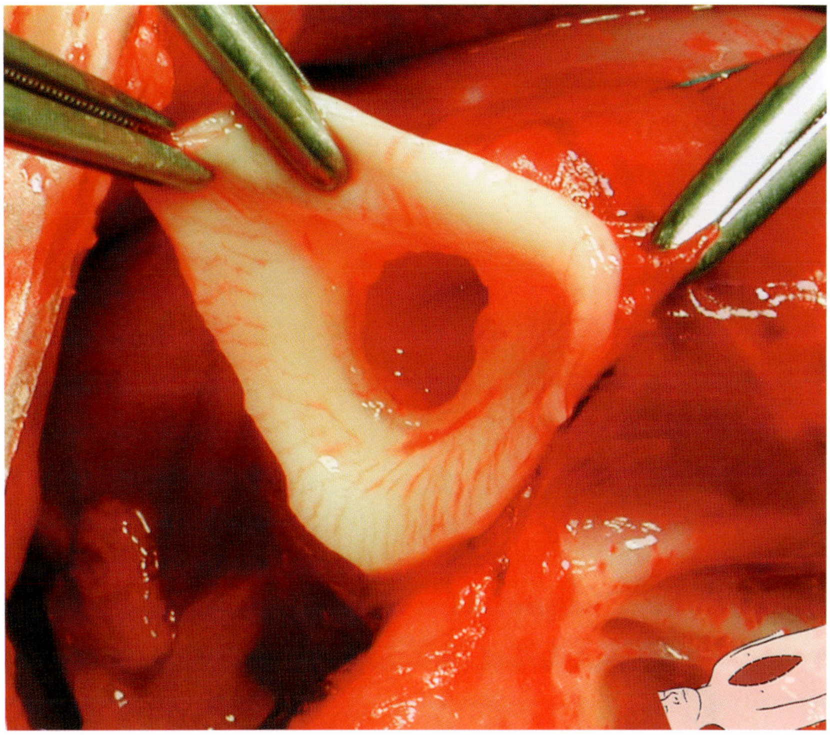

Figure 13.38. Close-up view of the same patient as in Figure 13.37. A small circumferential ridge representing rudimentary leaflets is seen at the pulmonary valve annulus.

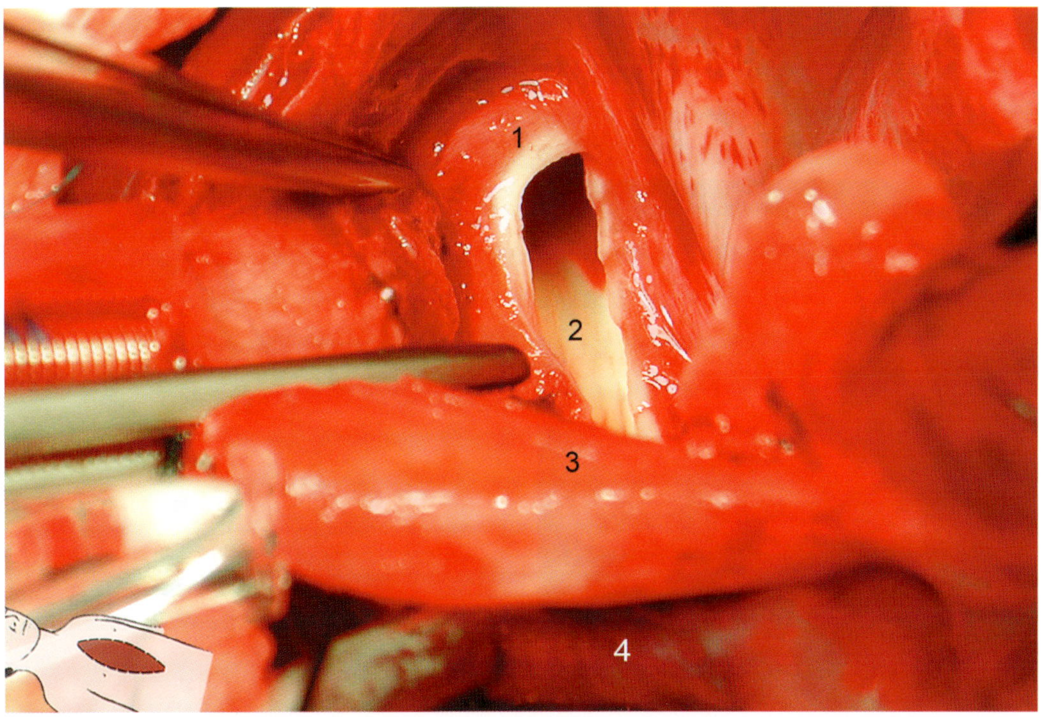

Figure 13.39. The same patient as in Figures 13.37 and 13.38 during repair. Part of the wall of the branch PAs was excised to reduce their size (the left PA is shown here). The VSD was closed, and a xenograft conduit (not shown) will be placed between the RV and the PAs.

1. Left PA
2. Lumen of left PA after excision of anterior wall
3. Ascending aorta
4. SVC

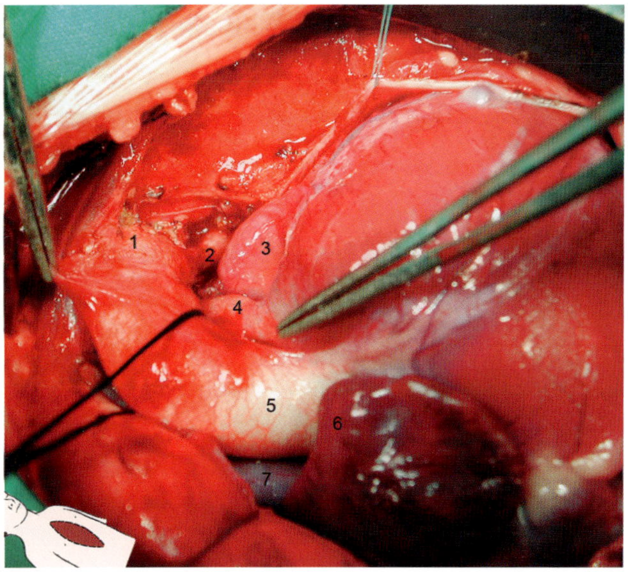

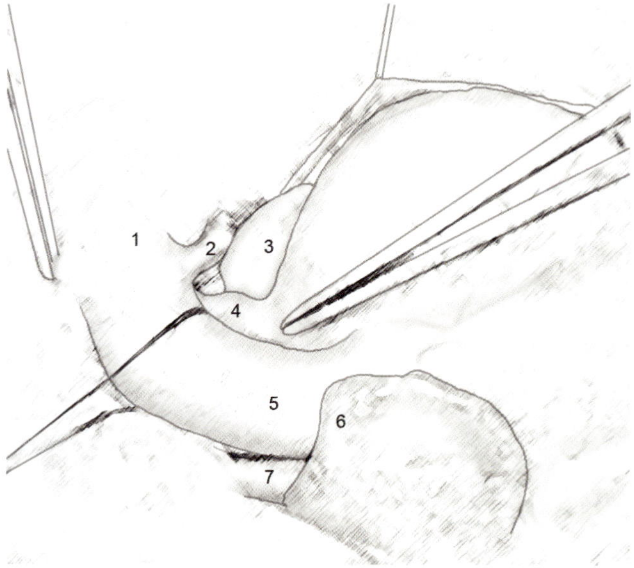

Figure 13.40 **Figure 13.41**

Median sternotomy view of a 2-month-old infant with TOF and absent pulmonary valve. Only the right PA originates from the MPA, whereas the left originates from the ductus arteriosus.

1. Transverse aortic arch
2. Ductus arteriosus
3. LAA
4. MPA
5. Ascending aorta
6. RAA
7. SVC

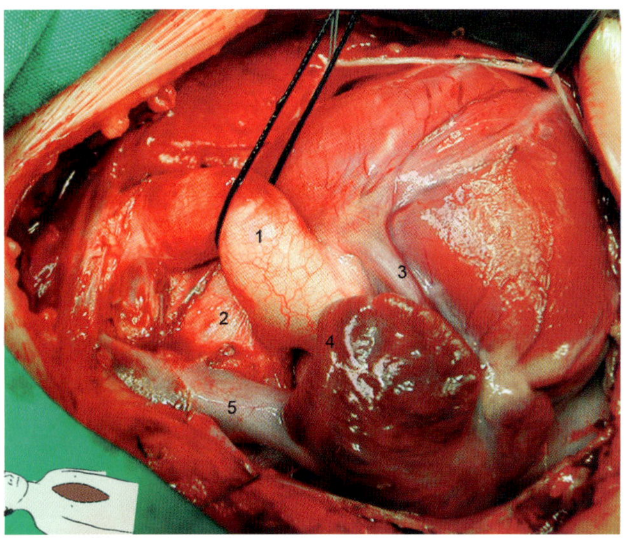

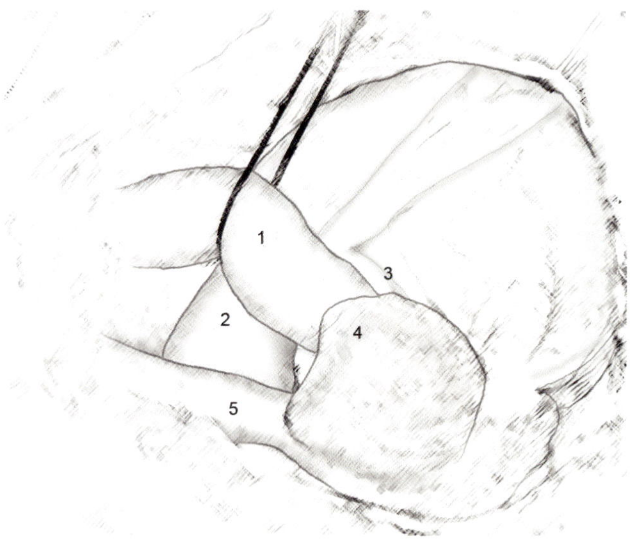

Figure 13.42 **Figure 13.43**

The same patient as in Figure 13.40. The aorta is retracted leftward to reveal the dilated right PA.

1. Ascending aorta
2. Right PA
3. Right coronary artery
4. RAA
5. SVC

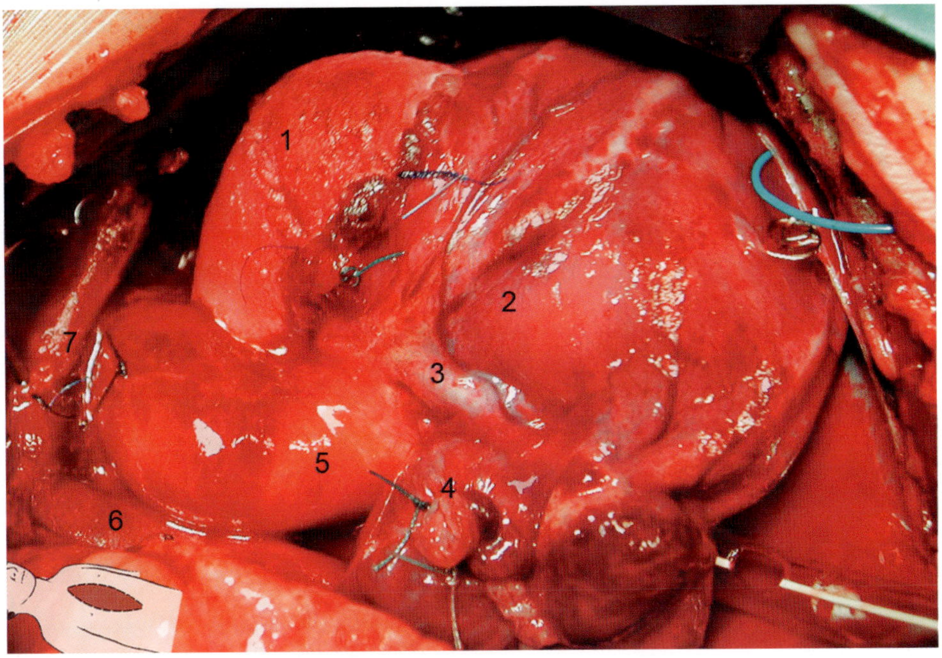

Figure 13.44. The same patient as in Figures 13.40 to 13.43, after repair. The 2 branch PAs were anastomosed to each other (not shown) to restore confluence. Then a xenograft conduit (12 mm Contegra) was placed between the RV and the PAs.

1. Conduit (12 mm Contegra)
2. RV
3. Right coronary artery
4. RAA
5. Ascending aorta
6. SVC
7. Innominate vein

Figure 13.45. TOF with absent pulmonary valve syndrome and nonconfluent PAs in a 3-week-old neonate. The left PA originates from the ductus arteriosus and is not dilated.

1. Transverse aortic arch
2. Ductus arteriosus giving rise to left PA
3. MPA giving rise to right PA only
4. RV outflow
5. RV
6. RAA
7. Ascending aorta
8. SVC

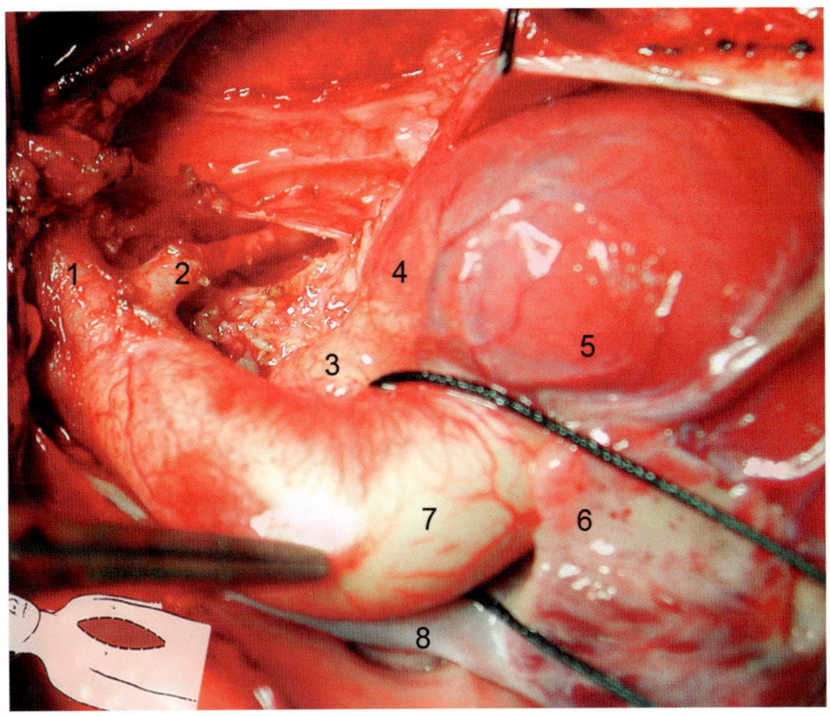

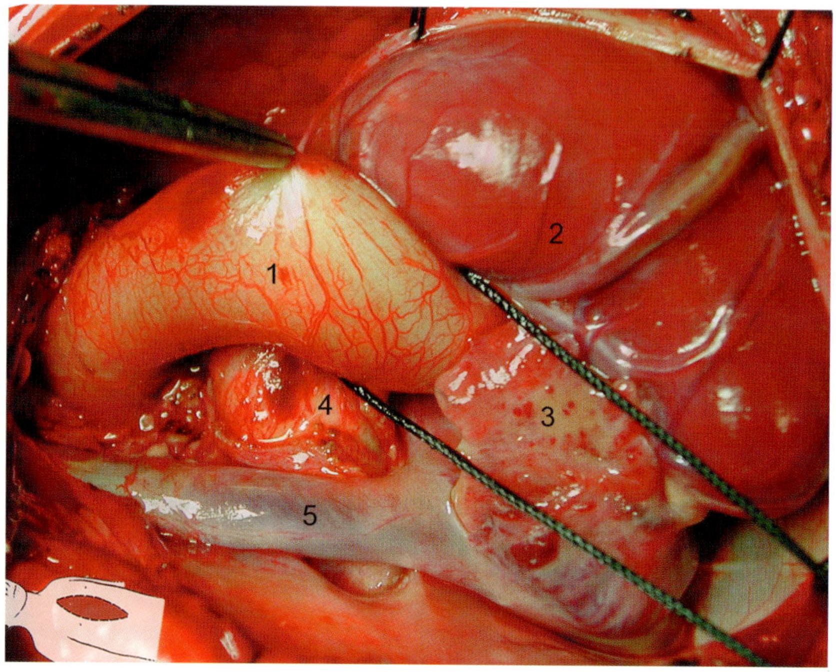

Figure 13.46. The same patient as in Figure 13.45, with aorta retracted to show the right PA, which is dilated.

1. Ascending aorta
2. RV
3. RAA
4. Right PA
5. SVC

REFERENCES

1. Nembhard W, Wang T, Loscalzo M, Salemi J. Variation in the prevalence of congenital heart defects by maternal race, ethnicity and infant sex. *J Pediatr.* 2010;156:259–264.
2. Kantorova A, Zbieranek K, Sauer H, et al. Primary early correction of tetralogy of Fallot irrespective of age. *Cardiol Young.* 2008;18:153–157.
3. Anderson R, Jacobs M. The anatomy of tetralogy of Fallot with pulmonary stenosis. *Cardiol Young.* 2008;18(Suppl. 3):12–21.
4. Rabinovitch M, Grady S, David I, et al. Compression of intrapulmonary bronchi by abnormally branching pulmonary arteries associated with absent pulmonary valves. *Am J Cardiol.* 1982;50:804–812.
5. Nørgaard M, Alphonso N, Newcomb A. Absent pulmonary valve syndrome. Surgical and clinical outcome with long-term follow-up. *Eur J Cardiothorac Surg.* 2006;29:682–687.

CHAPTER 14

Pulmonary Atresia

Two distinct entities have pulmonary atresia as a prominent feature: pulmonary atresia with intact ventricular septum, and pulmonary atresia with ventricular septal defect (VSD). The latter is considered an extreme form of tetralogy of Fallot (TOF). Both are cyanotic defects, but the morphology of the right ventricle (RV), coronary circulation, and pulmonary arterial tree is different in the 2 forms.[1] The choice of optimal treatment strategy should take into account these factors as well as other associated lesions. Major aortopulmonary collateral arteries (MAPCAs), or more accurately systemic-to-pulmonary collateral arteries, are common in pulmonary atresia with VSD,[2] and the RV is well developed. By contrast, coronary artery abnormalities, tricuspid valve stenosis, and hypoplastic RV are common in pulmonary atresia with intact septum.[3] See chapter 17 for single ventricle strategy.

A systemic-to-pulmonary shunt is often initially performed in these patients to provide blood flow to the lungs. The most commonly performed type of shunt in the current era is a modified Blalock-Taussig (BT) shunt. A tube graft of prosthetic material is implanted between the innominate or subclavian artery and the ipsilateral pulmonary artery (PA). See chapter 17 for further discussion on the BT shunt.

Figure 14.1 shows an operative view through a right thoracotomy in a 9-month-old infant with

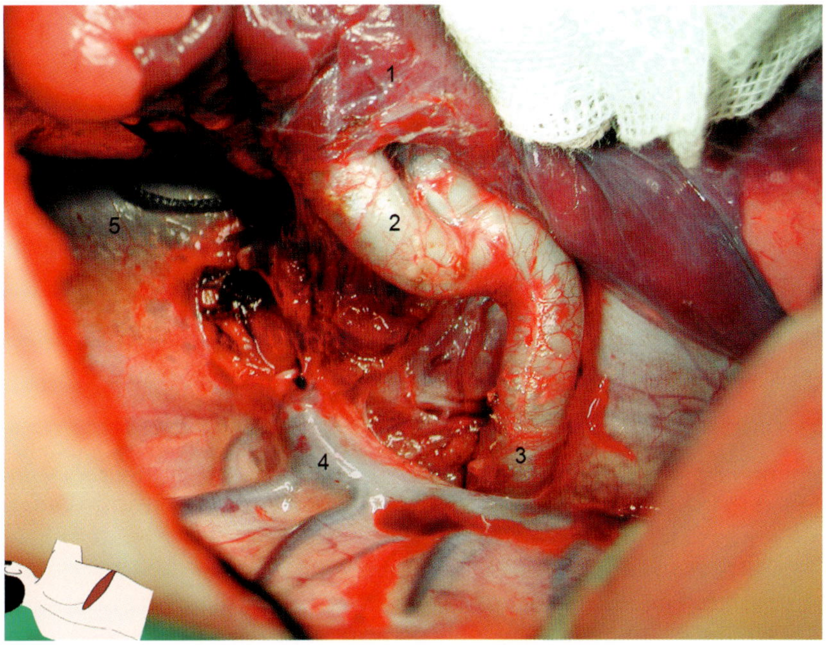

Figure 14.1. A right thoracotomy view of a 9-month-old infant with pulmonary atresia/VSD. A MAPCA arises from the descending thoracic aorta, supplying blood to the right lung.

1. Right lung
2. Distal end of MAPCA just before entering the right lung
3. Proximal part of MAPCA after originating from the descending aorta in the left hemithorax
4. Azygos vein
5. Superior vena cava (SVC)

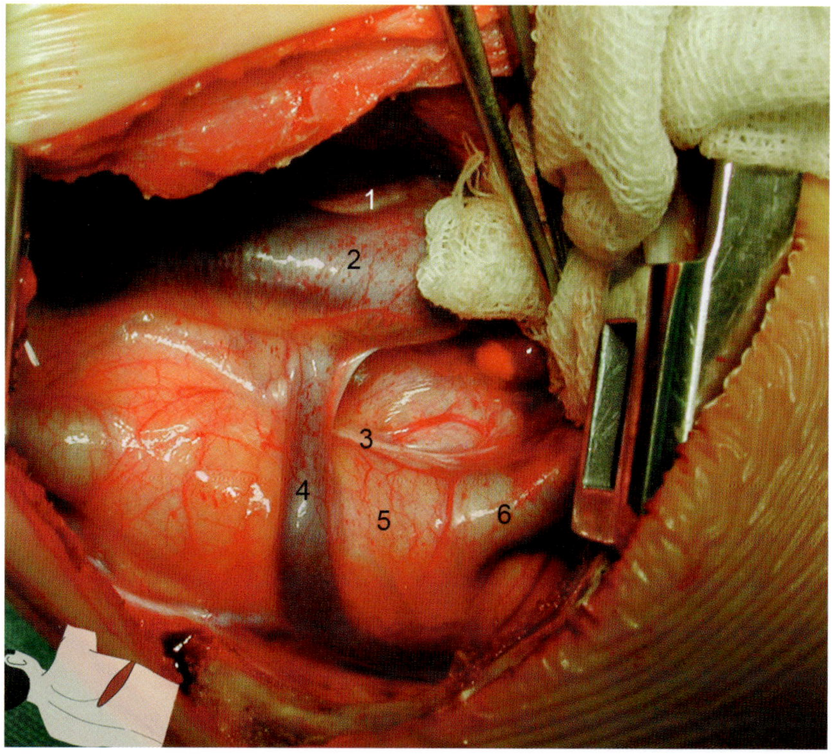

Figure 14.2. A right thoracotomy view of another 9-month-old infant with pulmonary atresia/VSD. This child has a right-sided aortic arch and a right-sided descending aorta that gives rise to a large MAPCA.

1. Right phrenic nerve
2. SVC
3. Right vagus nerve
4. Azygos vein
5. Descending thoracic aorta
6. MAPCA

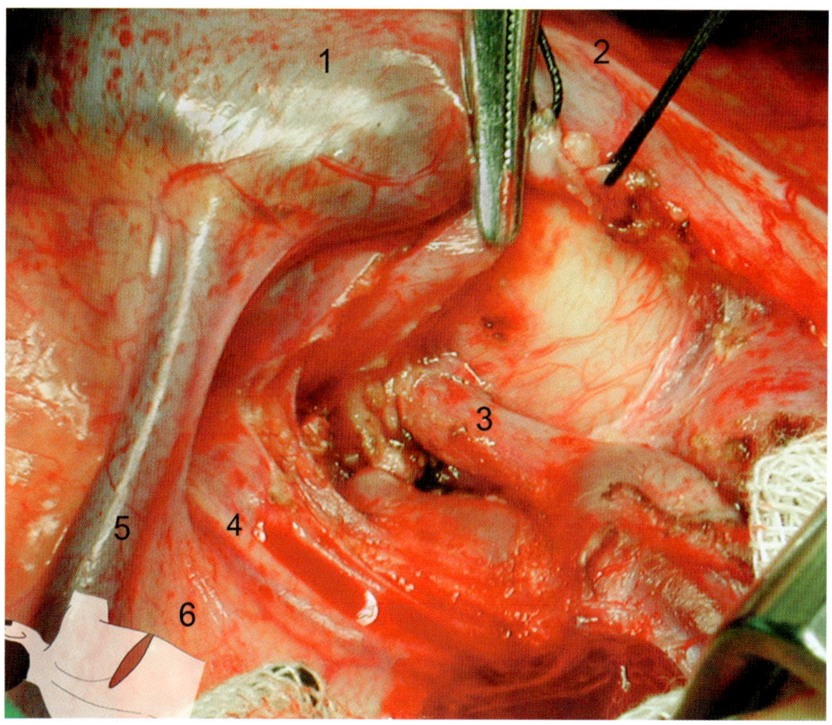

Figure 14.3. The same patient as in Figure 14.2. The parietal pleura has been dissected to reveal the MAPCA's connection to the right pulmonary arterial tree.

1. SVC
2. Right phrenic nerve
3. Right PA
4. Right vagus nerve
5. Azygos vein
6. Descending aorta

pulmonary atresia/VSD. A MAPCA is seen supplying blood to the right lung.

Figures 14.2 and 14.3 are from another infant with pulmonary atresia/VSD, MAPCA, and right-sided aortic arch. The MAPCA in this patient feeds the right PA. Unifocalization is a commonly performed procedure in these cases, whereby the collateral arteries are disconnected from the aorta, brought together, and connected to the main pulmonary artery (MPA), if it exists, or to a BT shunt (Figures 14.4 and 14.5).

Occasionally, the right internal mammary artery can be used to provide systemic-to-pulmonary blood in lieu of a BT shunt, as shown in Figures 14.6 and 14.7.

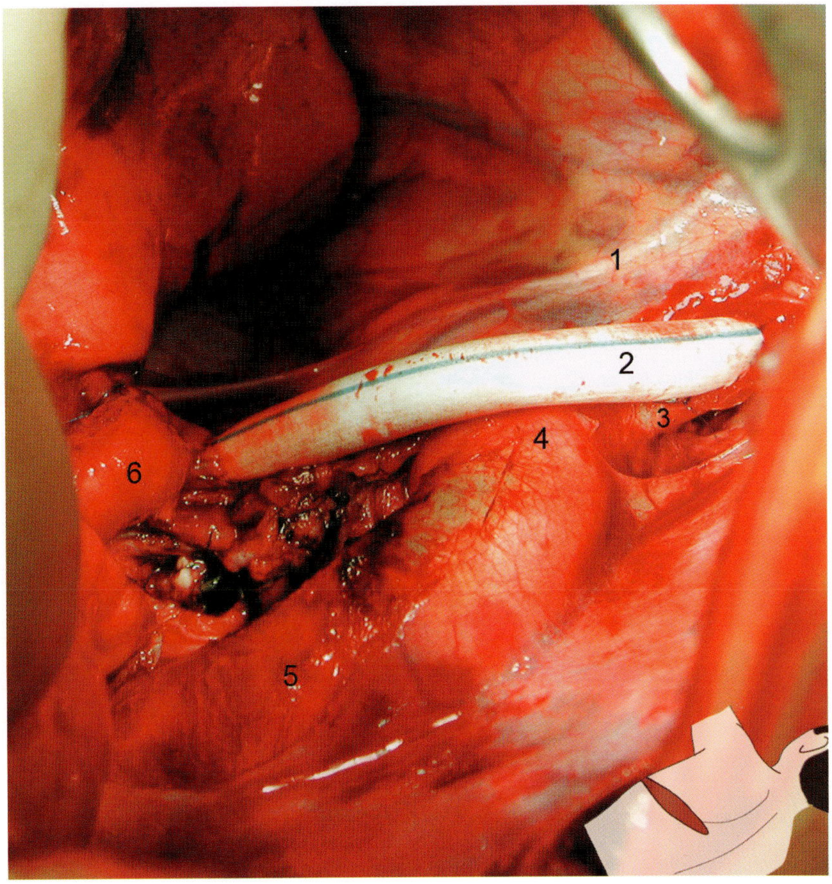

Figure 14.4. A left thoracotomy view of a 2.5-year-old child with pulmonary atresia/VSD and MAPCA. Unifocalization has been done, and a modified BT shunt has been placed between the left subclavian artery and the left PA (seen medial to the MAPCA).

1. Left vagus nerve
2. Modified BT shunt (5 mm)
3. Left subclavian artery
4. Transverse aortic arch
5. Descending thoracic aorta
6. Unifocalized MAPCA

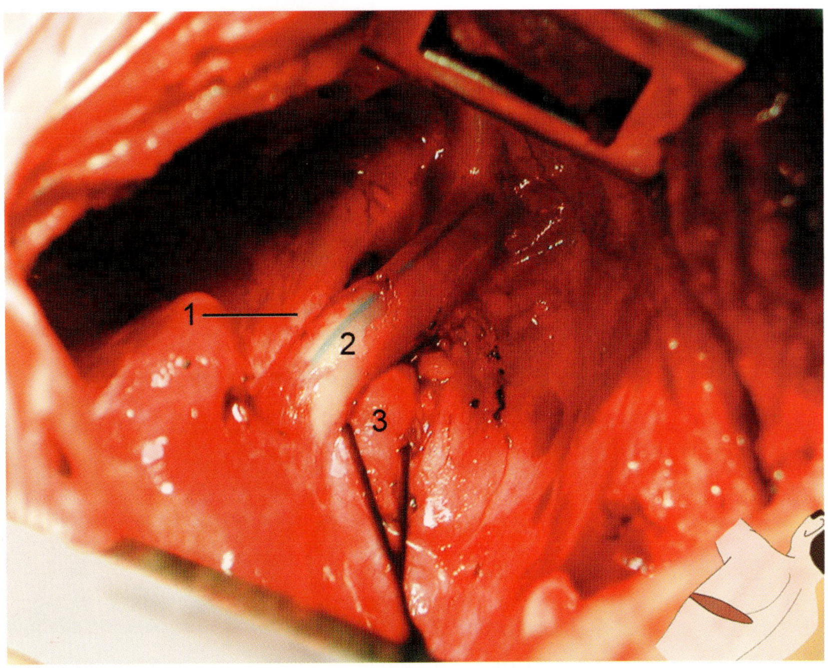

Figure 14.5. A redo left thoracotomy in a 5-month-old infant with pulmonary atresia/VSD. In the previous surgery, a left-modified BT shunt was placed and the patent ductus arteriosus (PDA) was left open. The latter did not close spontaneously, which led to pulmonary overflow and required surgical ligation. Note the vertical orientation of the PDA.

1. Left vagus nerve
2. Modified BT shunt
3. PDA

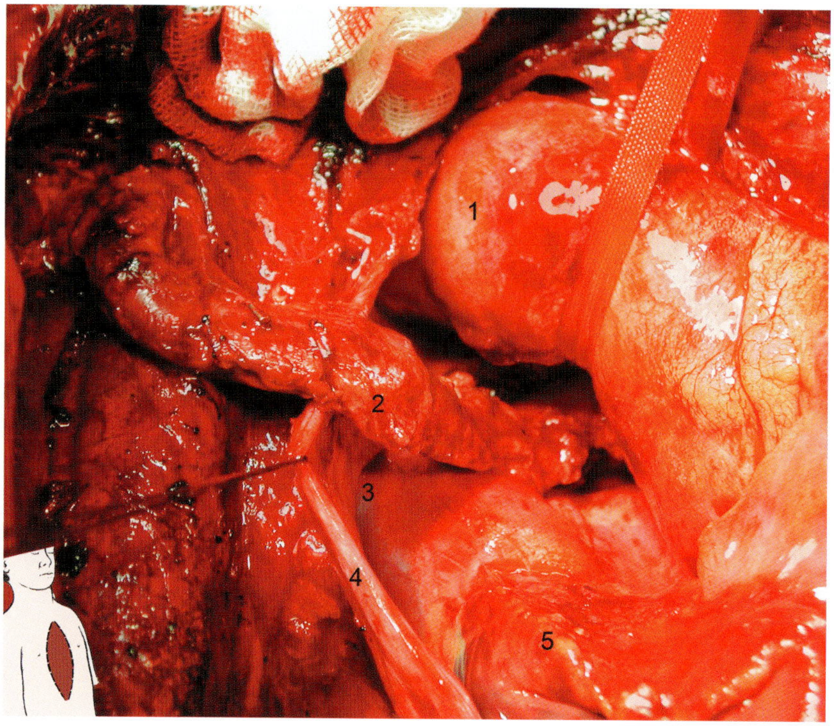

Figure 14.6. A median sternotomy view of an 18-year-old patient with pulmonary atresia/VSD. The branch PAs were confluent, and the MAPCAs were stenotic (not shown). A systemic-to-pulmonary artery shunt was established using the right internal mammary artery.

1. Ascending aorta
2. Right internal mammary artery
3. SVC
4. Pericardium
5. Right atrial appendage (RAA)

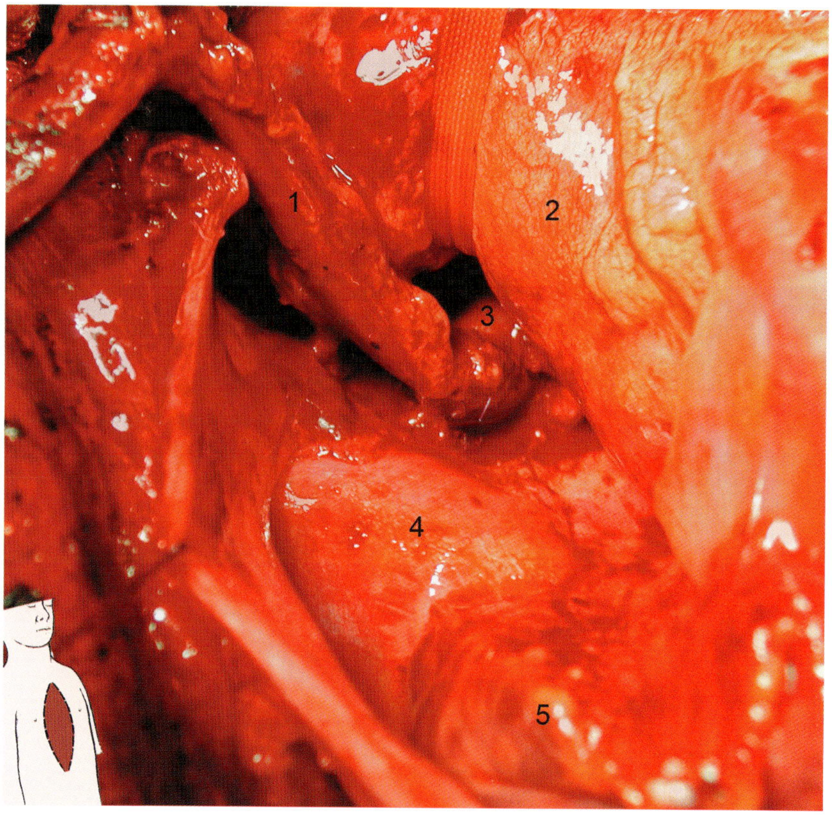

Figure 14.7. The same patient as in Figure 14.6 showing the anastomosis of the right internal mammary artery to the right PA.

1. Right internal mammary artery
2. Ascending aorta
3. Right PA
4. SVC
5. RAA

Completion of the repair is achieved by closing the VSD and implanting an RV-to-PA conduit. Two cases are shown in Figures 14.8 to 14.13. Occasionally, the intrapericardial segment of the pulmonary arterial tree is absent and the PAs are nonconfluent, as shown in Figures 14.14 to 14.23. In this patient, repair was achieved using a polytetrafluoroethylene (PTFE) tube graft to restore confluence of the PAs, and then a valved conduit was implanted between the PTFE tube graft and the RV.

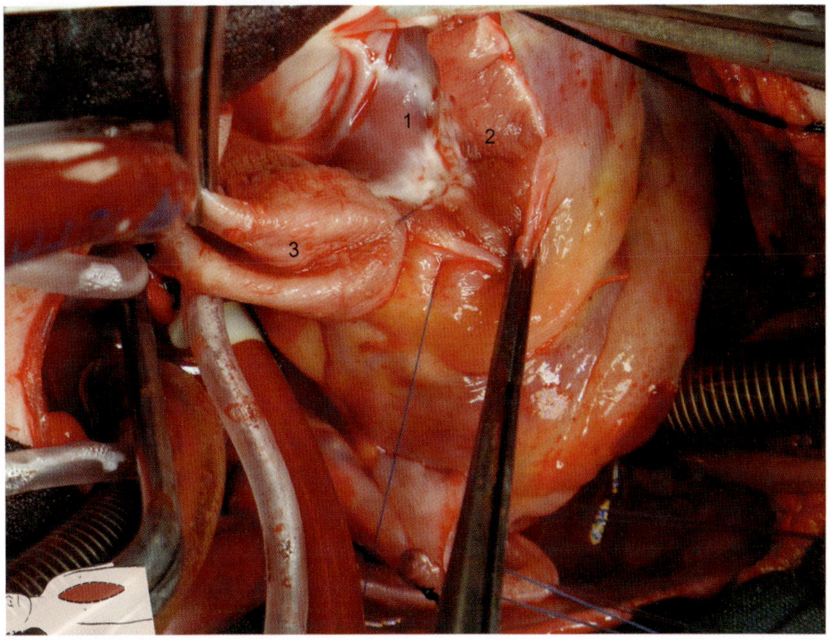

Figure 14.8. Median sternotomy view of a child with pulmonary atresia/VSD. The pulmonary valve is imperforate, so a valved conduit is being placed. The distal end of the conduit has already been anastomosed distally to the MPA. In this and the following figures, the proximal end is being sewn to the RV.

1. Outlet ventricular septum
2. Right ventriculotomy
3. Valved conduit

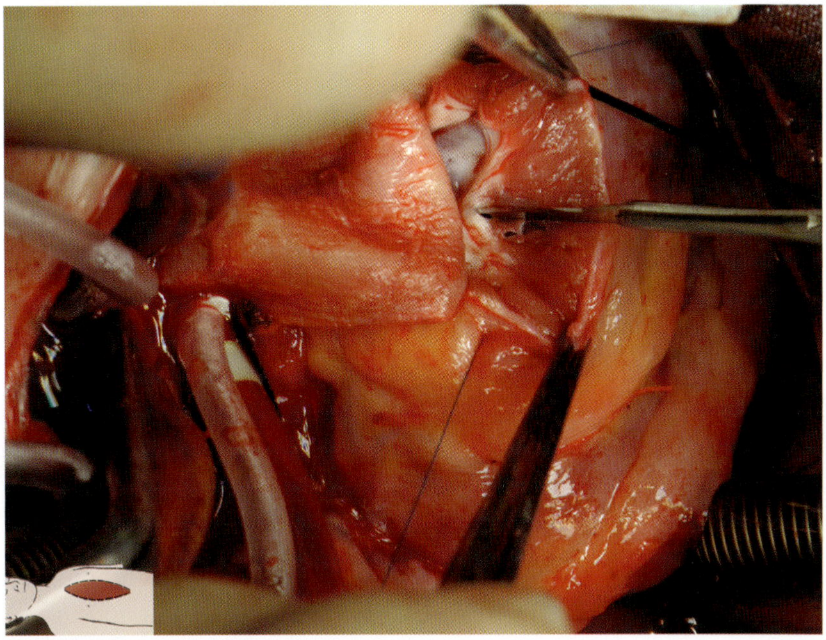

Figure 14.9. The same patient as in Figure 14.8. The right ventricular outflow tract (RVOT) is being cut open. Note the hypertrophied ventricular muscle.

Figure 14.10. The same patient as in Figures 14.8 and 14.9. An opening has been made in the RVOT.

1. RV free wall
2. Opening into outflow tract (surgically made)
3. Conduit

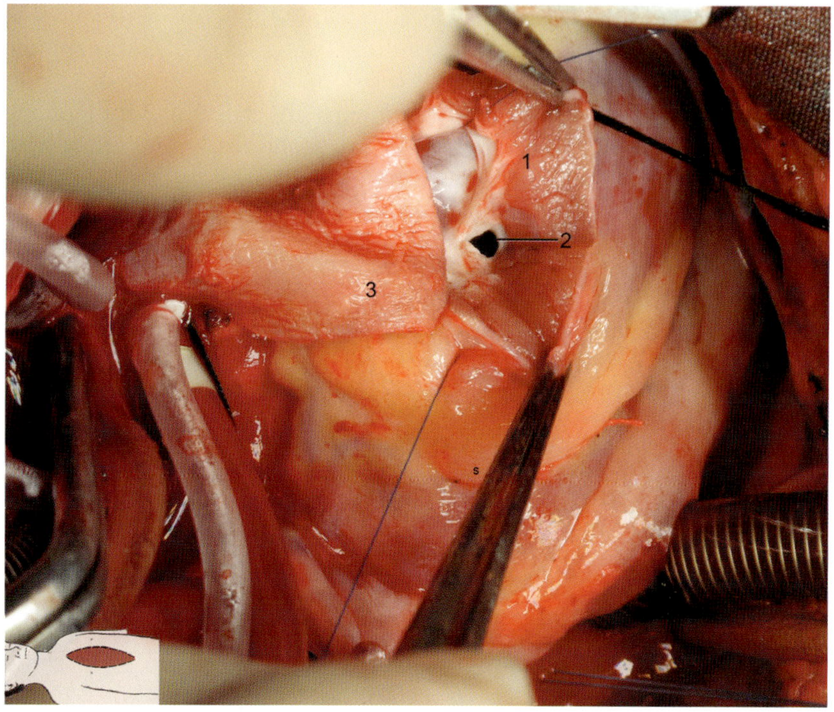

Figure 14.11. The same patient as in Figures 14.8 to 14.10. The opening to the RV has been enlarged. Note the pledget in the RV cavity that was used to close the VSD.

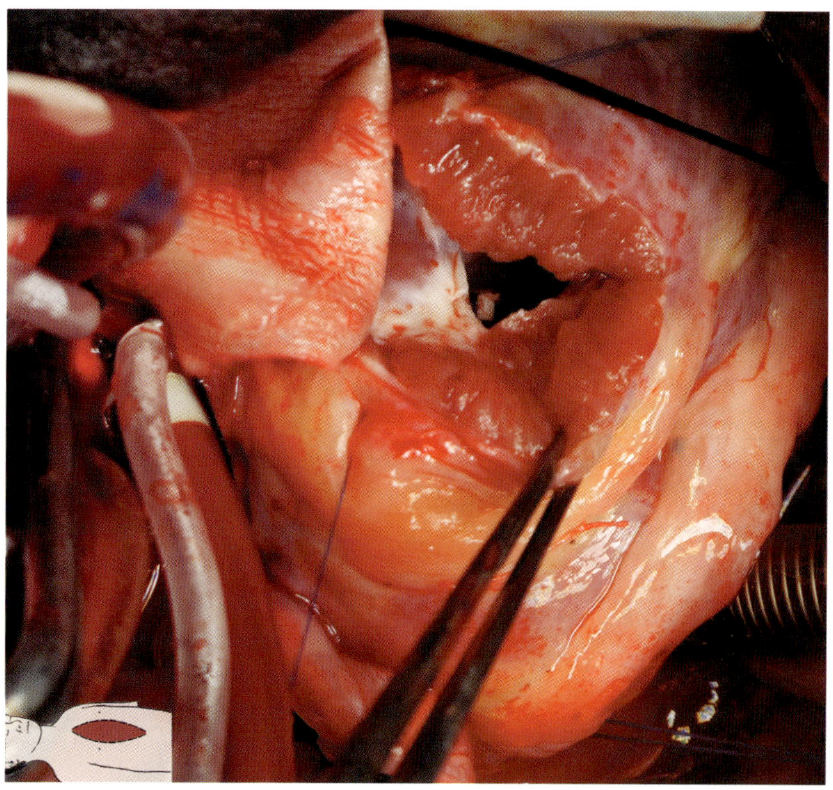

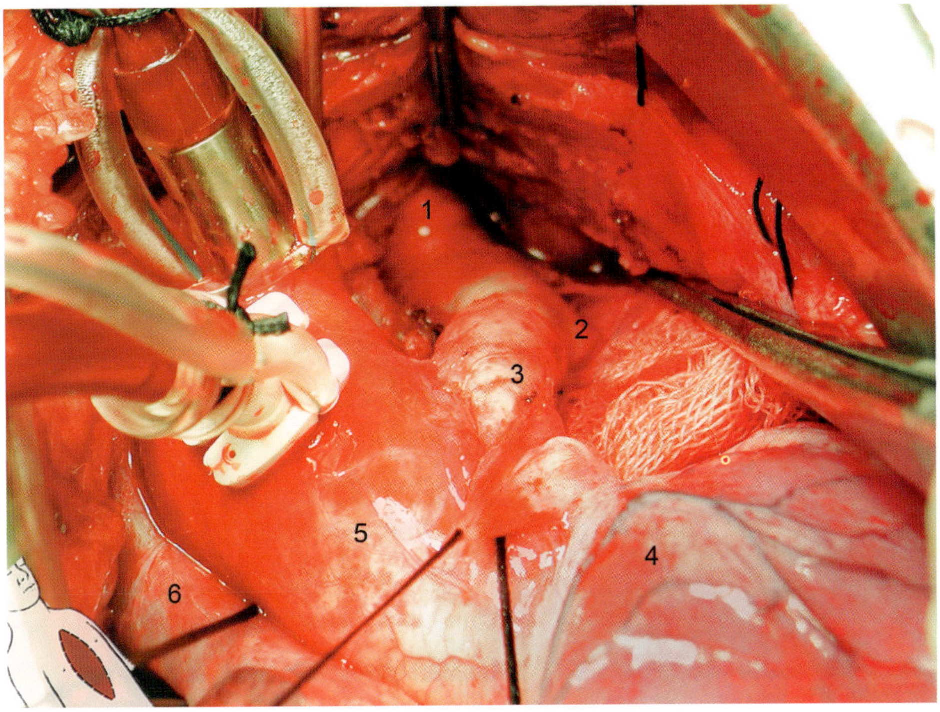

Figure 14.12. Median sternotomy view of a 10-month-old infant with pulmonary atresia/VSD and PDA.

1. PDA
2. Left PA
3. MPA
4. RV
5. Ascending aorta
6. SVC

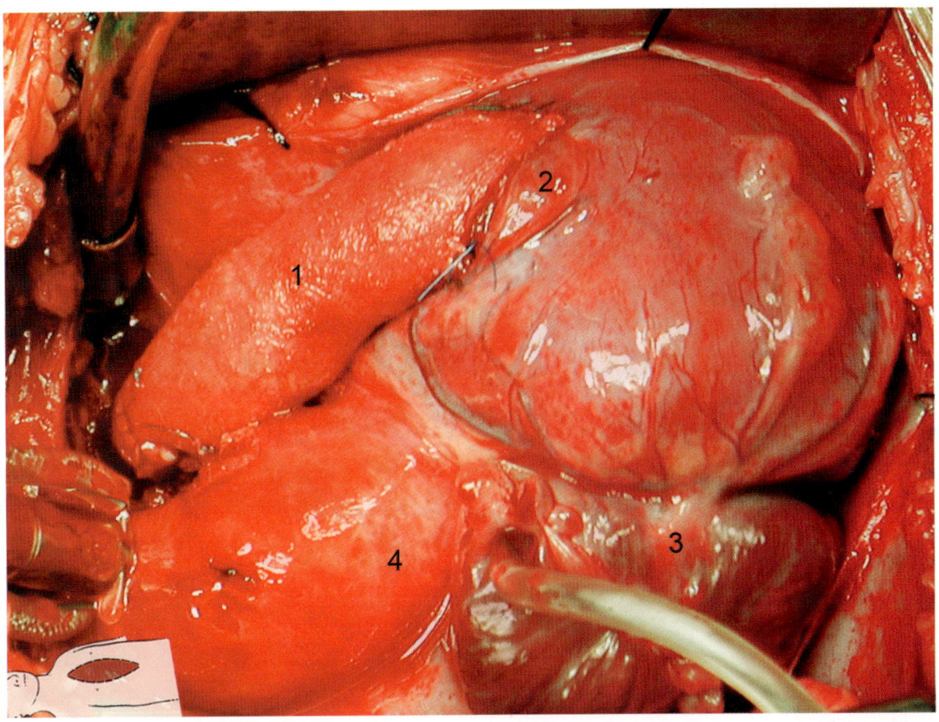

Figure 14.13. The same patient as in Figure 14.12, after repair. A 12 mm xenograft conduit (Contegra) has been implanted between the RV and the PA.

1. Xenograft conduit (Contegra)
2. RVOT
3. Right atrium
4. Ascending aorta

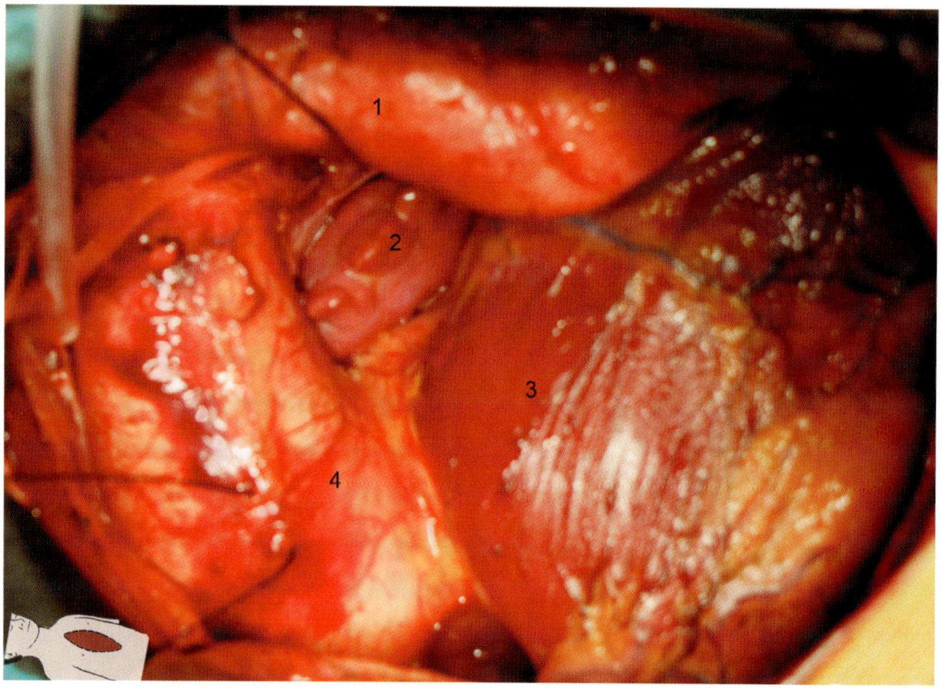

Figure 14.14. Pulmonary atresia, VSD, and nonconfluent PAs as seen through a median sternotomy. Note the absence of intrapericardial main and branch PAs. The lungs were supplied by collateral arteries, as shown in the next figures.

1. Left lung
2. Left atrium
3. RV
4. Ascending aorta

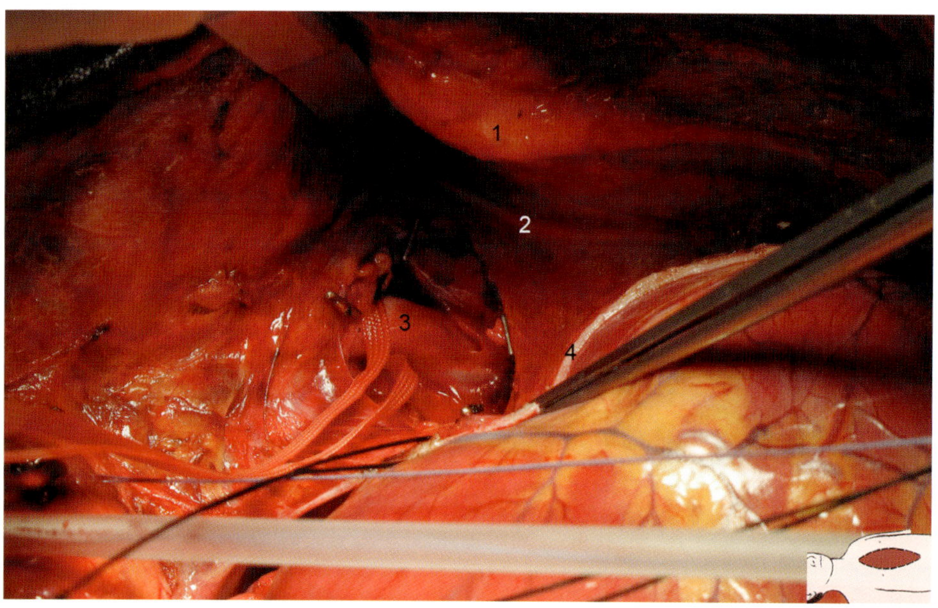

Figure 14.15. The same patient as in Figure 14.14. The left hilum is dissected. A MAPCA is seen.

1. Left lung
2. Left phrenic nerve
3. MAPCA
4. Pericardium

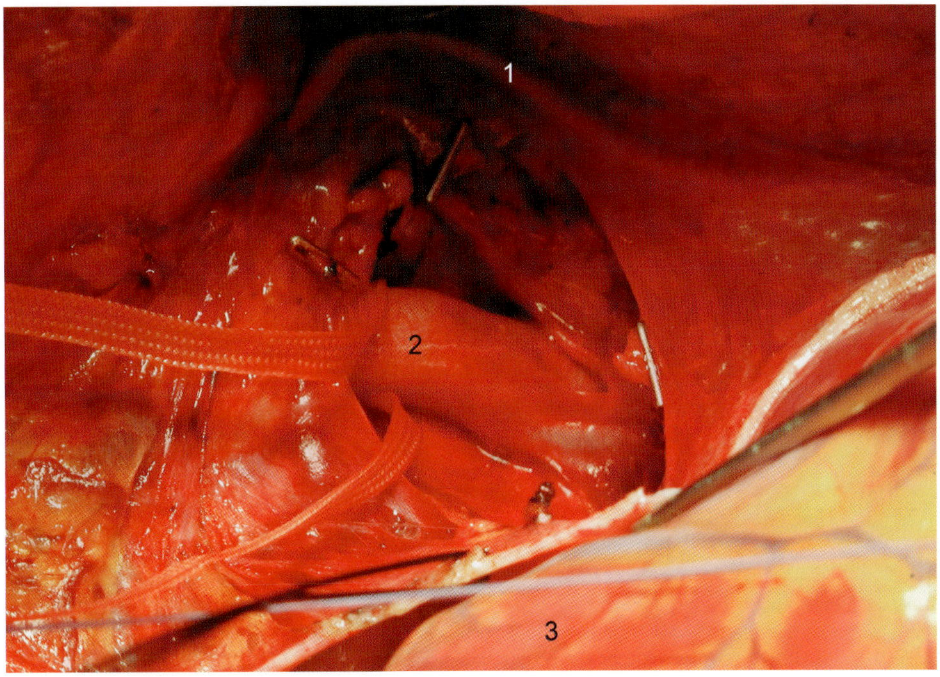

Figure 14.16. Close-up of the left hilar area of the same patient as in Figures 14.14 and 14.15. The left lung is supplied by a MAPCA.

1. Left phrenic nerve
2. MAPCA
3. Heart

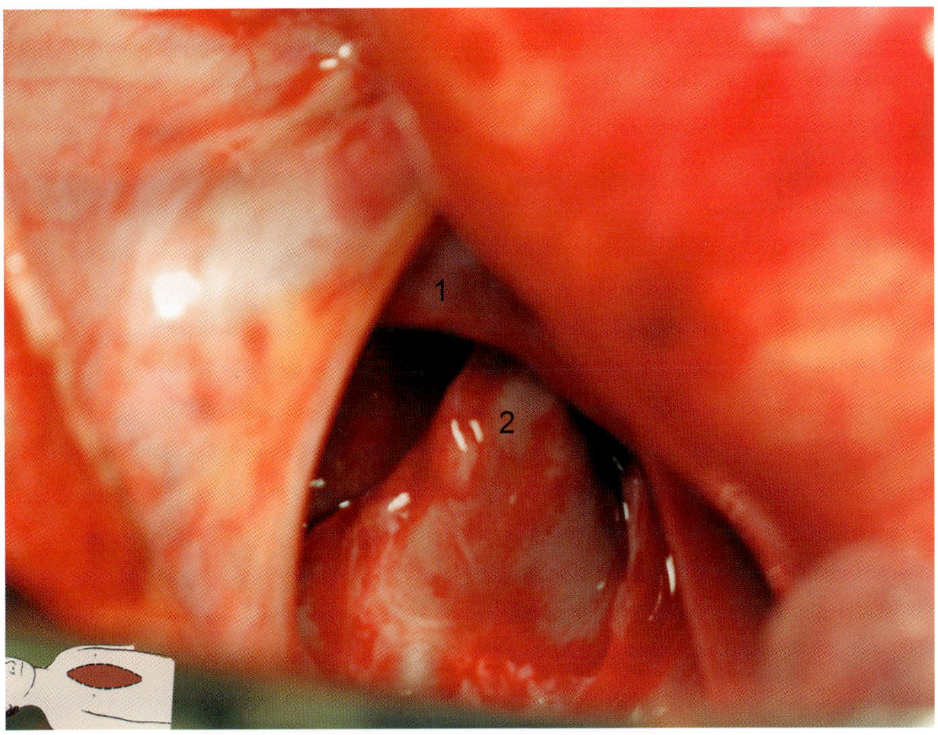

Figure 14.17. The same patient as in Figures 14.14 to 14.16 showing the right hilar area. A MAPCA is seen supplying the right lung.

1. SVC
2. MAPCA

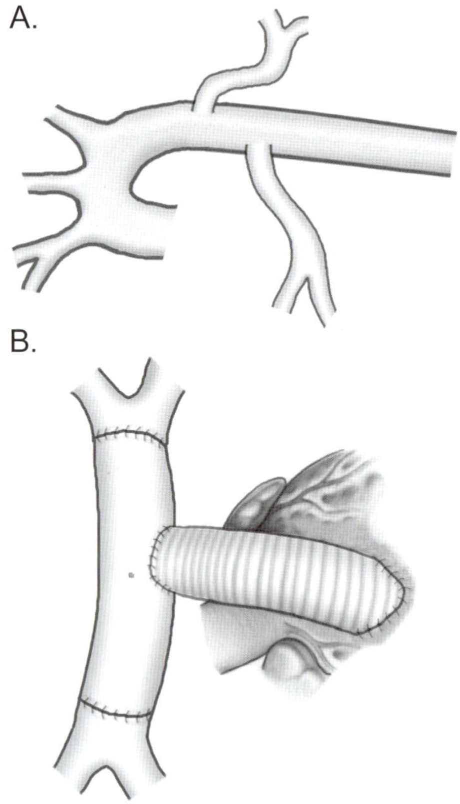

Figure 14.18. Diagrammatic illustration of the technique used to repair the lesions of the patient shown in Figures 14.14 to 14.17. The MAPCAs are centralized to the PTFE tube graft. Another graft, in this case, a stentless valved conduit, is used to connect the PTFE tube graft (which represents the central "PA") to the RV.

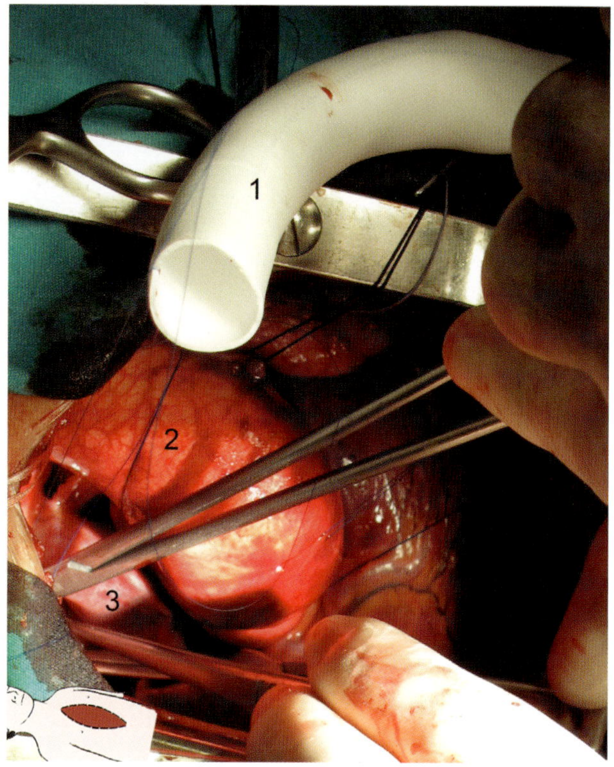

Figure 14.19. The same patient as in Figures 14.14 to 14.18. A PTFE tube graft will be used to connect the nonconfluent left and right PAs together.

1. PTFE tube graft
2. Ascending aorta
3. SVC

Figure 14.20. The same patient as in Figures 14.14 to 14.19. The tube graft has been anastomosed to the left and right PAs, restoring confluence. The tube graft will act as the central PA and will be connected to the RV.

1. Left lung
2. PTFE tube graft
3. Ascending aorta

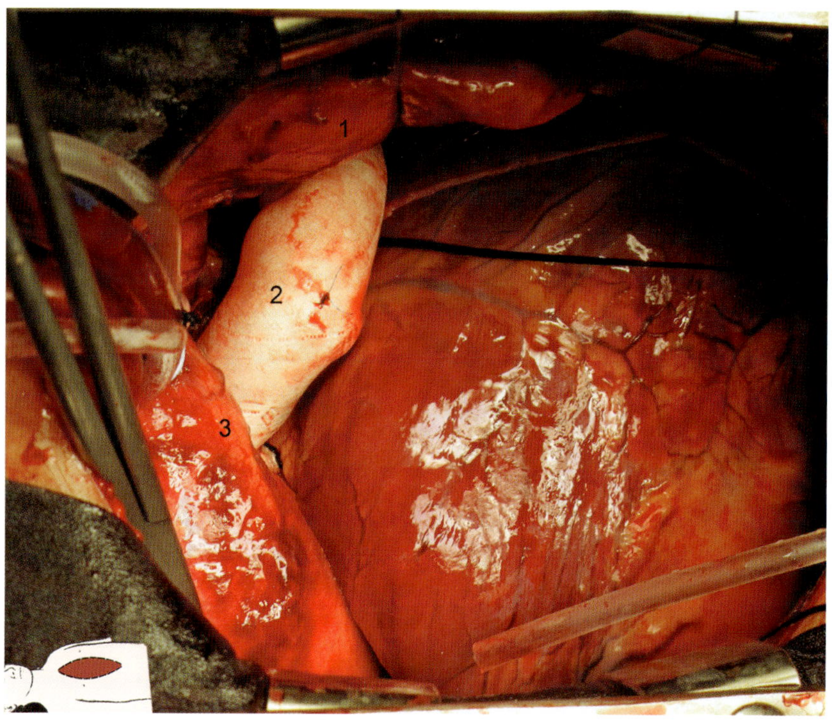

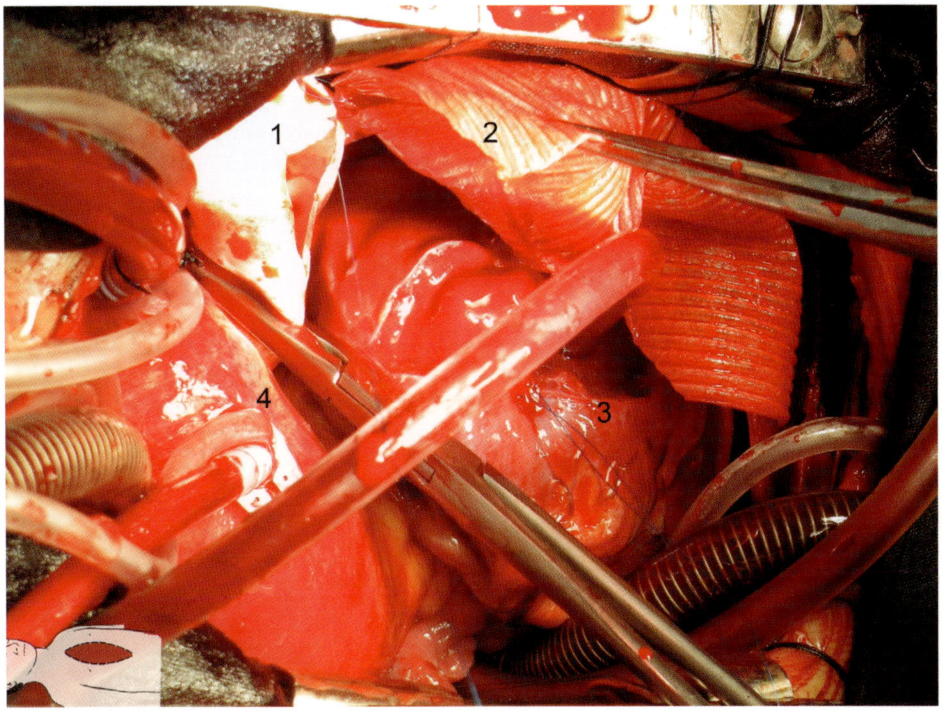

Figure 14.21. The same patient as in Figures 14.14 to 14.20. An incision has been made in the inferior aspect of the PTFE tube graft. A stentless valved conduit (Labcor) will be used to connect the PTFE tube graft (central PA) to the RV. Shown here is the distal end of the conduit being sutured to the PTFE tube graft.

1. PTFE tube graft
2. Stentless valved conduit
3. RV
4. Ascending aorta

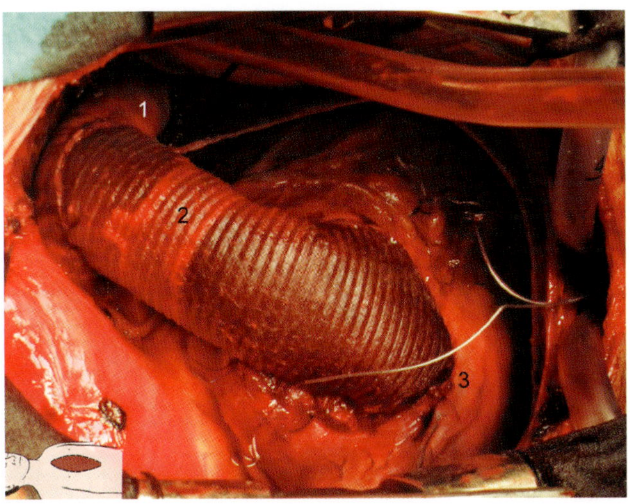

Figure 14.22

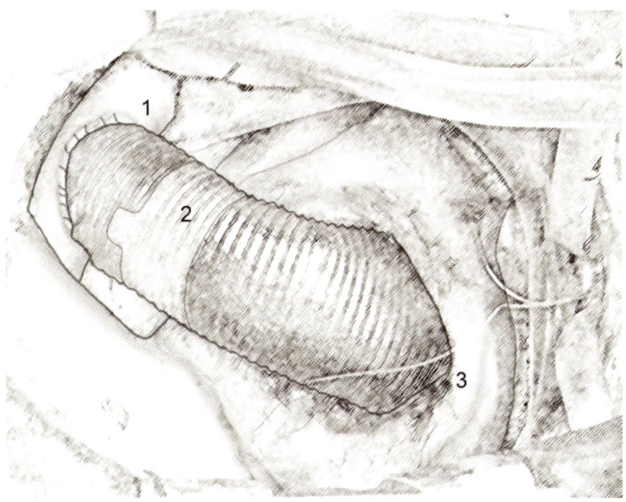

Figure 14.23

The same patient as in Figures 14.14 to 14.21. The repair has been completed by suturing the conduit in the RV. The VSD was closed with a patch (not shown). The number 2 overlies the area of the stentless valve.

1. PTFE tube graft
2. Stentless valved conduit (Labcor)
3. RV

REFERENCES

1. Leonard H, Derrick G, O'Sullivan J, Wren C. Natural and unnatural history of pulmonary atresia. *Heart.* 2000;84:499–503.
2. Hofbecka M, Rauchb A, Leipolda G, Singera H. Diagnosis and treatment of pulmonary atresia and ventricular septal defect. *Prog Pediatr Cardiol.* 1998;9:113–118.
3. Calder AL, Peebles CR, Occleshaw CJ. The prevalence of coronary arterial abnormalities in pulmonary atresia with intact ventricular septum and their influence on surgical results. *Cardiol Young.* 2007;17:387–396.

CHAPTER 15

Transposition of the Great Arteries

Complete transposition of the great arteries (TGA), also called d-TGA, is one of the common cyanotic heart diseases. There is usual or mirror-imaged atrial arrangement with concordant atrioventricular (AV) connections. However, the ventriculoarterial connections are discordant because the aorta arises from the right ventricle (RV), whereas the main pulmonary artery (MPA) arises from the left ventricle (LV). In about one-third of patients, there is an associated ventricular septal defect (VSD).[1] But in those with intact ventricular septum, the presence of an atrial septal defect (ASD) or patent ductus arteriosus (PDA) is crucial for postnatal survival. The coronary artery anatomy can be quite variable.[2]

TGA usually presents in the neonatal period with cyanosis. When mixing between the systemic and pulmonary circulations is limited, the cyanosis can be profound. Administering prostaglandin to keep the ductus arteriosus patent and creating an ASD by balloon atrial septostomy are carried out to alleviate the cyanosis and to act as a bridge to surgery. Double outlet right ventricle (DORV) with subpulmonic VSD (Taussig-Bing anomaly) shares the same pathophysiology with TGA and will be presented here.

In the current era, arterial switch is the operative procedure of choice for most patients and is undertaken in the early neonatal period.

Figures 15.1 to 15.12 are from a 3-day-old neonate with TGA. The gross anatomy of TGA and the coronary artery pattern are shown in Figures 15.1 to 15.3. The ductus arteriosus is shown in Figure 15.4. The subsequent figures show the steps of the arterial switch operation that was performed in this patient. The aorta and pulmonary artery (PA) were transected above the level of the valves. The coronary arteries were dissected and mobilized for a few millimeters. They were harvested from the aorta with a generous button of aortic wall (Figures 15.6–15.7). The coronary arteries were then transferred to their new locations on the PA (Figures 15.8–15.11). A Lecompte maneuver was performed by bringing the PA bifurcation in front of the neoaorta. The neoaorta was anastomosed to the ascending aorta. The neo-PA was reconstructed using autologous pericardium (Figure 15.12).

VARIATIONS IN ANATOMY

The anatomy of TGA can be quite variable. This includes different coronary arterial patterns, spatial arrangement of the great arteries, and the presence of associated lesions such as coarctation and septal defects.[3]

Figure 15.13 shows side-by-side arrangement of the great arteries. There is an accessory left anterior descending (LAD) coronary artery from the right coronary artery. In this patient, arterial switch was performed without the Lecompte maneuver. A single coronary artery system is shown in Figure 15.14.

Figures 15.15 and 15.16 are from a 14-day-old neonate with Taussig-Bing anomaly (DORV with subpulmonic VSD), coarctation, hypoplastic transverse aortic arch, a large PDA, and side-by-side arrangement of the great arteries.

Figures 15.17 and 15.18 show juxtaposition of the right atrial appendage (RAA). Figures 15.19 and 15.20 show an unusual systemic venous drainage in association with TGA. There were 2 innominate (brachiocephalic) veins; one passes behind and the other in front of the transverse aortic arch.

TGA with pulmonary stenosis is usually not amenable to arterial switch. When there is a VSD, a Rastelli procedure may be performed (Figures 15.21 and 15.22).

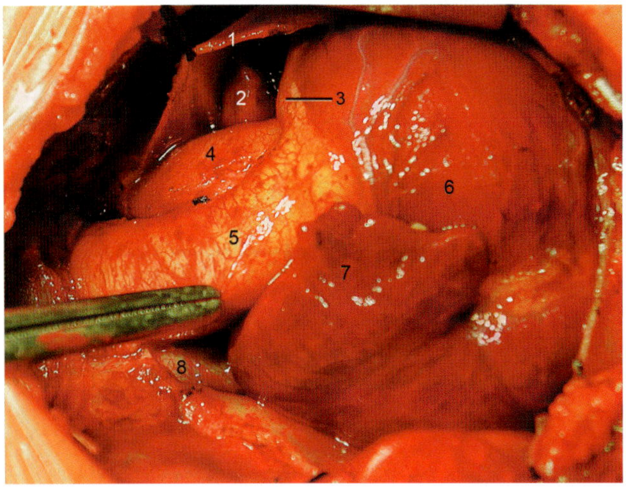

Figure 15.1

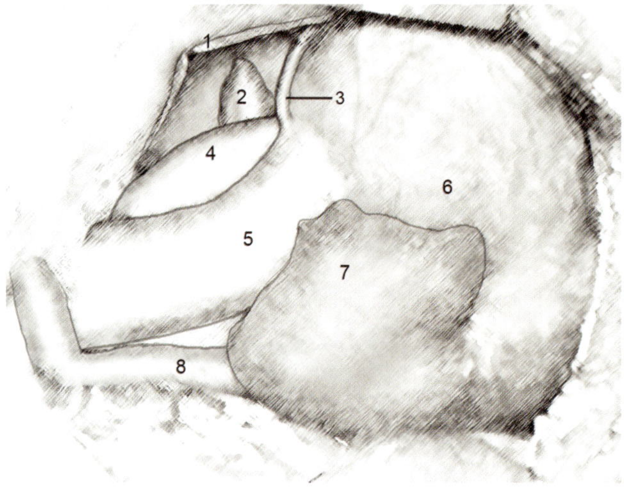

Figure 15.2

TGA as seen through a median sternotomy in a 3-day-old neonate. The aorta arises from the RV and is located anteriorly and to the right. The PA arises from the LV and is located posteriorly and to the left. The left coronary artery is shown.

1. Pericardium
2. Left atrial appendage (LAA)
3. Left coronary artery
4. MPA
5. Ascending aorta
6. RV
7. RAA
8. Superior vena cava (SVC)

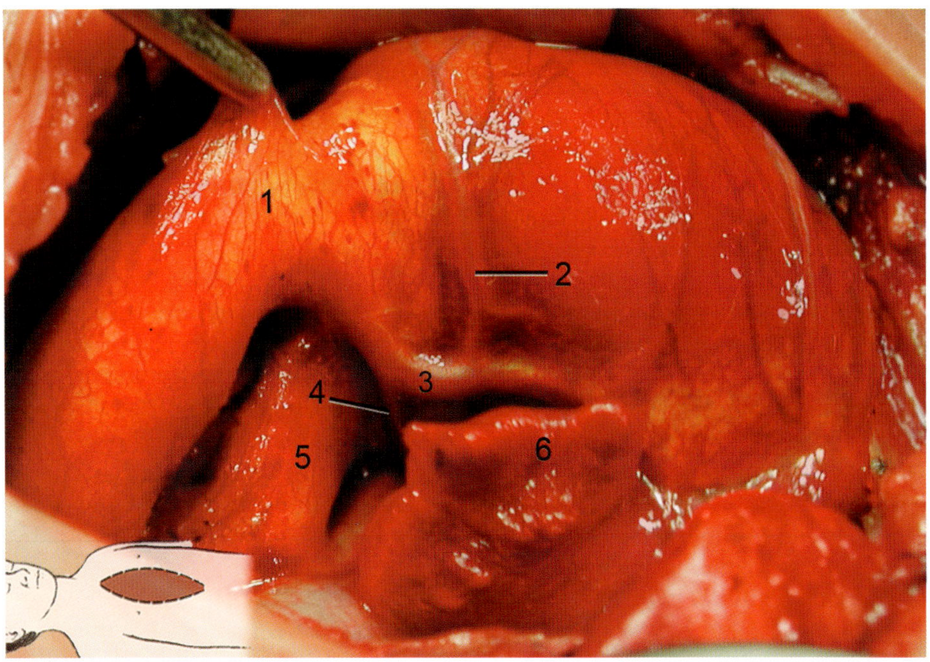

Figure 15.3. Same patient as in Figure 15.1. The right coronary artery and its proximal branches are shown. Note that in this patient, the circumflex artery arises from the right coronary artery.

1. Ascending aorta
2. Conal branch
3. Right coronary artery
4. Circumflex artery
5. Right PA
6. RAA

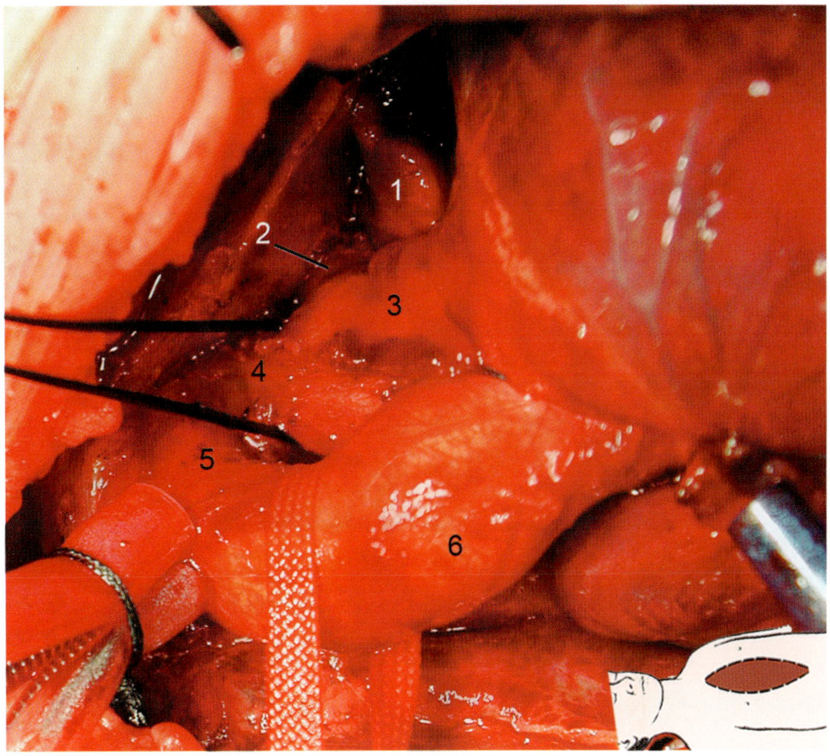

Figure 15.4. Same patient as in Figures 15.1 to 15.3. The aorta is retracted to the right to show the ductus arteriosus.

1. LAA
2. Left PA
3. MPA
4. Ductus arteriosus
5. Aortic arch
6. Ascending aorta

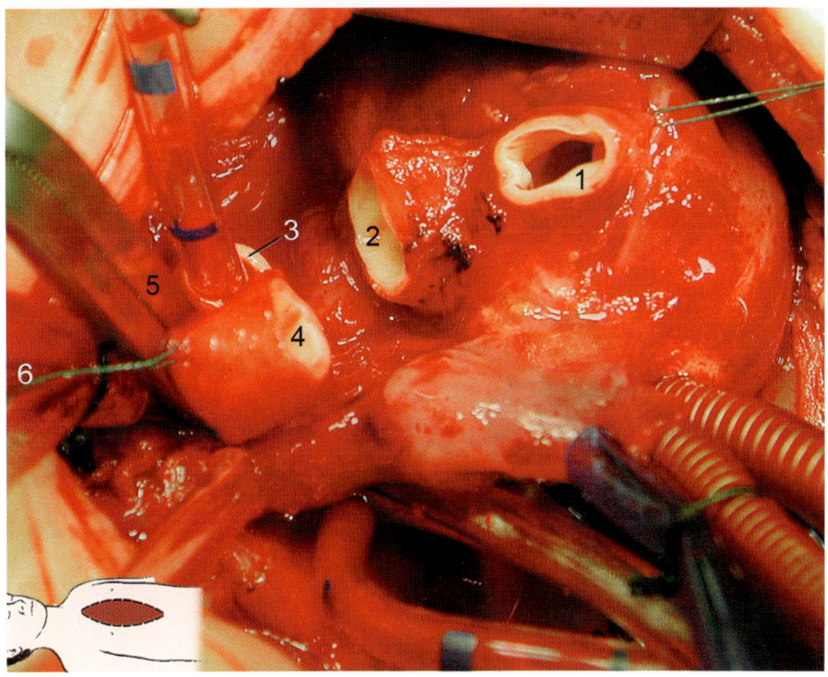

Figure 15.5. Same patient as in Figures 15.1 to 15.4, now on cardiopulmonary bypass, with aortic cross-clamping. The aorta and MPA have been transected above the valves.

1. Proximal transected end of aorta
2. Proximal transected end of MPA
3. Distal transected end of MPA
4. Distal transected end of aorta
5. Aortic cross-clamp
6. Aortic cannula

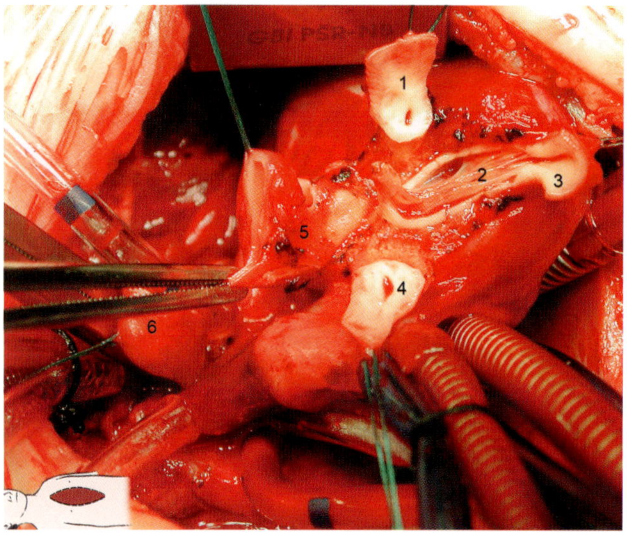

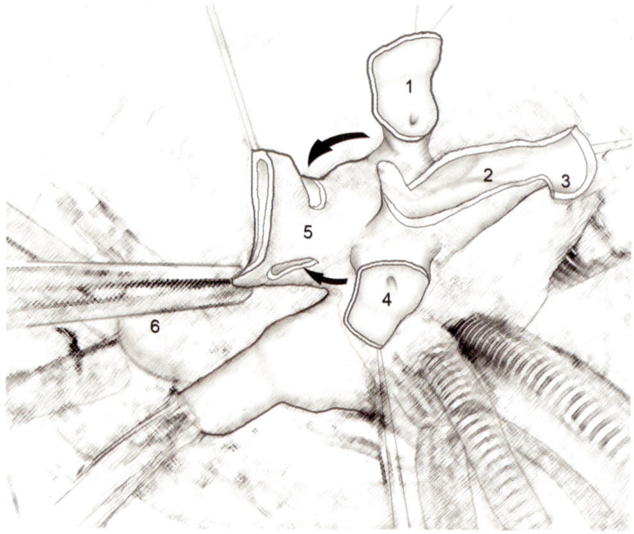

Figure 15.6

Figure 15.7

Same patient as in Figures 15.1 to 15.5. The coronary arteries have been dissected a few millimeters, and then cut off the aorta with a button of aortic wall. The arrows point to where they will be anastomosed in the PA wall, which will become the neoaorta.

1. Left coronary artery button
2. Aortic valve
3. Proximal transected end of aorta
4. Right coronary artery button
5. Proximal end of PA, the future neoaorta
6. Distal transected end of aorta

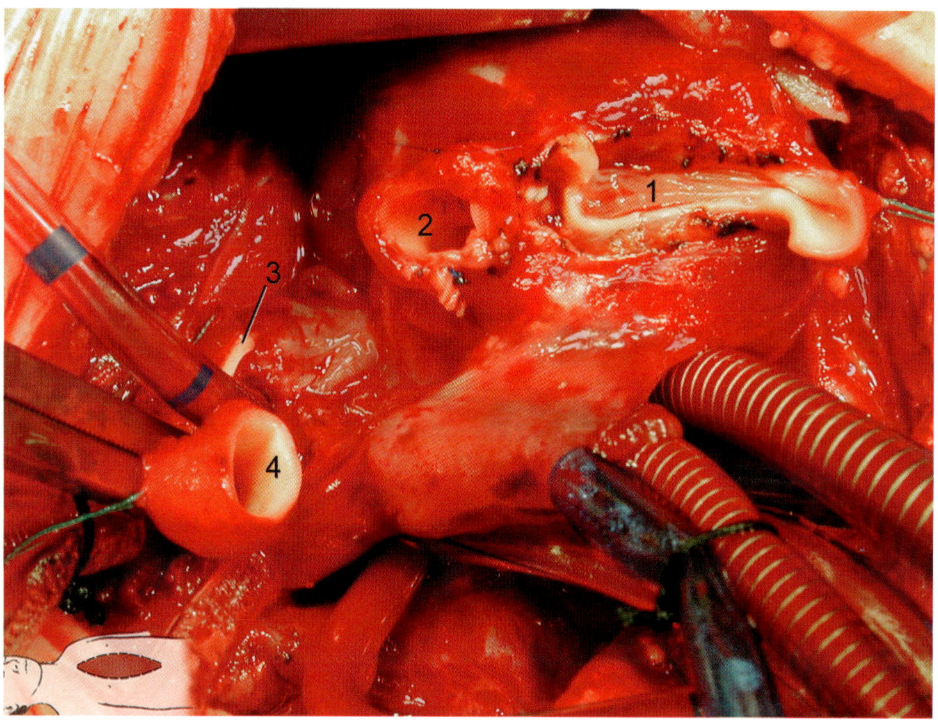

Figure 15.8. The same patient as in Figures 15.1 to 15.7. The coronary arteries have been anastomosed to their new locations on the PA (neoaorta).

1. Aortic valve
2. Transected proximal end of PA (neoaorta)
3. Transected distal end of PA
4. Transected distal end of aorta

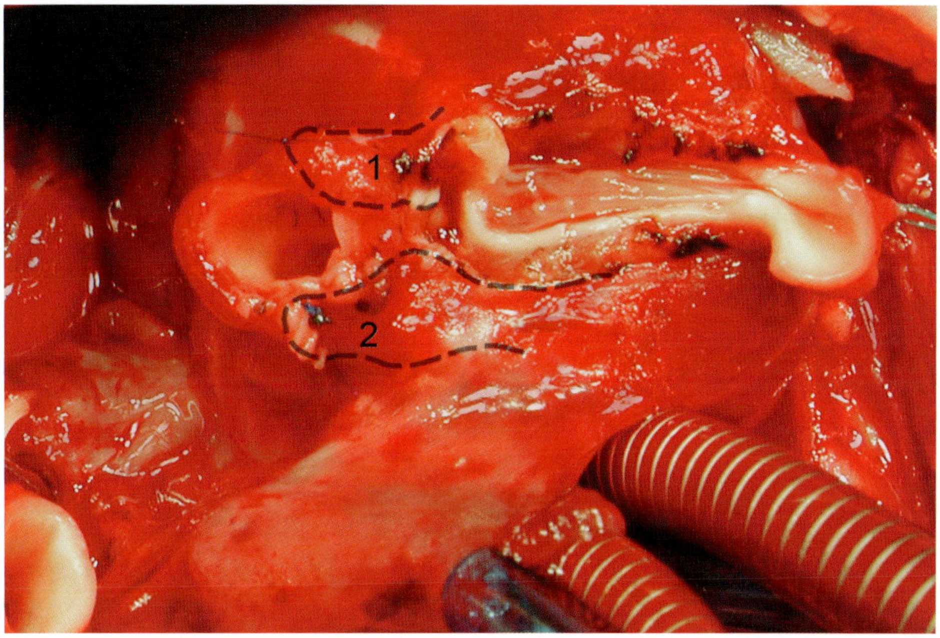

Figure 15.9. The same patient as in Figures 15.1 to 15.8. The coronary arteries buttons are outlined after being anastomosed to their new locations on the PA (neoaorta).

1. Left coronary artery
2. Right coronary artery

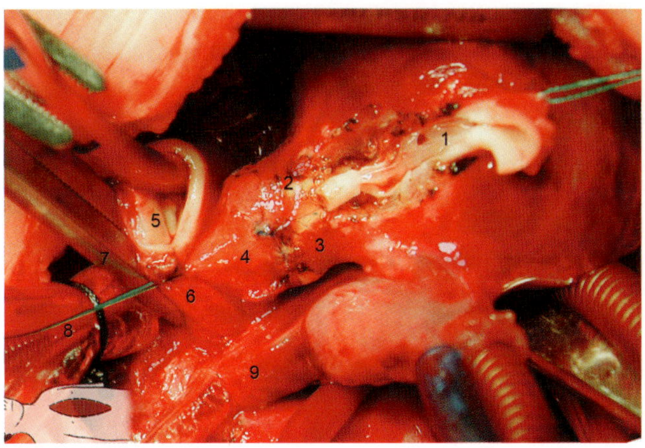

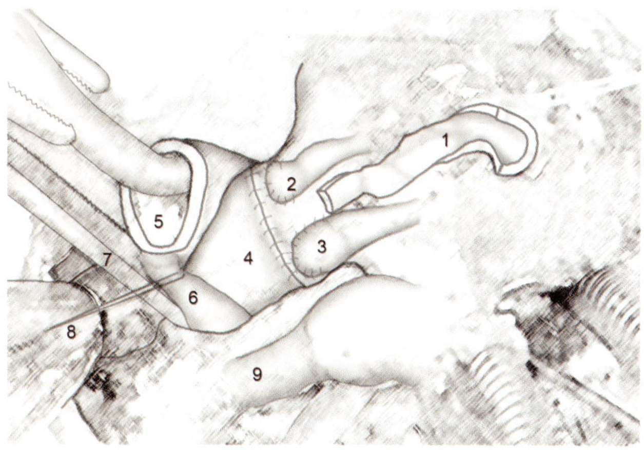

Figure 15.10 **Figure 15.11**

The same patient as in Figures 15.1 to 15.9. The transected distal end of the aorta has been anastomosed to the proximal neoaorta. Now the aorta arises from the LV. The MPA has been brought forward in front of the aorta (Lecompte maneuver).

1. Aortic valve (neopulmonary valve)
2. Left coronary artery
3. Right coronary artery
4. Ascending aorta
5. Transected distal end of MPA
6. Right PA
7. Aortic cross-clamp
8. Aortic cannula
9. SVC

Figure 15.12. The same patient as in Figures 15.1 to 15.11 after completion of the arterial switch. The PA has been reconstructed using autologous pericardium and now arises from the RV.

1. RV
2. Reconstructed PA
3. Right PA
4. Ascending aorta

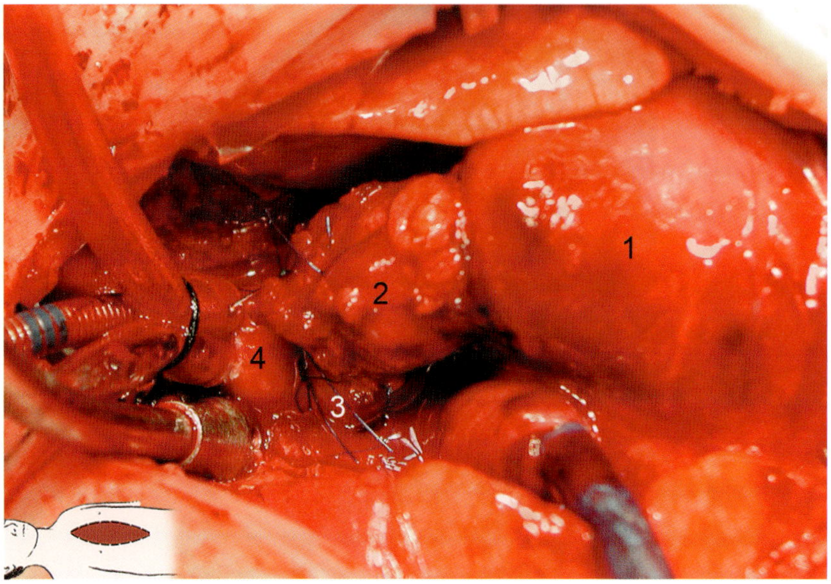

Figure 15.13. Surgical view through a median sternotomy in a 1-month-old neonate with Taussig-Bing anomaly. The great arteries are side-by-side. An accessory LAD coronary artery (4) is seen coming off the right coronary artery. The other LAD is not shown.

1. SVC
2. Ascending aorta
3. MPA
4. Accessory LAD coronary artery
5. Right coronary artery
6. RV
7. RAA

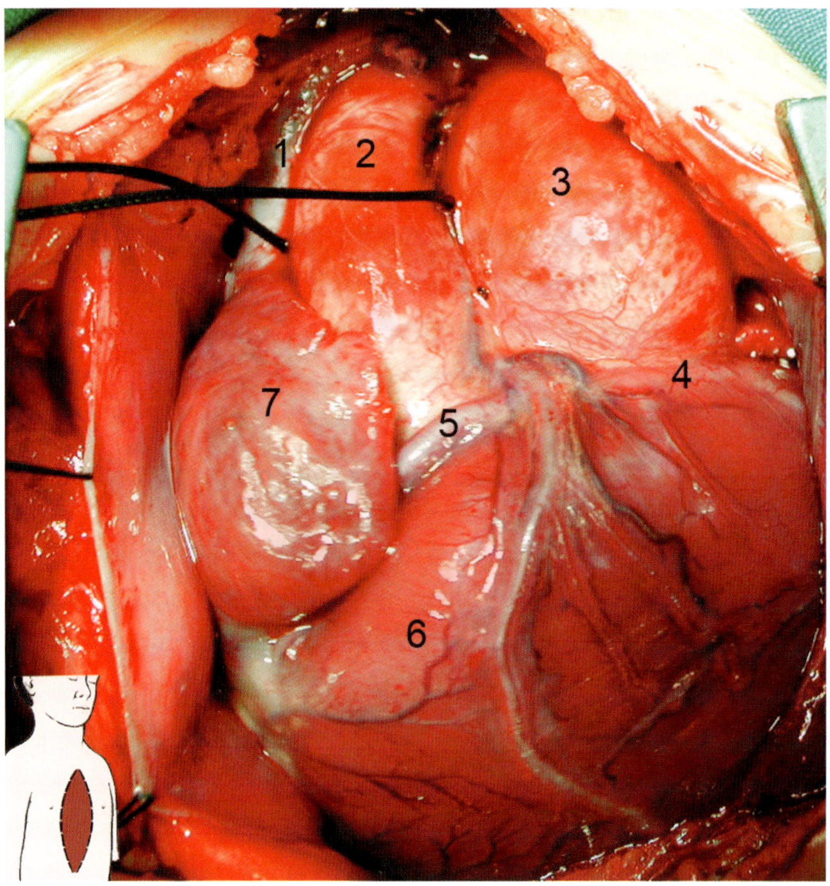

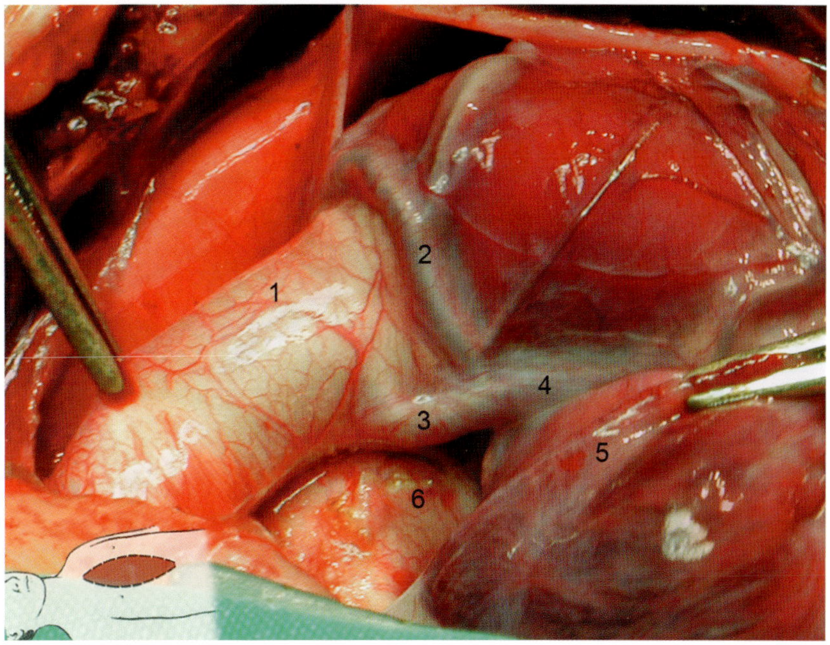

Figure 15.14. TGA as seen through a median sternotomy in a 2-day-old neonate. A single coronary artery arises from the right-facing sinus and branches into the left and right coronary arteries.

1. Ascending aorta
2. Left coronary artery
3. Main coronary artery
4. Right coronary artery
5. RAA
6. MPA

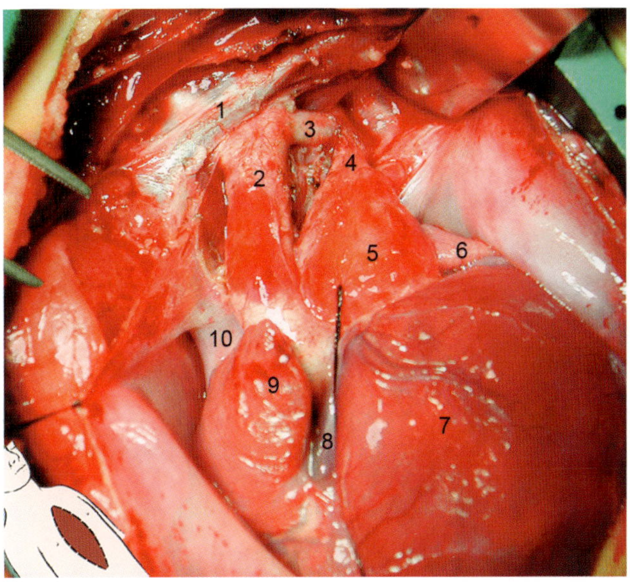

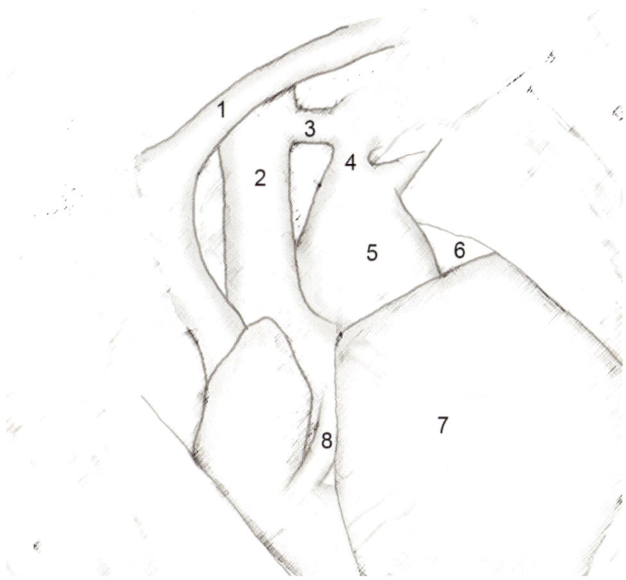

Figure 15.15 **Figure 15.16**

Taussig-Bing anomaly in a 14-day-old neonate. There is coarctation, hypoplastic transverse aortic arch, and a large PDA. The great arteries are arranged side-by-side. Repair was achieved by arch augmentation, coarctation repair, VSD closure, and arterial switch (not shown).

1. Innominate vein
2. Ascending aorta
3. Hypoplastic transverse aortic arch
4. PDA
5. MPA
6. LAA
7. RV
8. Right coronary artery
9. RAA
10. SVC

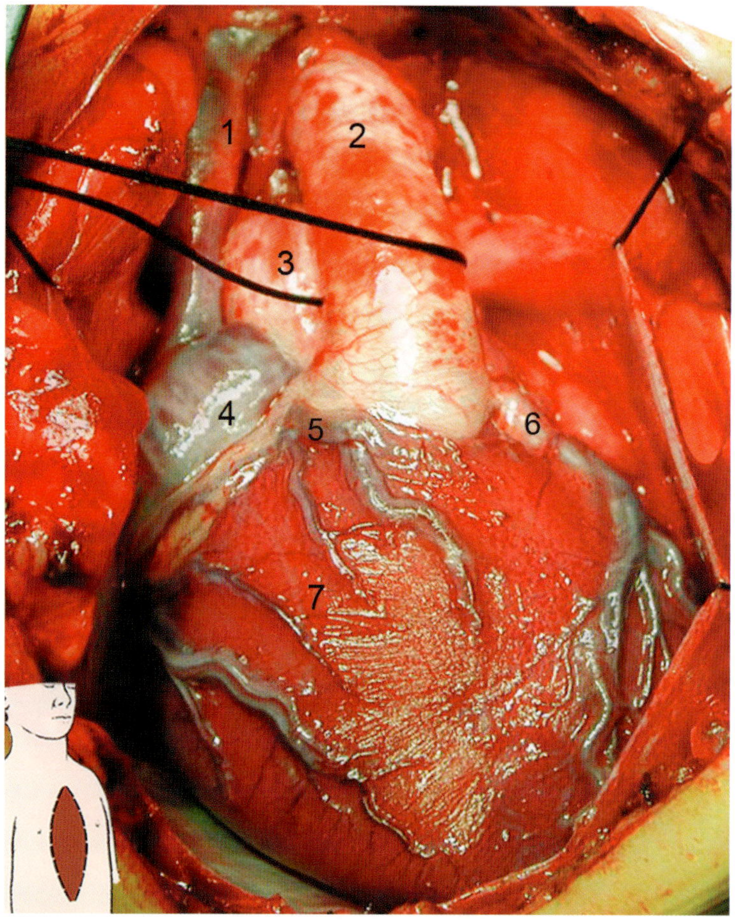

Figure 15.17. TGA in a 2-month-old infant as seen through a median sternotomy. Note that the RAA is not seen because of its juxtaposition behind the aorta.

1. SVC
2. Ascending aorta
3. MPA
4. Right atrium
5. Right coronary artery
6. Left coronary artery
7. RV

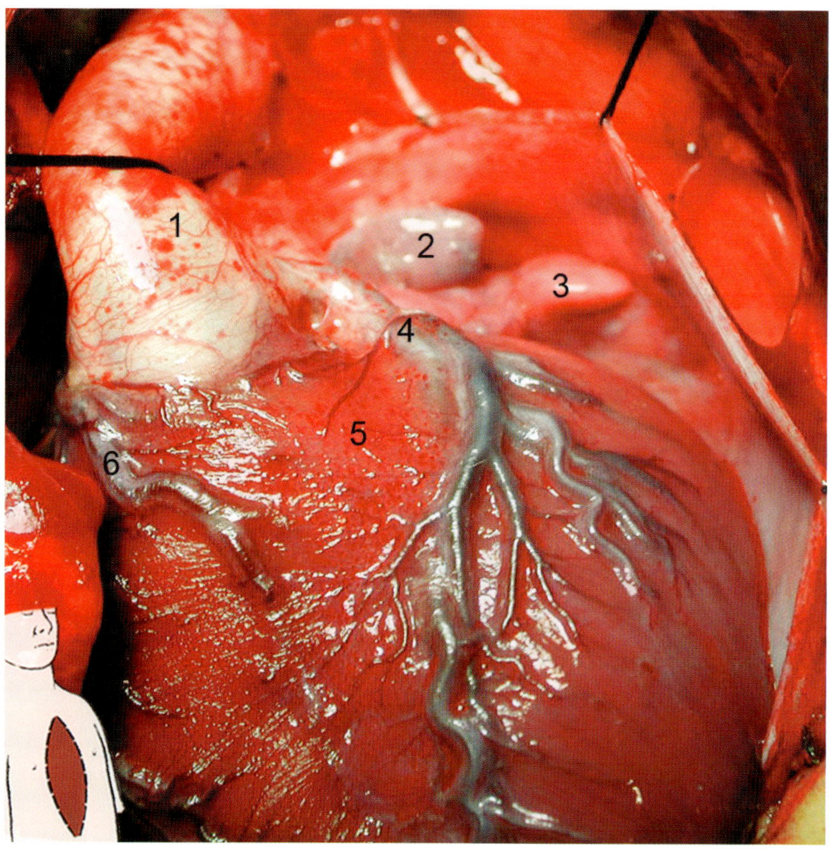

Figure 15.18. The same patient as in Figure 15.17. When the aorta is retracted to the right, the juxtaposed RAA becomes visible.

1. Ascending aorta
2. RAA
3. LAA
4. Left coronary artery
5. RV
6. Conal branch of right coronary artery

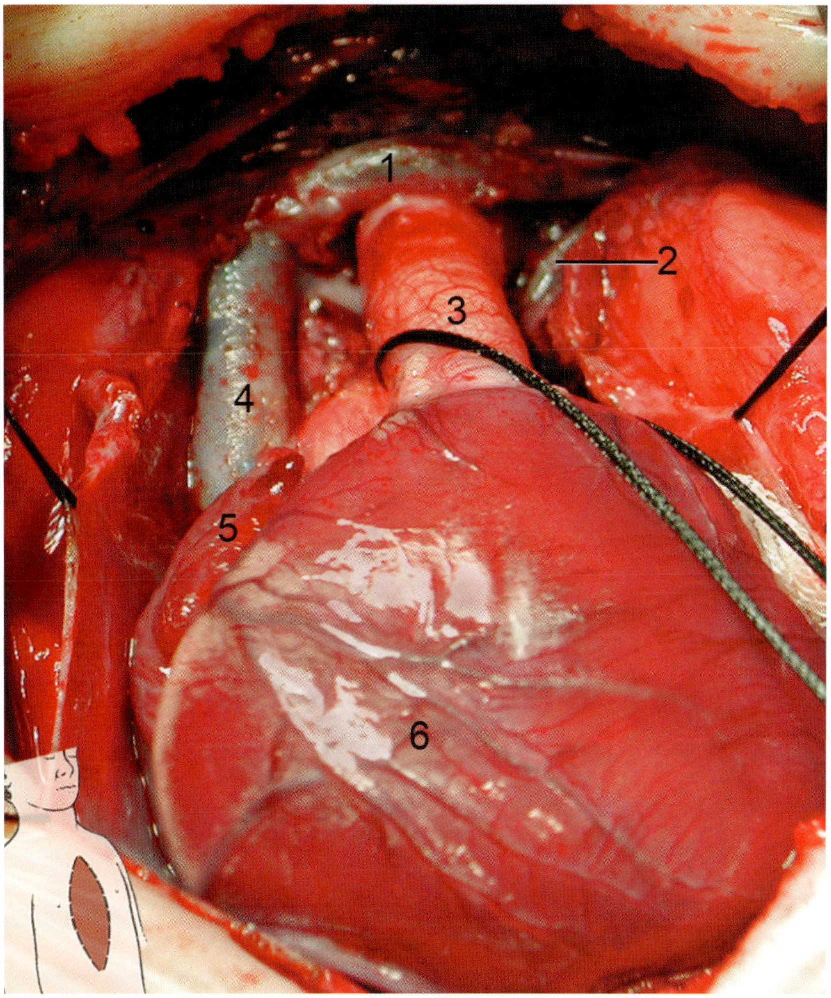

Figure 15.19. Median sternotomy view of a 15-day-old neonate with TGA. Note the double innominate vein, which has 2 components, running anterior to the aorta and retro-aortic.

1. Innominate vein
2. Retro-aortic innominate vein
3. Ascending aorta
4. SVC
5. RAA
6. RV

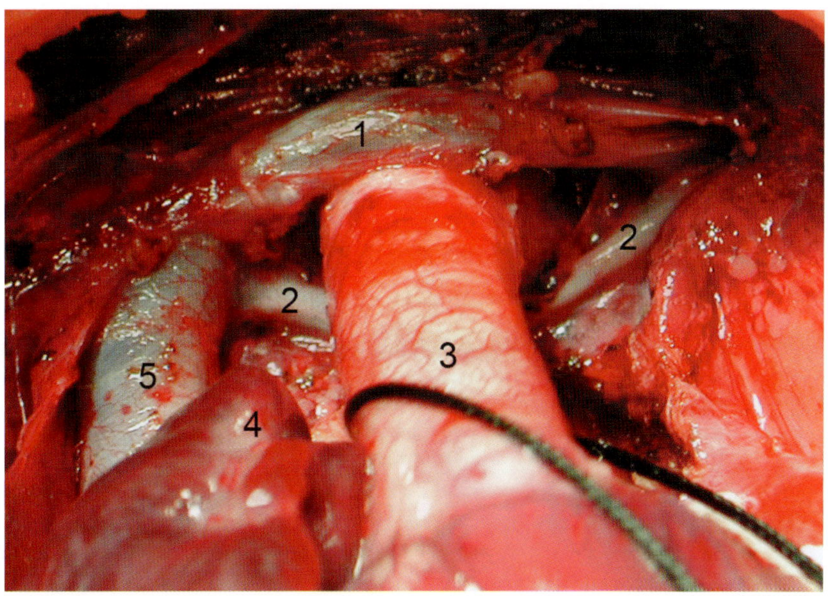

Figure 15.20. Close-up view of the same patient as in Figure 15.19. Again note the double innominate vein, embracing the aorta anteriorly and posteriorly.

1. Innominate vein
2. Retro-aortic innominate vein
3. Ascending aorta
4. RAA
5. SVC

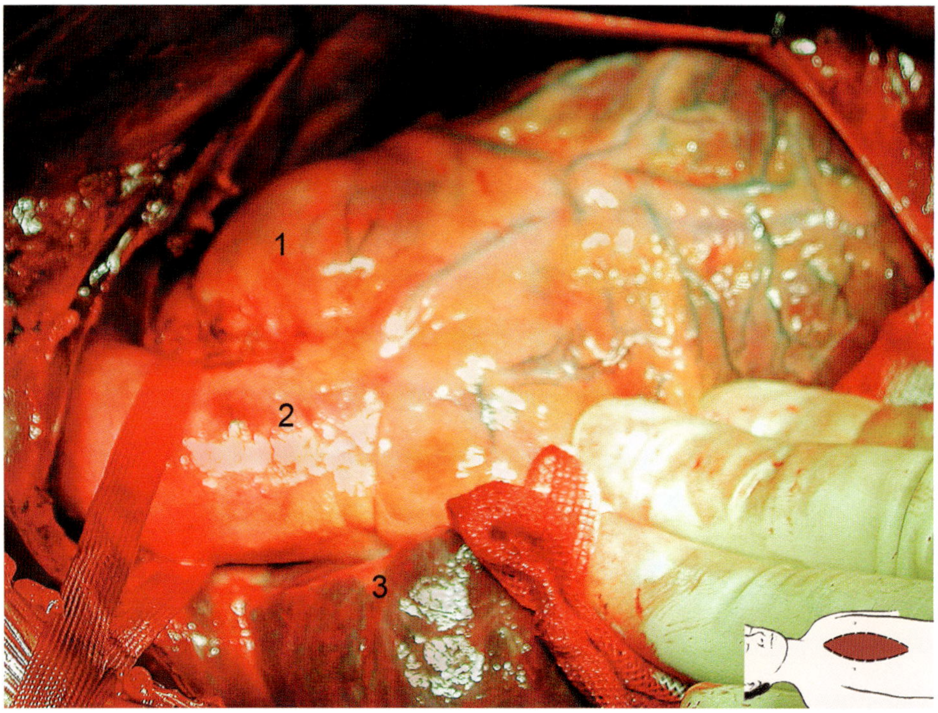

Figure 15.21. TGA with VSD and pulmonary stenosis in a 16-year-old patient. The great arteries are side-by-side.

1. MPA
2. Ascending aorta
3. RAA

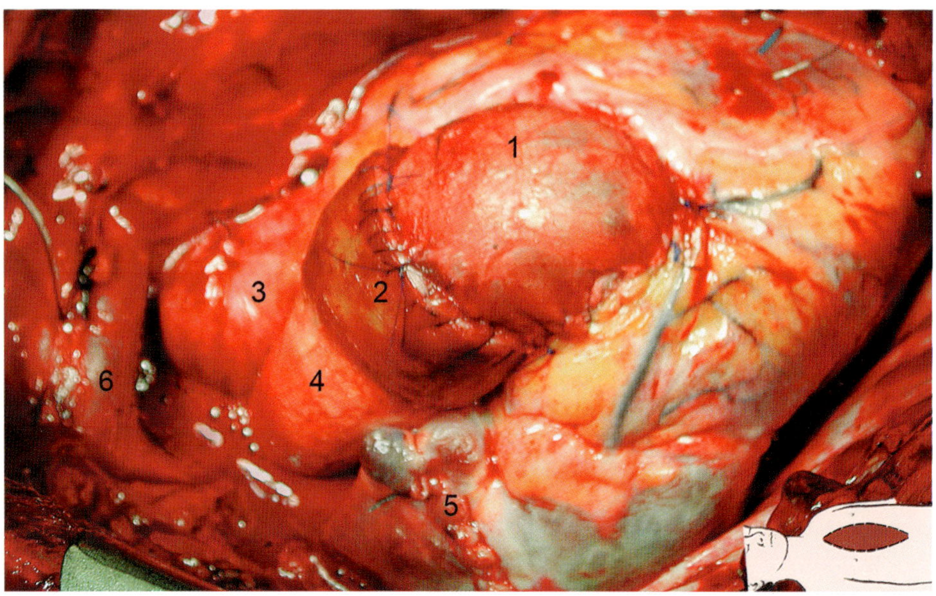

Figure 15.22. The same patient as in Figure 15.21, after Rastelli procedure. The left ventricular output was routed through the VSD (not shown) to the aorta. Continuity between the RV and the PA was established using a 21 mm Cryolife Ross conduit. It has been implanted into the RV to the right of the aorta.

1. Pericardial hood
2. Valved conduit (Cryolife Ross)
3. Ascending aorta
4. Distal end of conduit
5. RAA
6. Innominate vein

This entails routing the left ventricular outflow through the VSD to the aorta, and implanting an RV-to-PA conduit. Coronary artery transfer is not needed. Another procedure that can be used in such situations is arterial translocation (the Nikaidoh procedure),[4] which has the advantage of less long-term left ventricular outflow obstruction.[5] In this procedure, the aortic root, along with its valve, is completely explanted, the pulmonary trunk and valve are excised, and the outlet (conal) septum is removed. Then the aortic root is reimplanted in the left ventricular outflow tract (LVOT) in place of the excised pulmonary trunk, and the right ventricular outflow is reconstructed. Figures 15.23 to 15.37 are from a 3-year-old child who had TGA, VSD, and pulmonary stenosis. He also had a single coronary artery arising from the left-facing sinus and giving rise to the left and right coronary arteries, with the right branch coursing in front of the aortic root. Arterial translocation was done as shown in Figures 15.24 to 15.37. Figures 15.38 and 15.39 are from a child who had TGA with VSD and pulmonary stenosis. The main and branch PAs were hypoplastic, and there was near-complete obstruction of the left PA by an intraluminal fibrous shelf.

SENNING OPERATION

An occasional patient may not be a candidate for an arterial switch operation. Atrial-level switch (Senning or Mustard operations) would result in physiological rather than anatomic repair. The pulmonary venous return will be directed to the RV and from there to the aorta, whereas the systemic venous return will be directed to the LV and from there to the PA. Atrial switch is also employed as part of a double switch for corrected L-transposition of the great arteries (l-TGA).

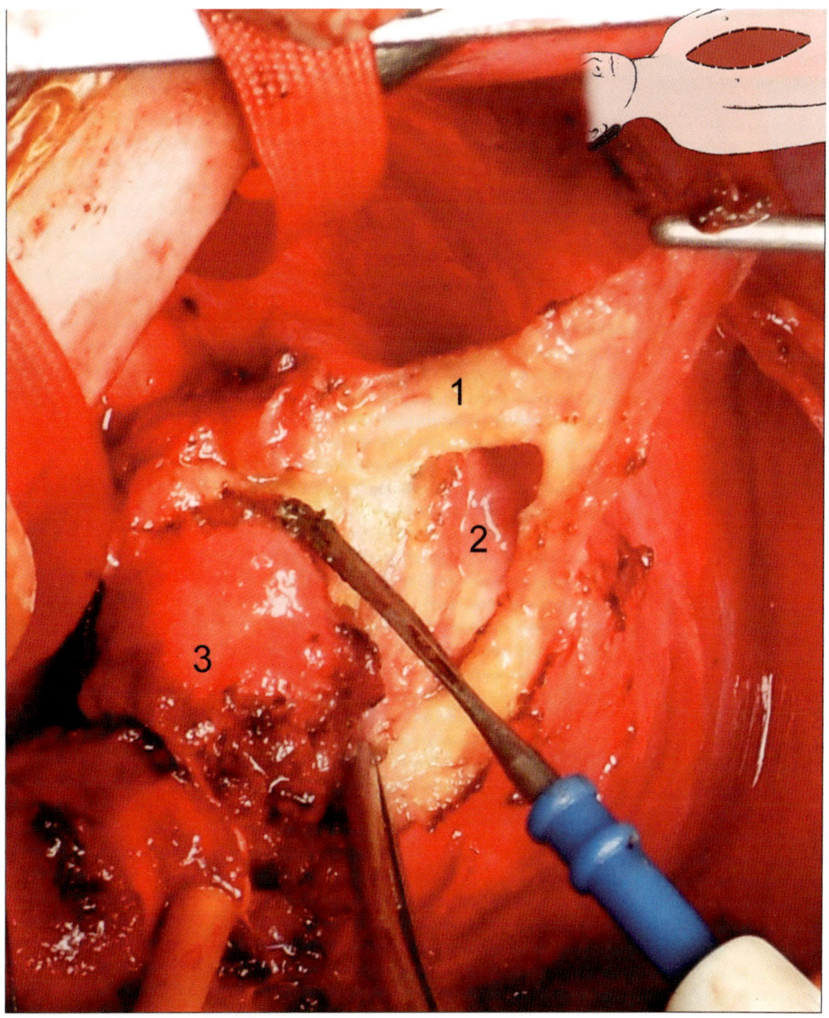

Figure 15.23. A median sternotomy view of a 3-year-old child with TGA, VSD, pulmonary stenosis, and single coronary artery. (This and the following photographs are taken with cranial angulations, from the anesthesia side of the operating table.) The right coronary artery is being dissected up to its origin from the main coronary artery, which arises from the left-facing sinus.

1. Right coronary artery
2. RV
3. Ascending aorta

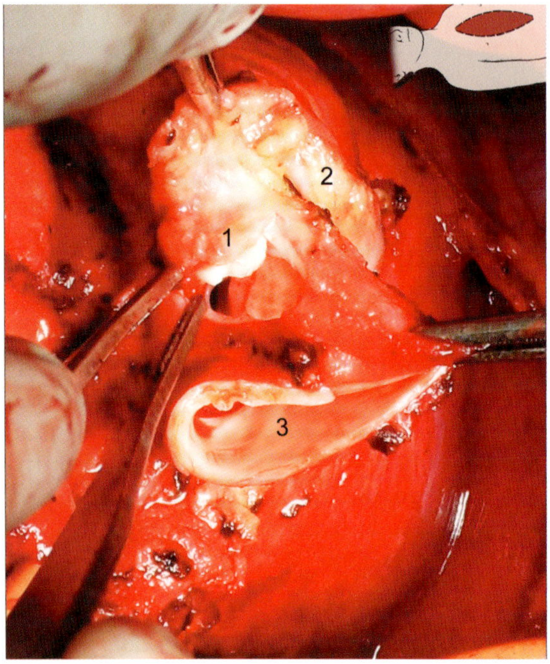

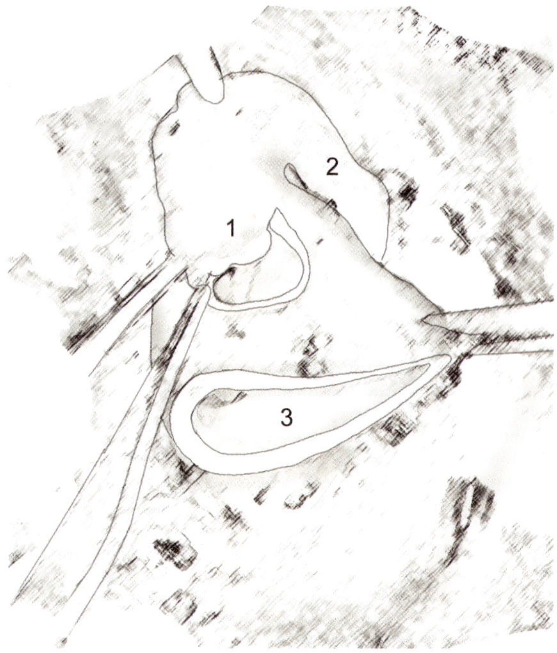

Figure 15.24 **Figure 15.25**

The same patient as in Figure 15.23, after transection of the ascending aorta above the sinotubular junction. The single coronary artery is being removed from the aortic root with a button of aortic wall.

1. Main coronary artery
2. Right coronary artery
3. Aortic root

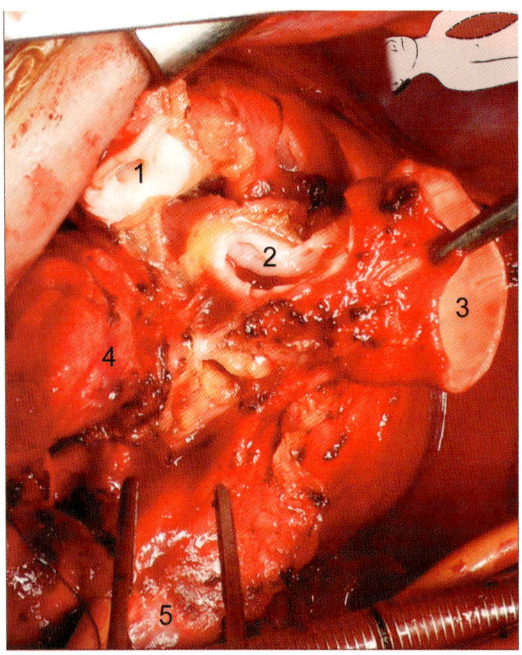

Figure 15.26. The same patient as in Figures 15.23 to 15.25. The main coronary artery has been completely freed from the aortic wall. The aortic root is retracted, revealing the PA.

1. Main coronary artery
2. Original site of coronary artery (now a defect in the aortic wall)
3. Aortic root
4. MPA
5. SVC–RA junction

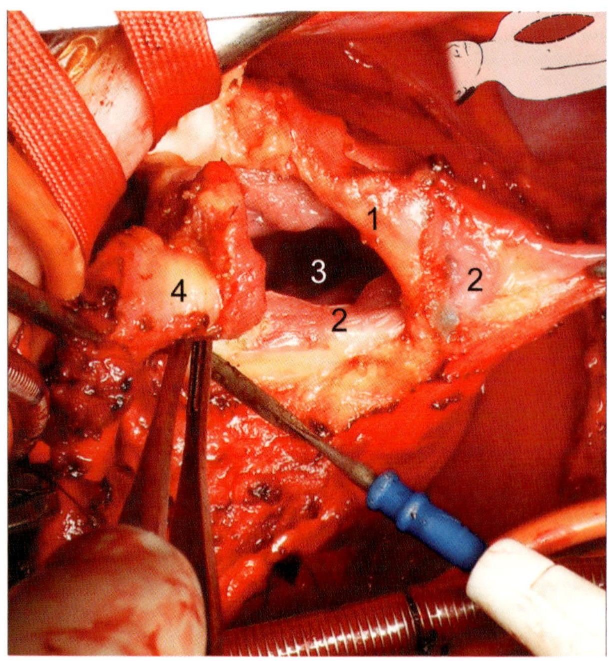

Figure 15.27. The same patient as in Figures 15.23 to 15.26. The aortic root is being explanted from the RV.

1. Right coronary artery
2. RV free wall
3. RV cavity
4. Aortic root

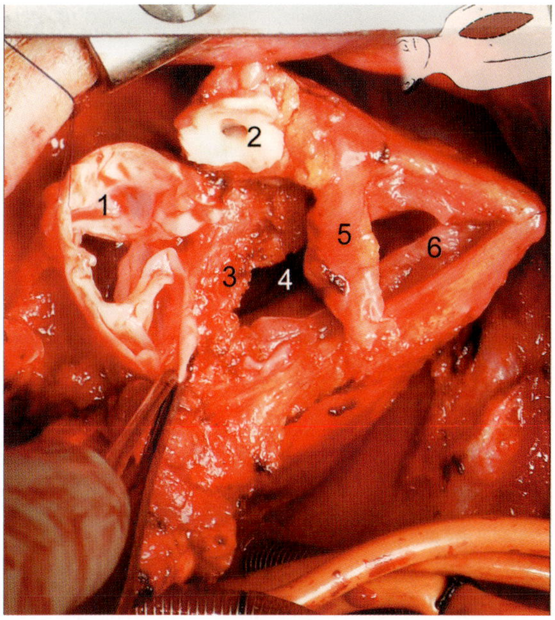

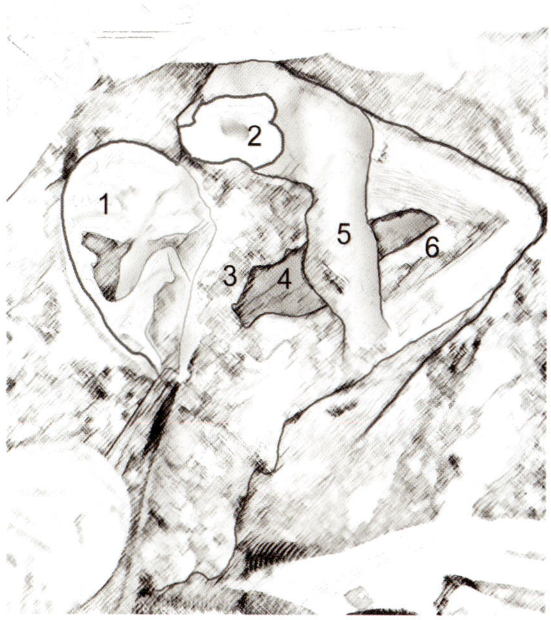

Figure 15.28 **Figure 15.29**

The same patient as in Figures 15.23 to 15.27 after mobilization of the aortic root and the MPA from their respective sites in the heart. Note the outlet (conal) septum (3) between the 2 ventricular outflows. This septum will be resected next.

1. Pulmonary valve
2. Main coronary artery
3. Outlet (conal) septum
4. RV cavity
5. Right coronary artery
6. RV free wall

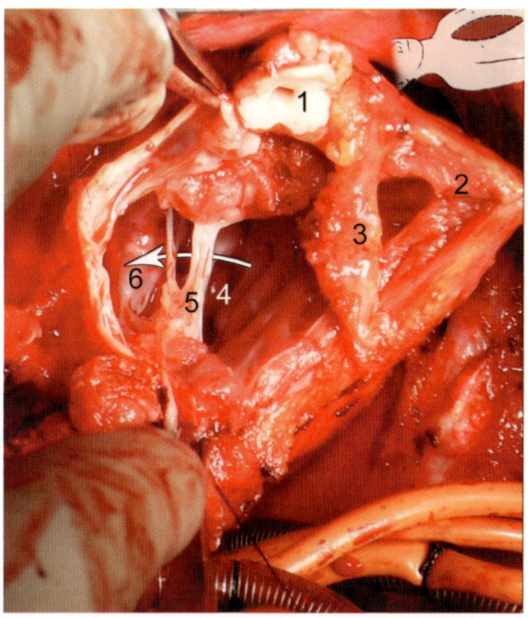

Figure 15.30. The same patient as in Figures 15.23 to 15.29. The outlet (conal) septum has been resected down to the VSD (the VSD is represented by the arrow).

1. Main coronary artery
2. RV free wall
3. Right coronary artery
4. RV cavity
5. Septal leaflet of tricuspid valve
6. Ventricular septum

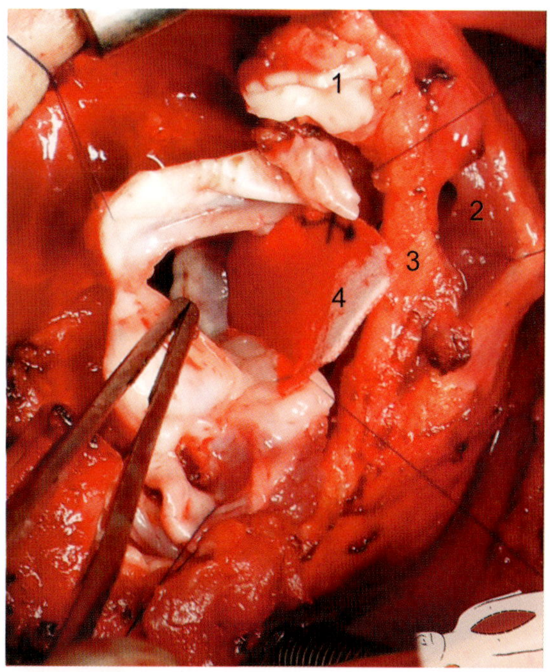

Figure 15.31. The same patient as in Figures 15.23 to 15.30. A Dacron patch has been placed to close the VSD and to act as the anterior (septal) wall for the enlarged LVOT.

1. Main coronary artery
2. RV free wall
3. Right coronary artery
4. Dacron patch

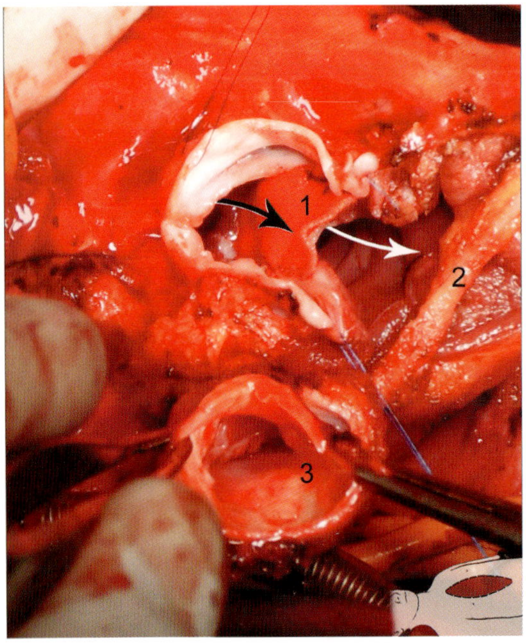

Figure 15.32. The same patient as in Figures 15.23 to 15.31 after placement of the Dacron patch. The black arrow represents the LVOT, whereas the white arrow represents the RVOT. The aortic root is brought into the surgical field and will next be implanted into the LV outflow position.

1. Dacron patch
2. Right coronary artery
3. Aortic root

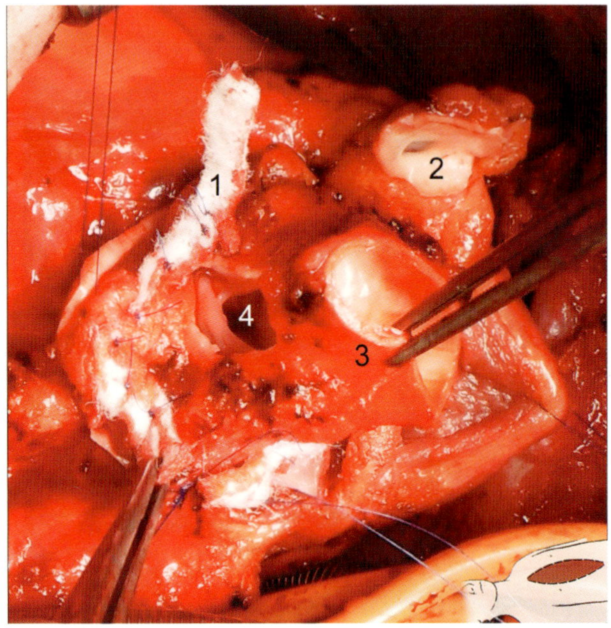

Figure 15.33. The same patient as in Figures 15.23 to 15.32. The aortic root is being implanted in its new location in the LVOT. A Teflon felt is used to support the anastomosis.

1. Teflon felt
2. Main coronary artery (button)
3. Aortic root
4. Defect in aortic wall (original site of coronary artery)

Figure 15.34. The same patient as in Figures 15.23 to 15.33. The aortic root is being anastomosed to the ascending aorta. The coronary artery has not been reimplanted yet.

1. Coronary artery
2. RV cavity
3. Aortic root
4. Ascending aorta

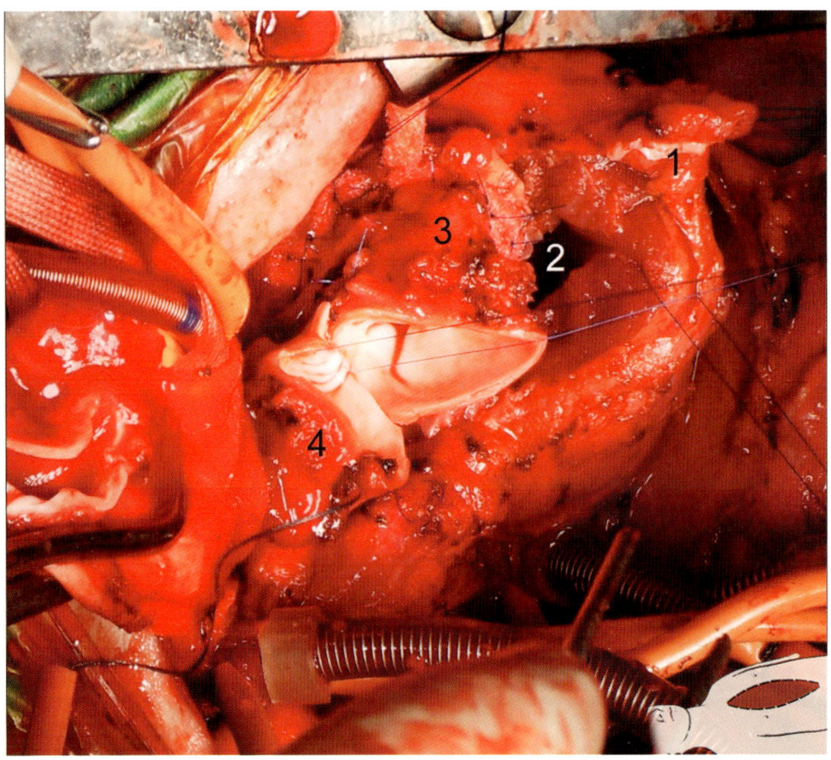

Figure 15.35. The same patient as in Figures 15.23 to 15.34. The coronary artery is being reimplanted into the aortic root.

1. Coronary artery button
2. Receiving site for the coronary artery
3. Aortic root

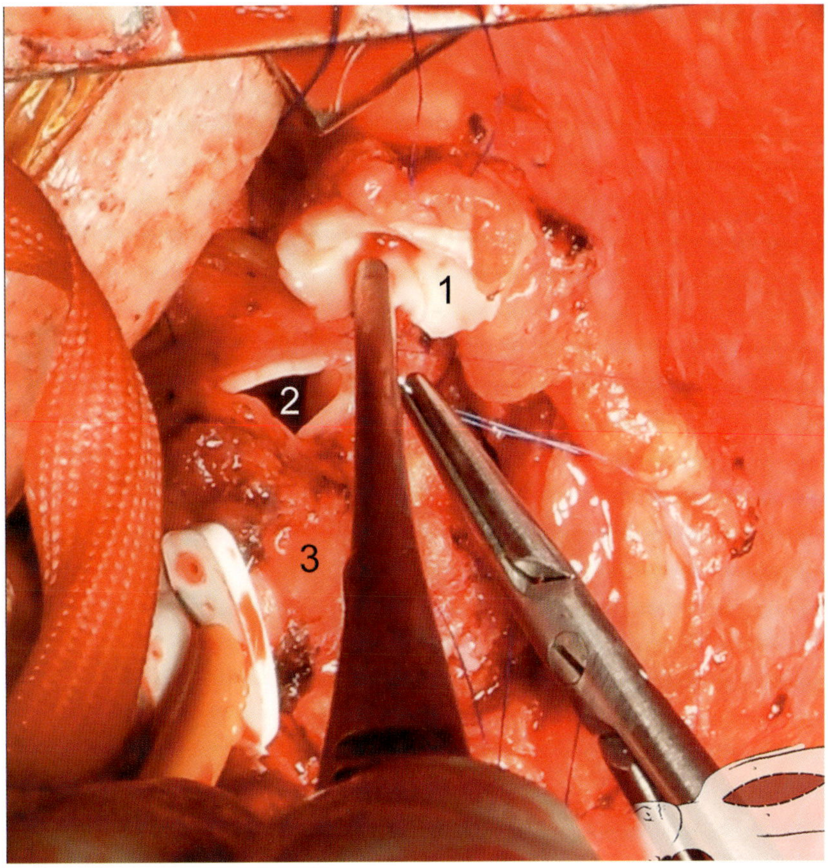

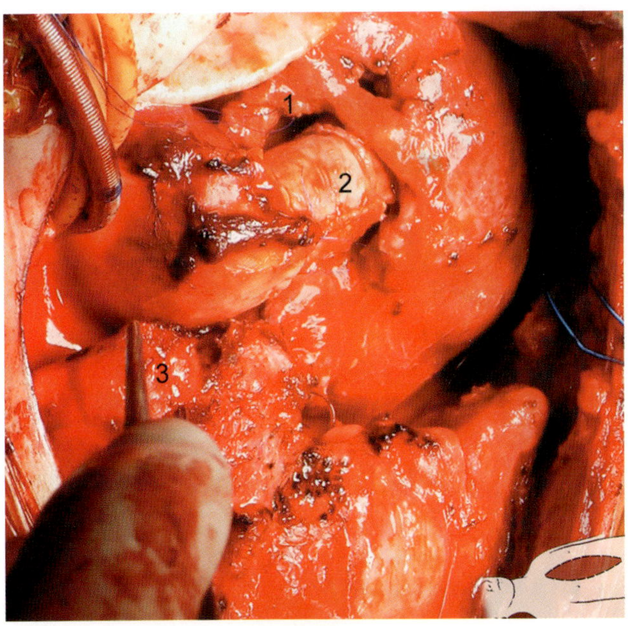

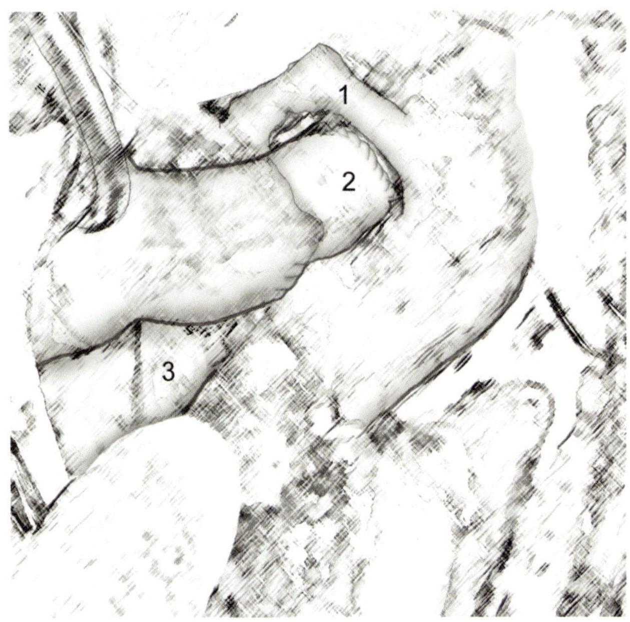

Figure 15.36 **Figure 15.37**

The same patient as in Figures 15.23 to 15.35 after completion of all anastomoses. A Shellhigh conduit was placed between the RV and the MPA.

1. Coronary artery
2. Shellhigh conduit
3. Ascending aorta

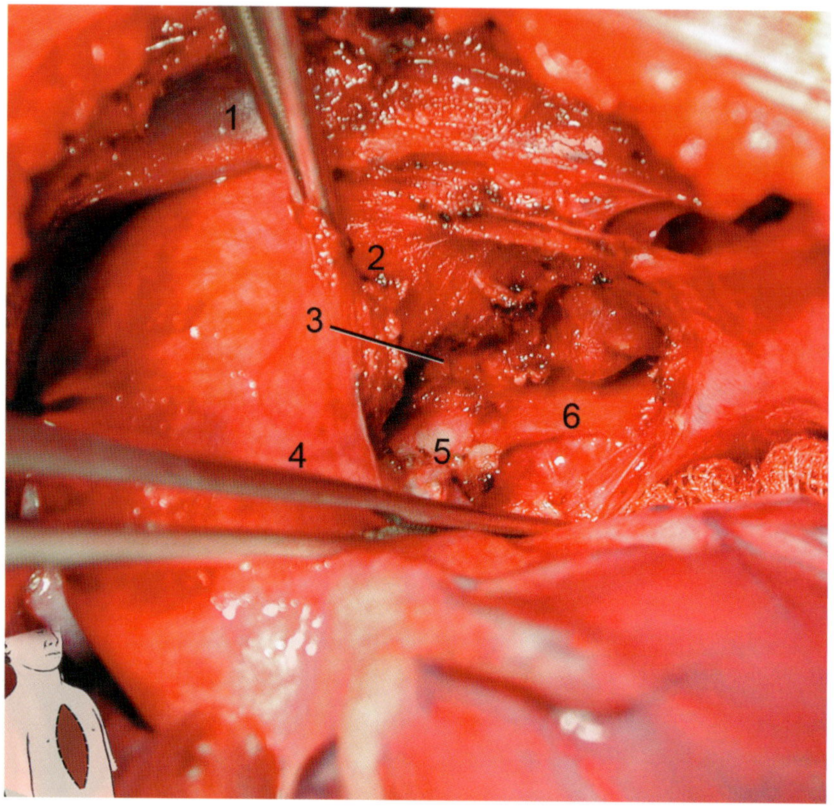

Figure 15.38. Median sternotomy view in a child with TGA, VSD, and pulmonary stenosis. The PA and its branches are hypoplastic.

1. Innominate vein
2. Aortic arch
3. Ductus arteriosus
4. Ascending aorta
5. Proximal left PA
6. Left PA

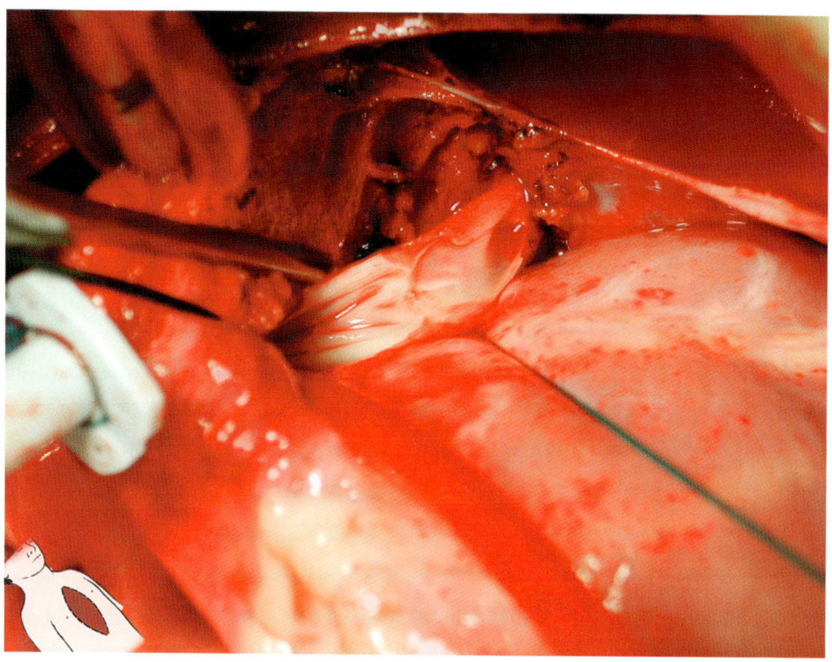

Figure 15.39. Same patient as in Figure 15.38. The left PA has been opened longitudinally. There is near-complete obstruction by an intraluminal fibromuscular shelf. Surgical repair was achieved by the Rastelli operation and patch augmentation of the PAs (not shown).

Figure 15.40 shows diagrammatically the technique of Senning surgery. Incisions are made in the right and left atria, and the atrial septum is opened by cutting along 3 sides, keeping the posterior portion attached to form a flap. This flap may need to be augmented with a pericardial patch to increase its size. The flap is sutured to the left atrial wall caudal to the PVs and cephalad to the opening of the LAA. Then the posterior wall of the right atrium is sutured to the margin of the opened interatrial septum. This will route the systemic venous return to the mitral valve. Then the left flap of the left atrial incision and the anterior wall of the right atrium are anastomosed together to form the new pulmonary venous atrium. This atrium often needs augmentation with a pericardial patch. At the end of the procedure, the pulmonary venous return is directed to the tricuspid valve.

Figures 15.41 to 15.52 are from a 5-month-old infant with TGA, a small VSD, and mild pulmonary stenosis who underwent a Senning operation.

LATE COMPLICATIONS

Postsurgical long-term follow-up is needed to detect complications. Pulmonary stenosis, usually supravalvar, is the most common long-term complication of arterial switch operation.[6] Figure 15.53 shows neopulmonary stenosis in a 30-month-old child who was born with TGA that was repaired with an arterial switch. A Lecompte maneuver was not used in this patient because of the side-by-side relationship of the great arteries. Figures 15.54 and 15.56 show another example of post–arterial switch pulmonary stenosis that required a transannular patch. The Lecompte maneuver can result in branch pulmonary stenosis caused by stretching of the branch PAs and mechanical compression by the aorta, as shown in Figures 15.57 and 15.58. Figures 15.59 and 15.60 are from a 12-year-old child who had TGA repaired by Senning operation and later developed pulmonary stenosis. A bovine jugular vein xenograft conduit (Contegra) was placed between the LV and the PA.

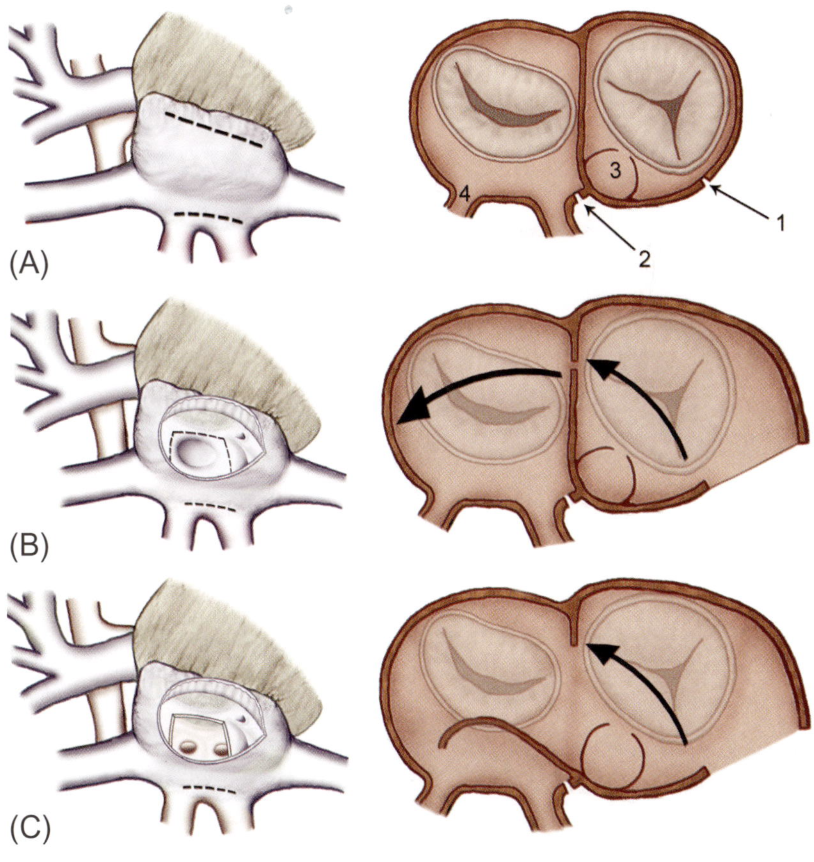

Figure 15.40. Diagramatic illustration of the technique of the Senning surgery. Incisions are made in the right and left atria (**A**). A flap is made of the interatrial septum by cutting the septum along 3 sides, keeping the posterior portion intact (**B** and **C**), thus allowing it to cover the pulmonary vein (PV) orifices. This flap may need to be augmented with a pericardial patch to increase its size and to close any ASD, if present.

1. Right atrial incision
2. Left atrial incision
3. Vena cava
4. PV

Figure 15.40 *(continued)*. The flap is sutured to the left atrial wall, thus separating the PVs from the mitral valve (**D**). The posterior edge of the right atrial incision is sutured to the anterior edge of the opened interatrial septum (D and **E**), thereby routing the systemic venous return to the mitral valve. Then the left margin of the left atrial incision and the anterior wall of the right atrium are anastomosed together to form the new pulmonary venous atrium (E). This atrium often needs augmentation with a pericardial patch (**F**). Now the pulmonary venous return is directed to the tricuspid valve.

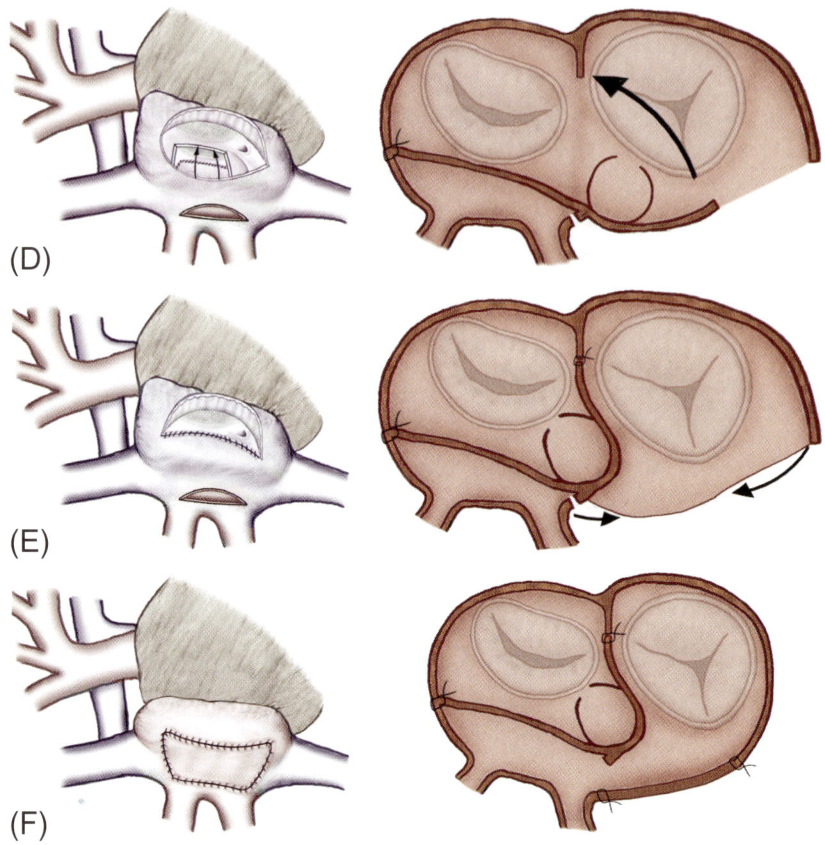

Figure 15.41. TGA in a 5-month-old infant as seen through a median sternotomy incision for a Senning operation. Picture shows the gross anatomy.

1. Left coronary artery
2. Ascending aorta
3. RV
4. Right coronary artery
5. RAA
6. Right coronary artery in the AV groove
7. Pericardium overlying the diaphragm
8. Right atrium
9. SVC
10. MPA
11. Innominate vein

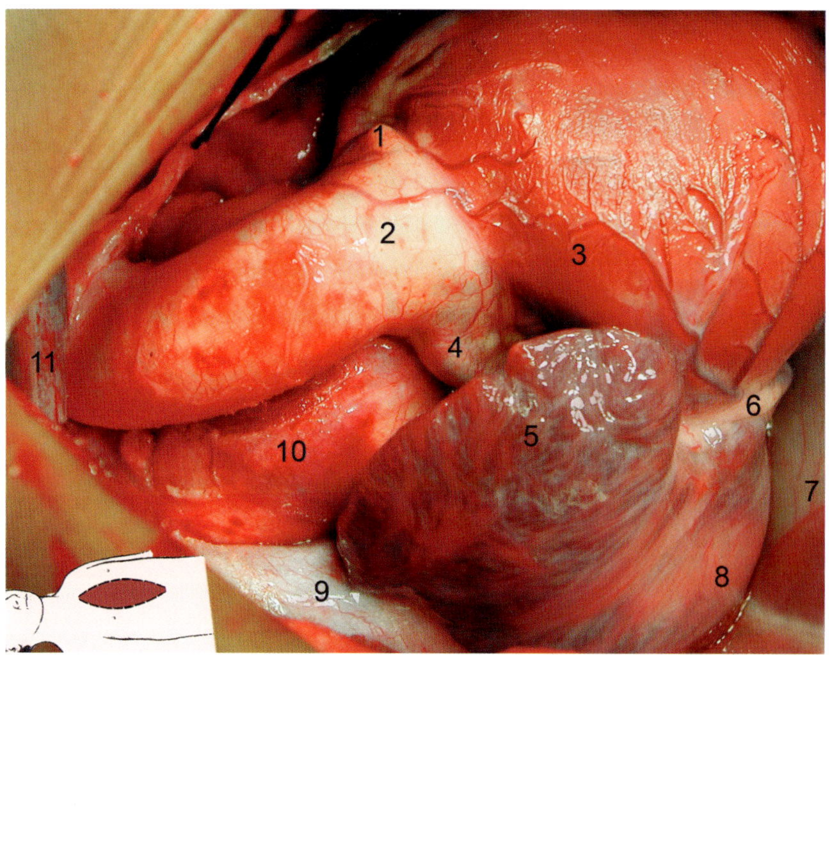

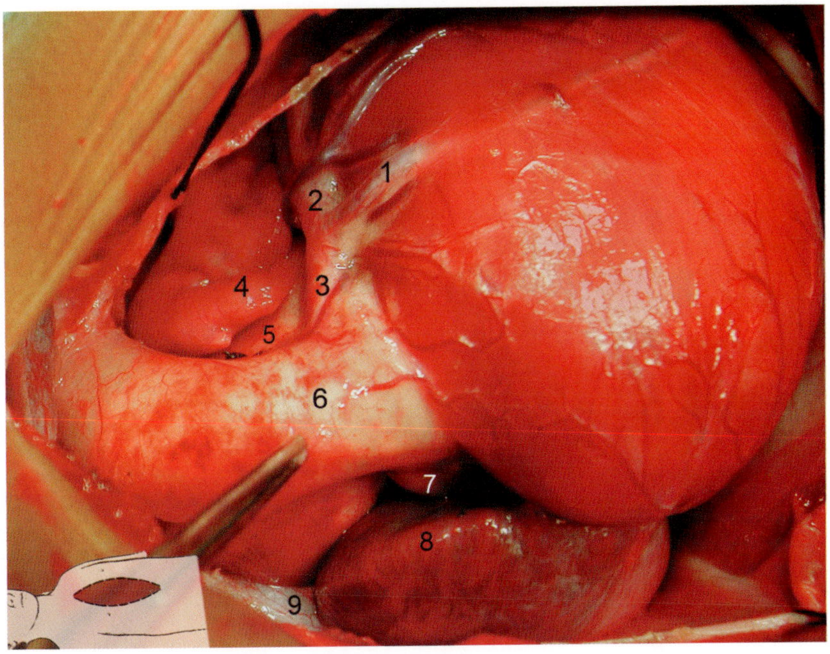

Figure 15.42. Same patient as in Figure 15.41. The aorta is retracted to the right to show the left coronary artery.

1. LAD coronary artery
2. Left circumflex coronary artery
3. Left main coronary artery
4. LAA
5. PA
6. Ascending aorta
7. Right coronary artery
8. RAA
9. SVC

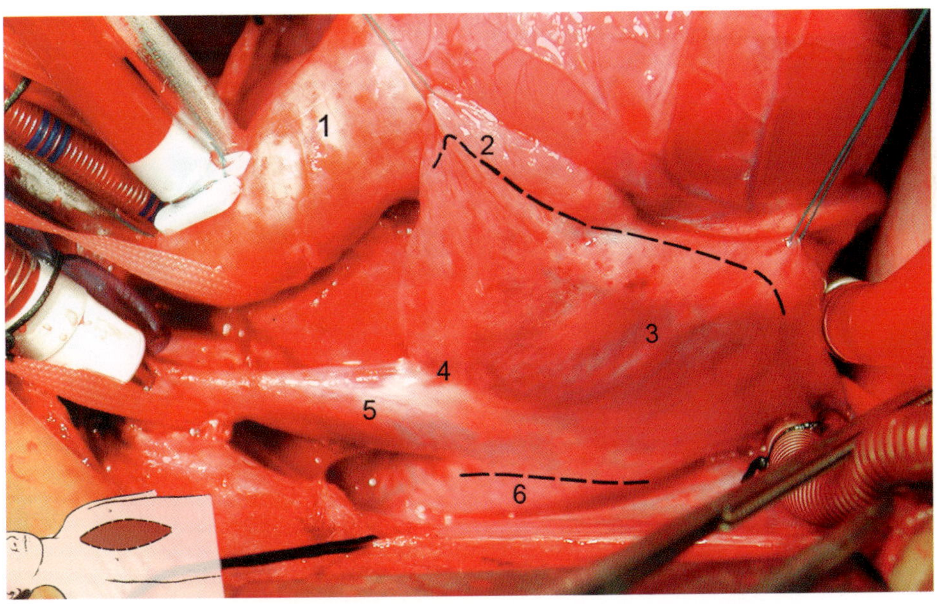

Figure 15.43. Same patient as in Figures 15.41 and 15.42, now on cardiopulmonary bypass. Interrupted lines mark the sites of incisions in right and left atria.

1. Ascending aorta
2. RAA
3. Right atrium
4. Sulcus terminalis
5. SVC
6. Left atrium

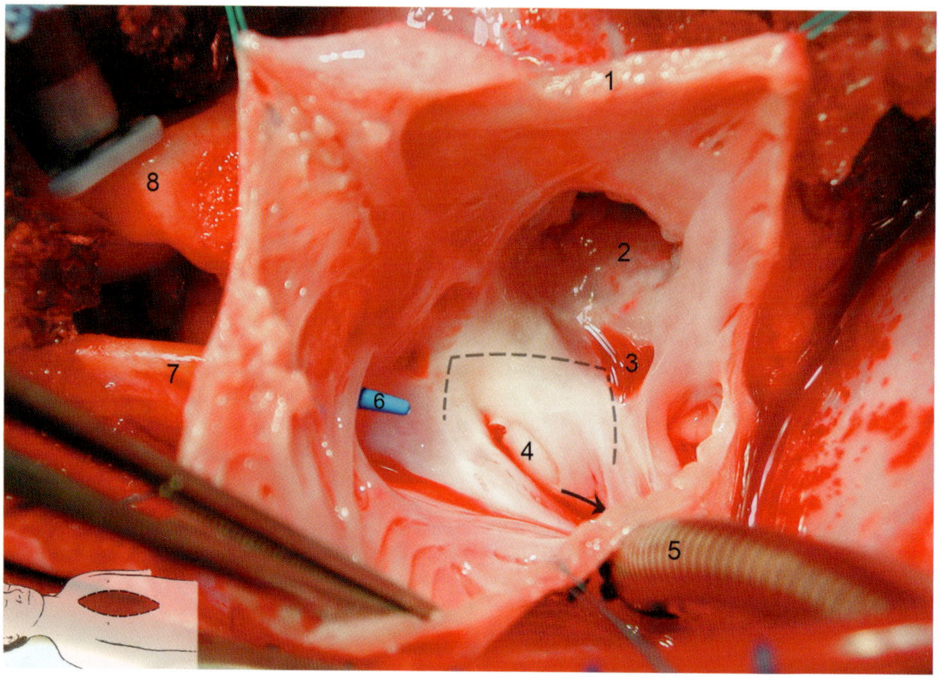

Figure 15.44. Same patient as in Figures 15.41 to 15.43 after right atriotomy. The internal right atrium anatomy is shown. The interrupted line shows approximate site for incision in the interatrial septum to make the septal flap. The arrow points to internal opening of IVC.

1. Free wall of right atrium
2. Tricuspid valve
3. Mouth of coronary sinus
4. Fossa ovalis
5. IVC cannula
6. Central venous catheter in SVC
7. SVC
8. Ascending aorta

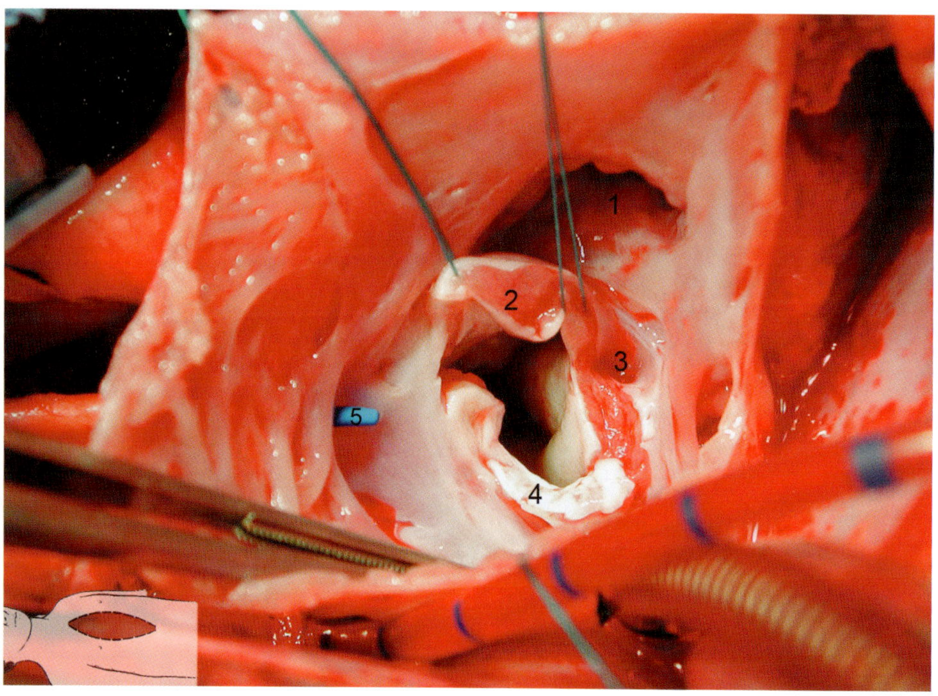

Figure 15.45. Same patient as in Figures 15.41 to 15.44. The atrial septum has been incised to make a flap (step C in Figure 15.40). The incision has been extended to involve part of the roof of the coronary sinus.

1. Tricuspid valve
2. Edge of atrial septal incision
3. Mouth of coronary sinus
4. Flap of atrial septum
5. Central venous catheter in SVC

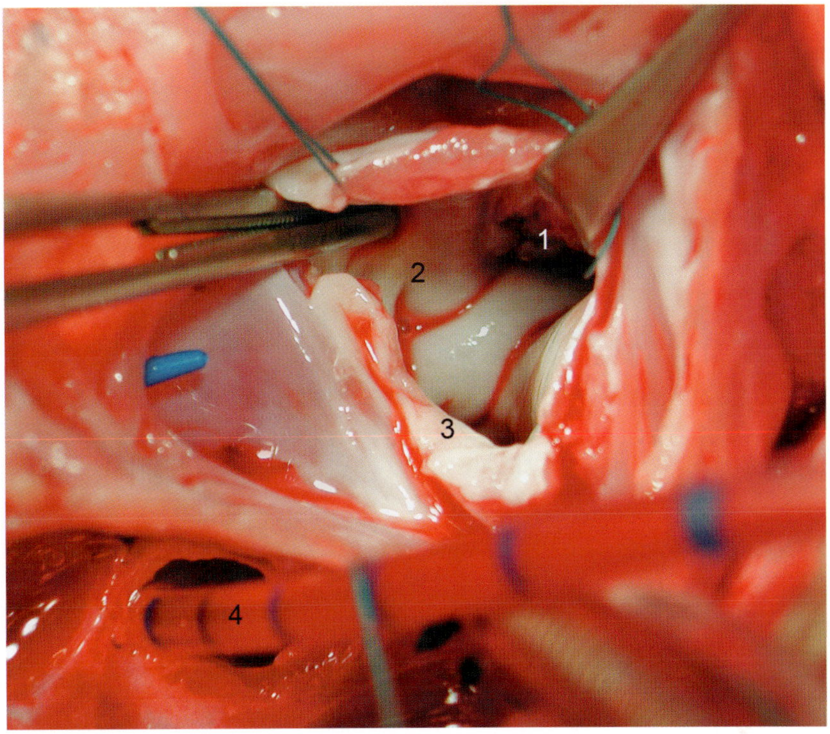

Figure 15.46. Same patient as in Figures 15.41 to 15.45. The left atrial cavity is seen through the surgically created ASD.

1. Mitral valve
2. Lateral wall of left atrium
3. Flap of atrial septum
4. Suction catheter passed through the left atriotomy to drain PVs

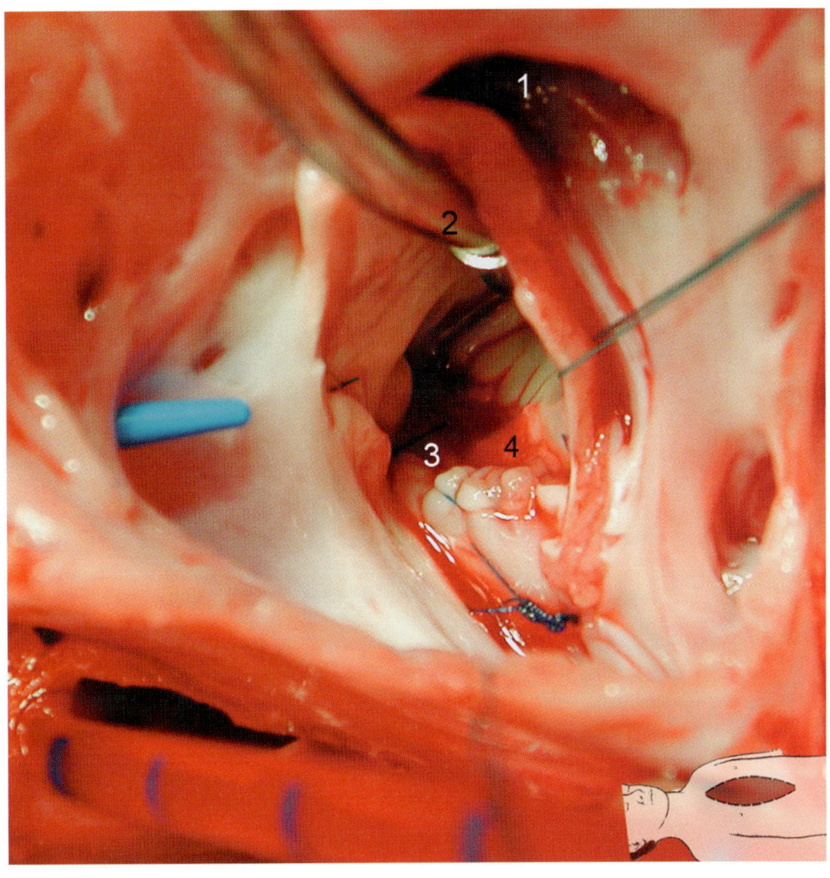

Figure 15.47. Same patient as in Figures 15.41 to 15.46. The atrial septal flap has been sutured to the left atrial wall. A patch of pericardium has been added to the flap to increase its size. At this stage, the pulmonary venous drainage has been separated from the mitral valve (step D in Figure 15.40).

1. Tricuspid valve
2. Suction catheter pointing to mitral valve
3. Atrial septal flap sutured to left atrial wall
4. Pericardial patch

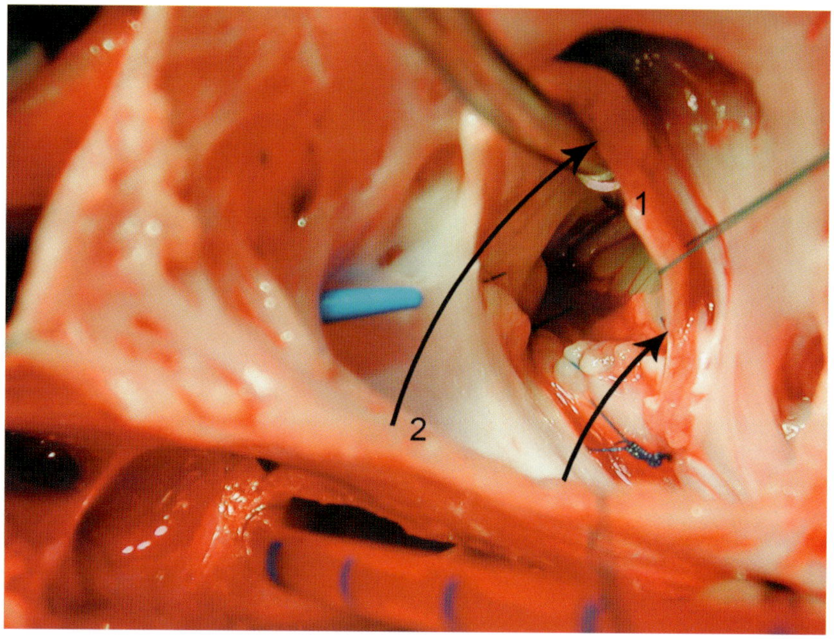

Figure 15.48. Same patient as in Figures 15.41 to 15.47. The next step in repair is to anastomose the posterior part of the right atrial free wall (2) to the anterior edge of the ASD (1). This corresponds to step D in Figure 15.40. The arrows show the direction of placement of the right atrial wall flap.

1. Edge of surgically created ASD
2. Posterior part of right atrial free wall

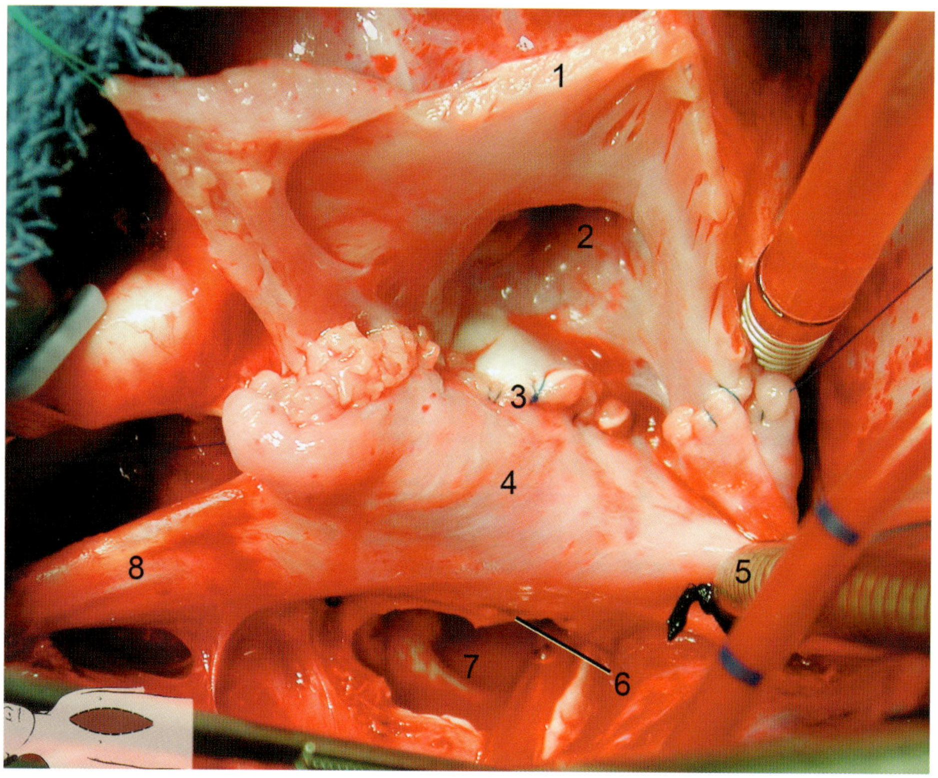

Figure 15.49. Same patient as in Figures 15.41 to 15.48. The systemic venous atrium (new right atrium) has been reconstructed by suturing the right atrial free wall to the edge of the atrial septum as shown in Figure 15.48. Now the vena cava blood is directed to the mitral valve and from there to the PA (step E in Figure 15.40).

1. Anterior part of right atrial free wall
2. Tricuspid valve
3. Suture line of ASD edge to posterior right atrial free wall
4. Systemic venous tunnel
5. IVC cannula
6. Incision into left atrium posterior wall
7. Left atrial cavity
8. SVC

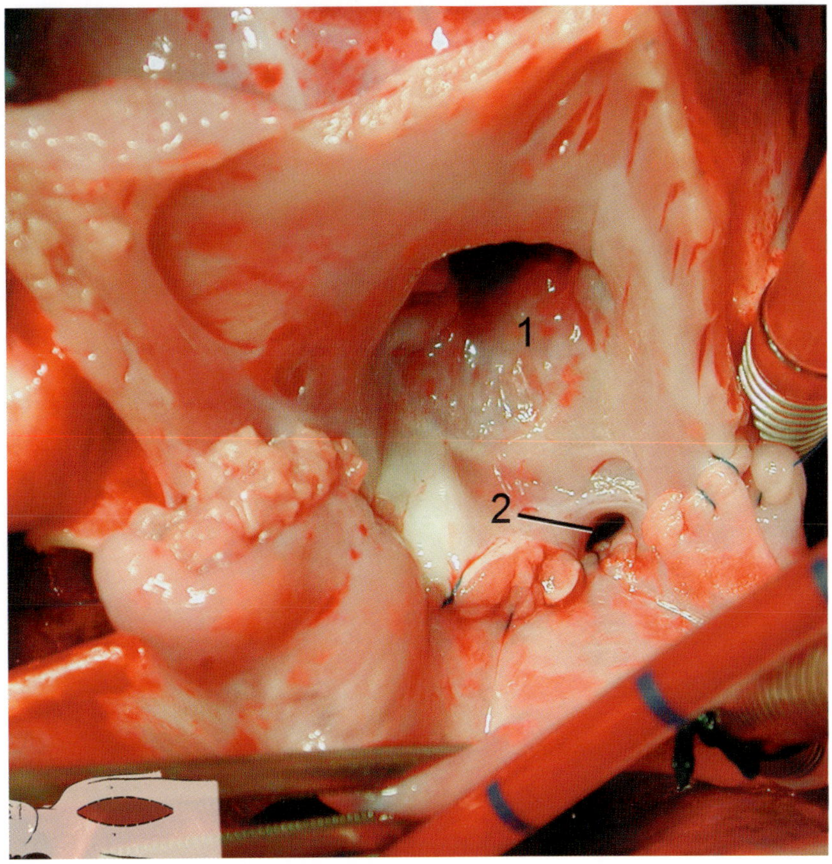

Figure 15.50. Same patient as in Figures 15.41 to 15.49. Close-up view of Figure 15.49. Note that the coronary sinus has been left to drain to the right side (the pulmonary venous atrium).

1. Tricuspid valve
2. Opening of coronary sinus

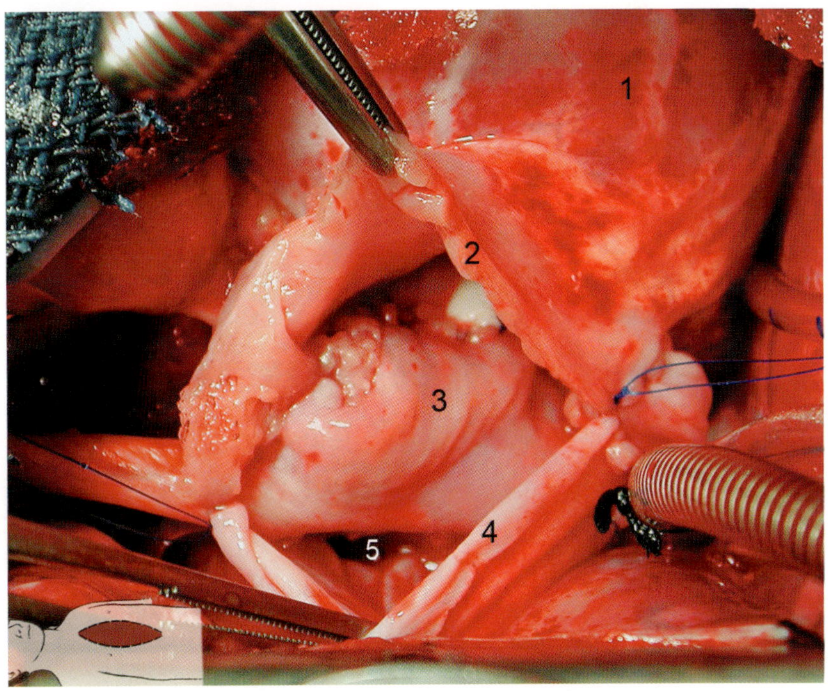

Figure 15.51. Same patient as in Figures 15.41 to 15.50. The wall of the pulmonary venous atrium has been augmented with a pericardial patch (4). The edge of this patch and the anterior edge of the right atriotomy will be anastomosed together to complete the repair (step E in Figure 15.40).

1. RV
2. Anterior part of right atrial free wall
3. Systemic venous tunnel
4. Pericardial patch augmenting the posterior wall of pulmonary venous atrium
5. PV opening into pulmonary venous atrium

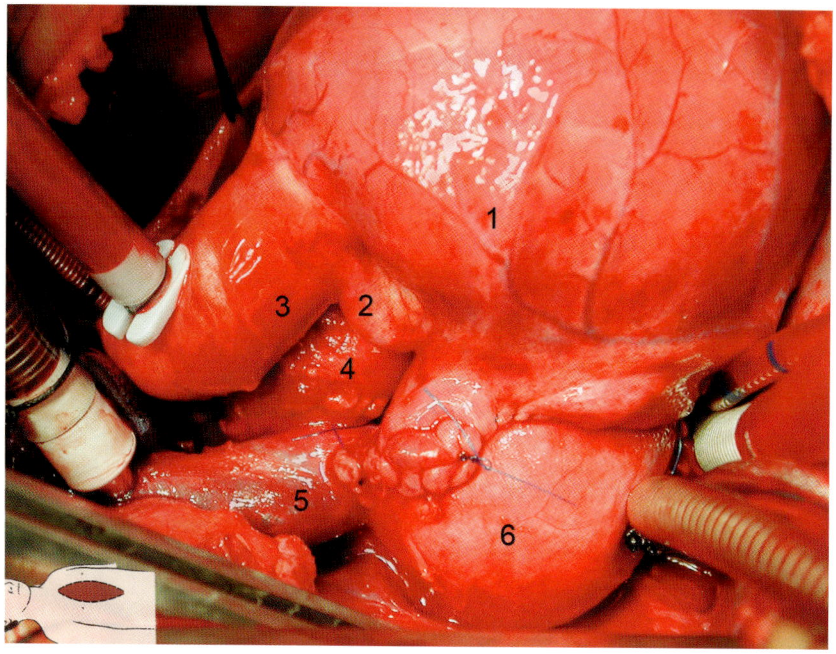

Figure 15.52. Same patient as in Figures 15.41 to 15.51 after completion of the Senning operation. This stage corresponds to step F in Figure 15.40.

1. RV
2. Right coronary artery
3. Aorta
4. MPA
5. SVC
6. Pulmonary venous atrium

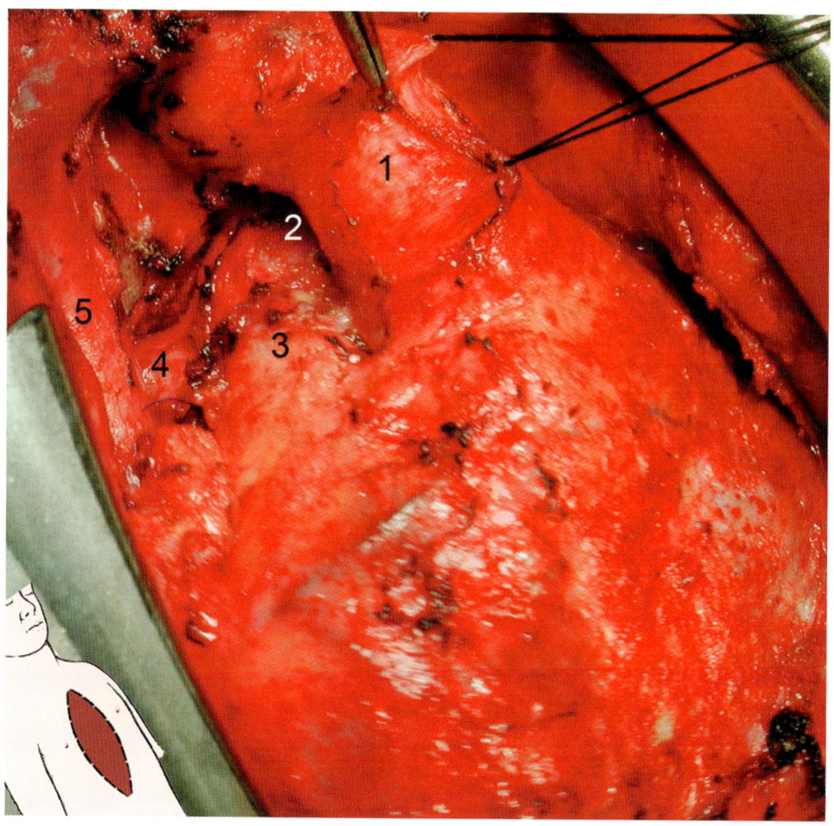

Figure 15.53. Median sternotomy view of a 30-month-old child with TGA repaired with arterial switch without a Lecompte maneuver because of the side-by-side relation of the great arteries. This photograph was taken during a reoperation to relieve pulmonary stenosis.

1. Ascending aorta
2. Left PA
3. MPA
4. Right PA
5. SVC

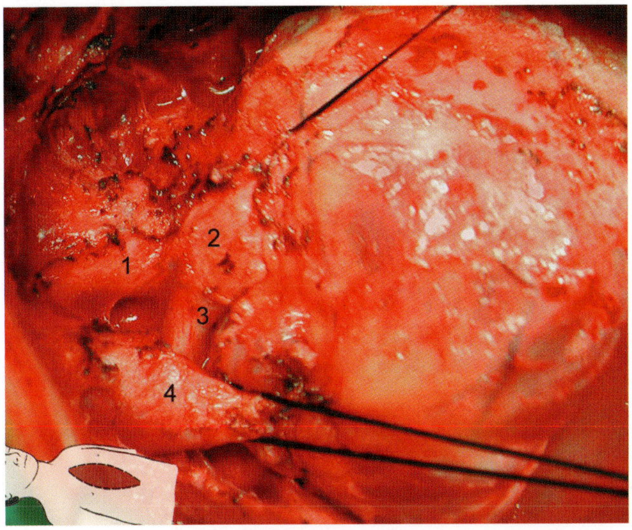

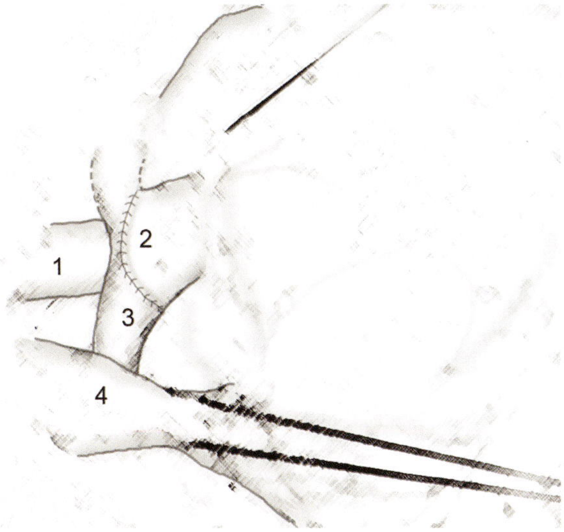

Figure 15.54 **Figure 15.55**

Redo sternotomy in a 2-year-old child with TGA that was repaired with an arterial switch. The MPA is anterior to the aorta because of the Lecompte maneuver. The reason for reoperation was stenosis at the valve level.

1. Ascending aorta
2. MPA
3. Right PA
4. SVC

Figure 15.56. Same patient as in Figure 15.54. The pulmonary valve stenosis was relieved by a transannular xenograft pericardial patch.

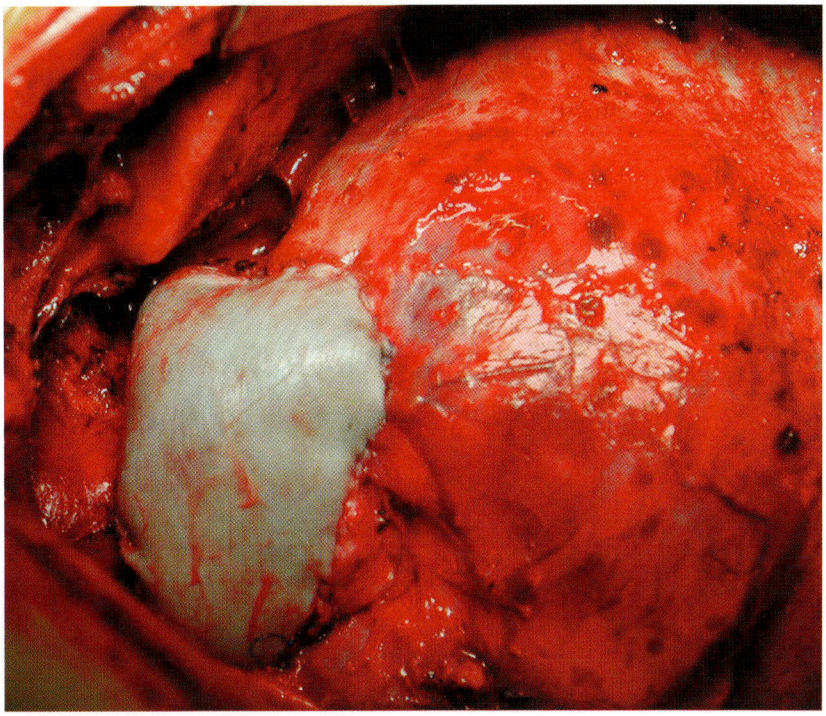

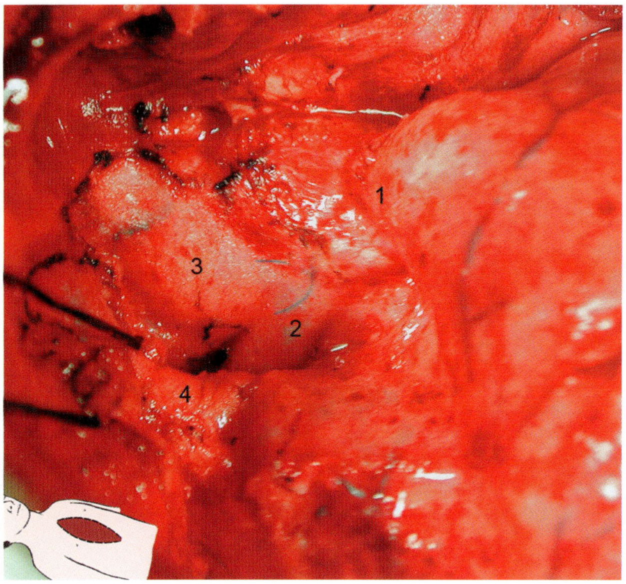

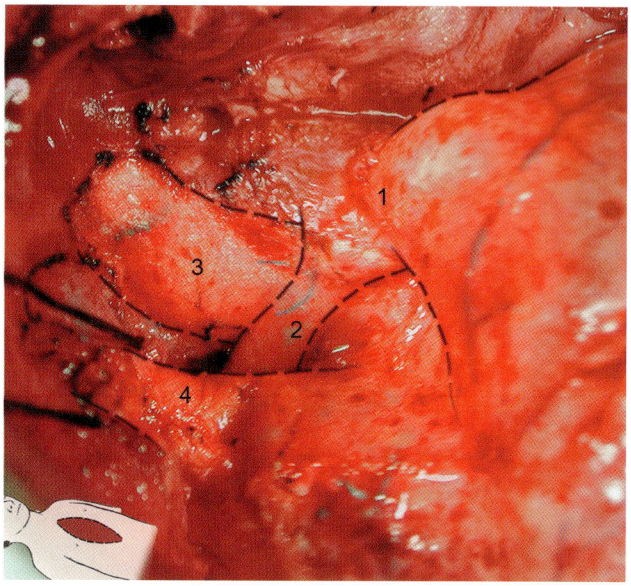

Figure 15.57 **Figure 15.58**

Redo sternotomy in a 2-year-old child with TGA that was repaired with an arterial switch and a Lecompte maneuver. Note the position of the MPA anterior to the aorta. There is stenosis of the right PA caused by compression by the underlying aorta. The structures are outlined in Figure 15.58.

1. MPA
2. Right PA
3. Ascending aorta
4. SVC

Figure 15.59. Median sternotomy view of a 12-year-old child who had TGA that was repaired with a Senning operation. The patient developed pulmonary stenosis. Left ventriculotomy has been performed in preparation for placement of a conduit between the LV and the PA. Note that the aorta (3) arises from the RV.

1. Left ventriculotomy
2. RV
3. Cardioplegia catheter in the aorta

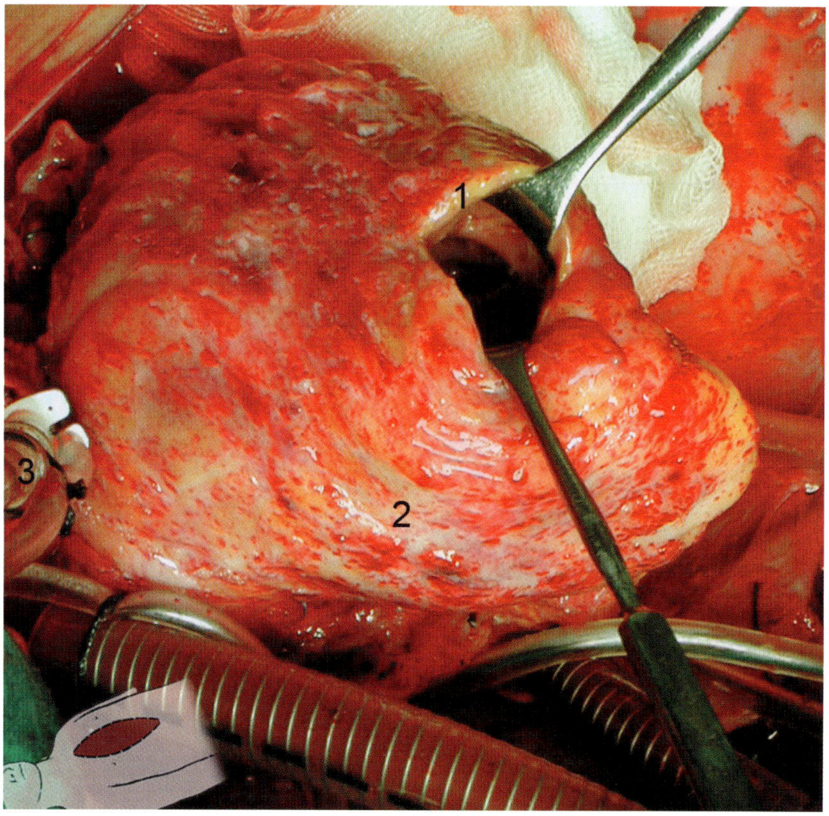

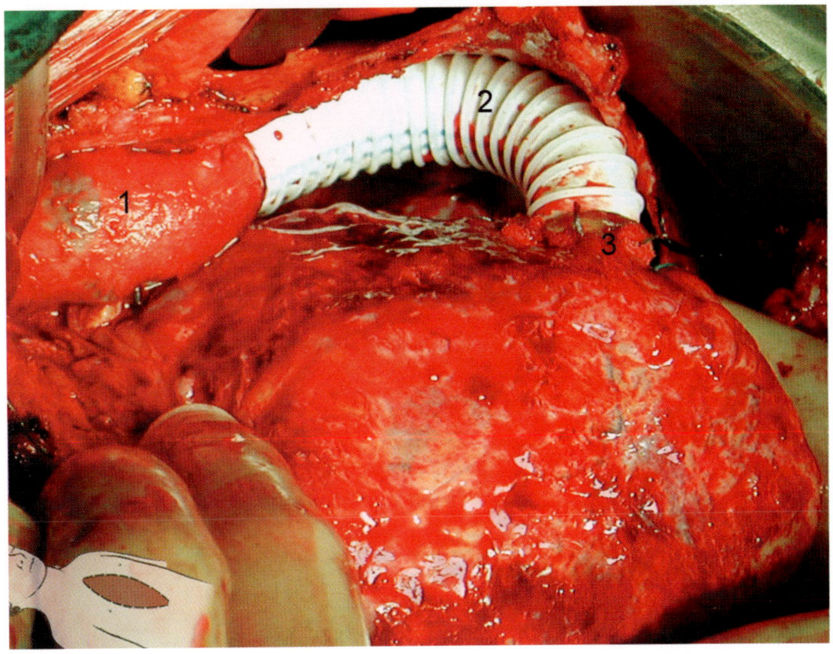

Figure 15.60. Same patient as in Figure 15.59. A conduit has been placed between the LV and the PA. Note that the conduit has 2 parts: a proximal ring Gore-Tex tube and a distal valved xenograft.

1. Valved xenograft conduit (Contegra, 16 mm)
2. Ring Gore-Tex tube graft (13 mm)
3. Ventriculotomy site

REFERENCES

1. Kirklin JW, Blackstone EH, Tchervenkov CI, Castaneda AR. Clinical outcomes after the arterial switch operation for transposition. Patient, support, procedural, and institutional risk factors. Congenital Heart Surgeons Society. *Circulation.* 1992;86:1501–1515.
2. Gremmels DB, Tacy TA, Brook MM, Silverman NH. Accuracy of coronary artery anatomy using two-dimensional echocardiography in d-transposition of great arteries using a two-reviewer method. *J Am Soc Echo.* 2004;17:454–460.
3. Freedom RM, Yoo, SJ, Williams WG. Complete transposition of the great arteries: history of palliation and atrial repair. In: *The Natural and Modified History of Congenital Heart Disease.* New York, NY: Futura; 2004:306–322.
4. Nikaidoh H. Aortic translocation and biventricular outflow tract reconstruction. A new surgical repair for transposition of the great arteries associated with ventricular septal defect and pulmonary stenosis. *J Thorac Cardiovasc Surg.* 1984;88:365–372.
5. Yeh T, Ramaciotti C, Leonard SR, Roy L, Nikaidoh H. The aortic translocation (Nikaidoh) procedure: midterm results superior to the Rastelli procedure. *J Thorac Cardiovasc Surg.* 2007;133:461–469.
6. van Beek E, Binkhorst M, de Hoog M, et al. Exercise performance and activity level in children with transposition of the great arteries treated by the arterial switch operation. *Am J Cardiol.* 2010;105:398–403.

CHAPTER 16

Congenitally Corrected Transposition of the Great Arteries

Congenitally corrected transposition of the great arteries (ccTGA) is also called double discordance or L-transposition of the great arteries (l-TGA). There is a discordant connection between the atria and the ventricles, *levo* looping of the ventricles, and a discordant connection between the ventricles and the great arteries. The systemic venous blood returns to the right atrium, passes through a mitral valve to the left ventricle (LV), and then to the main pulmonary artery (MPA). The pulmonary venous blood returns to the left atrium, passes through the tricuspid valve to the right ventricle (RV), and then goes to the aorta (Figure 16.1). Although anatomically the connections are "wrong," physiologically they are "correct," as blood flows from the systemic venous circulation to the lungs, and from the lungs to the systemic arteries. If no associated lesions exist, there will be no shunting or cyanosis.

ccTGA, however, rarely occurs in isolation, but most commonly has associated defects such as ventricular septal defect (VSD), pulmonary stenosis, and tricuspid valve abnormalities.[1] Complete heart block, tricuspid regurgitation, and failure of the systemic ventricle (morphologic RV) are common long-term complications.[2]

Malposition of the heart and viscera is relatively common, as ccTGA may be associated with levocardia, dextrocardia, situs solitus, situs inversus, or heterotaxy, although strictly speaking not in hearts with isomerism of the atrial appendages.

Importantly, the atrioventricular (AV) conduction system in a heart with the usual atrial arrangement is abnormally located. The AV node is displaced to an anterior location related to the anterior margin of the fibrous continuity between the mitral and pulmonary valves. From there, the penetrating bundle pierces the fibrous body to emerge on the ventricular side as a long AV bundle that passes anteriorly and cephalad in the musculature immediately beneath the pulmonary valve. The bundle then descends the anterior part of the ventricular septum or the anterior margin of the usual VSD branching to give origin to the left branch rightward and right branch leftward. With this abnormal course, the AV bundle is at risk when removing subvalvar tissue to relieve subpulmonary stenosis and when anchoring sutures to the antero-cephalad and anterior margins of a VSD. However, in hearts with mirror-imaged atrial arrangement (situs inversus), the conduction system reverts back to the regular posterior location.

Figure 16.2 shows the external appearance of the heart in a patient with ccTGA. Note that the apex is pointing to the right. Figures 16.3 and 16.4 are from an adult patient with ccTGA and atrial situs inversus.

Numerous small coronary artery branches are seen. Figures 16.5 and 16.6 are from an 11-month-old infant with ccTGA and hypoplastic morphologic LV and mitral valve.

CONVENTIONAL REPAIR

Conventional repair involves closing septal defects, relieving outflow obstruction, and repairing stenotic/regurgitant valves, but the morphologic RV remains the systemic ventricle.

A VSD is the most common lesion associated with ccTGA.[3] Closure is achieved by a patch, placing the sutures on the RV aspect of the septum, to avoid injuring the conduction system, which retains its

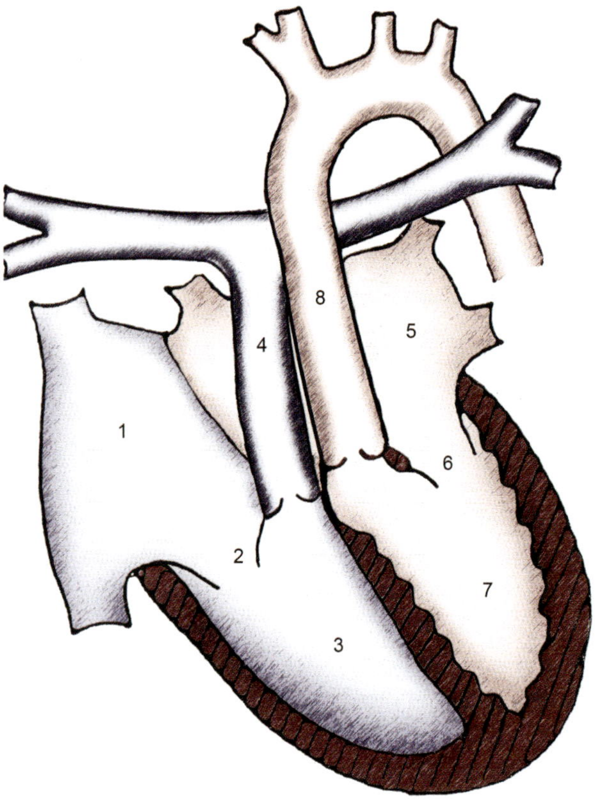

Figure 16.1A

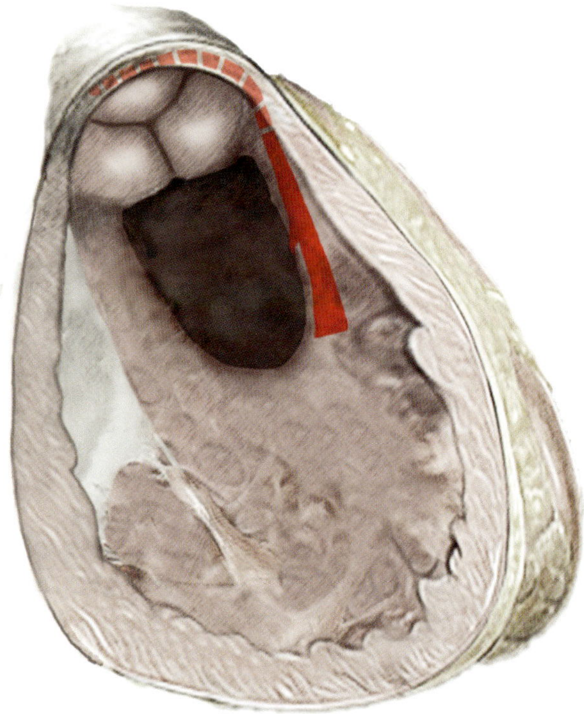

Figure 16.1B

Diagram illustrating ccTGA with the usual atrial arrangement (Figure 16.1A). The right atrium is connected to a mitral valve and the morphologic LV, albeit located on the right side. The MPA arises from the right-sided LV. The left atrium is connected to a tricuspid valve and the left-sided morphologic RV. The aorta arises from the left-sided RV. Figure 16.1B illustrates a view into the right-sided morphologic LV showing the relationship of the AV conduction system (colored red) to the pulmonary valve and the VSD (see text for explanation).

1. Right atrium
2. Mitral valve
3. Morphologic LV
4. MPA
5. Left atrium
6. Tricuspid valve
7. Morphologic RV
8. Aorta

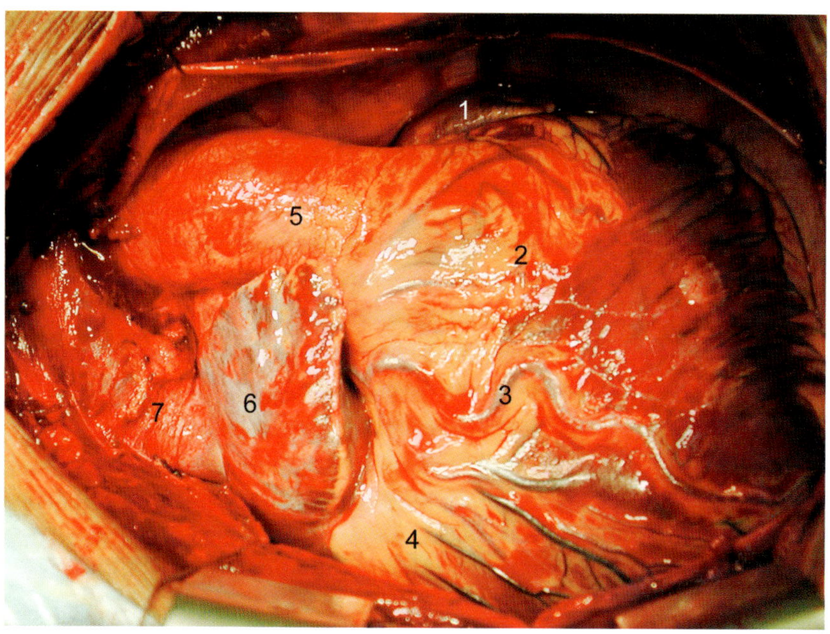

Figure 16.2. Median sternotomy view of a patient with ccTGA. The left atrium is on the left side, connected to a morphologic RV. The right atrium is located on the right side and is connected to a morphologic LV. Note that in this patient, the apex is pointing to the right.

1. Left atrial appendage (LAA)
2. Morphologic RV
3. LAD coronary artery
4. Morphologic LV
5. Ascending aorta
6. Right atrial appendage (RAA)
7. Superior vena cava (SVC)

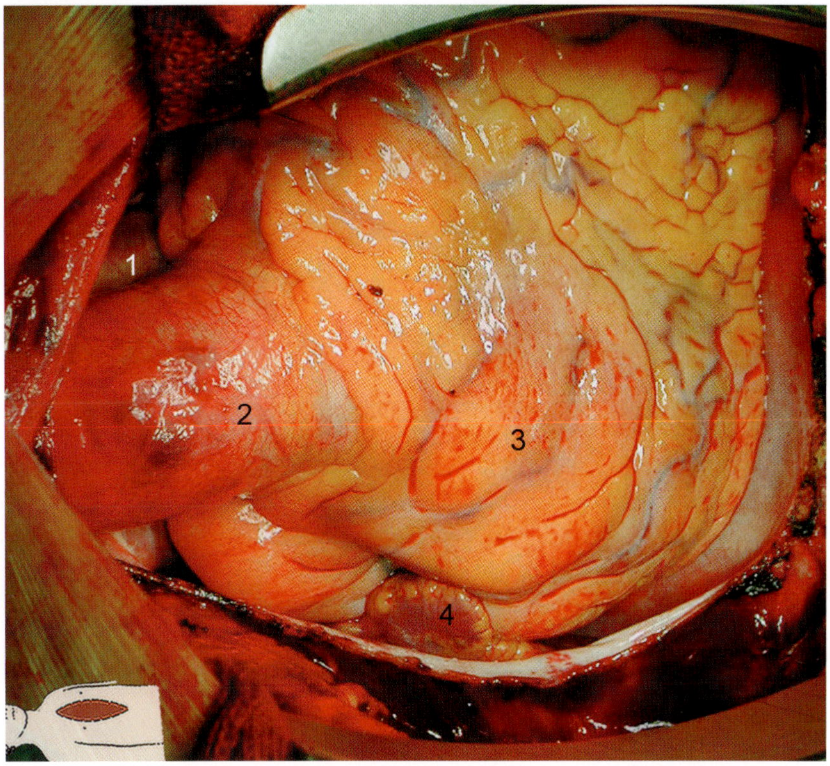

Figure 16.3. Median sternotomy view of another patient with ccTGA. There is atrial situs inversus, with levocardia. The right atrium is located on the left side but connects to a morphologic LV. The left atrium is located on the right and is connected to a morphologic RV. Also note the extensive network of small coronary artery branches.

1. Pulmonary artery
2. Ascending aorta
3. Morphologic RV
4. LAA

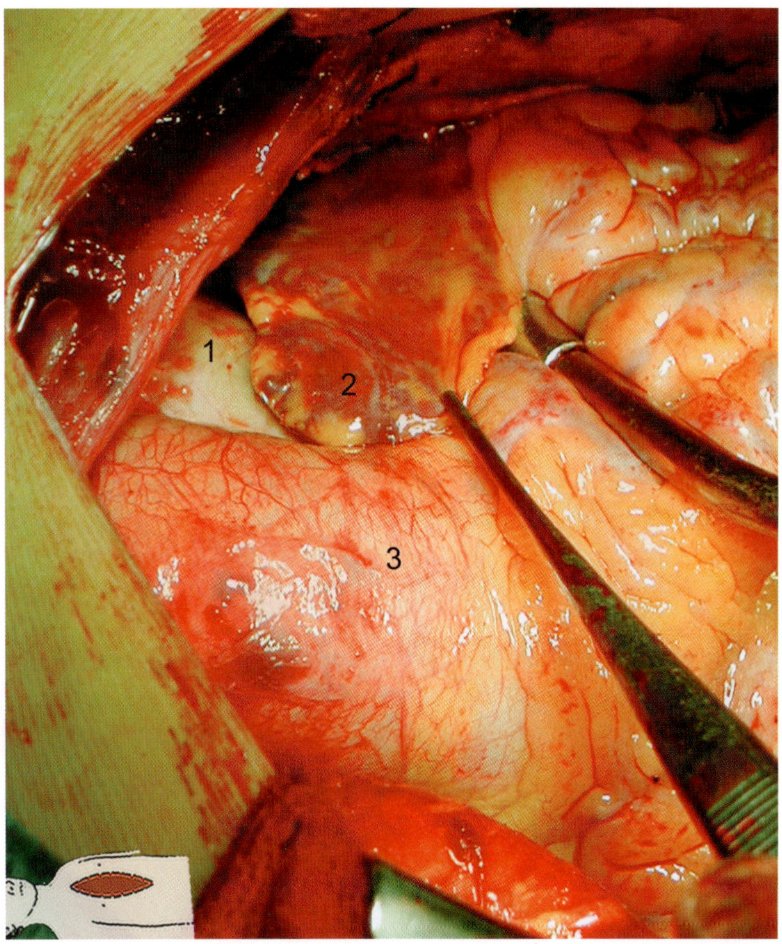

Figure 16.4. The same patient as in Figure 16.3 with the aorta retracted to the right to reveal the RAA.

1. MPA
2. RAA
3. Ascending aorta

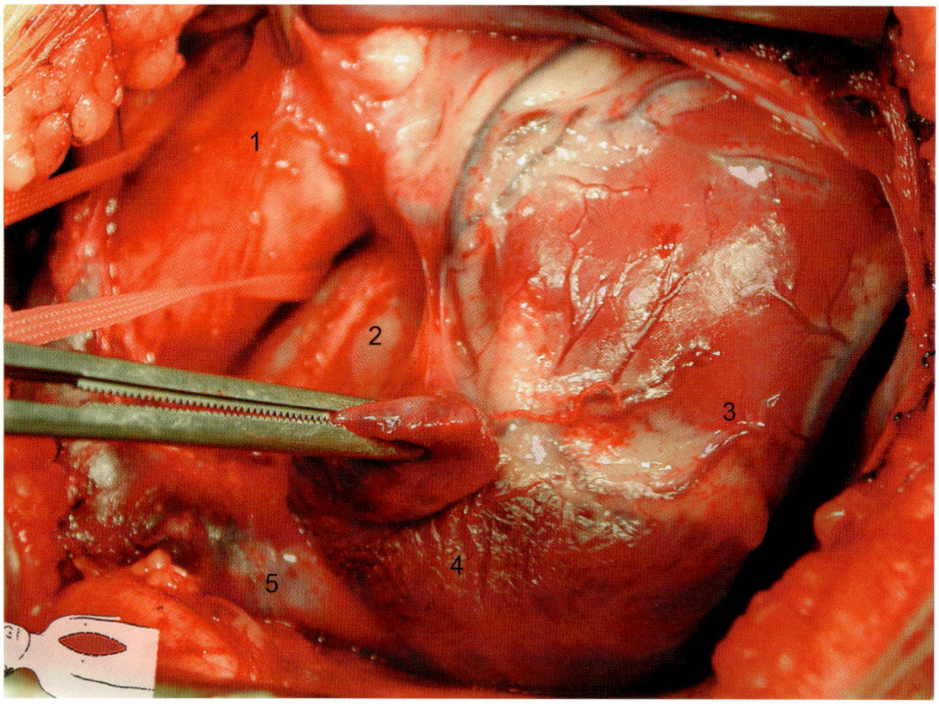

Figure 16.5. Median sternotomy view of an 11-month-old infant with ccTGA and hypoplastic LV. The aorta is left and anterior.

1. Ascending aorta
2. MPA
3. LV
4. Right atrium
5. SVC

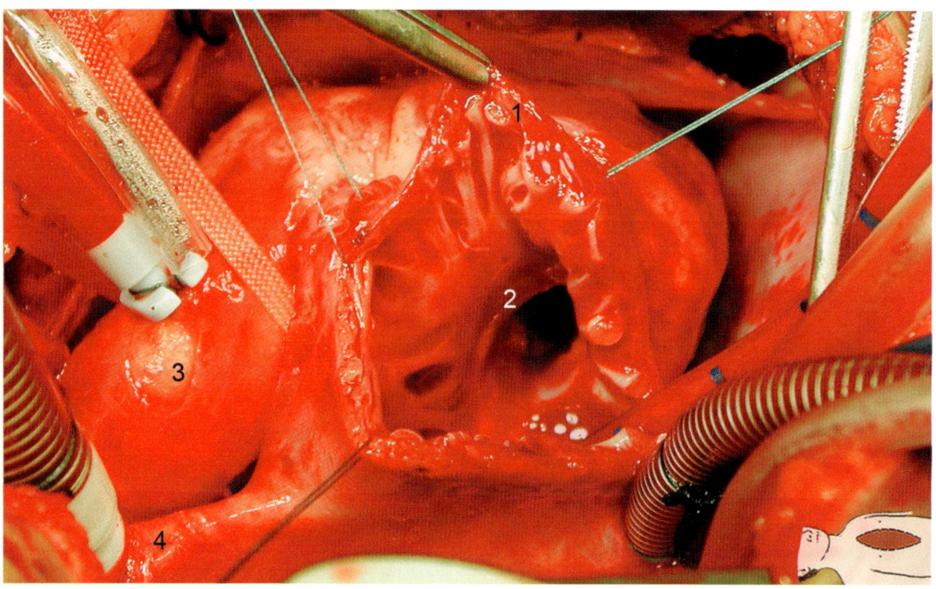

Figure 16.6. The same patient as in Figure 16.5 after cardiopulmonary bypass and right atriotomy. A hypoplastic mitral valve is seen.

1. Right atrial wall
2. Mitral valve
3. Ascending aorta
4. SVC

anatomic location on the LV aspect of the septum. Three examples of patients with VSD are shown in Figures 16.7 to 16.18. Another common association is pulmonic/subpulmonic stenosis. This can be relieved by valvotomy (Figures 16.19 and 16.20) or conduit implantation (Figures 16.21 to 16.23), depending on the anatomy and the severity of the obstruction.

ANATOMIC REPAIR

For many patients, the long-term outcome of conventional repair has been disappointing. Over time, the tricuspid valve and morphologic RV, which are kept on the systemic side of the circulation, tend to fail.[4]

Anatomic repair aims at switching the connections so that the morphologic LV pumps to the systemic circulation and the morphologic RV pumps to the pulmonary circulation. This is achieved by either a double-switch operation or a combination of atrial switch plus a Rastelli procedure.[5]

Figures 16.24 to 16.36 are from a child with ccTGA during a double-switch operation. This patient had a small RV that was deemed not capable of supporting full cardiac output, so a "1.5 ventricle" arrangement was elected, consisting of a "hemi-Mustard," an arterial switch, and a bidirectional Glenn shunt. At the conclusion of this procedure, the inferior vena cava (IVC) blood is directed via the Mustard baffle to the tricuspid valve and the morphologic RV on the left side, and from there to the PA. The SVC blood is shunted to the PA directly via a Glenn shunt. The pulmonary venous return is directed to the mitral valve and the morphologic LV, and from there to the aorta. Because heart block is common in ccTGA, permanent epicardial pacemaker leads (see Figures 16.35 and 16.36) may be implanted at the time of surgery for future use.

Another option when the anatomy is favorable and a VSD is present is to perform an atrial switch, plus a Rastelli procedure without having to switch the great arteries (Figures 16.37–16.39).

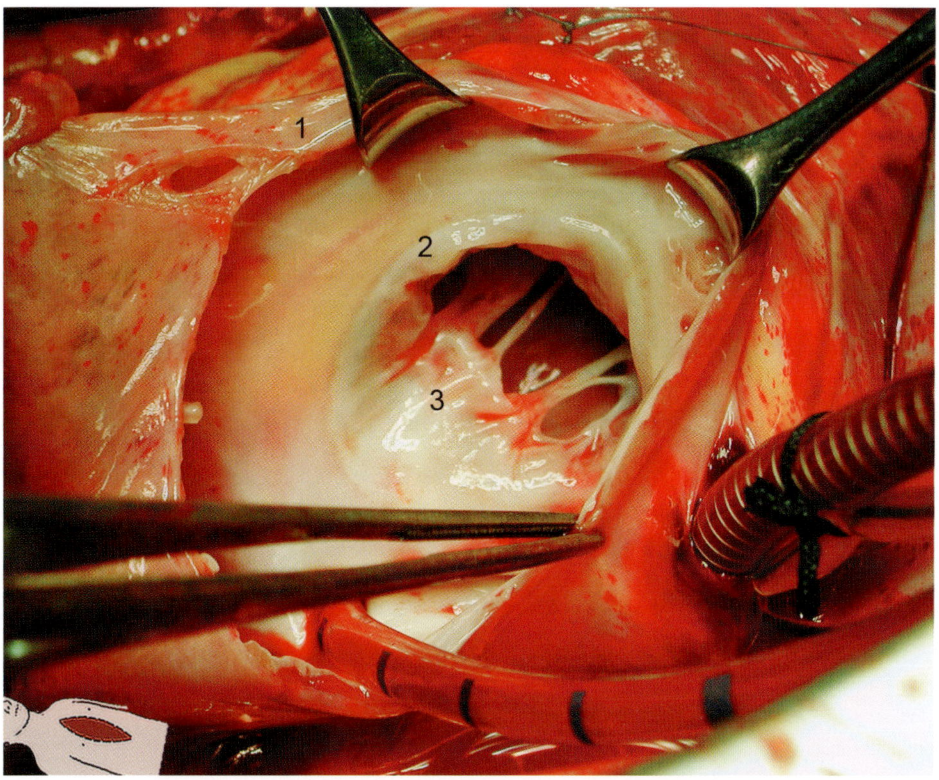

Figure 16.7. ccTGA with VSD in a 5-year-old child. A right atriotomy has been performed, showing the mitral valve. The VSD is located behind the posterior leaflet of the mitral valve; it is not visible in this view.

1. Right atrial wall
2. Annulus of the mitral valve
3. Posterior leaflet of the mitral valve

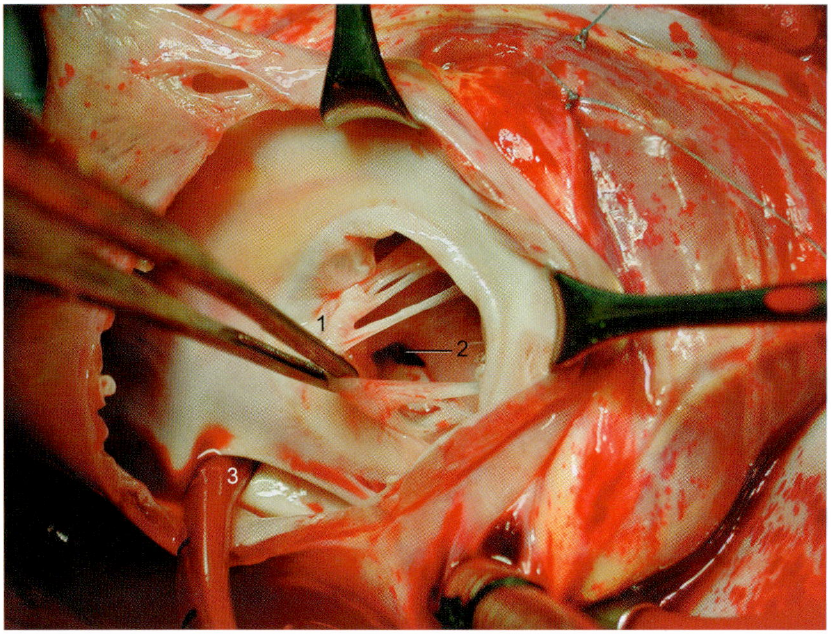

Figure 16.8. The same patient as in Figure 16.7 with the mitral valve retracted to reveal the VSD.

1. Posterior leaflet of mitral valve
2. VSD
3. Suction catheter passing through the patent foramen ovale

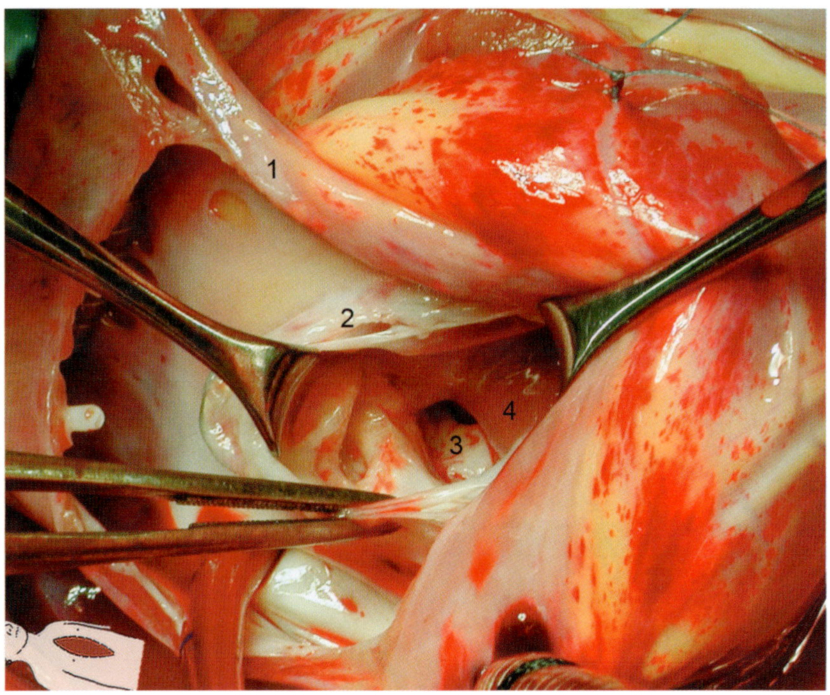

Figure 16.9. The same patient as in Figures 16.7 and 16.8. The tricuspid valve is seen through the VSD. The defect was closed by a patch sutured to the RV aspect of the septum (not shown) to avoid injuring the conduction system.

1. Right atrial wall
2. Annulus of mitral valve
3. Tricuspid valve
4. Ventricular septum

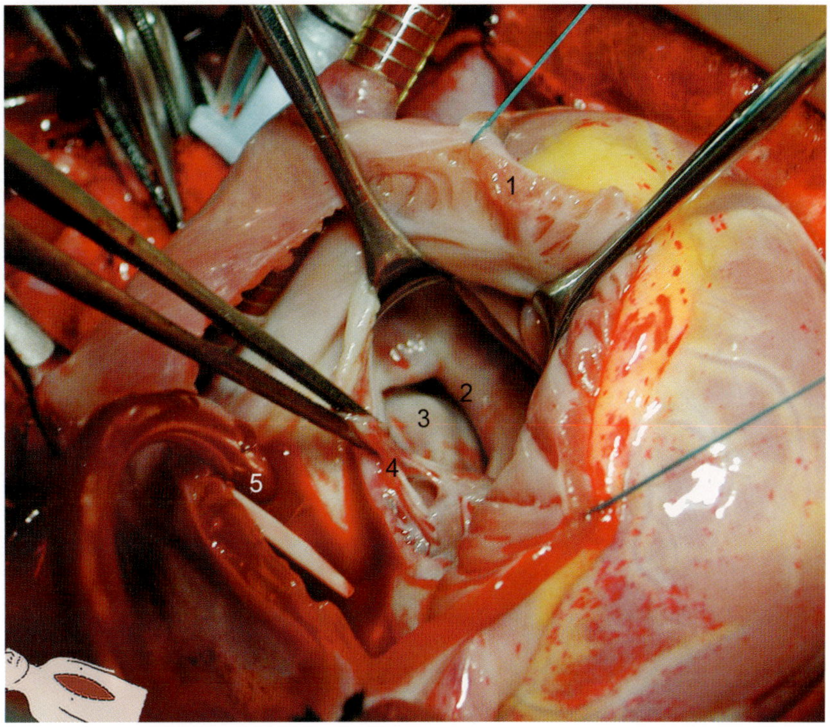

Figure 16.10. Right atriotomy view of another child, 3 years old, with ccTGA and a large VSD. The tricuspid valve is visible through the VSD.

1. Right atrial wall
2. Ventricular septum
3. Tricuspid valve
4. Mitral valve
5. Suction catheter passing through the patent foramen ovale

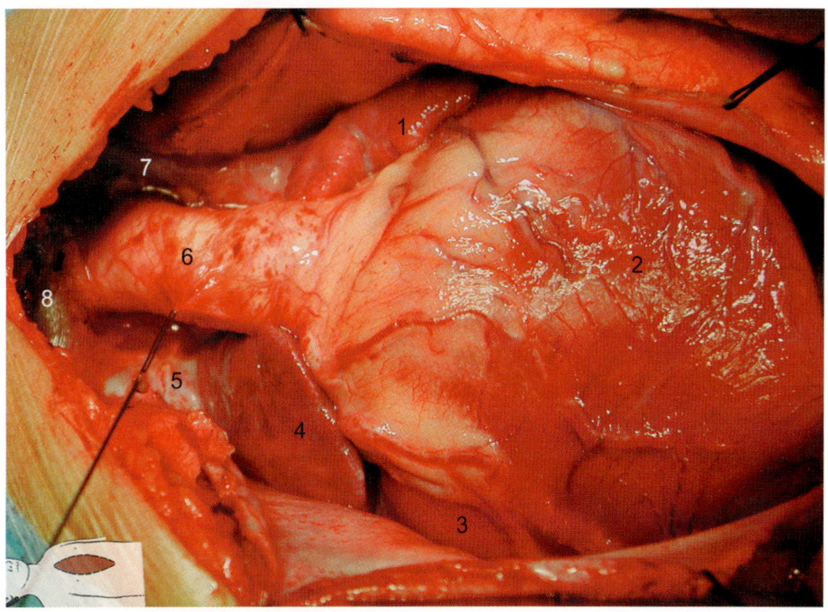

Figure 16.11. Median sternotomy view of a 1-year-old infant with situs solitus, dextrocardia, bilateral SVC, ccTGA, and VSD. The gross outside appearance of the heart is shown.

1. LAA
2. Morphologic RV
3. Morphologic LV
4. RAA
5. Right SVC
6. Ascending aorta
7. Left SVC
8. Innominate vein

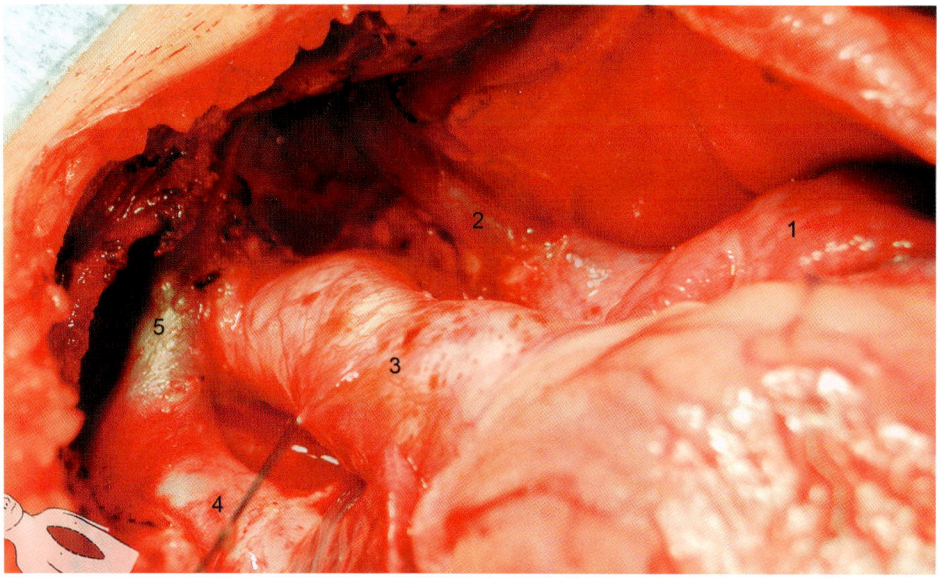

Figure 16.12. The same patient as in Figure 16.11 with the aorta retracted to show the left SVC.

1. LAA
2. Left SVC
3. Ascending aorta
4. Right SVC
5. Innominate vein

Figure 16.13. Right atriotomy view of the same patient as in Figures 16.11 and 16.12. A VSD is seen through a right atriotomy.

1. Aortic cross-clamp
2. Cardioplegia catheter
3. RAA
4. Ventricular septum
5. VSD
6. Mitral valve
7. Suction catheter in the foramen ovale

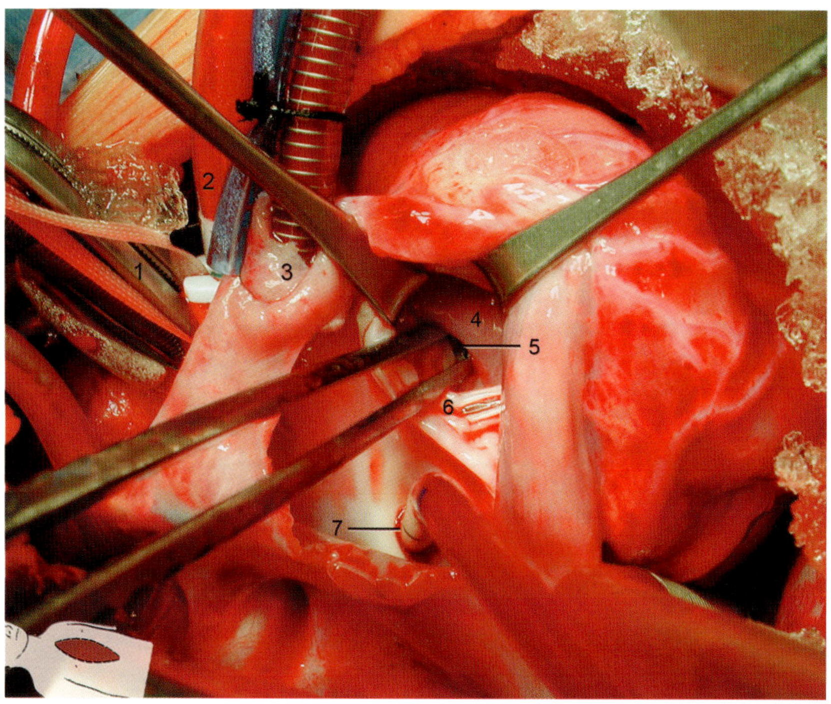

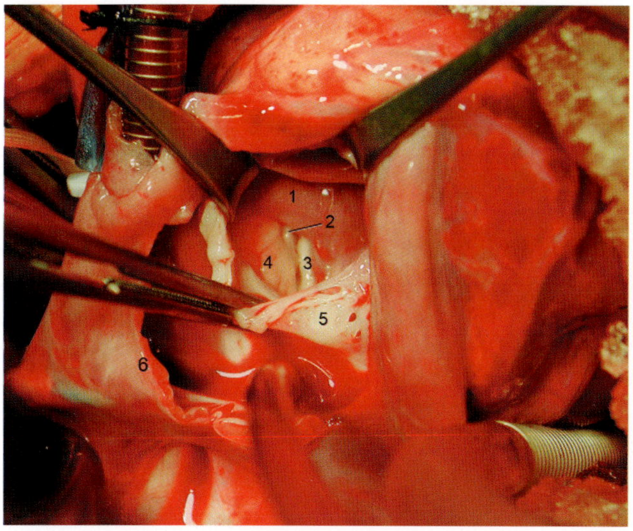

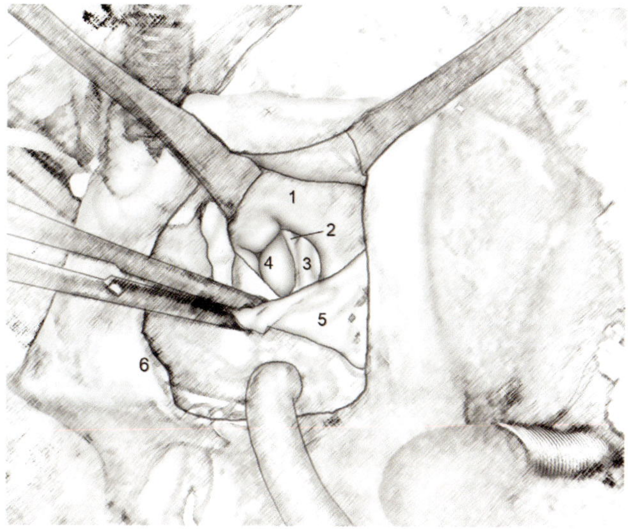

Figure 16.14 **Figure 16.15**

The same patient as in Figures 16.11 to 16.13. The mitral valve is retracted to show the VSD. The defect has no upper muscular rim and is doubly committed and juxtaarterial. Also note the mitral-pulmonary continuity.

1. Ventricular septum
2. Aortic valve leaflet
3. Fibrous tissue at edge of VSD
4. Pulmonary valve
5. Mitral valve
6. Right atrial wall

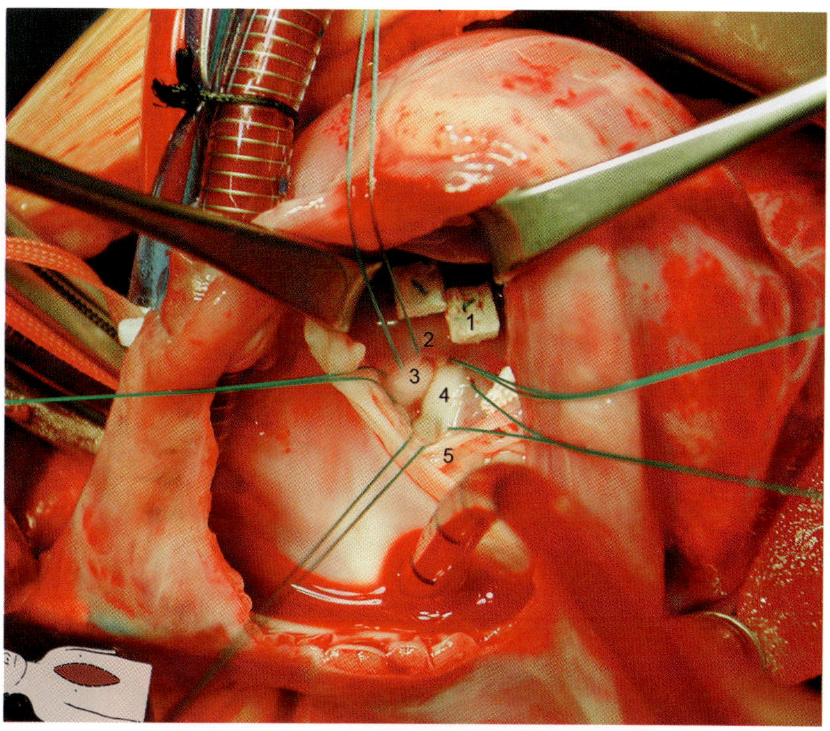

Figure 16.16. The same patient as in Figures 16.11 to 16.15 during closure of the VSD using interrupted pledget-supported mattress sutures and a patch. Because there is no upper muscular rim, 2 sutures, at the 7 and 9 o'clock positions, have been placed across the pulmonary valve leaflet. Note the aortic leaflet prolapsing through the VSD.

1. Teflon pledget
2. Interventricular septum
3. Aortic valve
4. Fibrous tissue at the edge of VSD
5. Mitral valve

Figure 16.17. Another view of the same patient as in Figures 16.11 to 16.16, showing placement of the sutures across the pulmonary valve. The pledgets could not be placed on the RV side of the septum, so they were placed on the LV side but at a distance from the edge of the VSD. Also note the Teflon pledget inside the pulmonary valve cusp (3).

1. Interventricular septum
2. Aortic valve
3. Pulmonary valve
4. Mitral valve

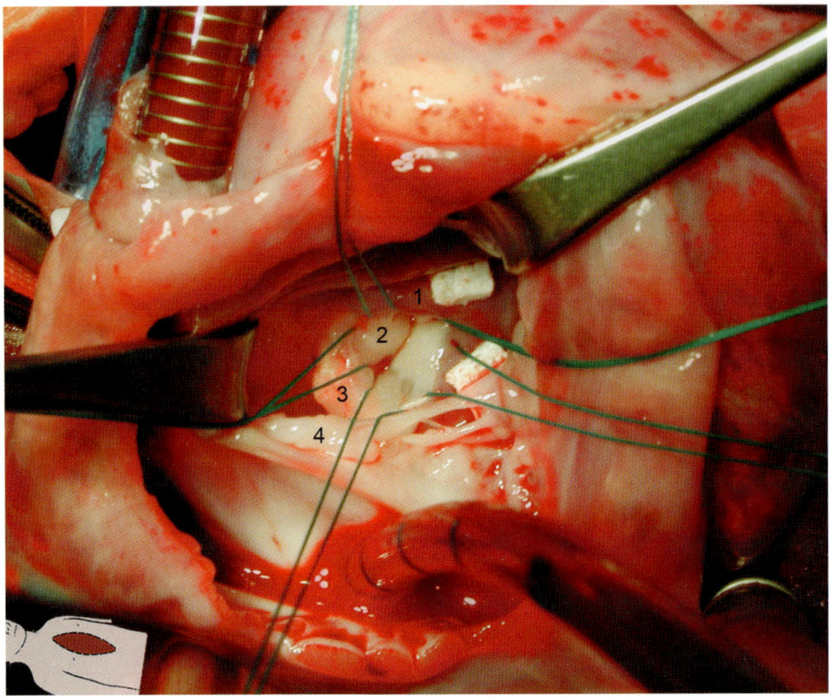

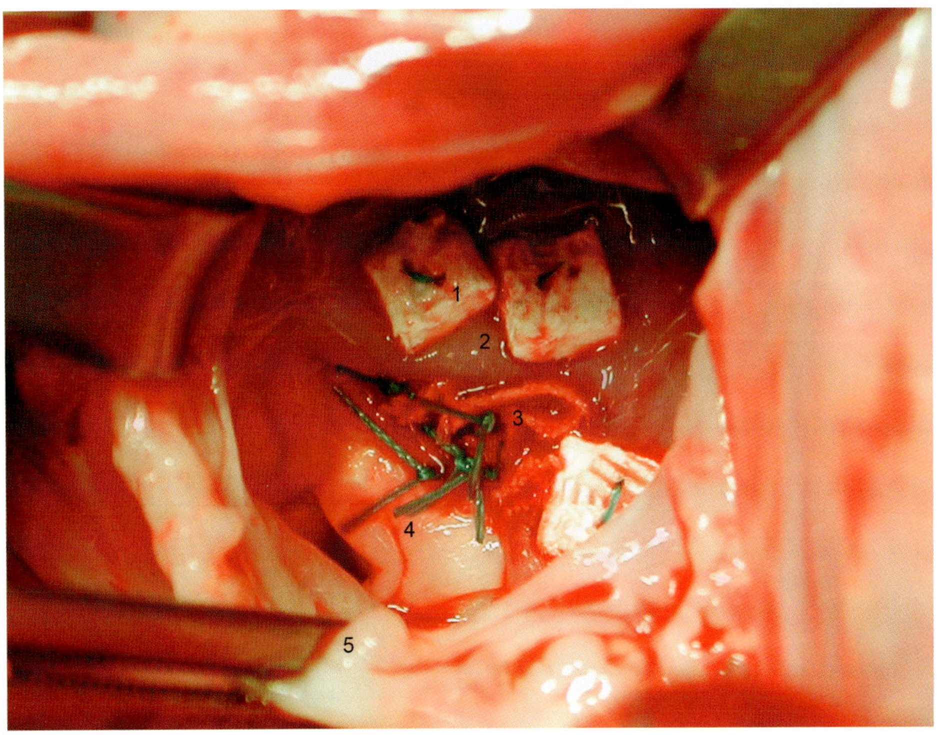

Figure 16.18. The same patient as in Figures 16.11 to 16.17 after closure of the VSD by a Dacron patch.

1. Teflon pledgets
2. Ventricular septum
3. Dacron patch
4. Pulmonary valve
5. Mitral valve

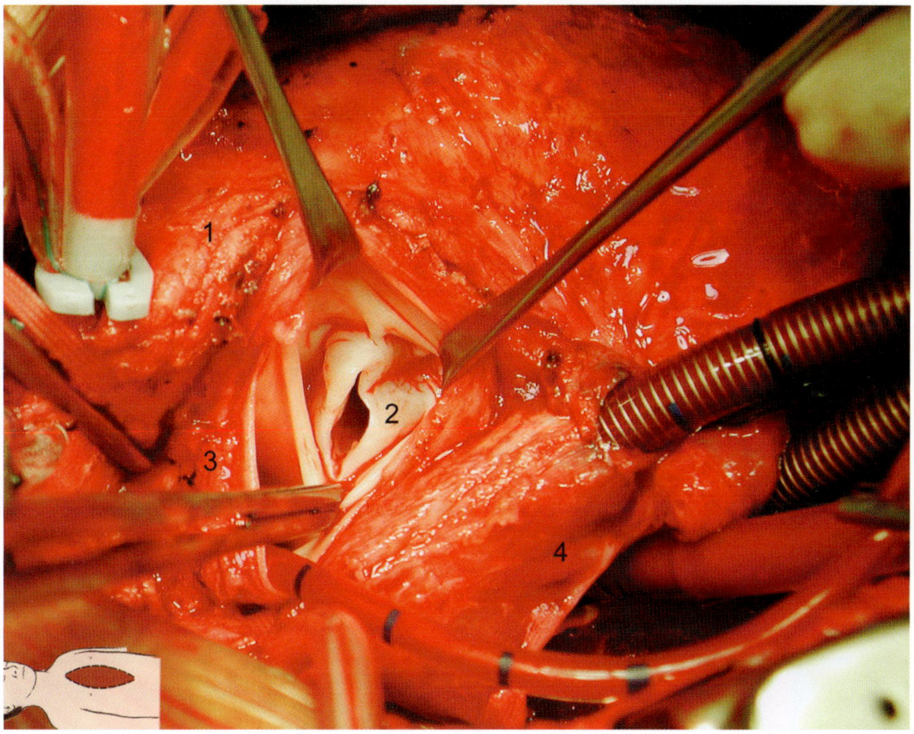

Figure 16.19. Median sternotomy view of a 5-year-old child with ccTGA, VSD, and pulmonary stenosis. The pulmonary valve is exposed via a pulmonary arteriotomy. It is bicuspid and stenotic. Note the usual arrangement of the arteries in ccTGA; the aorta is left and anterior, and the MPA is right and posterior.

1. Ascending aorta
2. Bicuspid pulmonary valve
3. MPA
4. Right atrium

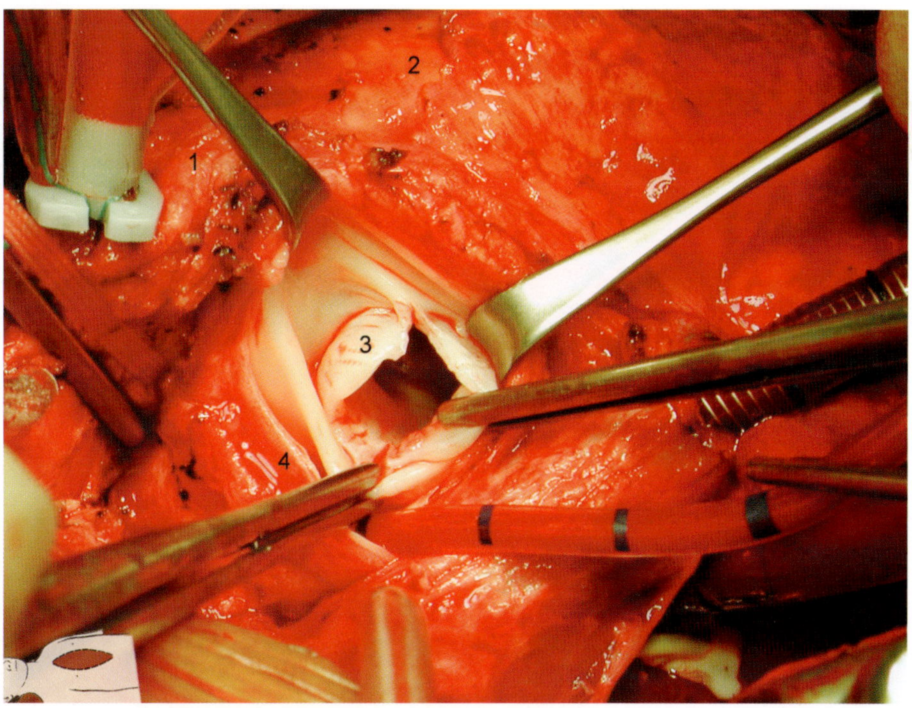

Figure 16.20. The same patient as in Figure 16.19. Pulmonary valve repair has been performed by commissurotomy at both commissures. The VSD was closed by a patch (not shown).

1. Ascending aorta
2. RV
3. Pulmonary valve
4. MPA

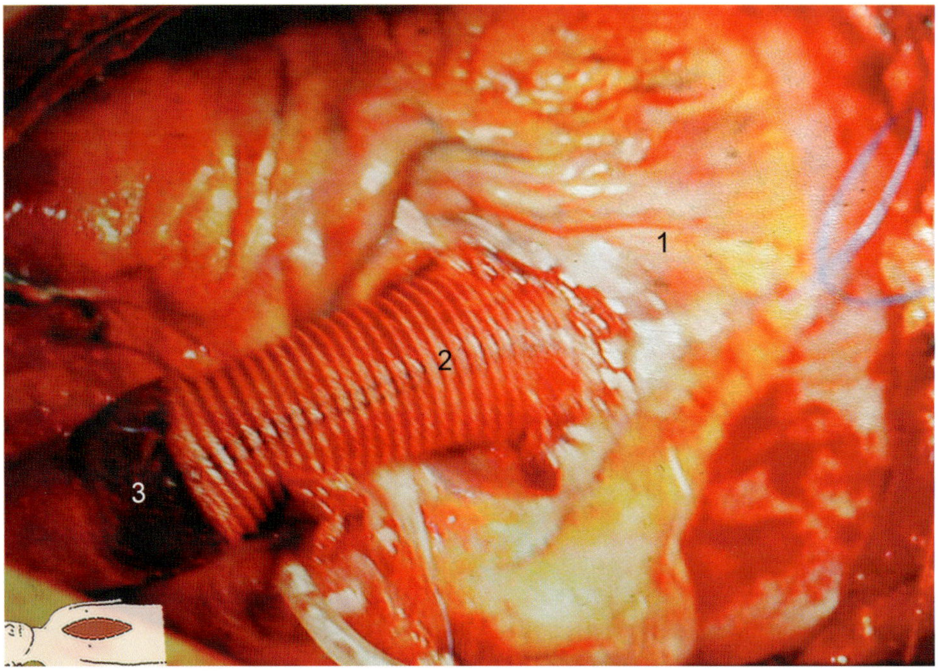

Figure 16.21. In another patient, the LV outflow/pulmonary stenosis was relieved by placing a conduit between the morphologic LV and the MPA. The conduit has 2 parts: a distal valved xenograft and a proximal Dacron tube.

1. Morphologic LV
2. Hemashield tube graft
3. Valved xenograft conduit

Figure 16.22. A redo sternotomy in a 20-year-old patient with ccTGA. The patient developed distal conduit stenosis and needed conduit replacement.

1. Morphologic LV
2. LV-to-PA conduit

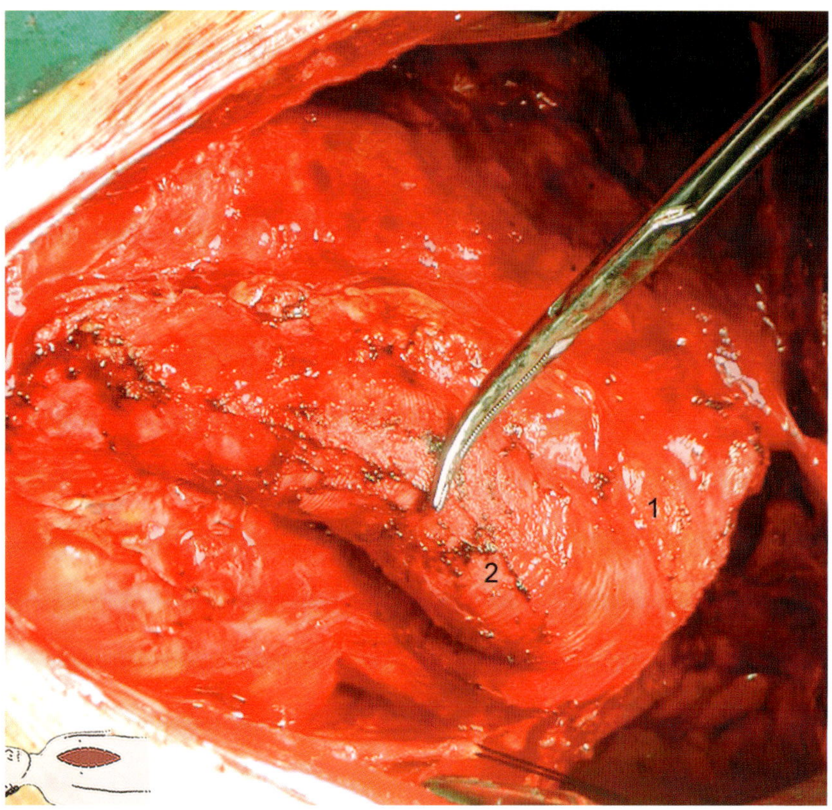

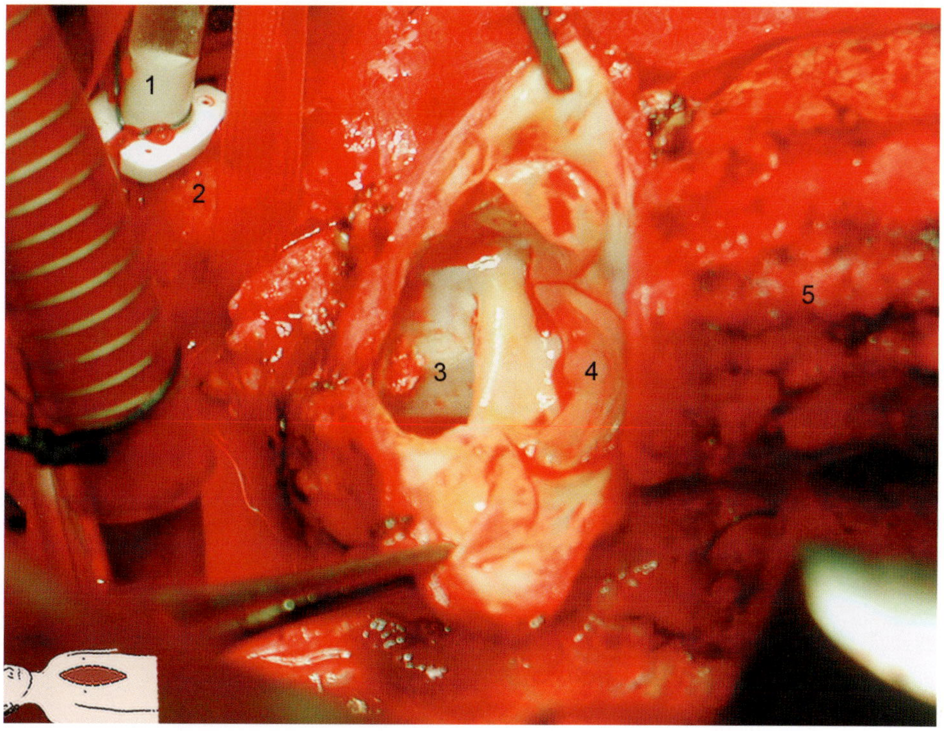

Figure 16.23. The same patient as in Figure 16.22 with the conduit open. The valve of the conduit is seen. The stenosis was distal at the anastomosis with native PAs.

1. Cardioplegia catheter
2. Ascending aorta
3. Distal part of the conduit
4. Valve of the conduit
5. Proximal part of the conduit

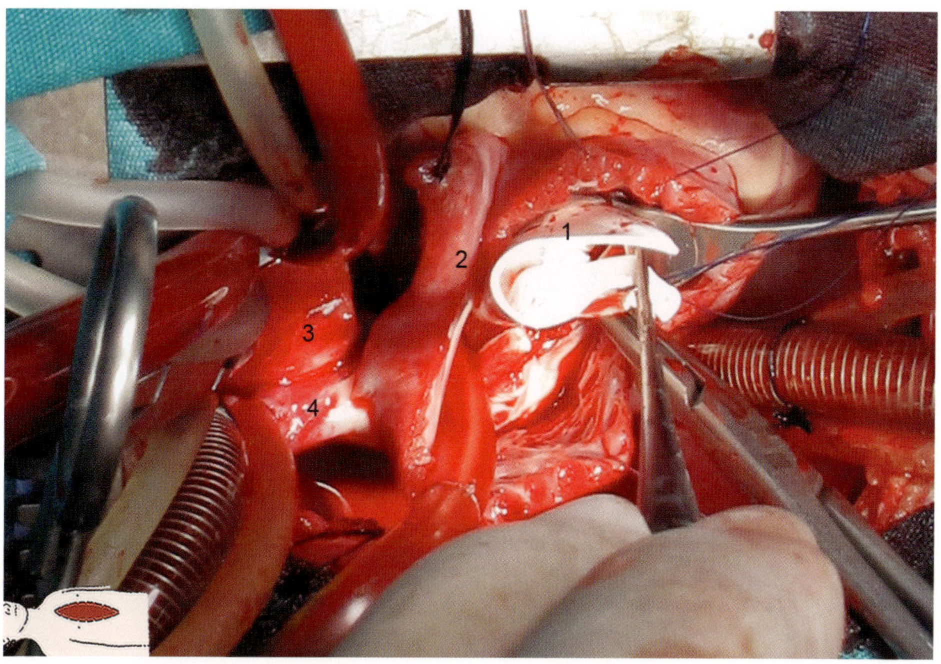

Figure 16.24. An intraoperative view of a child with ccTGA during a double-switch operation. A right atriotomy has been performed. The atrial septum has been excised. A polytetrafluoroethylene (PTFE) graft is cut to shape and is being placed to form the inferior leg of the Mustard baffle (see text).

1. PTFE patch of Mustard baffle
2. Right atrium
3. Ascending aorta
4. SVC

Figure 16.25. The same patient as in Figure 16.24. The patch is being sutured to the margin of the interatrial septum and the floor of the right atrium in such a way as to direct IVC blood to the left atrium.

1. Mitral valve
2. IVC venous cannula
3. Mustard IVC baffle
4. RAA
5. Ascending aorta

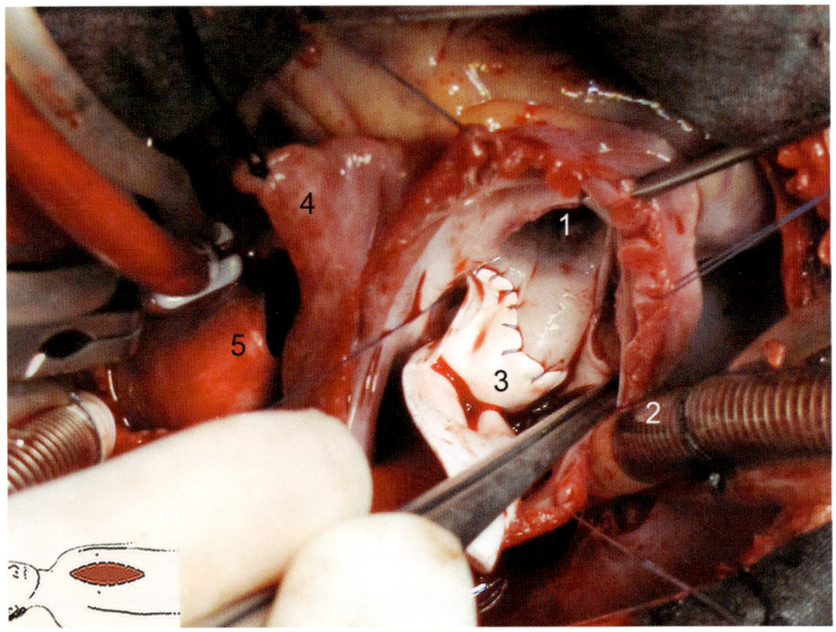

Figure 16.26. The same patient as in Figures 16.24 and 16.25 during arterial switching. The great arteries have been transected above the sinuses of Valsalva. The coronary arteries will next be transferred from the aorta to the PA.

1. Ascending aorta
2. MPA
3. RAA

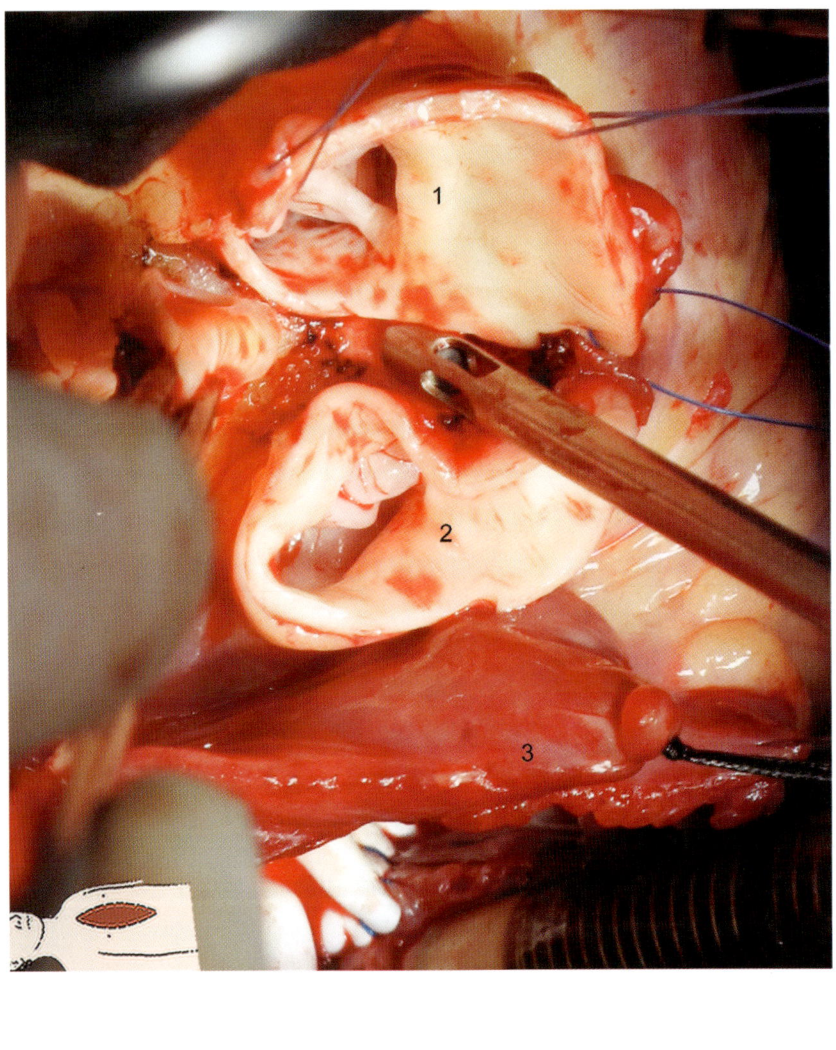

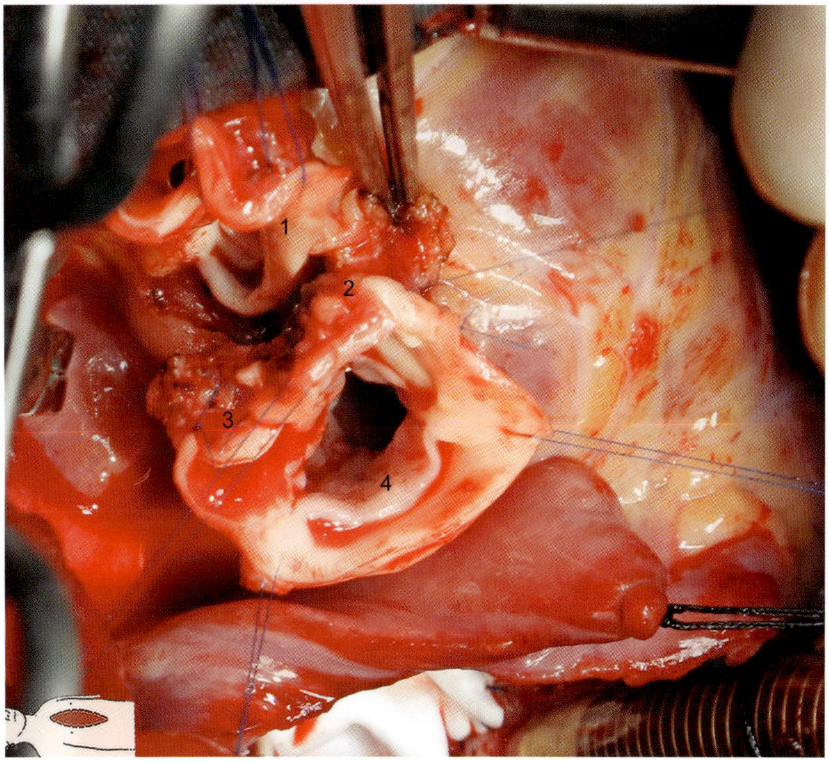

Figure 16.27. The same patient as in Figures 16.24 to 16.26. The left coronary artery has already been transferred, and the right is being sutured to its new location on the neoaorta.

1. Neo-PA (old aorta)
2. (Morphologic) left coronary artery
3. (Morphologic) right coronary artery
4. Neoaortic valve

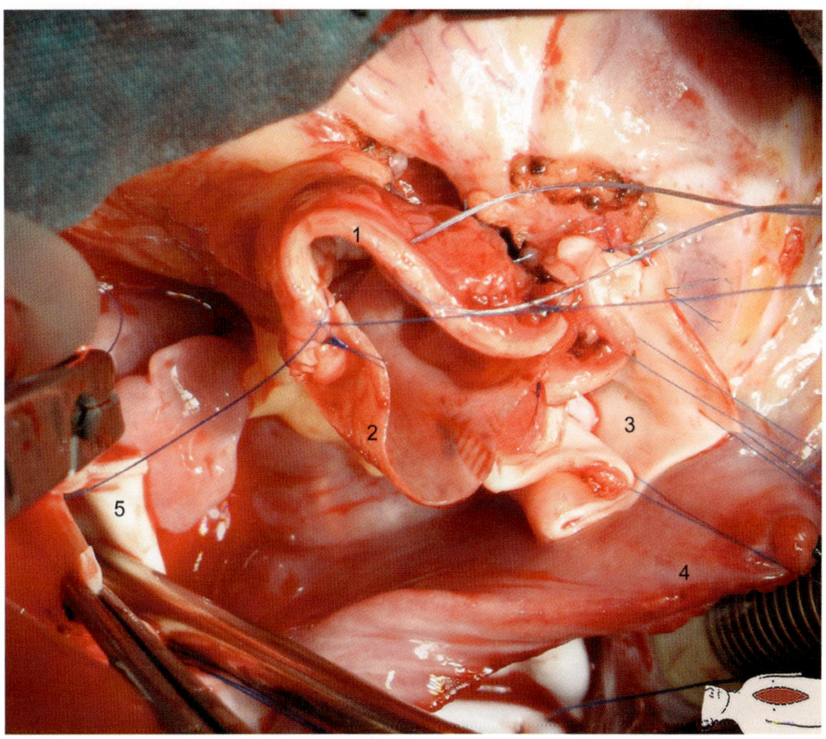

Figure 16.28. The same patient as in Figures 16.24 to 16.27. Coronary artery transfer has been completed. The defect at the original site of the coronary arteries on the old aorta is being patched with a piece of pericardium. The reconstructed proximal neo-PA will next be sutured to the distal PA.

1. Neo-PA (old aorta)
2. Pericardial patch
3. Neoaorta (old PA)
4. RAA
5. Distal MPA

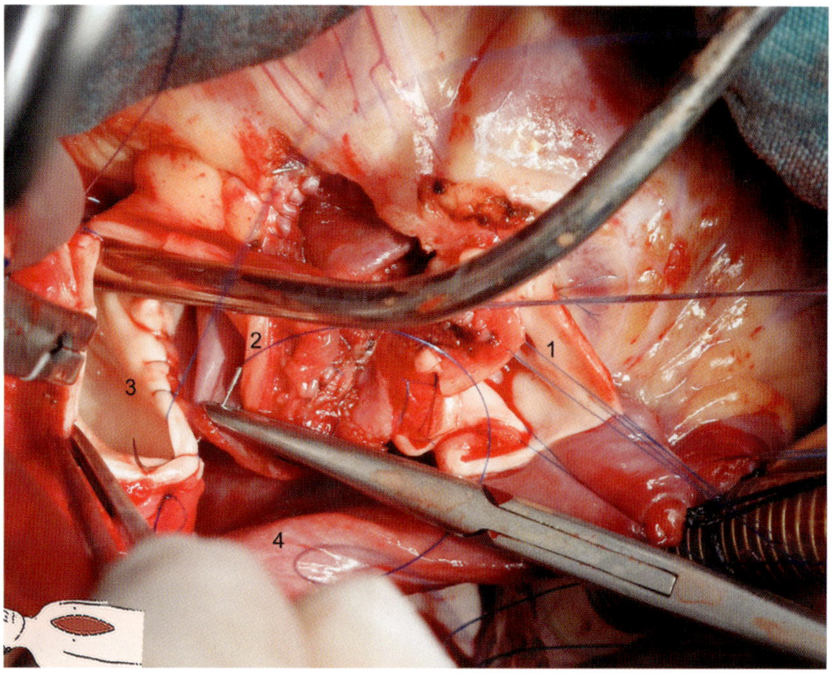

Figure 16.29. The same patient as in Figures 16.24 to 16.28. The proximal neo-PA is being sutured to the distal PA, without a Lecompte maneuver.

1. Neoaorta
2. Proximal neo-PA
3. Distal MPA
4. SVC

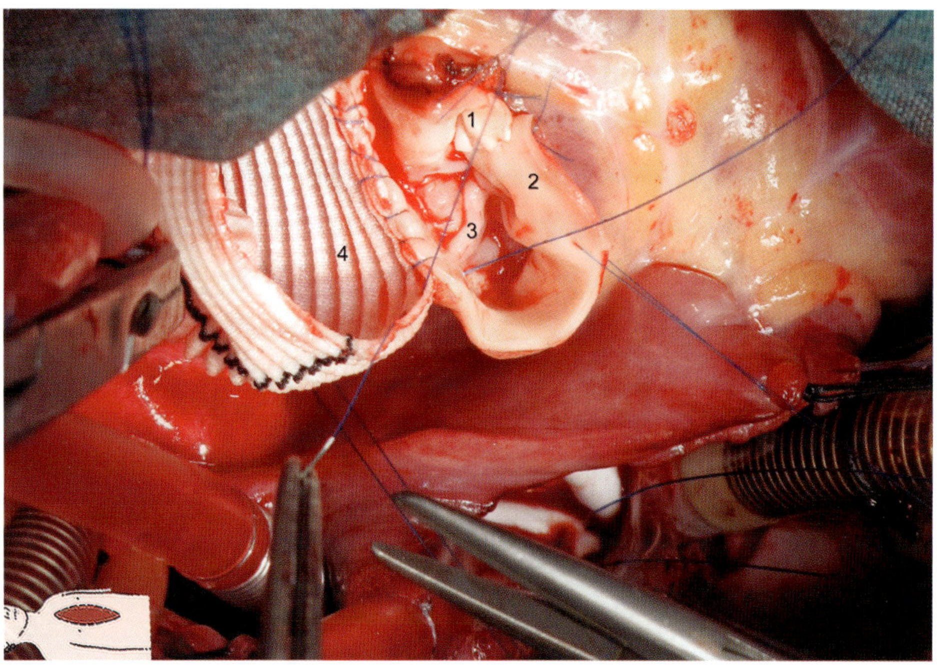

Figure 16.30. The same patient as in Figures 16.24 to 16.29. An interposition Dacron tubular graft is being placed between the proximal neoaorta and the distal aorta.

1. Coronary artery button
2. Neoaorta
3. Neoaortic valve
4. Dacron tubular graft

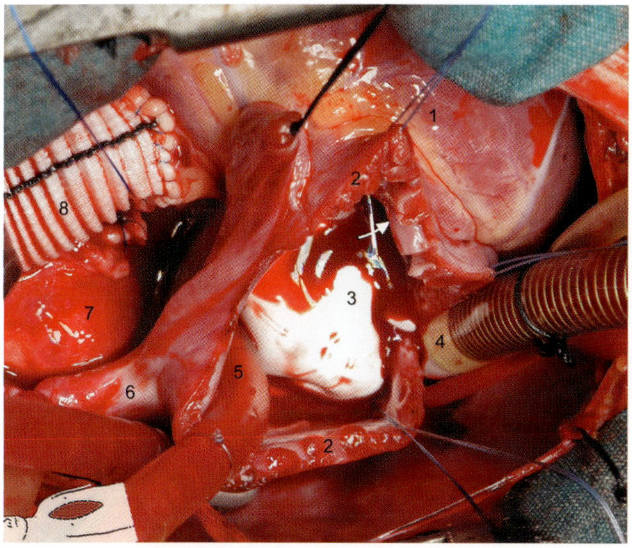

Figure 16.31

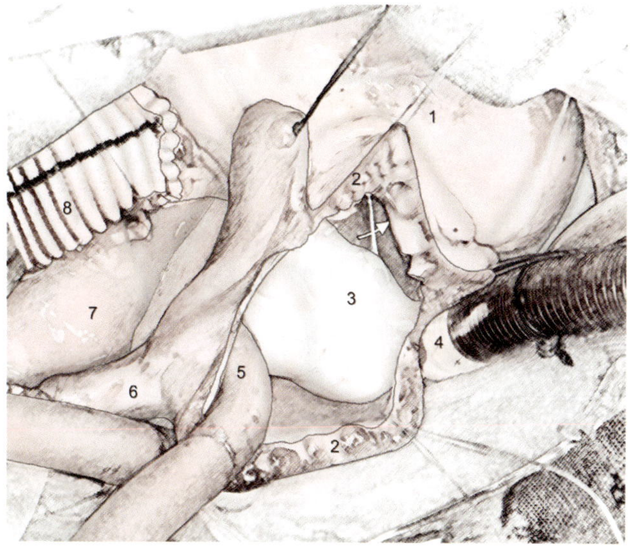

Figure 16.32

The same patient as in Figures 16.24 to 16.30 after completion of the arterial switch. The "hemi-Mustard" is also shown (the baffle between the IVC and the left-sided tricuspid valve). The arrow points to the mitral valve.

1. Morphologic LV
2. Right atrial wall
3. Hemi-Mustard baffle
4. IVC venous cannula
5. Suction catheter to the left atrium
6. SVC
7. Neo-PA
8. Reconstructed neoaorta

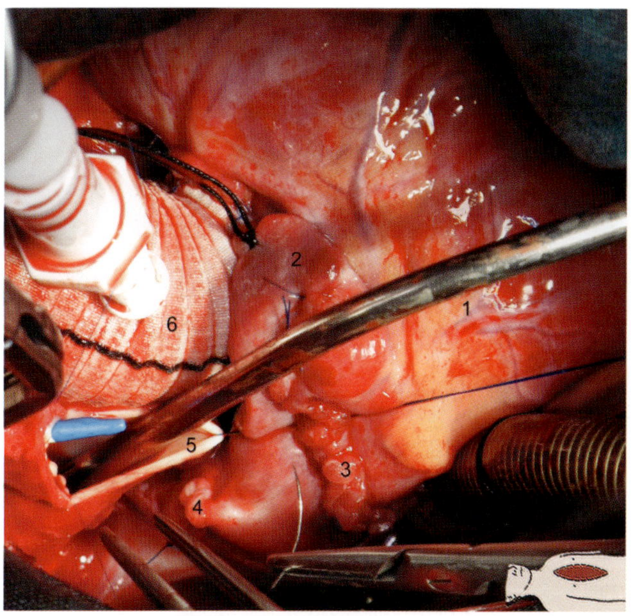

Figure 16.33

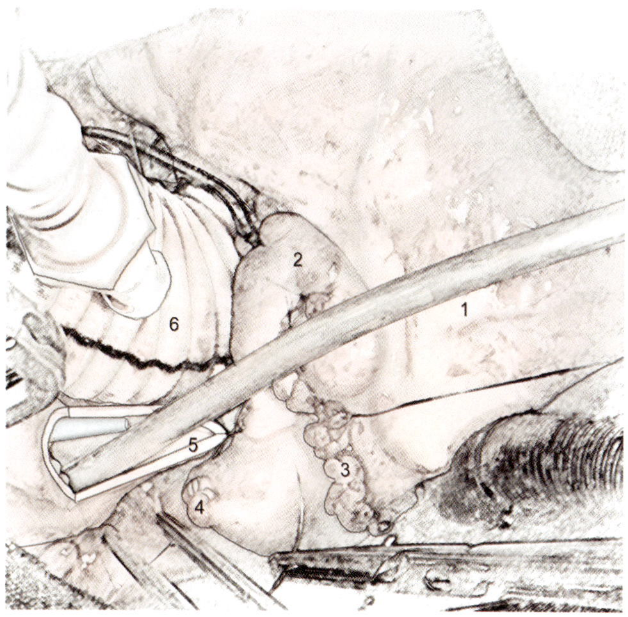

Figure 16.34

The same patient as in Figures 16.24 to 16.32 during the final part of the surgery for a Glenn shunt. The SVC has been incised open and is being anastomosed to the right PA (5). The tip of a central venous catheter is seen in the SVC. The right atrial end of the SVC (4) has been oversewn.

1. Morphologic LV
2. RAA
3. Right atriotomy incision (closed)
4. Oversewn RA–SVC junction
5. Right PA
6. Reconstructed neoaorta

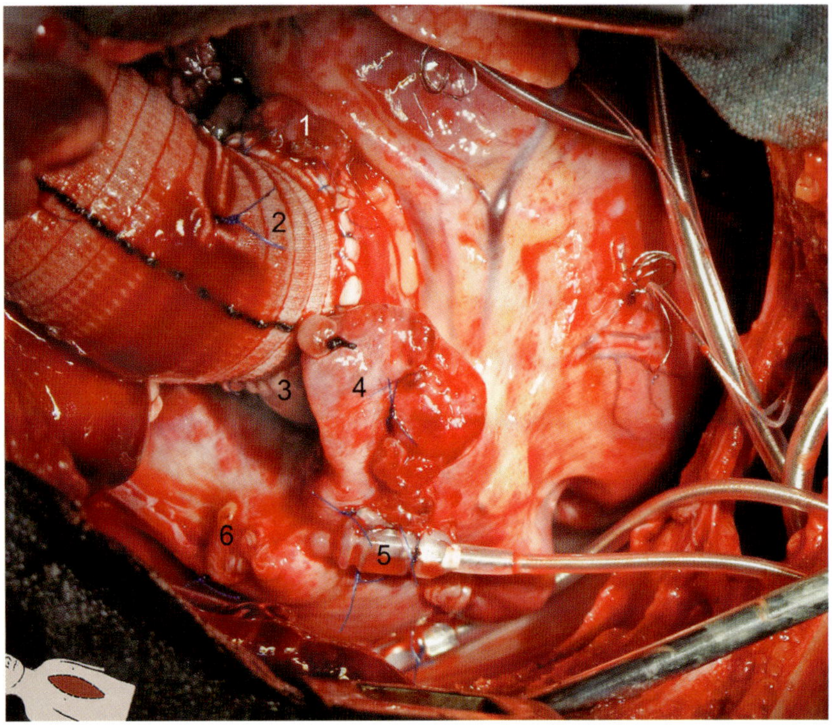

Figure 16.35. The same patient as in Figures 16.24 to 16.34 after completion of the repair. See Figure 16.36 for a close-up view of the Glenn shunt. Permanent epicardial pacemaker leads have also been implanted.

1. (Morphologic) right coronary artery button
2. Neoaorta
3. (Morphologic) left coronary artery button
4. RAA
5. Permanent atrial epicardial pacemaker lead
6. Oversewn RA–SVC junction

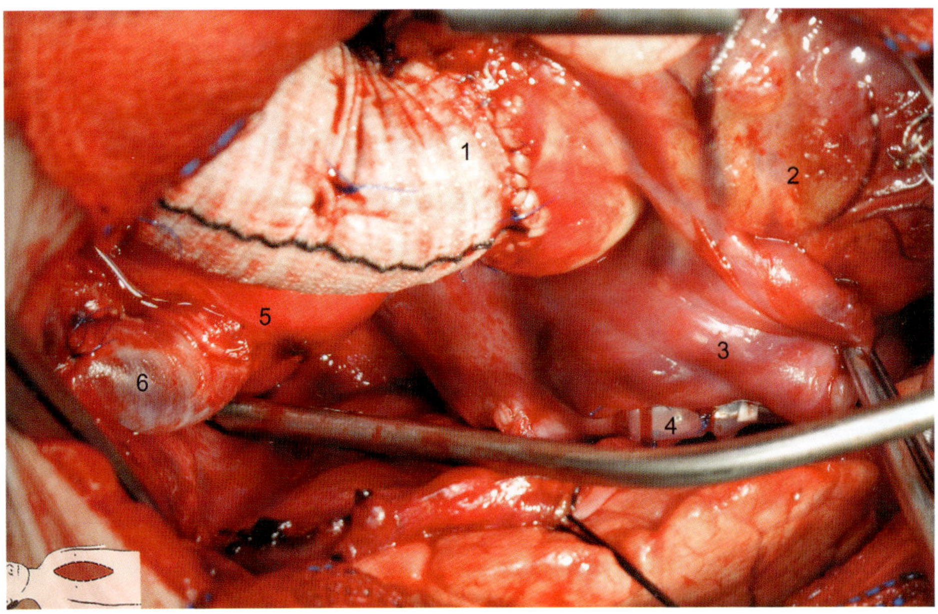

Figure 16.36. The same patient as in Figures 16.24 to 16.35 with structures retracted to show the Glenn anastomosis.

1. Neoaorta
2. Morphologic LV
3. Right atrium
4. Permanent atrial epicardial pacemaker lead
5. Right PA
6. SVC

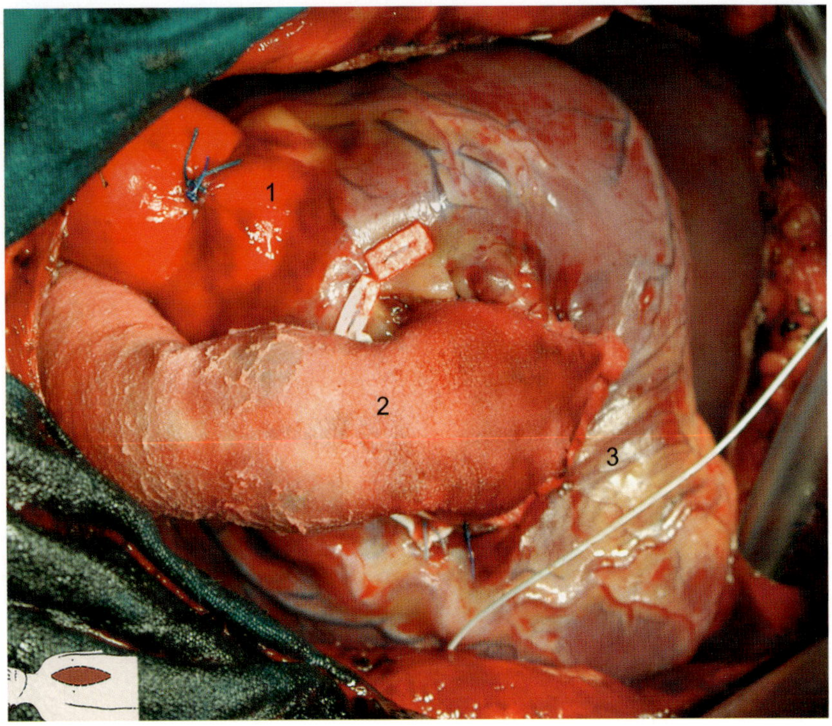

Figure 16.37. Median sternotomy view of a patient who had ccTGA, after an atrial switch and a Rastelli procedure. Shown here is the completed operation, with a conduit placed between the RV and the PA.

1. Ascending aorta
2. RV–PA conduit
3. RV

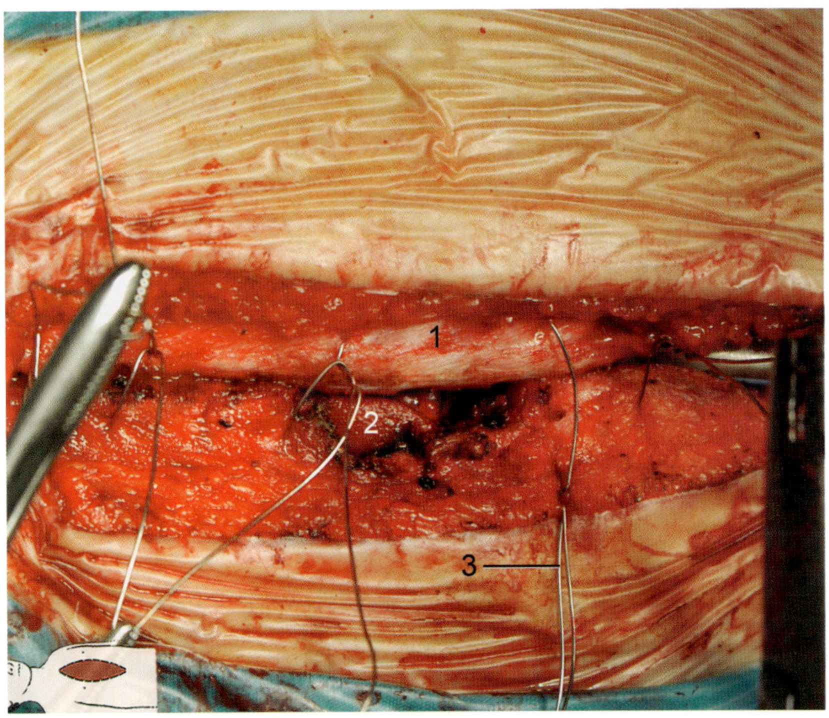

Figure 16.38. The same patient as in Figure 16.37 during sternal closure. The conduit lies immediately beneath the sternum and is subject to compression, so a small portion of the overlying bone was excised.

1. Sternum
2. RV–PA conduit
3. Sternal wires

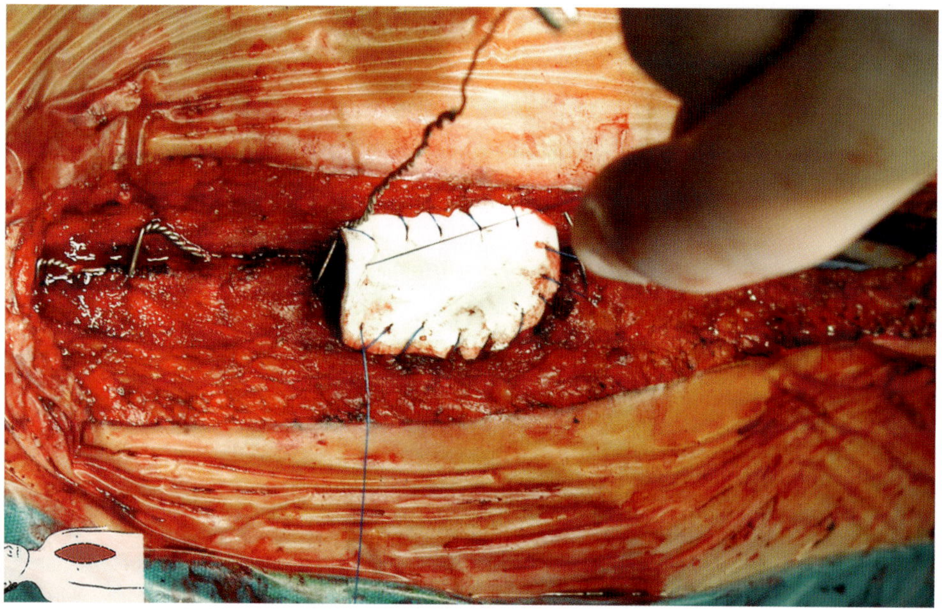

Figure 16.39. The same patient as in Figures 16.37 and 16.38 during sternal closure. The defect in the sternum is being patched with a piece of PTFE.

REFERENCES

1. Shin'oka T, Kurosawa H, Imai Y, et al. Outcomes of definitive surgical repair for congenitally corrected transposition of the great arteries or double outlet right ventricle with discordant atrioventricular connections: risk analyses in 189 patients. *J Thorac Cardiovasc Surg.* 2007;133(15):1318–1324.
2. Graham TP, Bernard YD, Mellen BG. Long-term outcome in congenitally corrected transposition of the great arteries: a multi-institutional study. *J Am Coll Cardiol.* 2000;36:255–261.
3. Mahle W, Marx G, Anderson R. Anatomy and echocardiography of discordant atrioventricular connections. *Cardiol Young.* 2006;16(Suppl. 3):65–71.
4. Voskuil M, Hazekamp MG, Kroft LJ, et al. Postsurgical course of patients with congenitally corrected transposition of the great arteries. *Am J Cardiol.* 1999;83:558–562.
5. Sharma R, Talwar S, Marwah A. Anatomic repair for congenitally corrected transposition of the great arteries. *J Thorac Cardiovasc Surg.* 2009;137:404–412.

CHAPTER 17

Single Ventricle

Congenital heart diseases that are characterized by a so-called single ventricle are those in which one ventricle is functionally dominant, resulting in single-ventricle physiology. The malformations include tricuspid valve atresia, hypoplastic left heart syndrome (HLHS), hypoplastic right ventricle (RV), double inlet left ventricle (DILV), unbalanced atrioventricular septal defect (AVSD), and some forms of double outlet right ventricle (DORV) and pulmonary atresia; the heart with a truly single ventricle is rare. These hearts commonly require a so-called univentricular instead of biventricular "repair."

Patients afflicted with these complex diseases typically undergo a series of staged surgeries that do not aim at correcting the underlying anomalies, but rather aim at improving oxygen saturation and optimizing hemodynamics. The conclusion of this single-ventricle palliation pathway is a total cavopulmonary connection (Fontan surgery).

STAGE 1 PROCEDURES

The purpose of a first-stage procedure is to regulate pulmonary and systemic blood flow in order to achieve "balanced circulation," alleviate cyanosis, and/or relieve systemic outflow obstruction. Depending on the underlying pathology, an initial palliative procedure may be required to augment pulmonary blood flow such as a Blalock-Taussig (BT) shunt, or to limit pulmonary blood flow such as pulmonary artery (PA) banding. Figure 17.1 shows a left-modified BT shunt along with PA banding in an infant with tricuspid atresia. Other examples of BT shunt are presented in the chapters on tetralogy of Fallot (TOF) and pulmonary atresia.

The Norwood procedure is usually the first-stage surgery for HLHS. An example of HLHS is shown in Figures 17.2 to 17.4. Note the diffusely hypoplastic ascending aorta. Figures 17.5 to 17.7 show other examples of neonates with HLHS. The Norwood procedure is shown in Figures 17.8 and 17.9. After complex surgeries such as the Norwood procedure, the sternum is often left open, and the skin is covered with Silastic or similar material (Figure 17.10). An open sternum prevents cardiac compression caused by mediastinal and myocardial edema, improves diastolic function, and facilitates ventilation.[1] Damus-Kaye-Stansel (DKS) surgery has similarities to the Norwood procedure and is used to bypass systemic outflow obstruction in single-ventricle patients (Figures 17.11 to 17.14).

BIDIRECTIONAL GLENN SHUNT

Bidirectional Glenn shunt, also called superior bidirectional cavopulmonary connection, is commonly performed as a bridge to total cavopulmonary connection (Fontan surgery). It entails routing the venous return from the superior vena cava (SVC) to the PA tree directly, without passing through the heart. The venous pressure acts as the driving force for blood flow. An illustrative case is shown in Figures 17.15 to 17.20. The SVC is transected above the cavoatrial junction. The cardiac end of the SVC is oversewn, and the cephalad end is anastomosed end-to-side to the superior aspect of the right PA.

Figures 17.21 and 17.22 are from a 8-month-old infant with transposition of the great arteries (TGA), ventricular septal defect (VSD), pulmonary stenosis, and hypoplastic RV. Because of the size of the RV, biventricular repair could not be done, and the

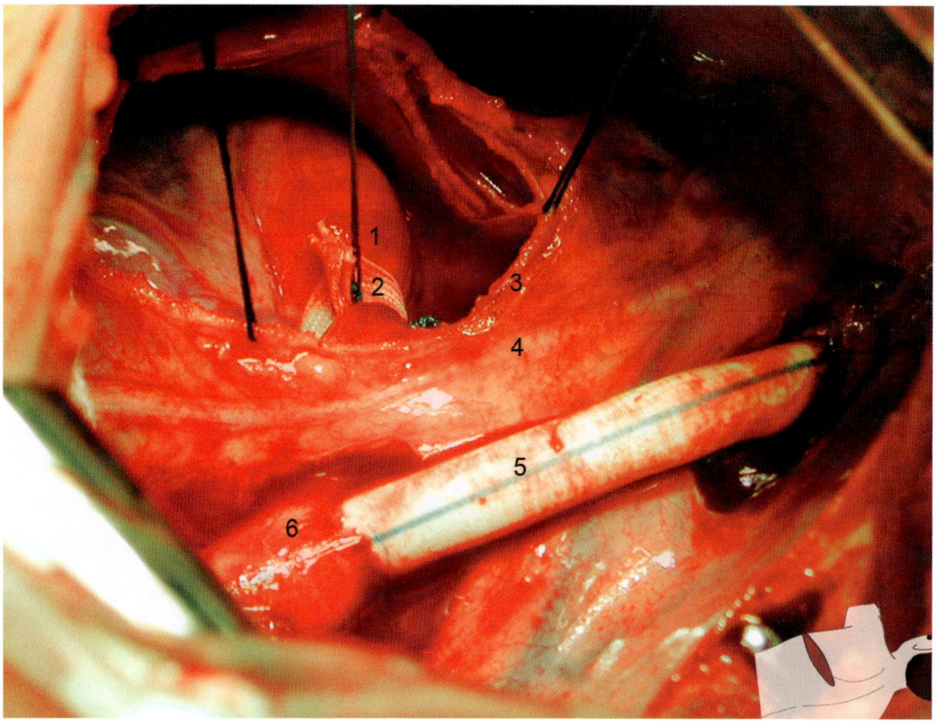

Figure 17.1. Left lateral thoracotomy view of a 6-month-old infant with tricuspid atresia, VSD, and pulmonary hypertension. PA banding and left BT shunt (4 mm Gore-Tex) were performed as a first step in single-ventricle palliation that will culminate in the Fontan operation.

1. Main pulmonary artery (MPA)
2. PA band
3. Pericardium
4. Left phrenic nerve
5. BT shunt (4 mm Gore-Tex graft)
6. Left PA

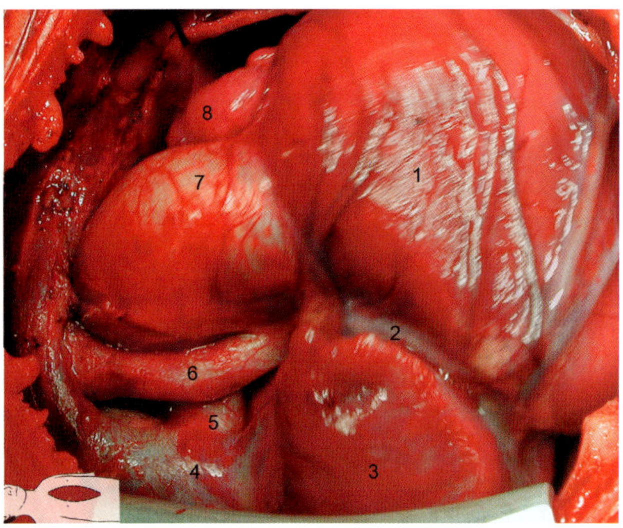

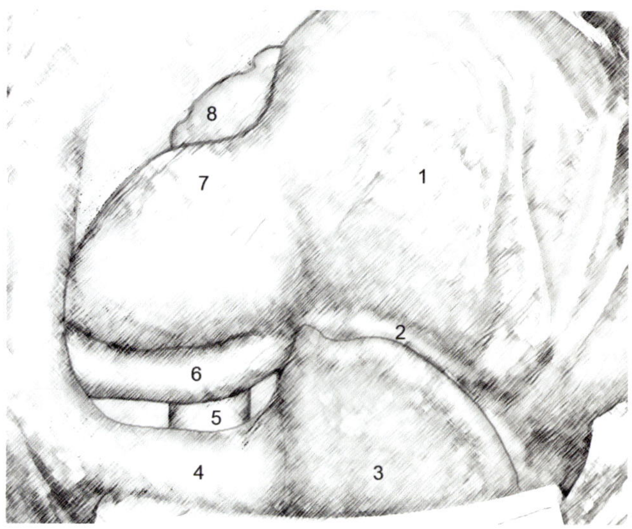

Figure 17.2 **Figure 17.3**

Median sternotomy view of a 1-day-old neonate with HLHS. Note the relative sizes of the MPA and the hypoplastic ascending aorta.

1. RV
2. Right coronary artery
3. Right atrium
4. SVC
5. Right PA
6. Ascending aorta
7. MPA
8. Left atrial appendage (LAA)

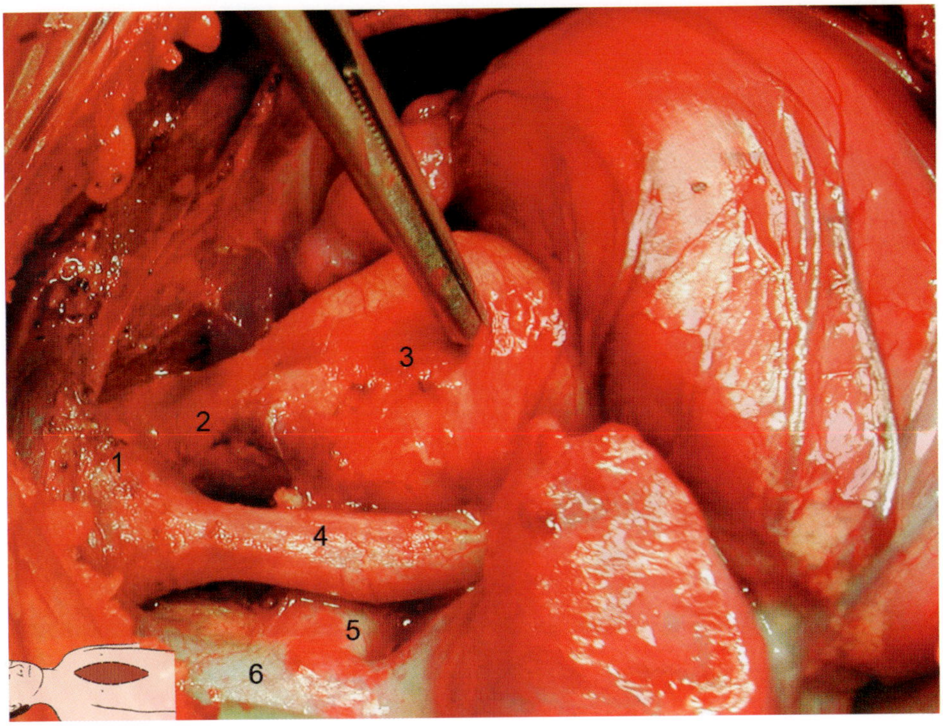

Figure 17.4. The same patient as in Figure 17.2. The MPA is retracted to reveal the ductus arteriosus. Note that the transverse arch is larger than the ascending aorta.

1. Transverse arch
2. Ductus arteriosus
3. MPA
4. Ascending aorta
5. Right PA
6. SVC

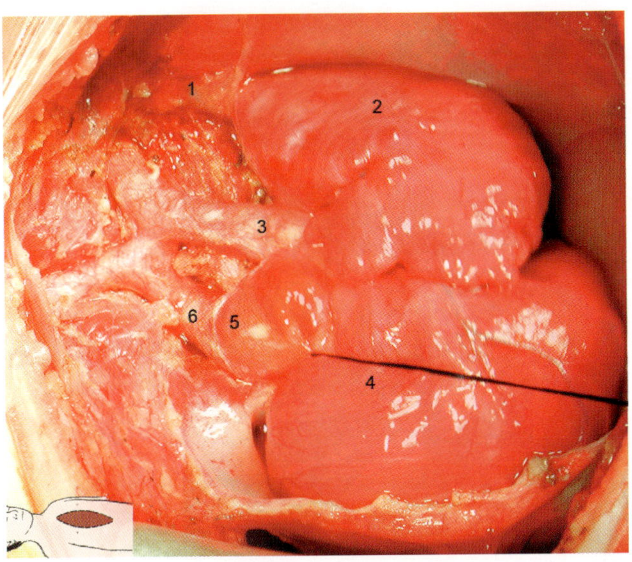

Figure 17.5

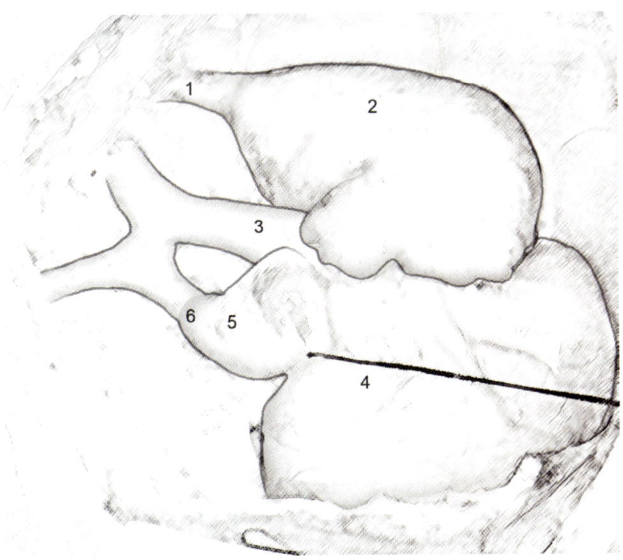

Figure 17.6

A 7-day-old neonate with HLHS in the setting of mirror-imaged atrial arrangement, with the heart in the right chest and the apex pointing rightward, as seen through a median sternotomy. The aortic arch is diffusely hypoplastic.

1. SVC
2. Left-sided right atrium
3. Ascending aorta
4. Right ventricle
5. PA
6. Ductus arteriosus

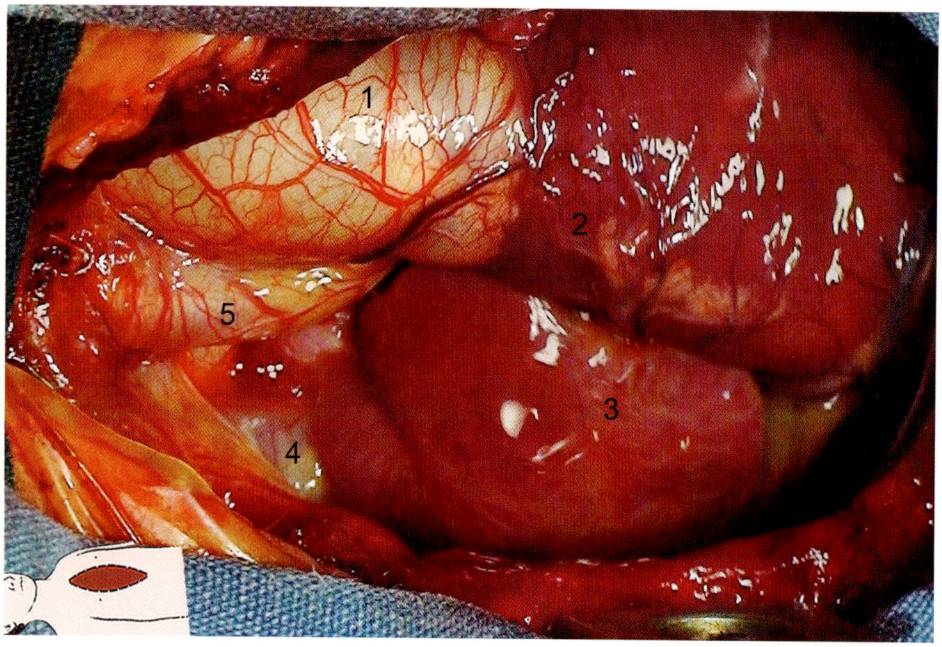

Figure 17.7. Another patient, 5 days old, with HLHS as seen through a median sternotomy. The gross anatomy is shown. Again note the relative sizes of the MPA and the ascending aorta.

1. MPA
2. Outflow part of RV
3. Right atrium
4. SVC
5. Ascending aorta

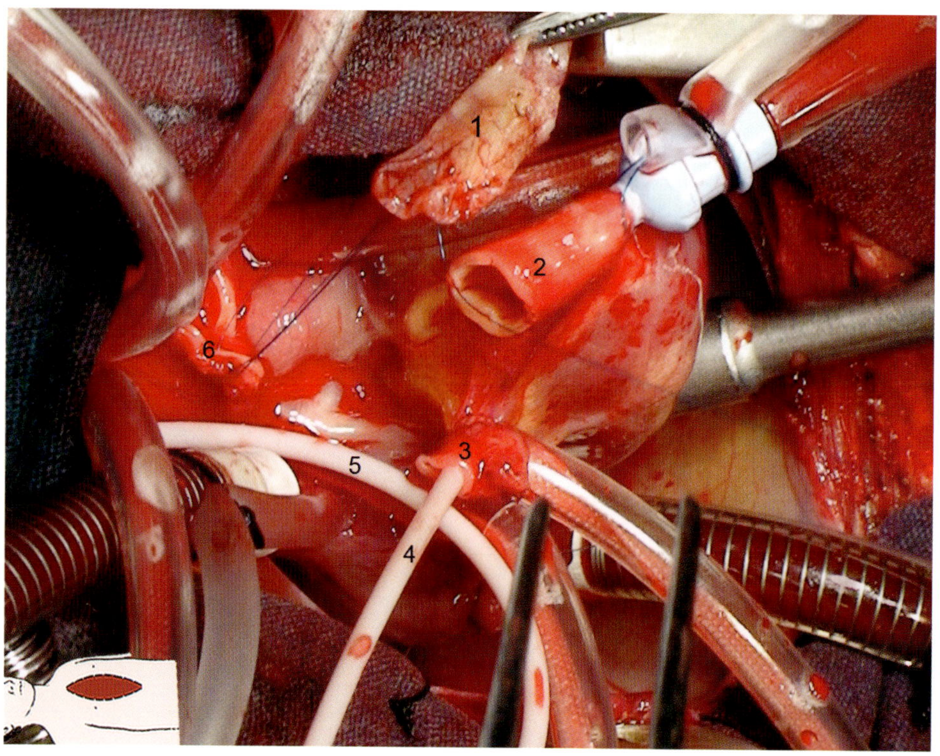

Figure 17.8. The same patient as in Figure 17.7 during the Norwood procedure under circulatory arrest, with cerebral perfusion. The great arteries have been transected. A pericardial patch is being sutured to the distal PA.

1. Autologous pericardial patch
2. MPA
3. Proximal ascending aorta
4. Coronary perfusion catheter
5. Cerebral perfusion catheter
6. Distal PA

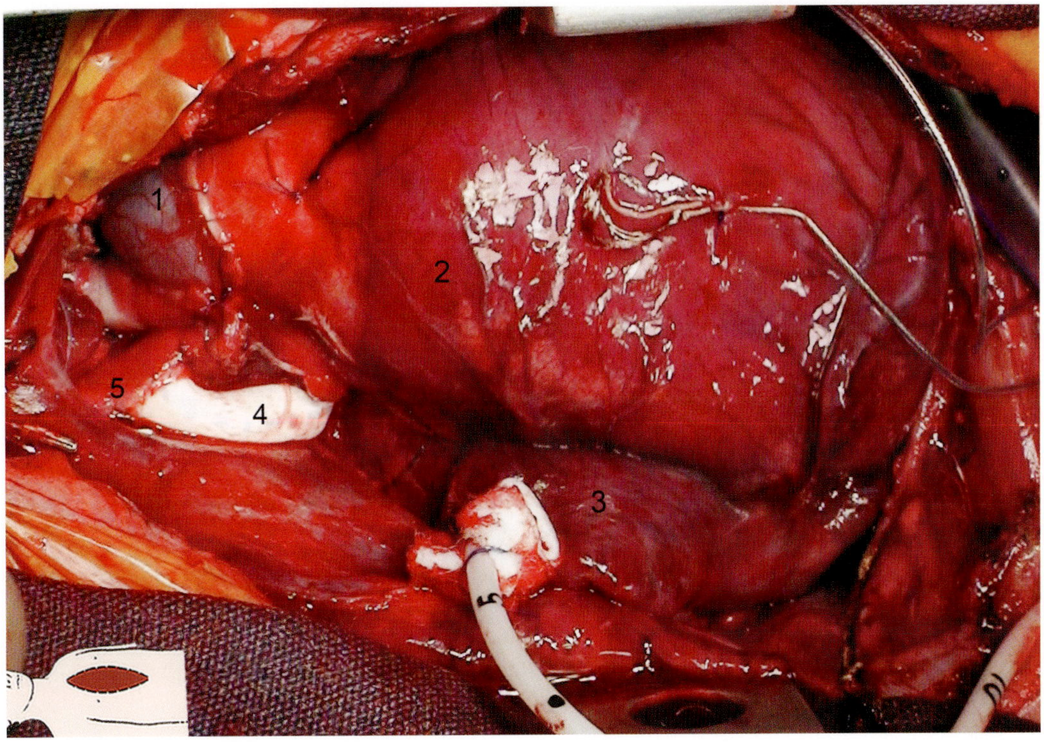

Figure 17.9. The same patient as in Figures 17.7 and 17.8 after completion of the Norwood procedure. The neoaorta has been reconstructed by side-to-side anastomosis with the PA. Pulmonary blood flow is provided by a right-modified BT shunt.

1. Neoaorta
2. RV
3. Right atrium
4. Right-modified BT shunt
5. Innominate artery

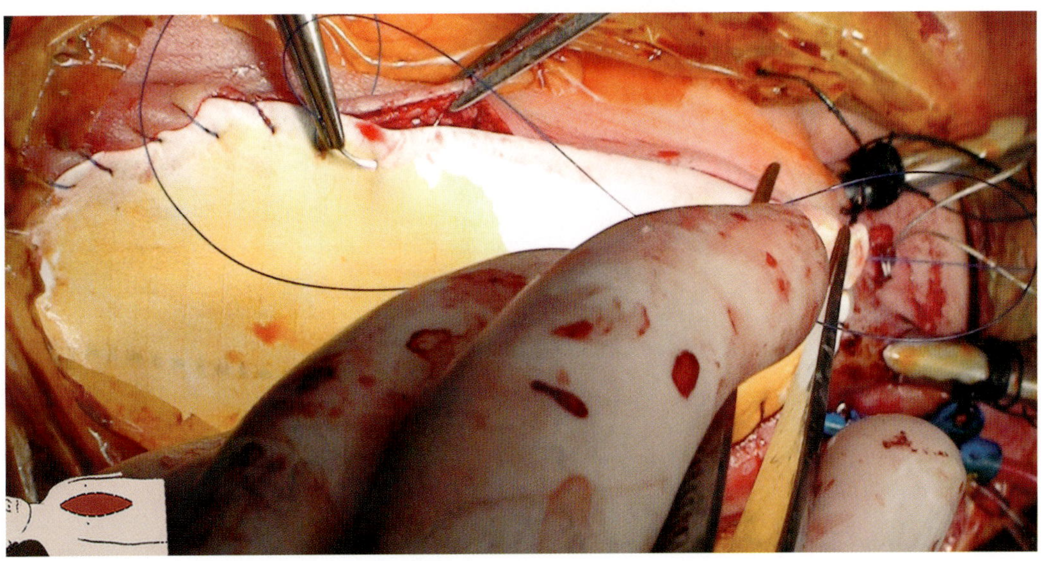

Figure 17.10. The same patient as in Figures 17.7 to 17.9 after completion of the Norwood procedure. The sternum was left open, and the skin was covered with a patch. The sternum is usually closed 2 to 3 days postoperatively.

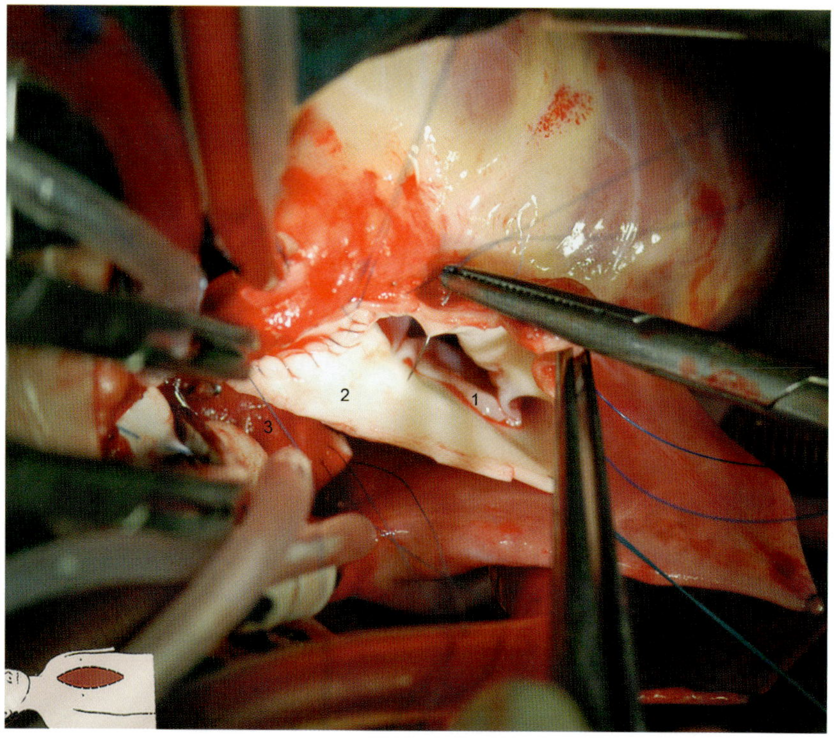

Figure 17.11. Median sternotomy view of a child with TGA, restrictive VSD, and hypoplastic RV. A DKS operation is performed to direct LV blood to the aorta. In this picture, the MPA is being anastomosed to the aorta.

1. Pulmonary valve
2. MPA
3. Ascending aorta

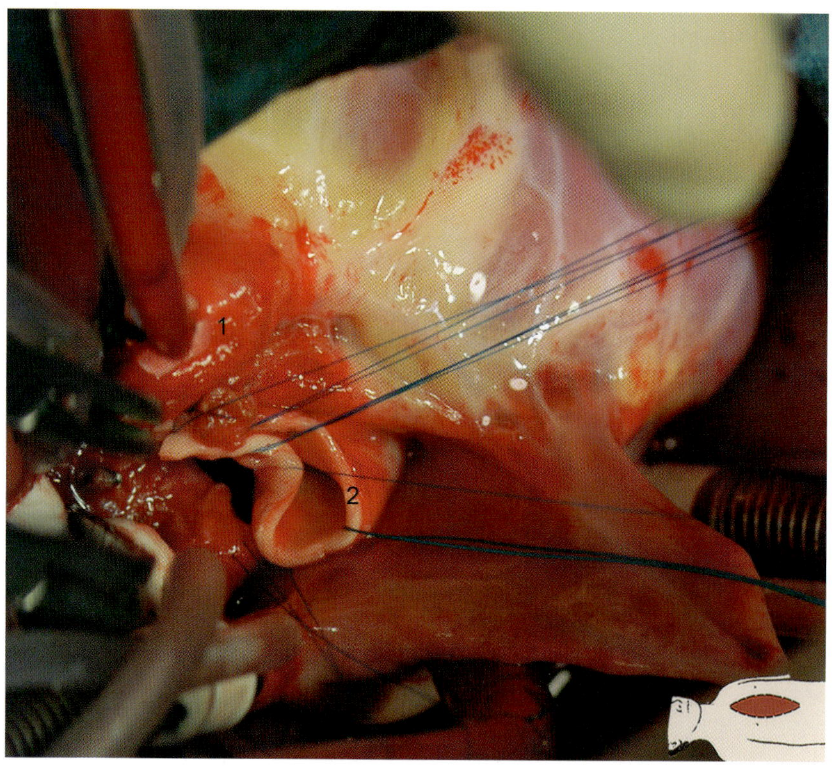

Figure 17.12. The same patient as in Figure 17.11. The MPA has been anastomosed to the side of the aorta. The superior part of the pulmonary arteriotomy will be covered with a patch.

1. Ascending aorta
2. MPA

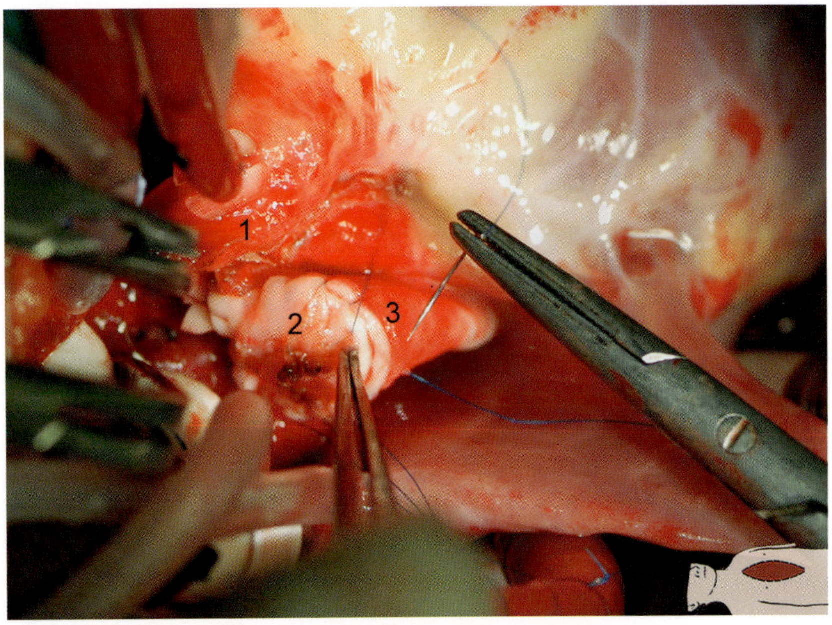

Figure 17.13. The same patient as in Figures 17.11 and 17.12. The superior part of the MPA is closed with a patch hood.

1. Ascending aorta
2. A patch closing the upper part of the MPA
3. MPA

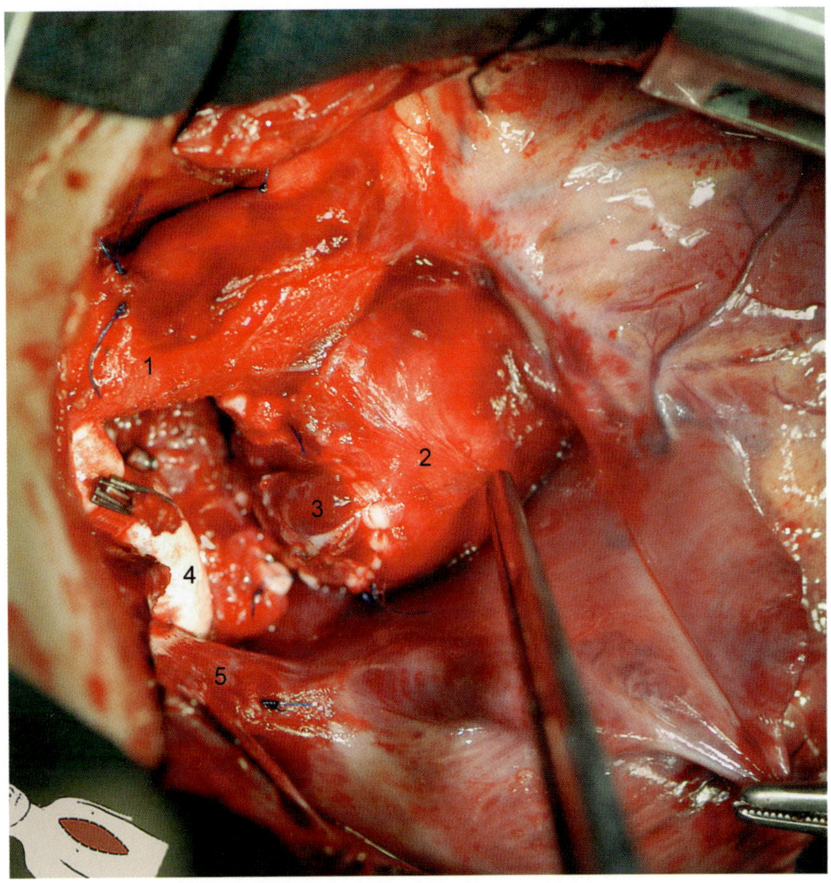

Figure 17.14. The same patient as in Figures 17.11 to 17.13 after completion of the DKS procedure. The MPA is anastomosed to the side of the ascending aorta. Pulmonary blood flow is supplied by a right BT shunt. An oversized BT shunt was implanted, so a band was placed around it to limit pulmonary blood flow.

1. Ascending aorta
2. MPA
3. Roof of the MPA
4. Right-modified BT shunt
5. SVC

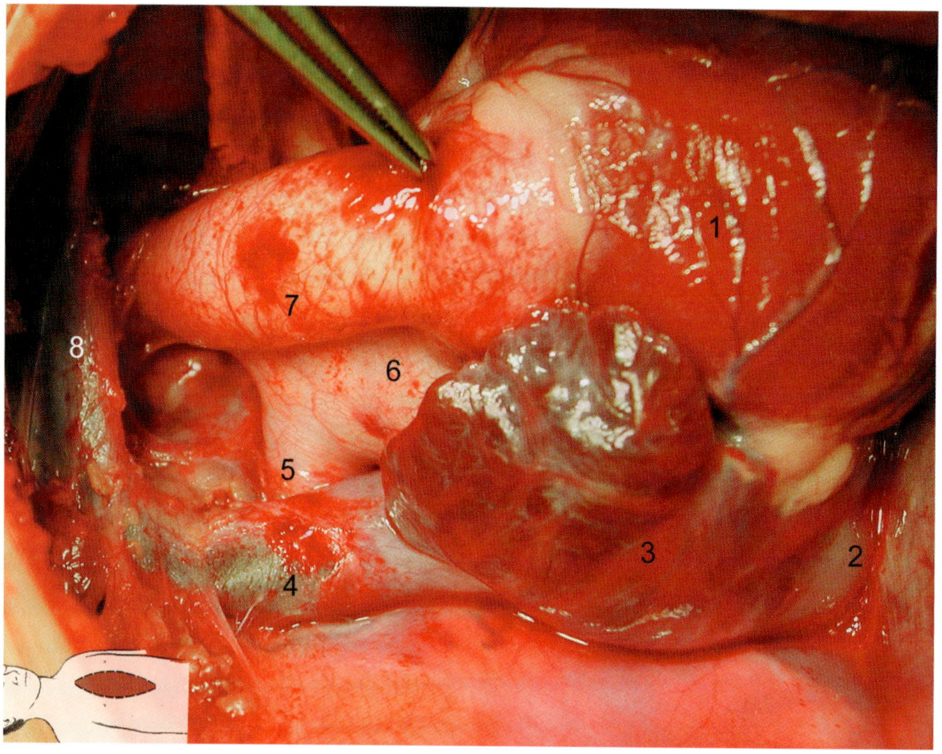

Figure 17.15. Median sternotomy view of a 6-month-old infant with discordant ventriculoarterial connections, DILV, hypoplastic RV, and pulmonary stenosis. The child is undergoing a Glenn shunt procedure.

1. RV
2. Inferior vena cava (IVC)
3. Right atrium
4. SVC
5. Right PA
6. MPA
7. Ascending aorta
8. Innominate vein

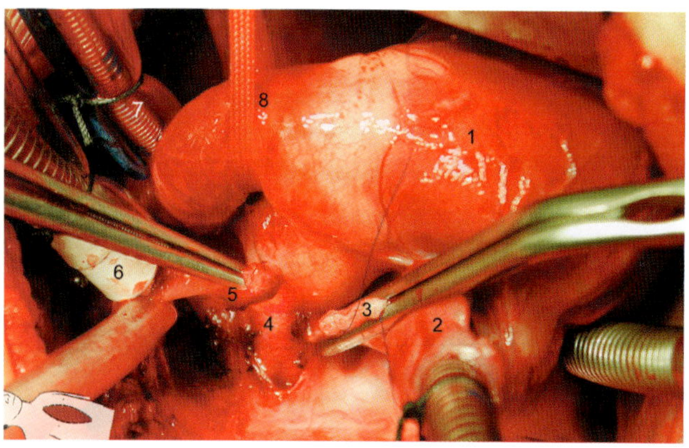

Figure 17.16

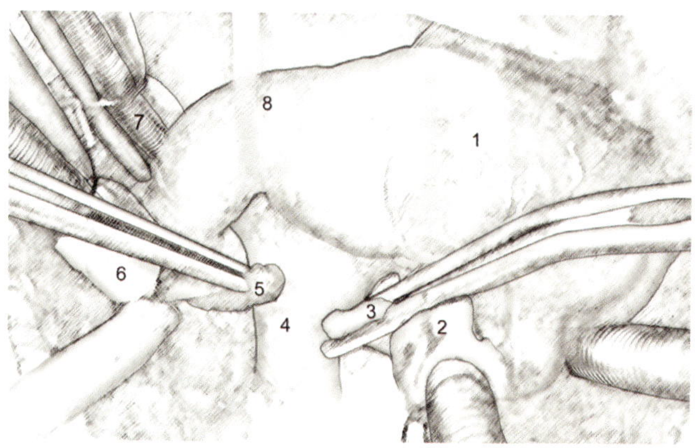

Figure 17.17

The same patient as in Figure 17.15, now on cardiopulmonary bypass. The SVC is cannulated high, the IVC is cannulated through the right atrium, and the aorta is cannulated in the usual manner but with no cardioplegia or cross-clamping. The SVC has been transected above the cavoatrial junction. The cardiac end will be oversewn, while the upper end will be anastomosed to the right PA (Figure 17.18).

1. RV
2. Right atrial appendage (RAA)
3. Cardiac end of SVC
4. Right PA
5. Cephalad end of SVC
6. SVC venous cannula
7. Aortic cannula
8. Ascending aorta

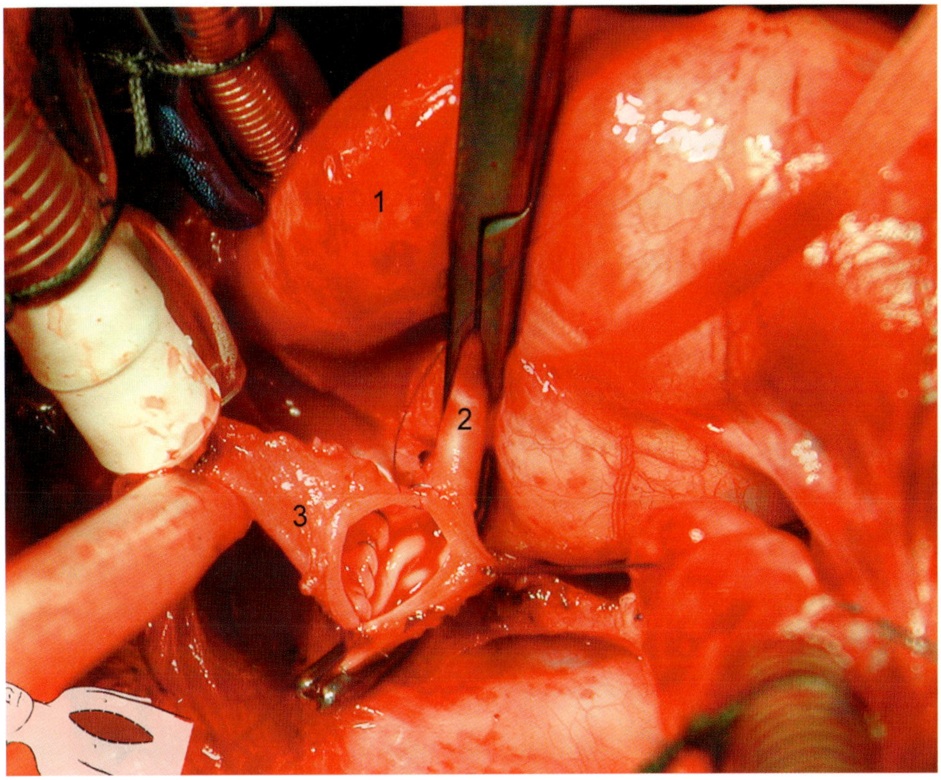

Figure 17.18. The same patient as in Figures 17.15 to 17.17. The SVC is being sutured end-to-side to the right PA.

1. Ascending aorta
2. Right PA
3. SVC

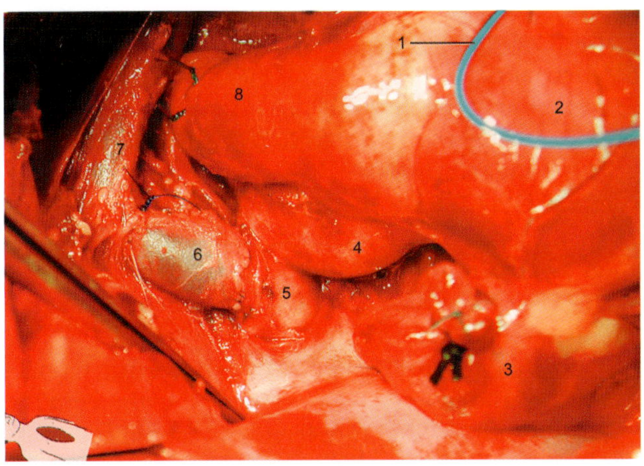

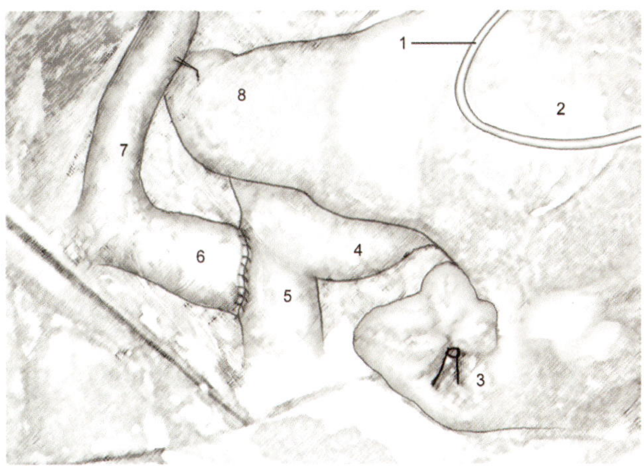

Figure 17.19 **Figure 17.20**

The same patient as in Figures 17.15 to 17.18 after completion of the cavopulmonary (Glenn) anastomosis. The SVC has been anastomosed to the right PA. Thus, the blood return from the upper body goes directly to the lungs without having to pass through the heart.

1. Temporary pacing wire
2. RV
3. Right atrium
4. MPA
5. Right PA
6. SVC
7. Innominate vein
8. Ascending aorta

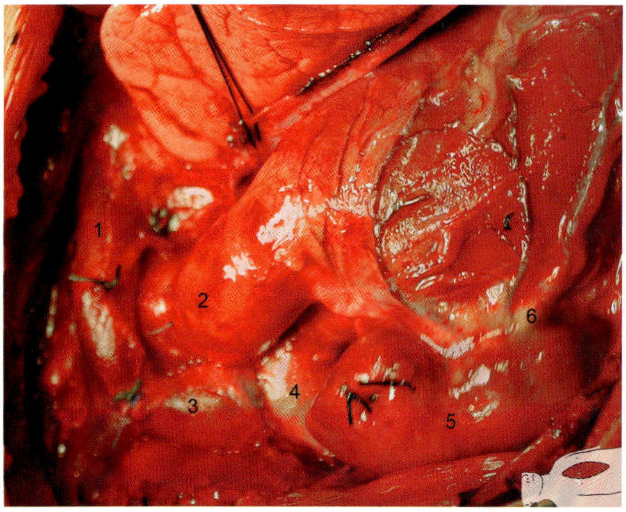

Figure 17.21

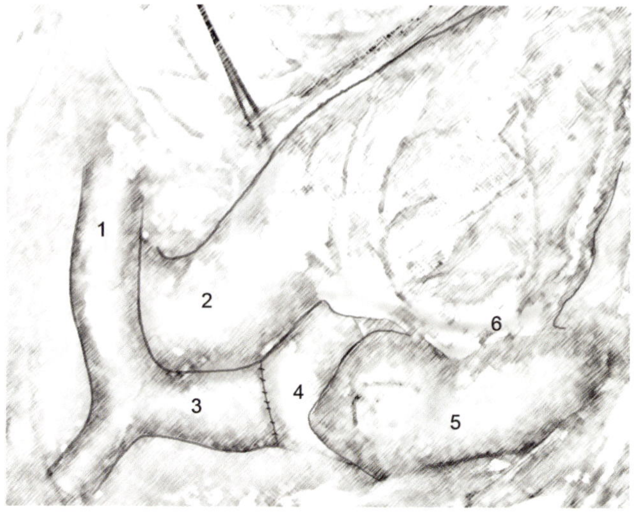

Figure 17.22

Median sternotomy view of an 8-month-old infant with TGA, VSD, pulmonary stenosis, and hypoplastic RV. A bidirectional Glenn shunt has just been completed. The SVC is connected to the right PA, with end-to-side anastomosis.

1. Innominate vein
2. Ascending aorta
3. SVC
4. Right PA
5. Right atrium
6. Right coronary artery

patient underwent single-ventricle palliation. The systemic and pulmonary circulations were "balanced" so an initial procedure to augment or limit pulmonary blood flow was not needed. A bidirectional Glenn shunt was performed at 8 months of age. Figure 17.23 is a median sternotomy view of another child with tricuspid atresia who had a Glenn shunt at an earlier stage.

FONTAN SURGERY

This final step in univentricular palliation is usually performed in a patient who has already had a Glenn shunt. The IVC blood is directed to the PA without passing through the RV. After Fontan surgery, essentially all systemic venous return bypasses the heart and goes directly to the lungs, thus avoiding intracardiac mixing and achieving separation of systemic and pulmonary circulations. Ever since it was first conceived and performed by Fontan and Baudet,[2] many modifications of this procedure have been introduced. Of the various forms of this procedure, the most popular now are the lateral tunnel and the extracardiac conduit,[3] with or without fenestration.

Figures 17.23 to 17.33 are intraoperative pictures of a 3.5-year-old child with tricuspid valve atresia. The patient previously had 2 surgical procedures: initially PA banding, then a bidirectional Glenn shunt. An intracardiac lateral tunnel Fontan procedure is performed using the patient's own atrial wall to create the intracardiac tunnel. Alternatively, a patch of polytetrafluoroethylene (PTFE) may be used to construct the intracardiac baffle. In extracardiac Fontan, a tube graft is used to connect the IVC to the right PA. Figures 17.34 to 17.39 are from a 4-year-old child with tricuspid atresia who has already had a Glenn shunt. Another example is shown in Figure 17.40.

Figure 17.23. Median sternotomy view of a 3.5-year-old child with absence of right AV connection (tricuspid atresia). Initially, PA banding was performed to limit pulmonary blood flow. Then a bidirectional Glenn shunt was performed and is seen here.

1. Ascending aorta
2. SVC
3. Right PA
4. Right atrium

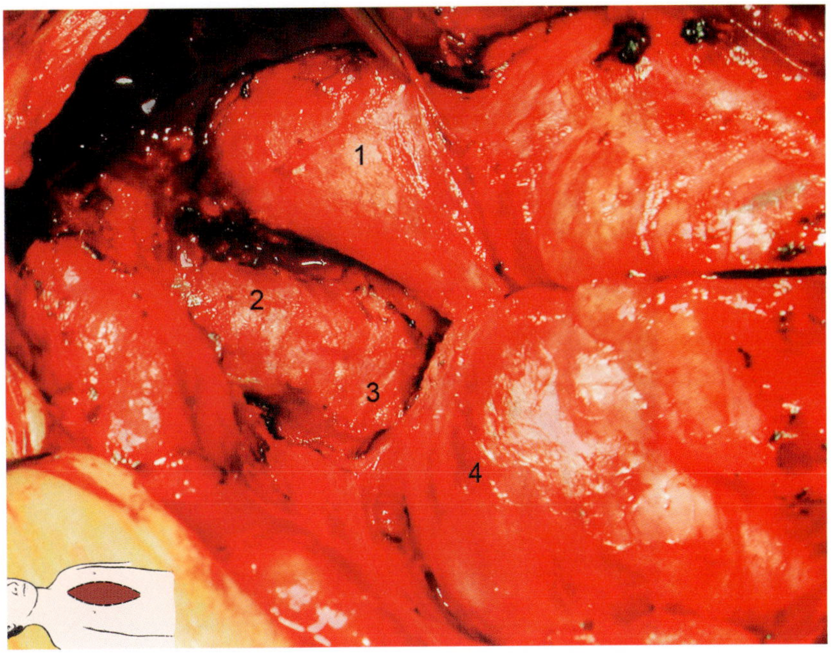

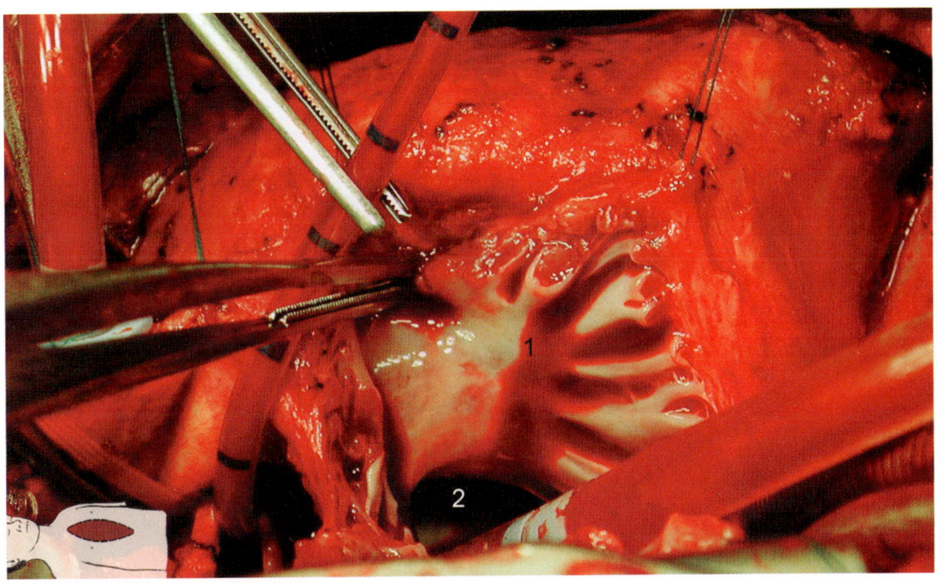

Figure 17.24. The same patient as in Figure 17.23 after right atriotomy on cardiopulmonary bypass. Note the absence of the tricuspid valve.

1. Floor of right atrium, no tricuspid valve
2. Atrial septal defect (ASD)

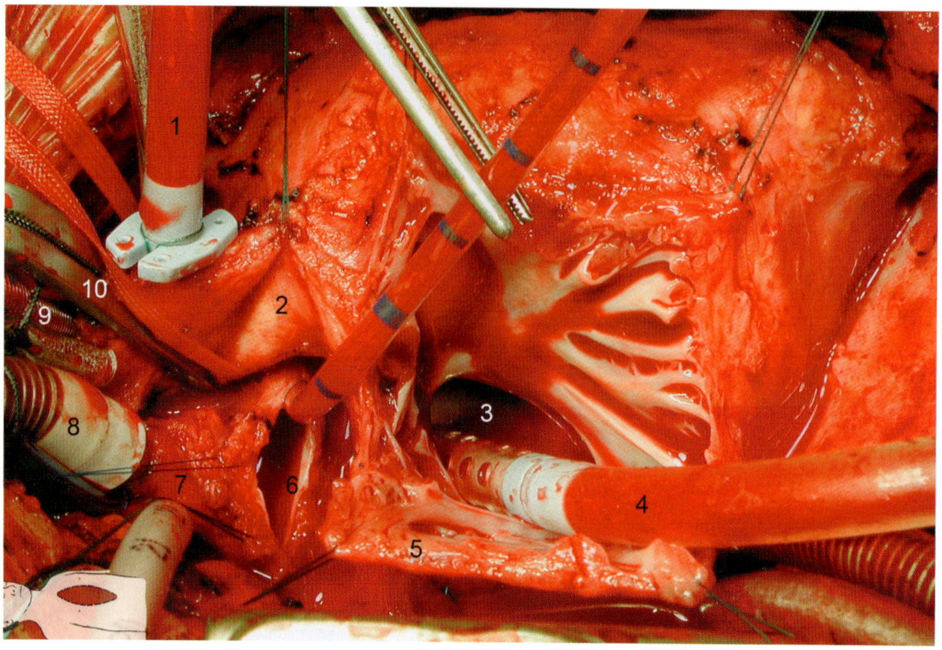

Figure 17.25. The same patient as in Figures 17.23 and 17.24. The cannulation setup is also shown. An incision has been made in the inferior aspect of the right PA (6), opposite the site of SVC anastomosis.

1. Cardioplegia catheter
2. Ascending aorta
3. ASD
4. Catheter draining left atrium
5. Right atrial free wall
6. Incision in right PA
7. SVC
8. SVC cannula
9. Arterial cannula
10. Aortic cross-clamp

Figure 17.26. The same patient as in Figures 17.23 to 17.25. An opening has been made in the roof of the right atrium just opposite the incision in the right PA.

1. Ascending aorta
2. Atrial septum
3. Left atrial cavity seen through ASD
4. Opening in roof of right atrium
5. SVC

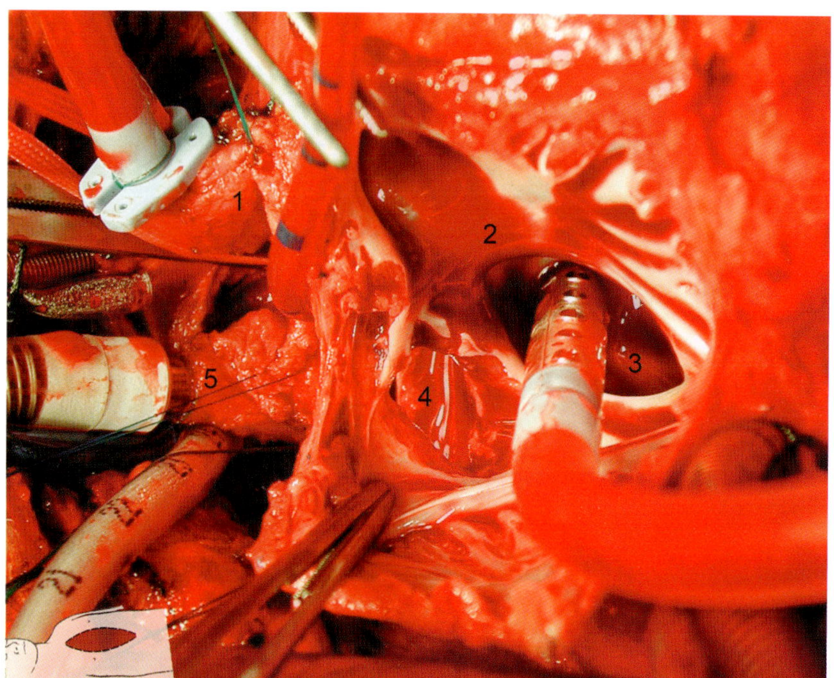

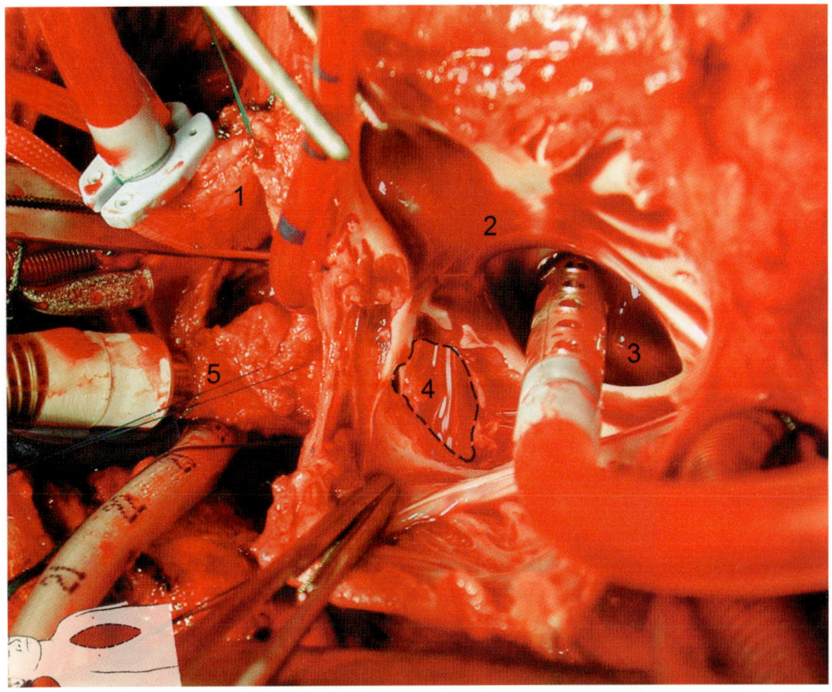

Figure 17.27. The same picture as Figure 17.26; the opening in the roof of the right atrium (4) is outlined.

1. Ascending aorta
2. Atrial septum
3. Left atrial cavity seen through ASD
4. Opening in roof of right atrium
5. SVC

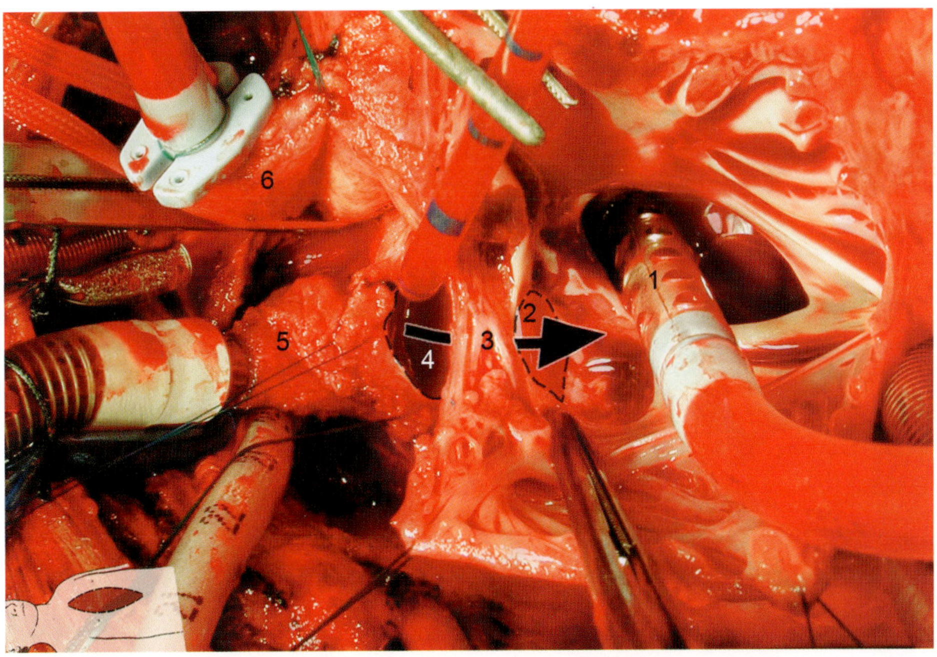

Figure 17.28. The same patient as in Figures 17.23 to 17.27. The 2 incisions (in the right PA and the right atrium) are shown opposite each other. The arrow passes through the opening in the superior wall of the right atrium.

1. Catheter draining left atrium
2. Opening in roof of right atrium
3. Roof of right atrium
4. Incision in right PA
5. SVC
6. Ascending aorta

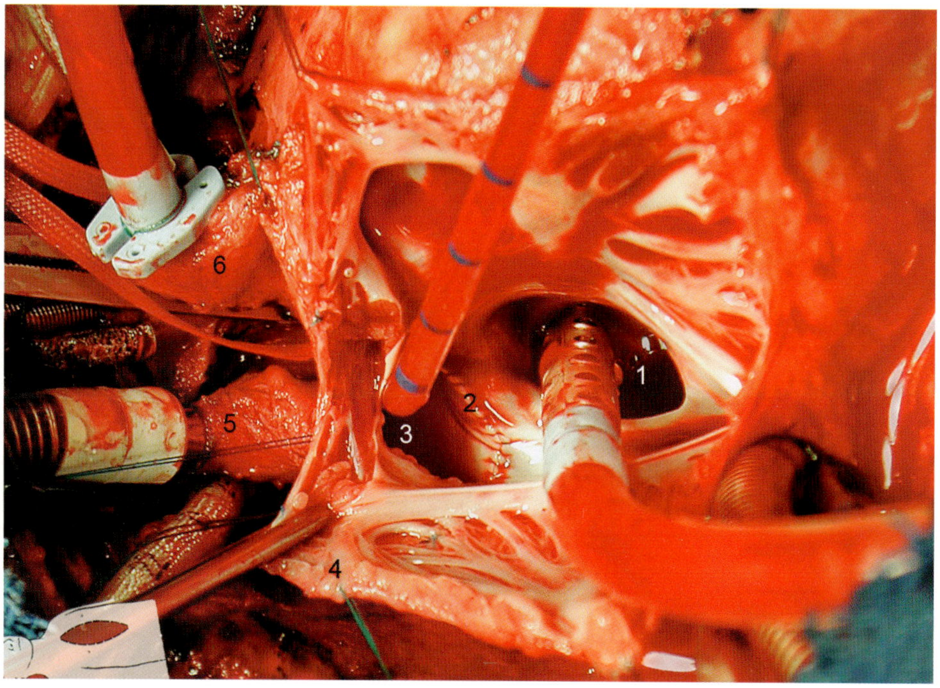

Figure 17.29. The same patient as in Figures 17.23 to 17.28. The right atrial superior wall has been anastomosed to the PA at the site where the incision was made. Now the right atrium communicates directly with the right PA.

1. ASD
2. Anastomosis between right atrium and right PA
3. Right PA lumen
4. Right atrial free wall
5. SVC
6. Ascending aorta

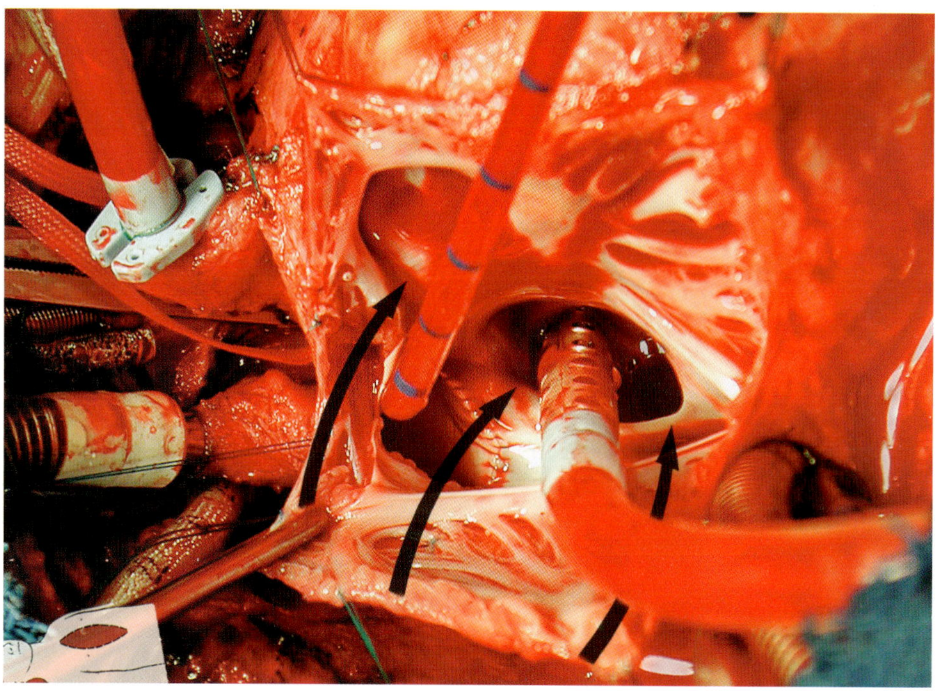

Figure 17.30. The same patient as in Figures 17.23 to 17.29. The next step will be turning in the flap of the right atrial free wall as shown by the arrows. This will create a tunnel from the IVC to the right PA.

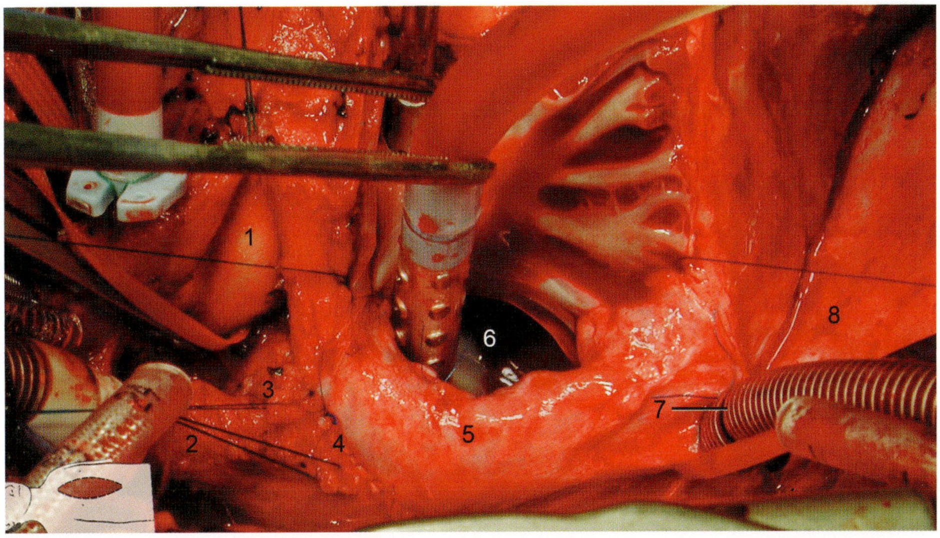

Figure 17.31. The same patient as in Figures 17.23 to 17.30. The flap of the right atrial free wall has been anastomosed to the inner aspect of the right atrium as illustrated in Figure 17.30. Using the patient's own atrial wall, an intracardiac lateral tunnel has thus been created from the IVC to the right PA.

1. Ascending aorta
2. SVC
3. Right PA
4. Anastomosis of right atrium to right PA
5. Intracardiac lateral tunnel
6. ASD
7. IVC venous cannula
8. Pericardium overlying the diaphragm

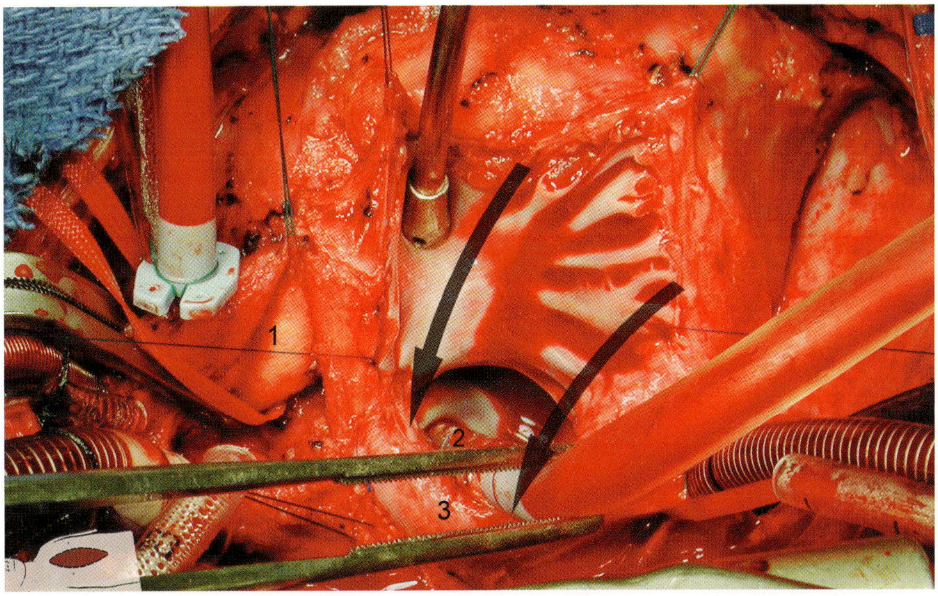

Figure 17.32. The same patient as in Figures 17.23 to 17.31. The next step will be closing the right atrium as shown by the arrows. After closure, the remaining right atrial cavity will be functionally part of the left atrium.

1. Ascending aorta
2. Catheter draining a pulmonary vein (PV)
3. Intracardiac lateral tunnel

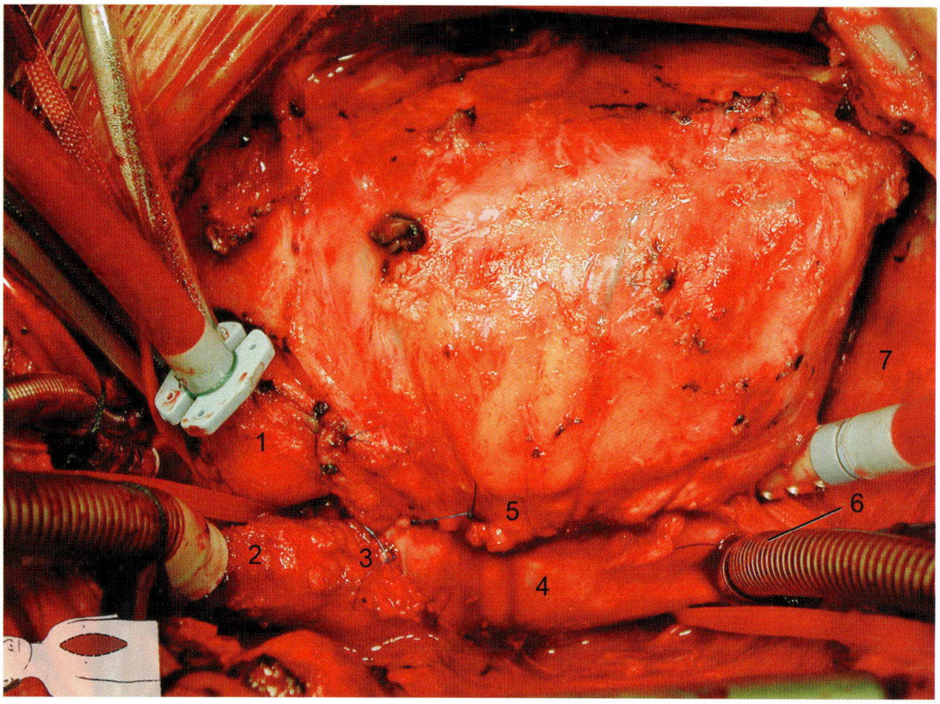

Figure 17.33. Same patient as in Figures 17.23 to 17.32 after completion of the Fontan surgery. The SVC and IVC blood goes directly to the PA, avoiding intracardiac mixing, and achieving separation of systemic and pulmonary circulations.

1. Ascending aorta
2. SVC
3. Right PA
4. Intracardiac lateral tunnel
5. Old right atrium, now an extension of left atrium
6. IVC cannula
7. Pericardium overlying the diaphragm

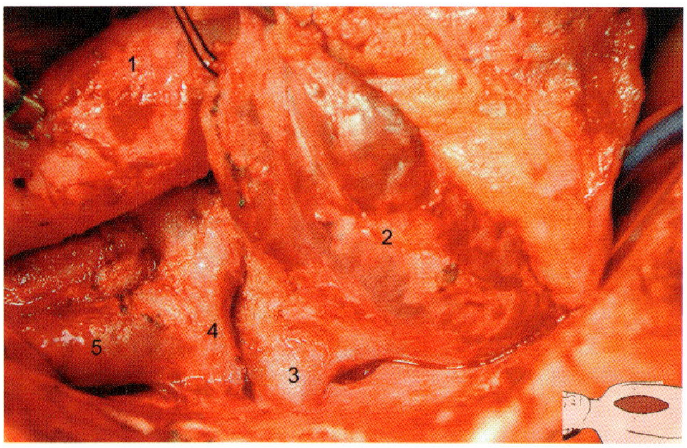

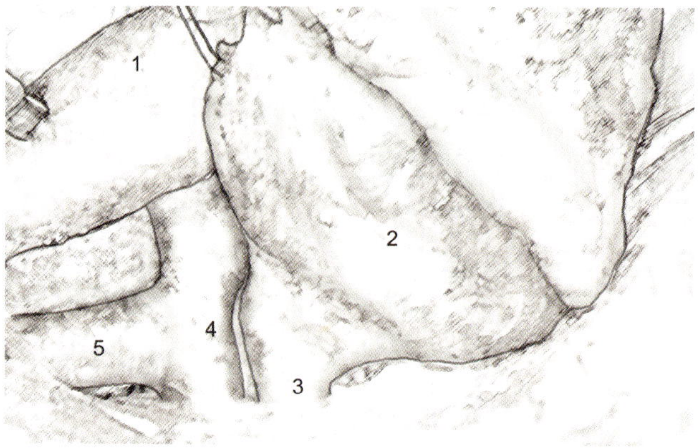

Figure 17.34 **Figure 17.35**

Median sternotomy view of a 4-year-old child with tricuspid atresia and hypoplastic RV. He has previously undergone a Glenn shunt, shown here. Now he is being operated on for a total cavopulmonary connection (extracardiac conduit).

1. Ascending aorta
2. Right atrium
3. Right PV
4. Right PA
5. SVC

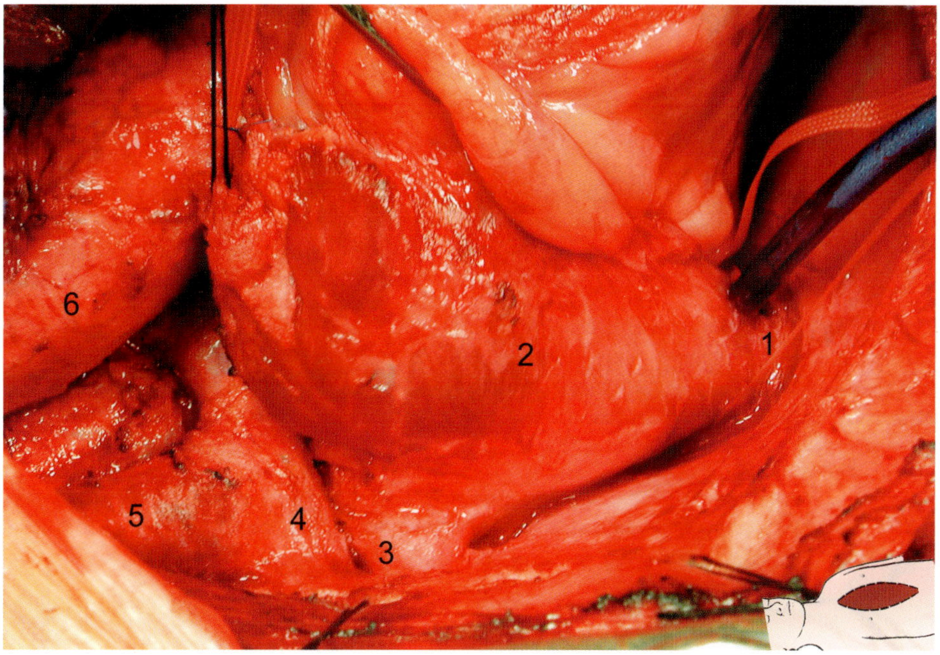

Figure 17.36. The same patient as in Figures 17.34 and 17.35. The right atrium is retracted to reveal the junction of the IVC with the right atrium.

1. IVC
2. Right atrium
3. Right PV
4. Right PA
5. SVC
6. Ascending aorta

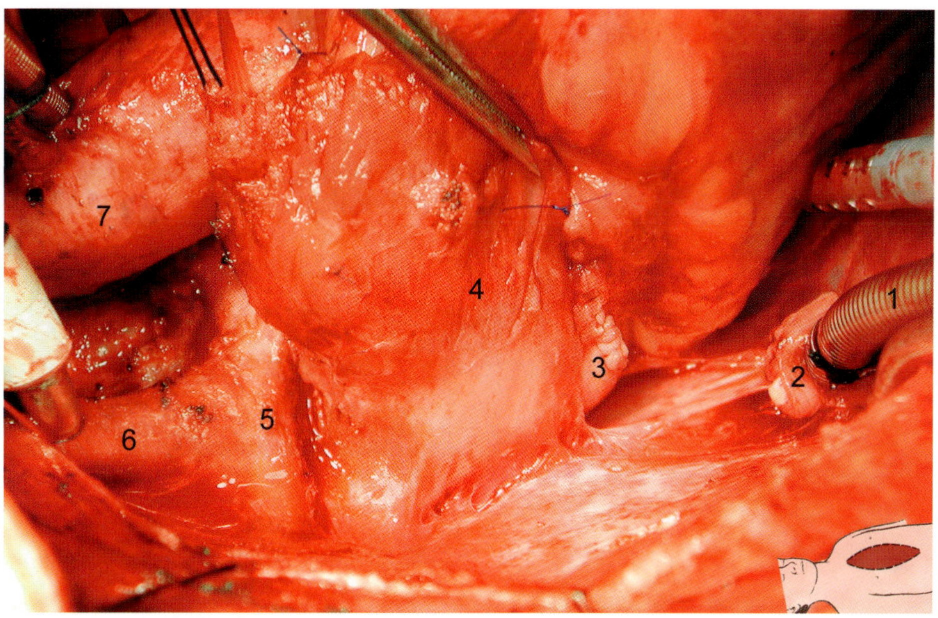

Figure 17.37. The same patient as in Figures 17.34 to 17.36 after transection of the IVC at its junction with the right atrium. The opening into the right atrium has been closed with sutures. The IVC has also been temporarily closed. The procedure is being performed on cardiopulmonary bypass, so venous cannulae were placed in the IVC and SVC, and an arterial cannula was placed in the ascending aorta.

1. IVC cannula
2. IVC
3. IVC–right atrium junction (sutured)
4. Right atrium
5. Right PA
6. SVC
7. Ascending aorta

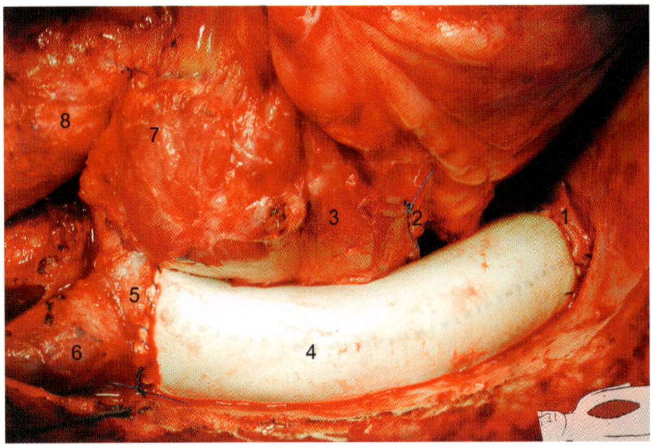

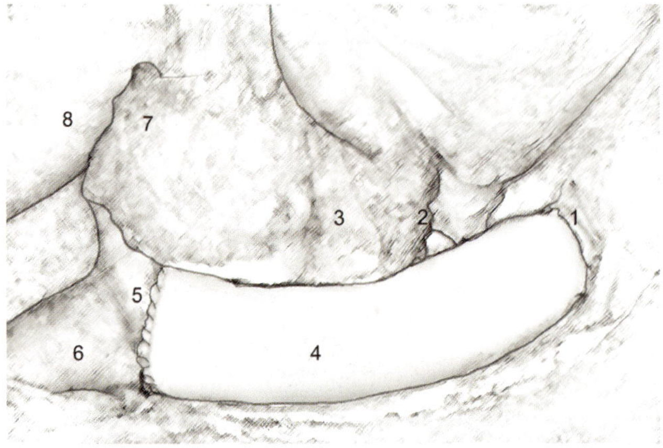

Figure 17.38 **Figure 17.39**

The same patient as in Figures 17.34 to 17.37 after completion of a nonfenestrated extracardiac Fontan surgery. A 16 mm PTFE (Gore-Tex) tube graft was used as a conduit between the IVC and the right PA.

1. IVC
2. Site of previous IVC–right atrium junction
3. Right atrium
4. PTFE tube graft (16 mm)
5. Right PA
6. SVC
7. RAA
8. Ascending aorta

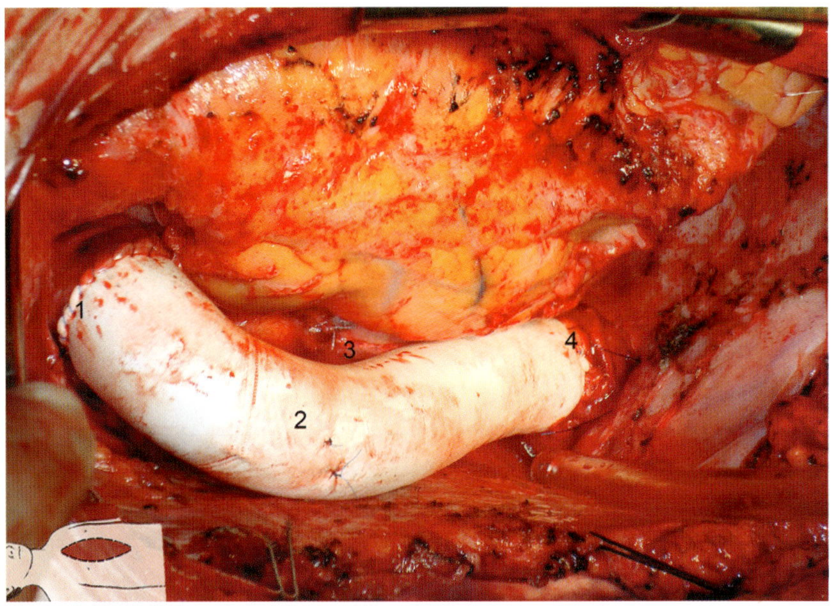

Figure 17.40. Extracardiac conduit Fontan in a patient who has tricuspid atresia. A 20 mm PTFE (Gore-Tex) tube graft was used.

1. Anastomosis to PA
2. PTFE tube graft (20 mm)
3. Right atrium
4. Anastomosis of IVC

REFERENCES

1. Nigro J, Bart P, Starnes V. Mitral valve diseases. In: Nichols D, Ross M, Ungerleider RM, Spevak PJ, eds. *Nichols: Critical Heart Disease in Infants and Children.* (2nd ed.) Philadelphia, PA: Mosby; 2006:140.
2. Fontan F, Baudet E. Surgical repair of tricuspid atresia. *Thorax.* 1971;26:240–248.
3. Anderson P, Sleeper L, Mahony L, et al. Contemporary outcomes after the Fontan procedure: a pediatric heart network multicenter study. *JACC.* 2008;52:85–98.

CHAPTER 18

Double Outlet Right Ventricle

Double outlet right ventricle (DORV) encompasses a heterogeneous group of anomalies unified by the fact that the great arteries arise, wholly or predominantly, from the right ventricle (RV).[1] In this chapter, we discuss the hearts with usual or mirror-imaged atrial arrangement and concordant atrioventricular connections. In these, DORV ranges from a variant similar to tetralogy of Fallot (TOF) with extreme aortic override to transposition of the great arteries (TGA) as in Taussig-Bing anomaly.[2] The latter is discussed along with TGA in chapter 15. The location of the ventricular septal defect (VSD) is used to classify DORV into 4 types (Figure 18.1). This is important in understanding

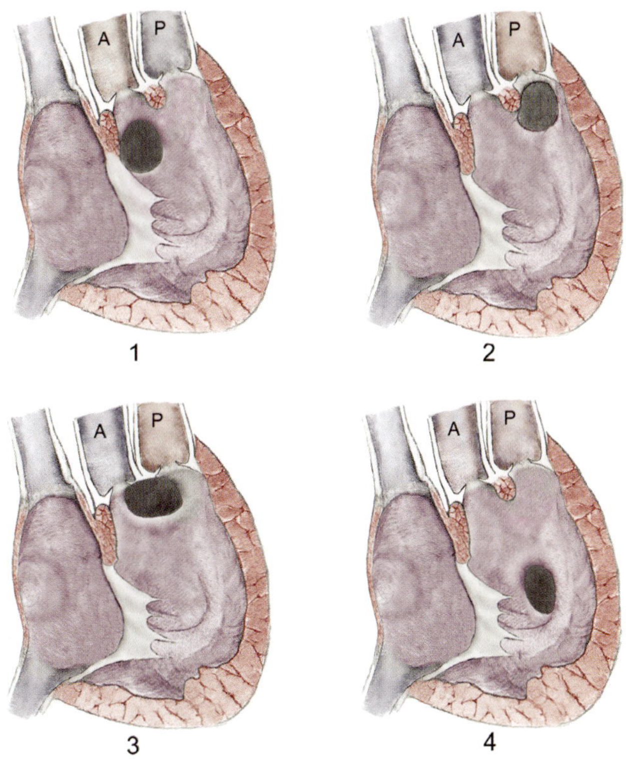

Figure 18.1. Schematic diagram of the classification of DORV based on the location of the VSD in relation to the great arteries. (**A**) DORV with subaortic VSD. (**B**) DORV with subpulmonic VSD. (**C**) DORV with doubly committed and juxtaarterial VSD. (**D**) DORV with noncommitted (remote) VSD. A, aorta; P, pulmonary artery (PA).

Congenital Heart Disease: A Surgical Color Atlas © 2015 A. Sukru Mercan, Zakariya Hubail, S. Yen Ho.
Cardiotext Publishing, ISBN: 978-1-935395-90-4.

the pathophysiology and in deciding on management options.

Figures 18.2 to 18.13 are from a 7-month-old infant with DORV, subaortic VSD, and additional muscular VSDs. There was a large subpulmonic infundibulum (conus) but with no pulmonary or subpulmonary stenosis. Through a right ventriculotomy the outlet (conal) septum was excised, and through a right

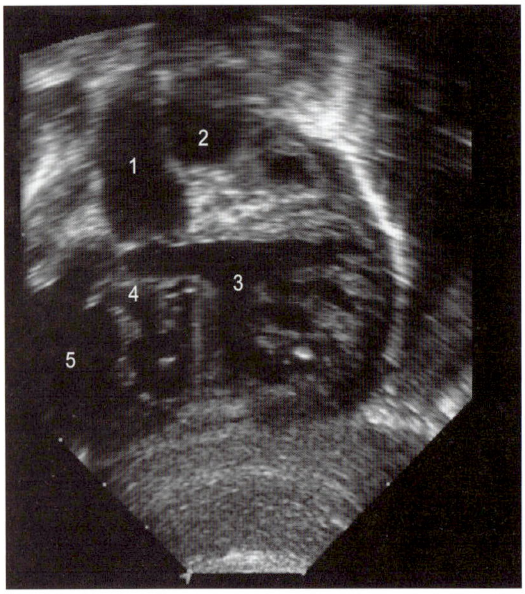

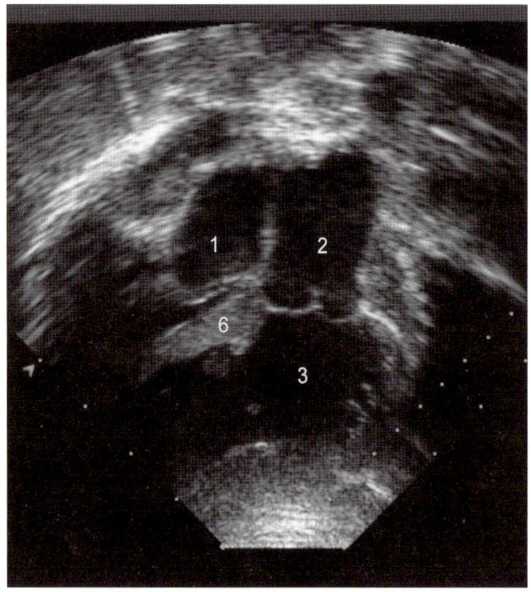

Figure 18.2 **Figure 18.3**

An echocardiogram still frame for a 7-month-old infant with DORV and subaortic VSD. These are modified, angled sagittal subcostal views; the cut in Figure 18.3 is at a more anterior level. Both arteries are seen arising from the RV. The great arteries are side-by-side but with the aorta slightly posterior and the PA slightly anterior. There is a prominent outlet (conal) septum with no subpulmonic stenosis. The patient also had an additional muscular VSD (not shown).

1. Ascending aorta
2. Main pulmonary artery (MPA)
3. RV
4. Tricuspid valve
5. Right atrium
6. Outlet (conal) septum

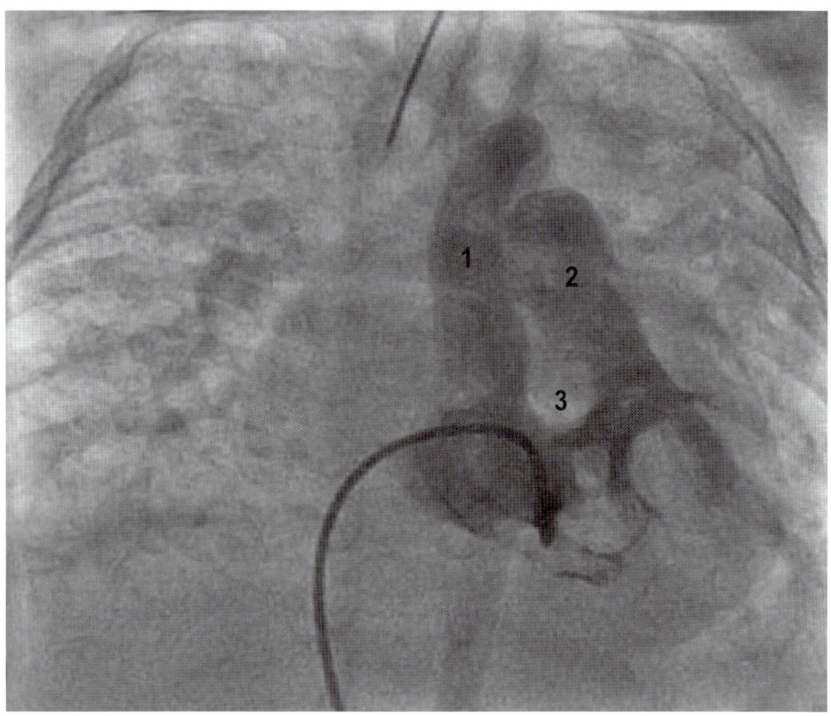

Figure 18.4. An angiogram of the same patient whose echocardiogram is shown in Figures 18.2 and 18.3. Contrast medium has been injected in the RV. Note the arrangement of the great arteries and the prominent outlet (conal) septum.

1. Ascending aorta
2. MPA
3. Outlet (conal) septum

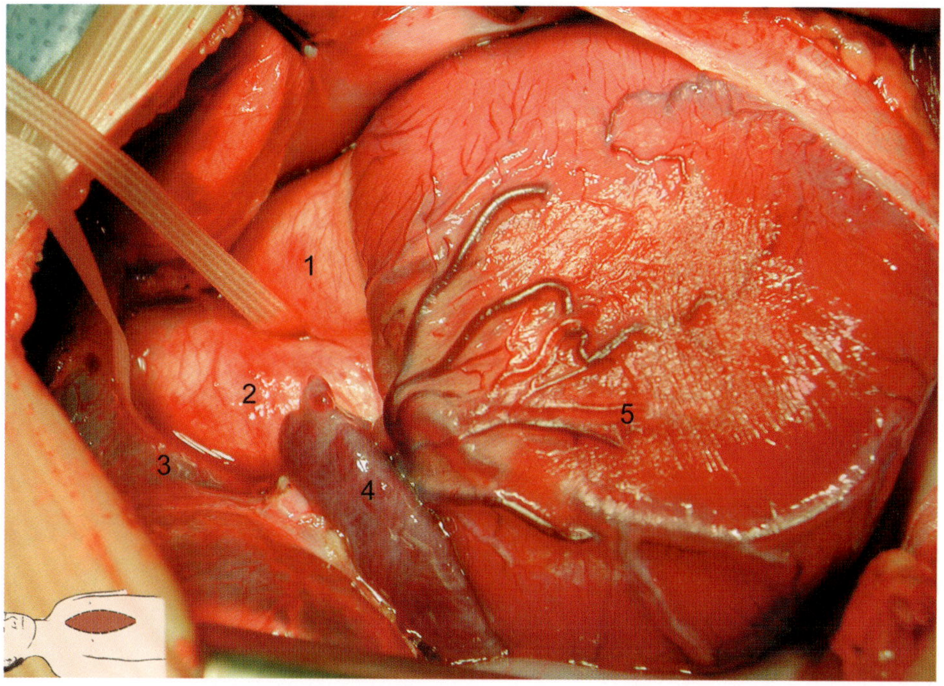

Figure 18.5. The same patient as in Figures 18.2 to 18.4 during surgery. On gross inspection, the aorta and the MPA arise from the RV, arranged side-by-side.

1. MPA
2. Ascending aorta
3. Superior vena cava (SVC)
4. Right atrial appendage (RAA)
5. RV

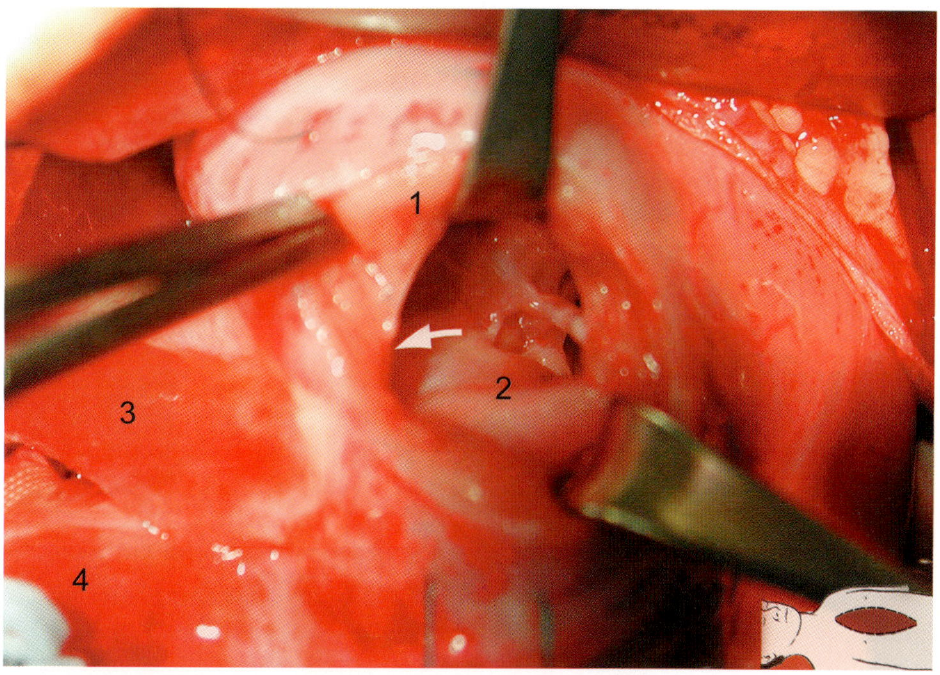

Figure 18.6. The same patient as in Figures 18.2 to 18.5. A right ventriculotomy has been performed. The hypertrophied outlet septum is seen. The arrow points to the direction of the pulmonary valve (subpulmonic RVOT is further shown in Figures 18.8 and 18.9).

1. Right ventriculotomy
2. Outlet (conal) septum
3. MPA
4. Ascending aorta

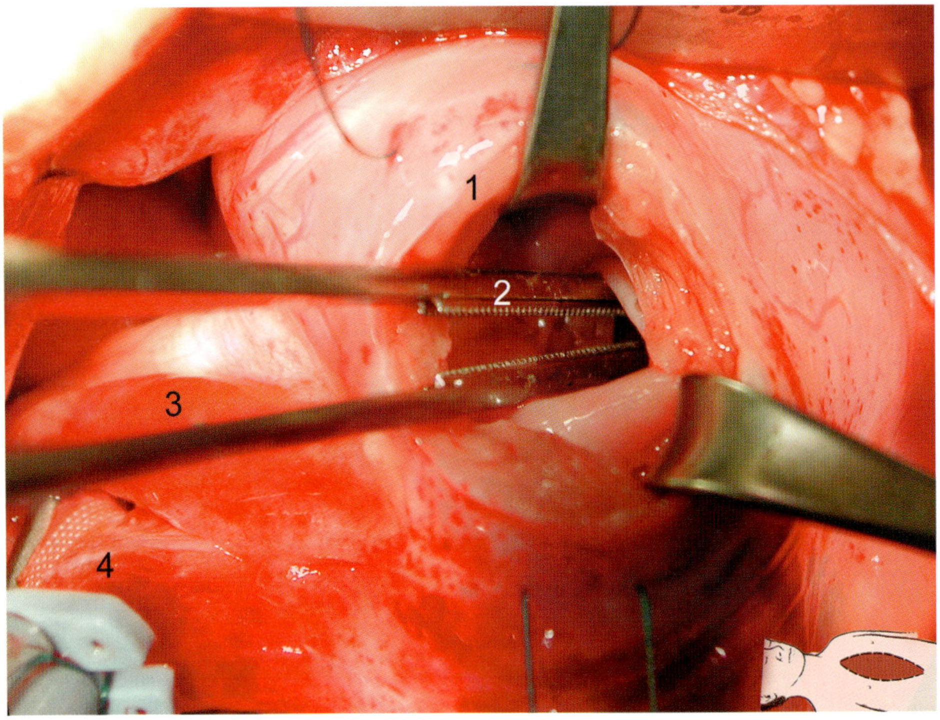

Figure 18.7. The same patient as in Figures 18.2 to 18.6. The forceps are passed through the RV outflow (from the infundibulum to the RV main cavity).

1. Right ventriculotomy
2. Forceps passed through RV outflow
3. MPA
4. Ascending aorta

Figure 18.8. The same patient as in Figures 18.2 to 18.7. The hypertrophied outlet septum is shown; the forceps passed underneath one of the muscle bundles.

1. Right ventriculotomy
2. Ascending aorta

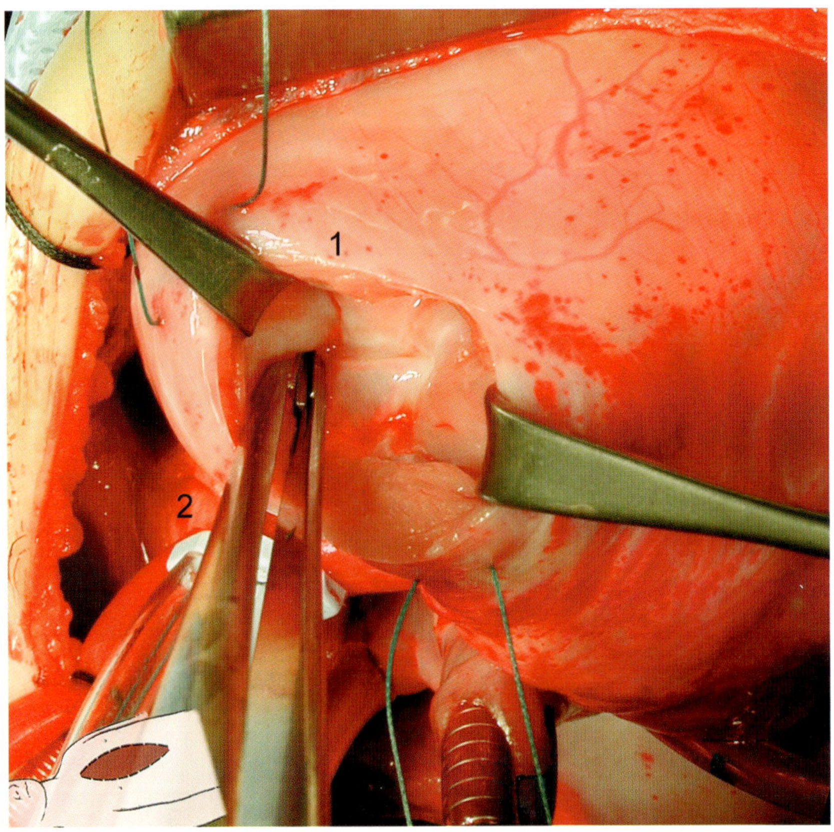

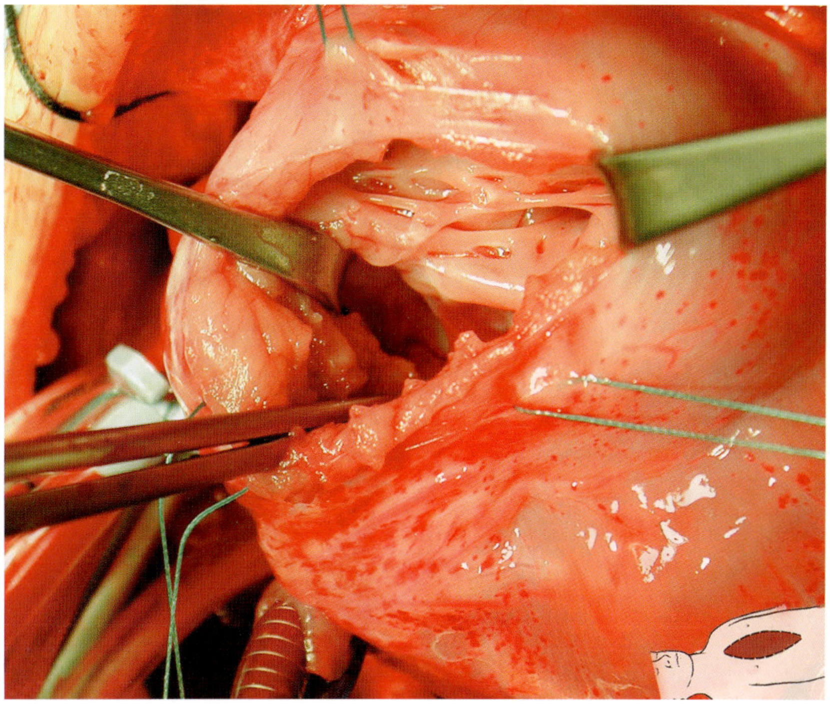

Figure 18.9. The same patient as in Figures 18.2 to 18.8, after resection of part of the outlet (conal) septum.

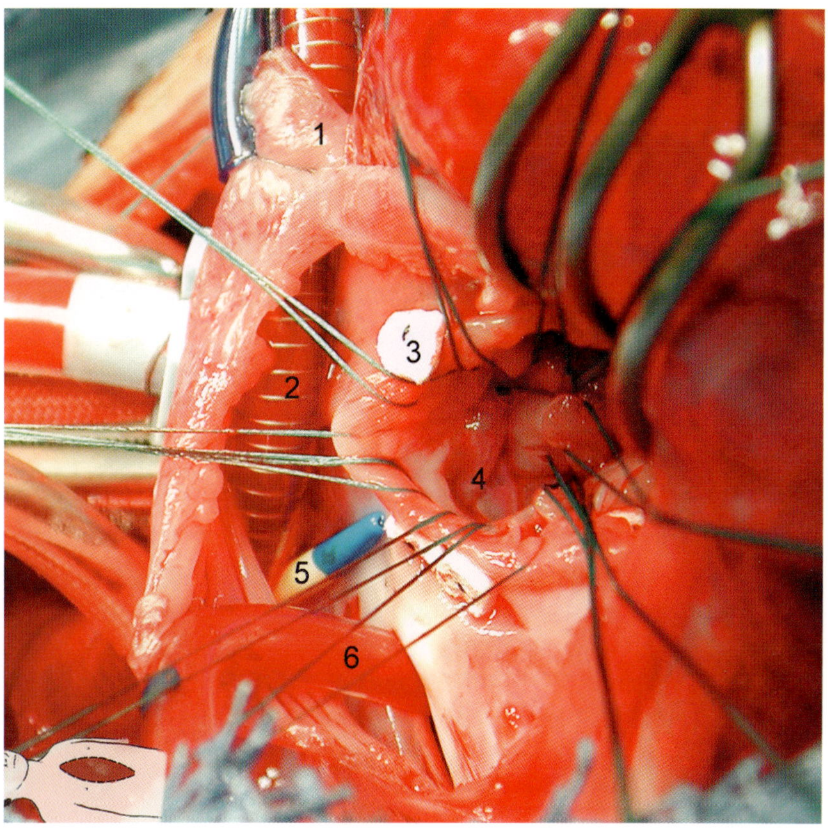

Figure 18.10. The same patient as in Figures 18.2 to 18.9. The VSD will be closed via a right atriotomy. Teflon pledgets have been placed around the subaortic VSD. Some of the pledgets have been placed across the tricuspid valve on the floor of the right atrium. The VSD itself is not seen here but is shown in Figure 18.11. Note the aortic valve arising from the RV.

1. RAA
2. SVC venous cannula
3. Teflon pledget
4. Aortic valve
5. Central venous catheter
6. Suction catheter passing through atrial septal defect (ASD)

Figure 18.11. The same patient as in Figures 18.2 to 18.10. The subaortic VSD is probed by forceps. The patch, when placed, will act as an intracardiac baffle that directs the blood exiting the VSD toward the aorta.

1. RAA
2. Teflon pledget
3. Base of conal septum after resection
4. Forceps through VSD
5. Suction catheter passing through ASD
6. Central venous catheter

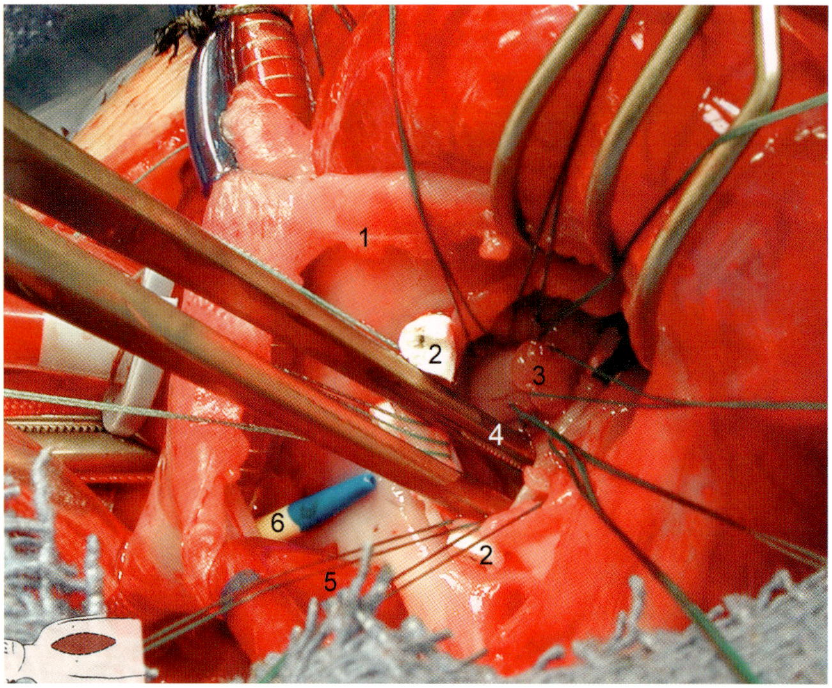

Figure 18.12. The same patient as in Figures 18.2 to 18.11. A Dacron patch has been placed using pledget-supported interrupted sutures. Now the aorta is separated from the RV and receives blood only from the left ventricle (LV) via the VSD.

1. RAA
2. Teflon pledgets
3. Dacron patch
4. ASD

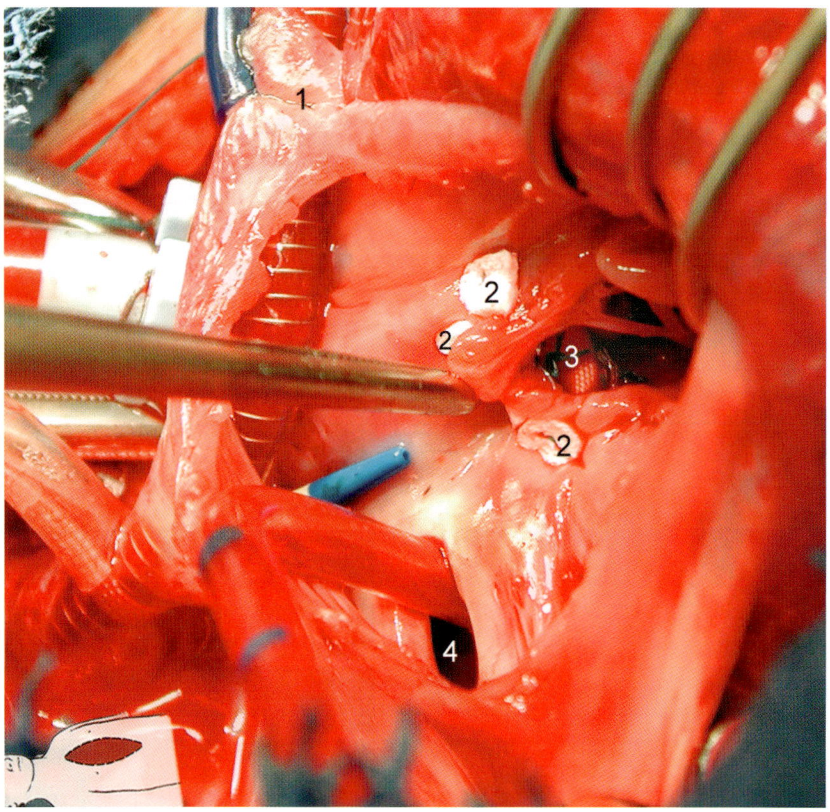

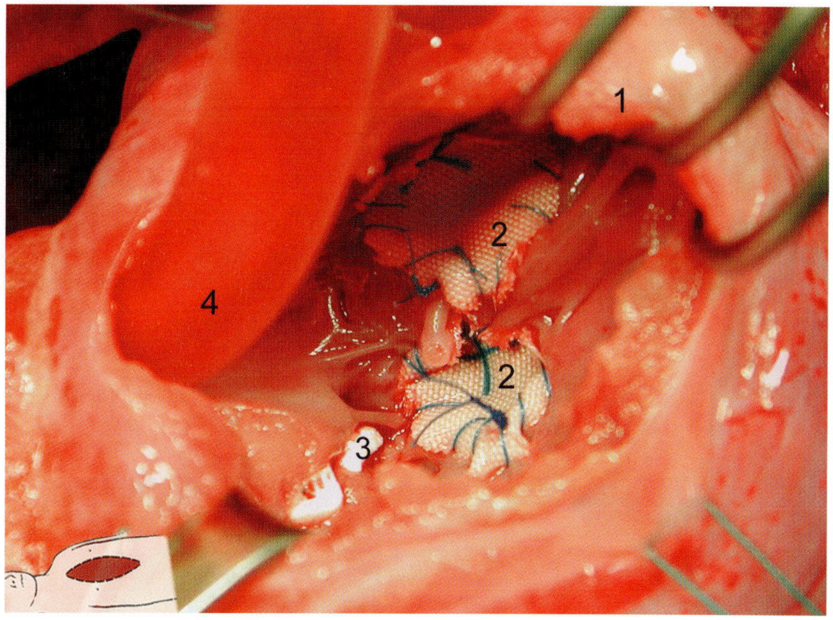

Figure 18.13. The same patient as in Figures 18.2 to 18.12. Through the right ventriculotomy incision, the muscular VSDs have been accessed and closed using Dacron patches.

1. Right ventriculotomy
2. Dacron patches
3. Teflon pledget of the subaortic VSD
4. Suction catheter going to PA

atriotomy, the VSDs were closed. The subaortic VSD was "closed" with a Dacron patch in a way that directed blood from the LV through the VSD to the aorta. In this way, the patch acted as an intracardiac baffle.

Figures 18.14 and 18.15 are from another patient with DORV. The VSD was closed through a pulmonary atriotomy approach using a polytetrafluoroethylene (PTFE) patch.

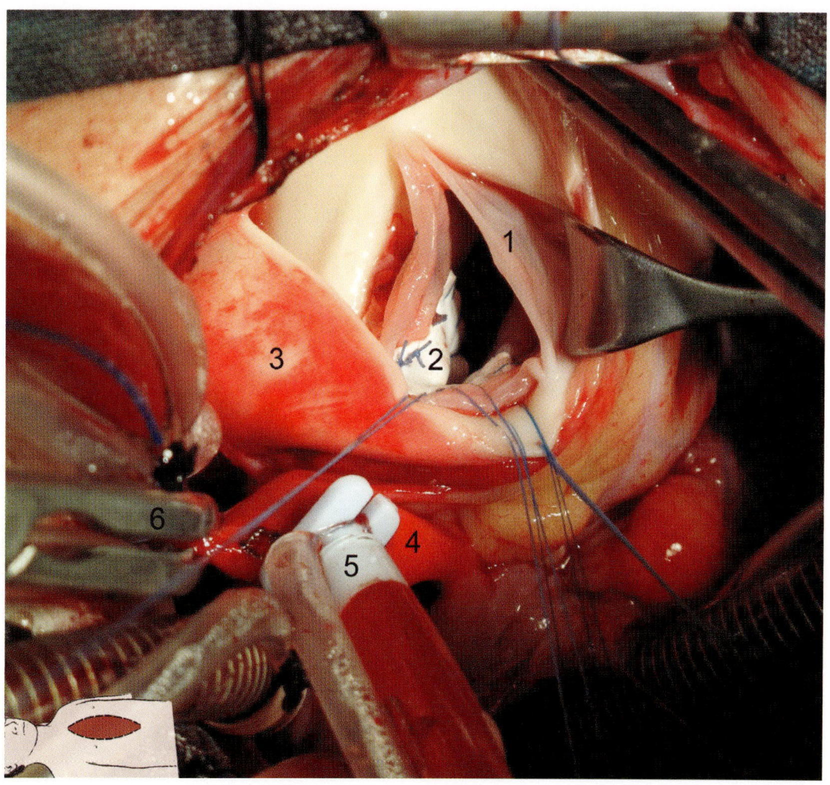

Figure 18.14. Intraoperative median sternotomy view of a patient with DORV. The VSD has been closed via a transpulmonary approach.

1. Pulmonary valve
2. PTFE patch closing the VSD
3. MPA
4. Ascending aorta
5. Cardioplegia catheter
6. Aortic cross-clamp

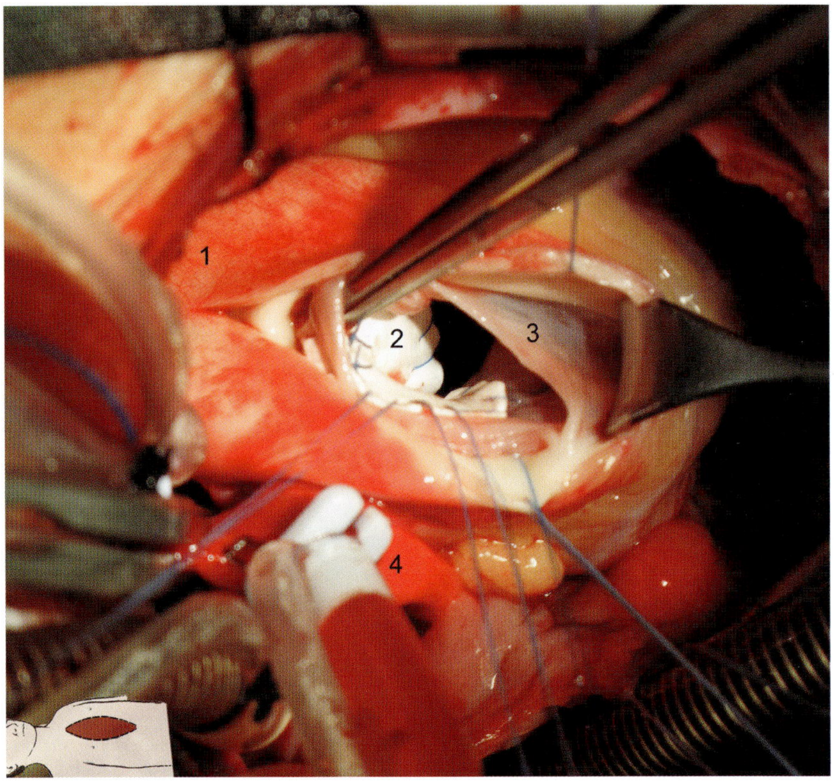

Figure 18.15. The same patient as in Figure 18.14. The extent of the VSD patch is shown.

1. MPA
2. PTFE patch closing the VSD
3. Pulmonary valve
4. Ascending aorta

REFERENCES

1. Mahle WT, Martinez R, Silverman N, et al. Anatomy, echocardiography, and surgical approach to double outlet right ventricle. *Cardiol Young.* 2008;18(Suppl. 3):39–51.
2. Griselli M, McGuirk SP, Ko C, et al. Arterial switch operation in patients with Taussig–Bing anomaly—influence of staged repair and coronary anatomy on outcome. *Eur J Cardiothoracic Surg.* 2007;31:229–235.

CHAPTER 19

Aortic Valve

In this chapter, aortic valve disease is discussed, whereas chapter 20 deals with diseases of other cardiac valves.

SUBAORTIC STENOSIS

Subaortic stenosis is caused by a fibrous or fibromuscular membrane, or by septal hypertrophy. The membrane, commonly having the appearance of a ridge, may occur sporadically or may accompany congenital heart disease, especially ventricular septal defect (VSD) and coarctation of the aorta.[1] Medical management and interventional catheterization have limited roles; the mainstay of treatment is surgical intervention.

The procedure consists of membrane resection, often with additional myectomy. Figures 19.1 to 19.10 are intraoperative examples of patients with a subaortic membrane. Surgical treatment was achieved by resection of the membrane. In some patients, myectomy was also necessary to relieve the left ventricular (LV) outflow narrowing. The membrane may be close to the valve leaflets, as seen in Figures 19.11 to 19.15, which requires utmost care not to injure the aortic valve during repair. Subaortic stenosis is also seen in asymmetric septal hypertrophy and is relieved by myectomy, as shown in Figure 19.16. In all cases, the proximity of the atrioventricular conduction bundle to the subvalvar area between the right and noncoronary leaflets must be borne in mind when

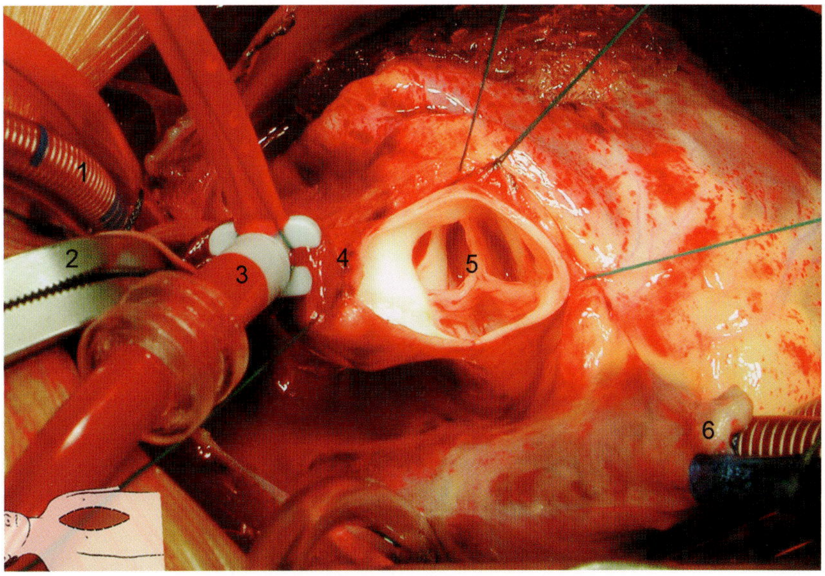

Figure 19.1. Median sternotomy view of a 4-year-old child with subaortic stenosis. The aortic valve is seen through an aortotomy. The valve is in the closed position and has normal anatomy. The cannulation setup is also shown. See Figure 19.2 for a close-up view.

1. Aortic cannula
2. Aortic cross-clamp
3. Cardioplegia catheter
4. Ascending aorta
5. Aortic valve
6. Superior vena cava (SVC) cannula in right atrial appendage (RAA)

Figure 19.2. Close-up view of the aortic valve of the same patient shown in Figure 19.1. The arrows point to the orifices of the coronary arteries.

1. Aortotomy incision
2. Left coronary leaflet
3. Right coronary leaflet
4. Noncoronary leaflet

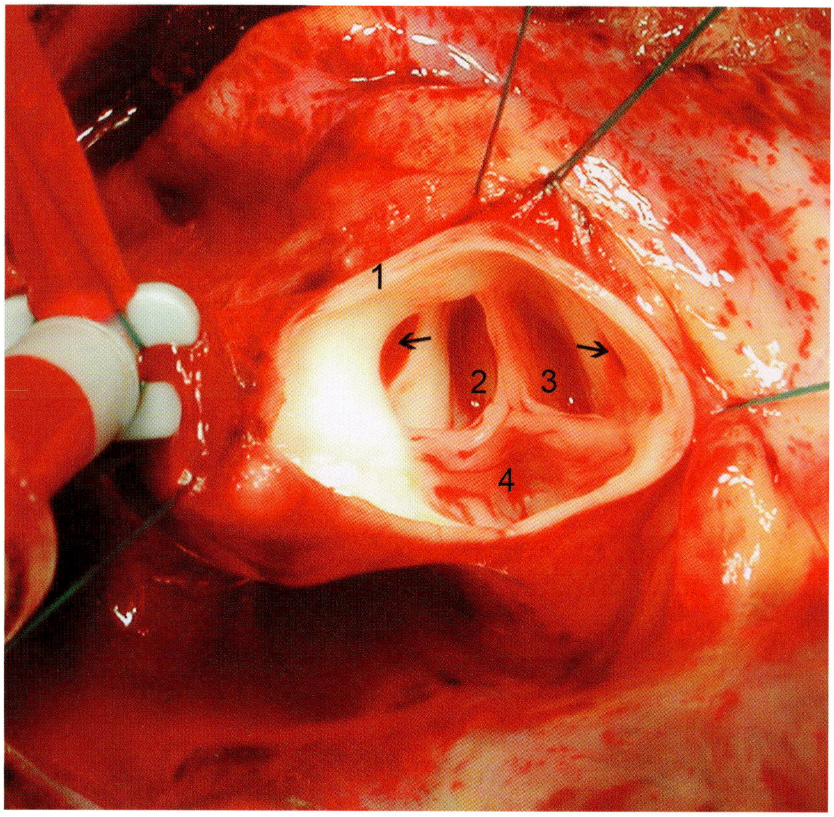

Figure 19.3. The same patient as in Figures 19.1 and 19.2. The aortic valve leaflets are retracted to show the subvalvar area. A crescent-shaped membrane is visible under the right and left cusps.

1. Subaortic membrane
2. Left coronary leaflet

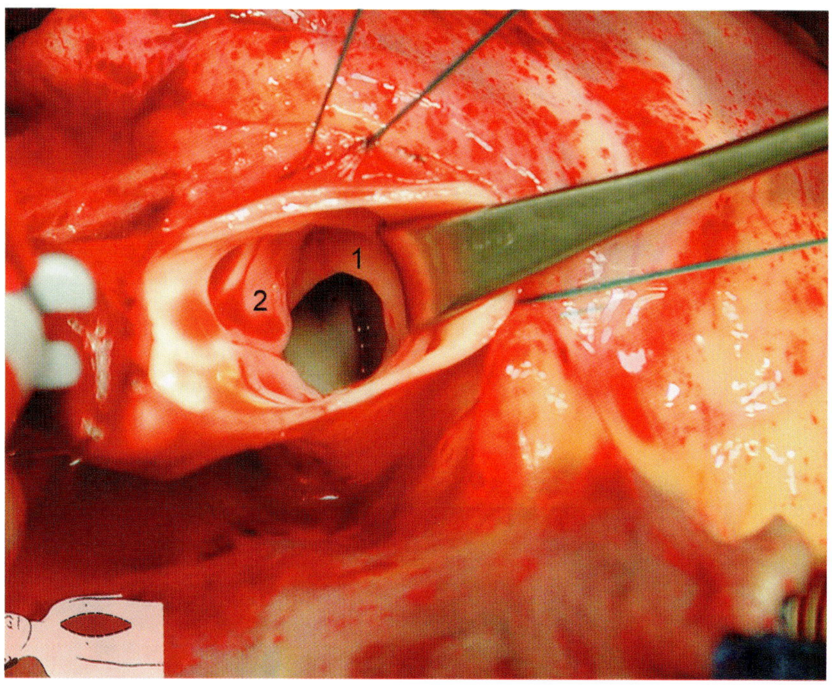

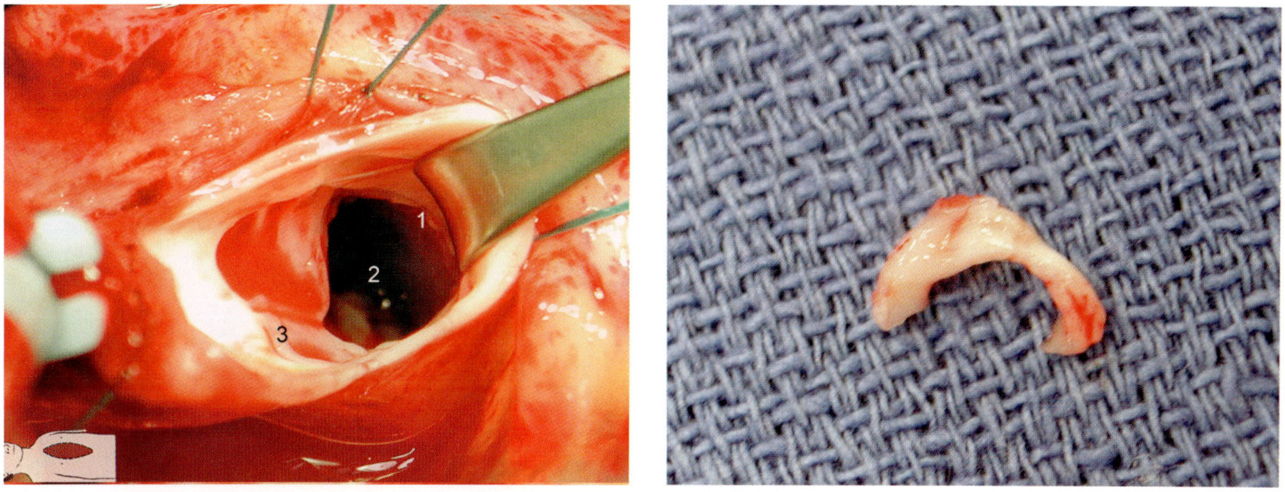

Figure 19.4. The same patient as in Figures 19.1 to 19.3 after resection of the subaortic membrane. The photo on the right shows the resected membrane.

1. Site of the resected subaortic membrane
2. Left ventricular outflow tract (LVOT), now wide open
3. Aortic valve leaflet

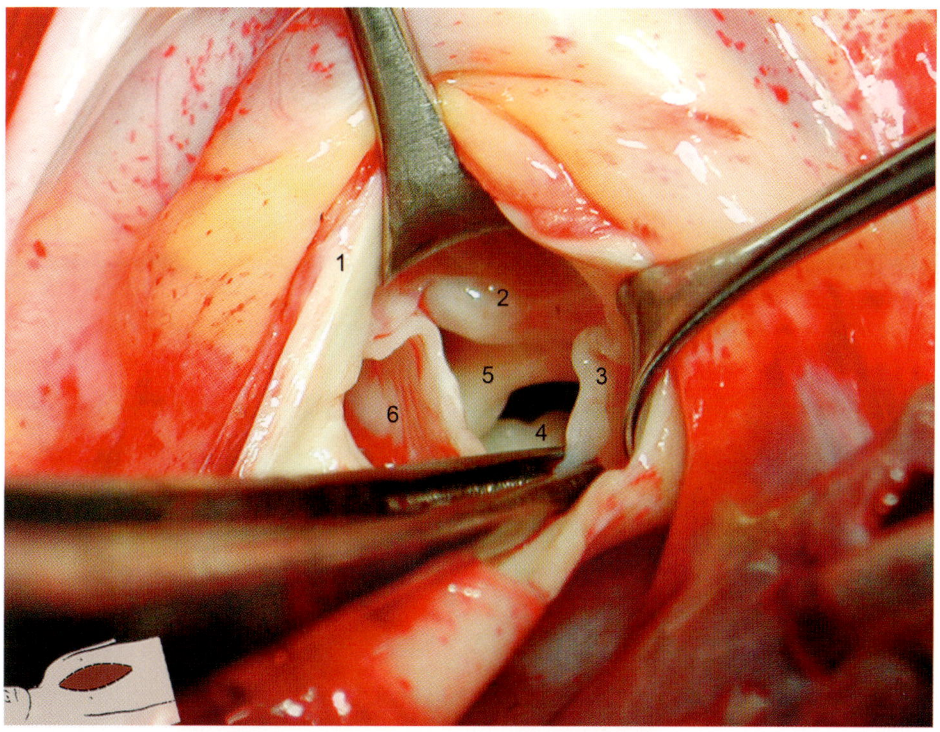

Figure 19.5. Another example of a subaortic membrane in a 10-year-old child.

1. Aortotomy incision
2. Right coronary leaflet
3. Noncoronary leaflet
4. Anterior leaflet of mitral valve
5. Subaortic membrane
6. Left coronary leaflet

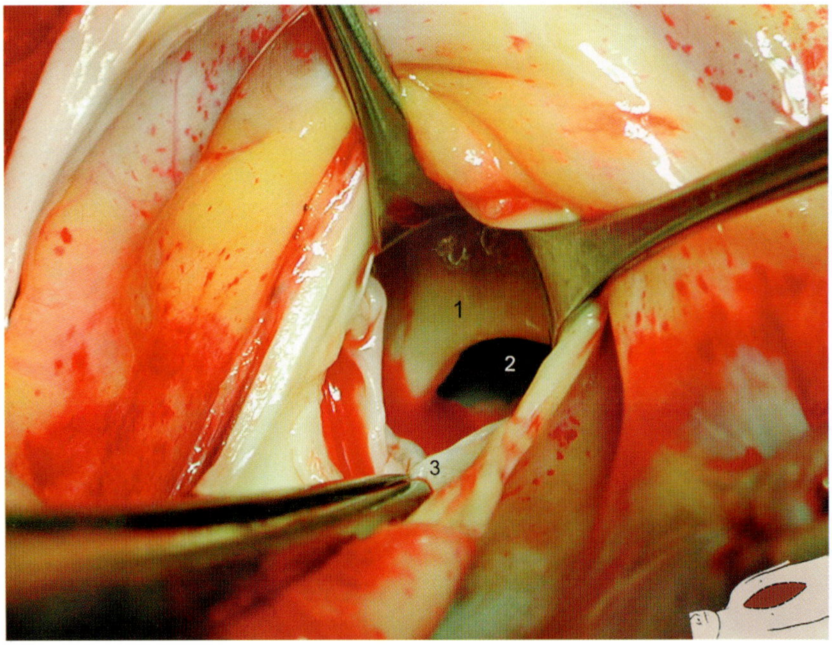

Figure 19.6. The same patient as shown in Figure 19.5. The aortic leaflets are retracted to show the extent of the subaortic membrane.

1. Subaortic membrane
2. LVOT
3. Noncoronary leaflet

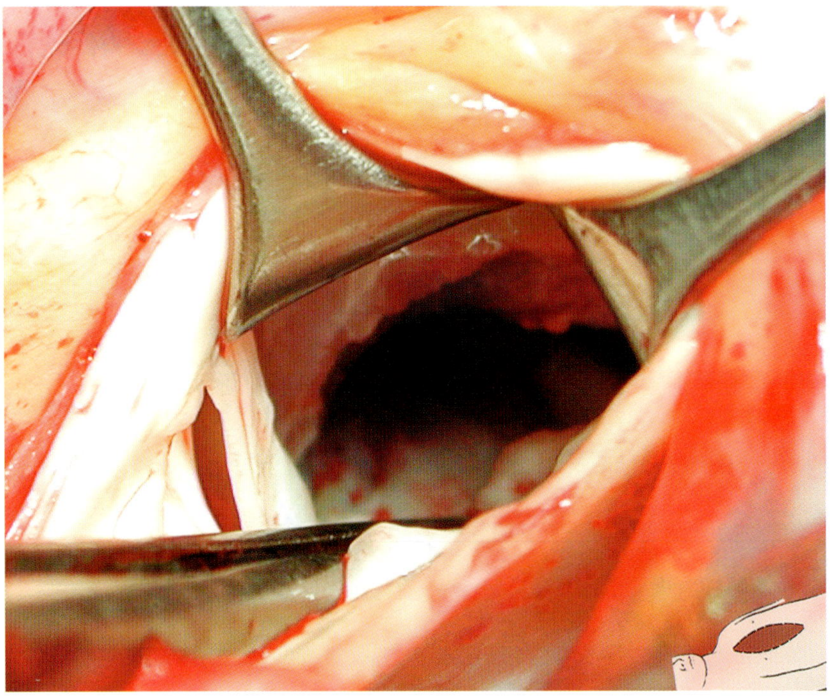

Figure 19.7. The same patient as shown in Figures 19.5 and 19.6 after resection of the subaortic membrane and myectomy.

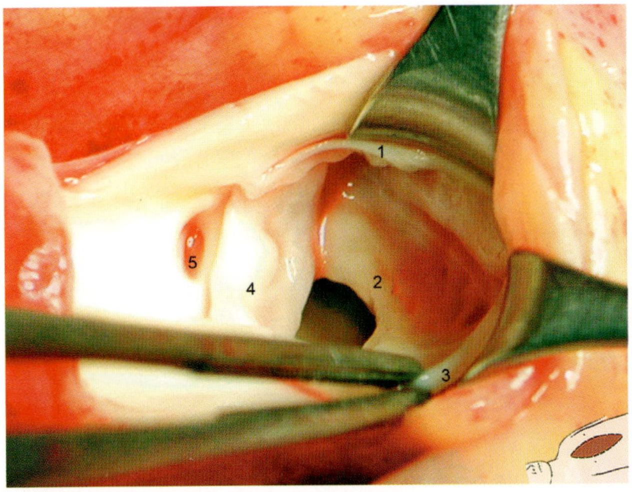

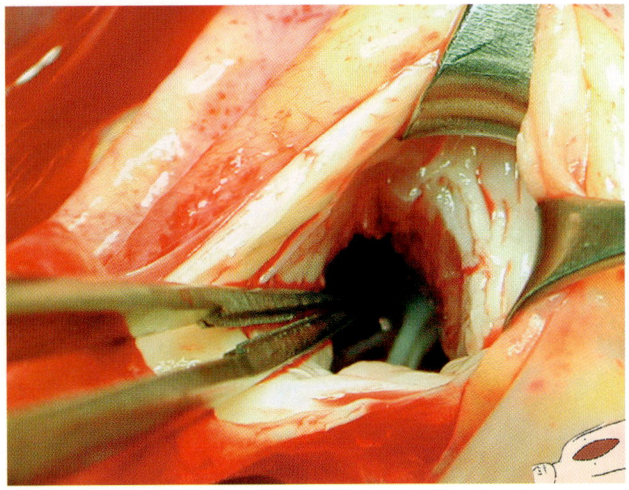

Figure 19.8 **Figure 19.9**

Aortotomy view of the subvalvar area in a 6-year-old child. A subaortic membrane is seen in the LVOT. Treatment was achieved by resection of the membrane, along with myectomy, as shown in Figure 19.9.

1. Right coronary leaflet
2. Subaortic membrane
3. Noncoronary leaflet
4. Left coronary leaflet
5. Orifice of left coronary artery

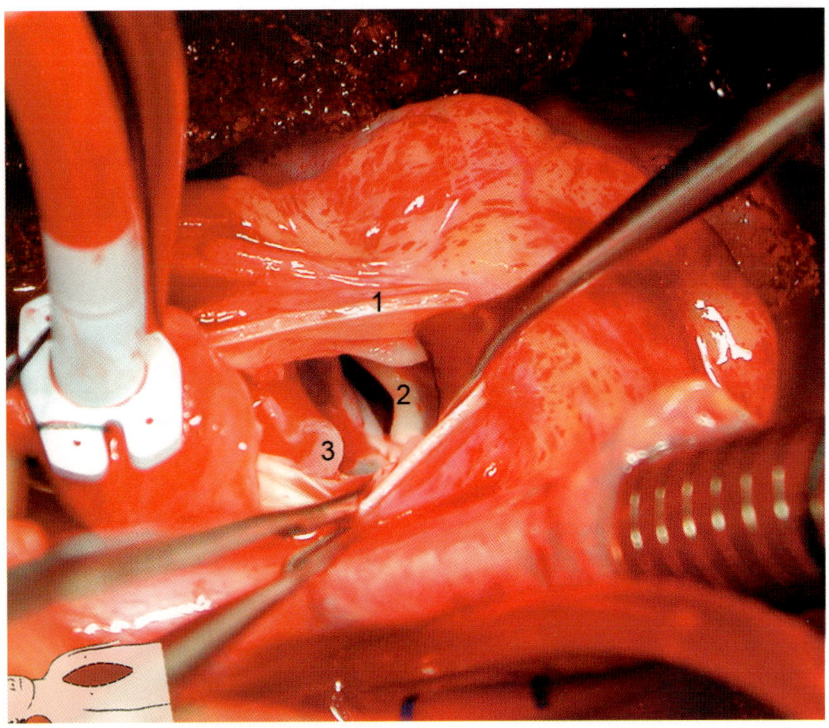

Figure 19.10. Subaortic membrane in an 8-year-old child as seen through an aortotomy. The membrane is located some distance beneath the valve, leaving a slit-like opening as outflow of the LV.

1. Aortotomy
2. Subaortic membrane
3. Aortic valve

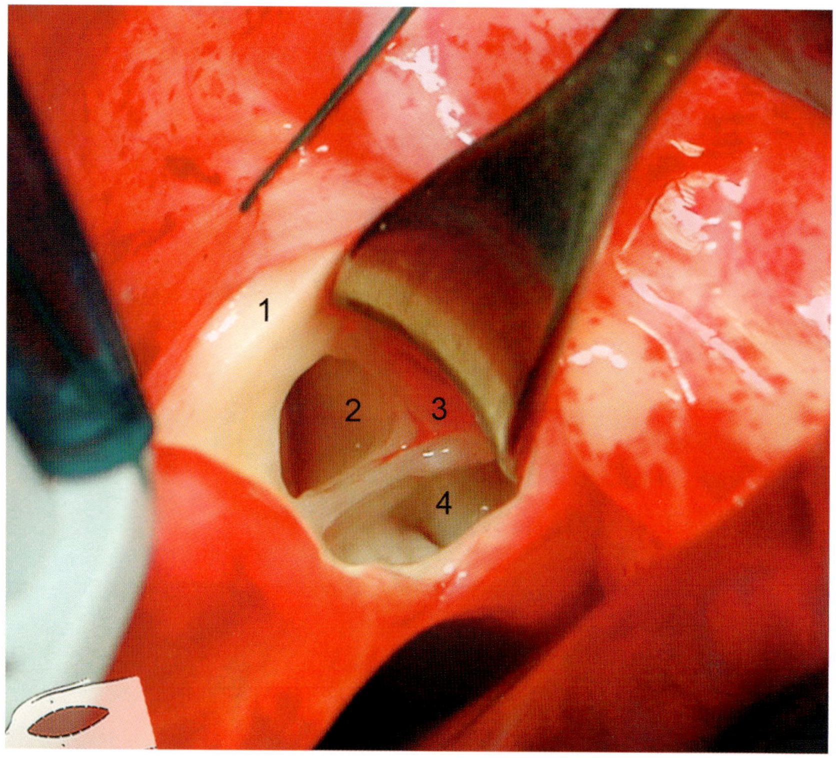

Figure 19.11. Aortotomy view of the aortic valve during surgery for subaortic membrane resection in a 1-year-old infant.

1. Aortotomy incision
2. Left coronary leaflet
3. Right coronary leaflet
4. Noncoronary leaflet

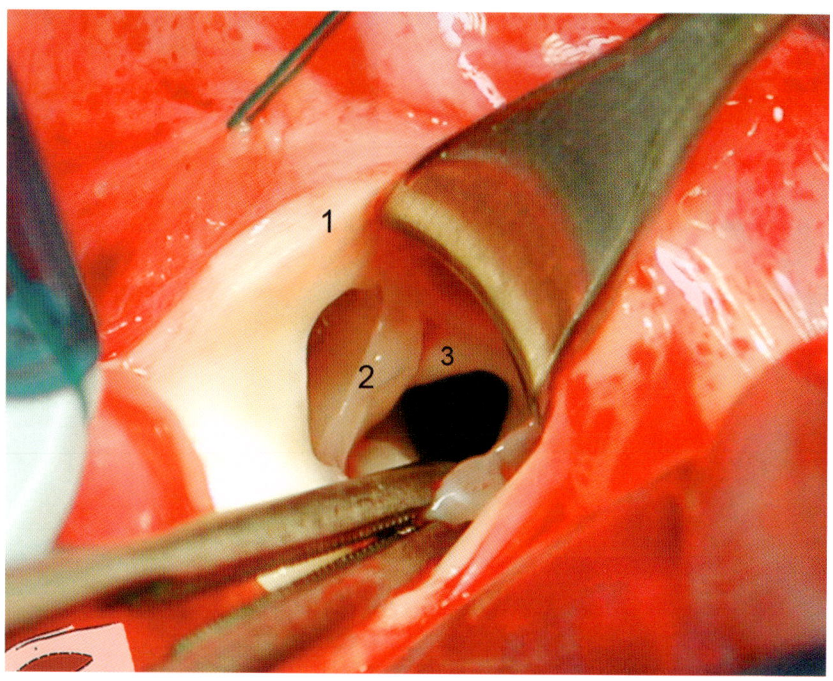

Figure 19.12. The same patient as in Figure 19.11. The subaortic membrane is abutting the valve leaflets. Very careful resection was done to avoid injury to the aortic valve.

1. Aortotomy incision
2. Left coronary leaflet
3. Subaortic membrane

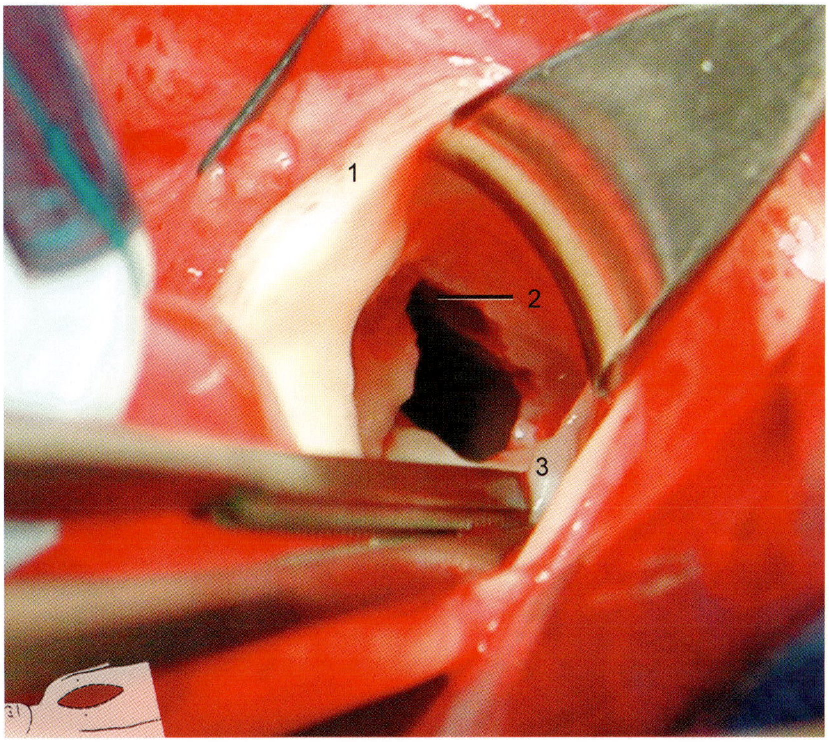

Figure 19.13. The same patient as in Figures 19.11 and 19.12 after resection of the subaortic membrane.

1. Aortotomy incision
2. Area of the resected membrane
3. Noncoronary leaflet

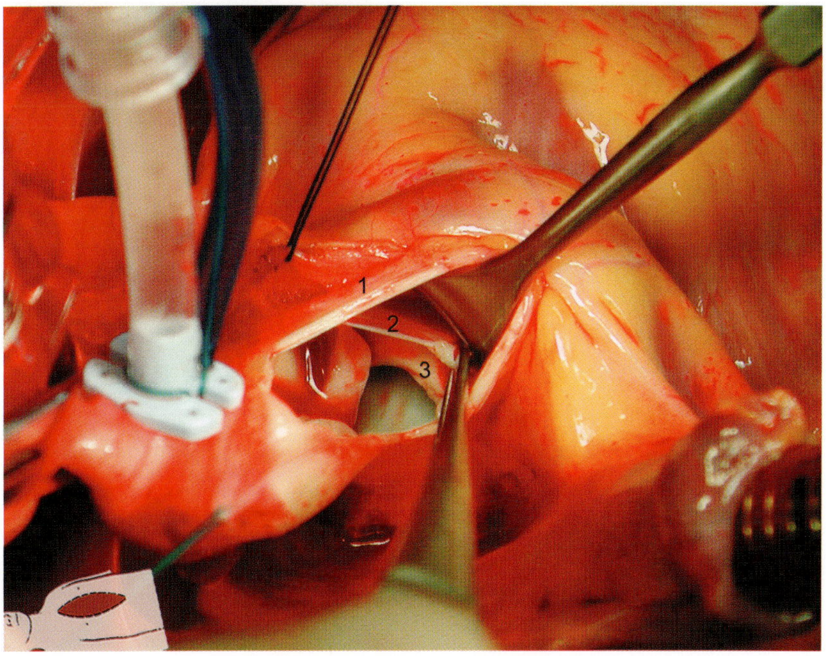

Figure 19.14. Aortotomy view of the aortic valve and subaortic membrane in a 13-year-old child. The membrane is very close to the valve leaflets.

1. Aortotomy incision
2. Right coronary leaflet
3. Subaortic membrane

Figure 19.15. The same patient as in Figure 19.14 after resection of the membrane and myectomy.

1. Right coronary leaflet
2. Remnant of resected membrane
3. Left coronary leaflet
4. Ascending aorta

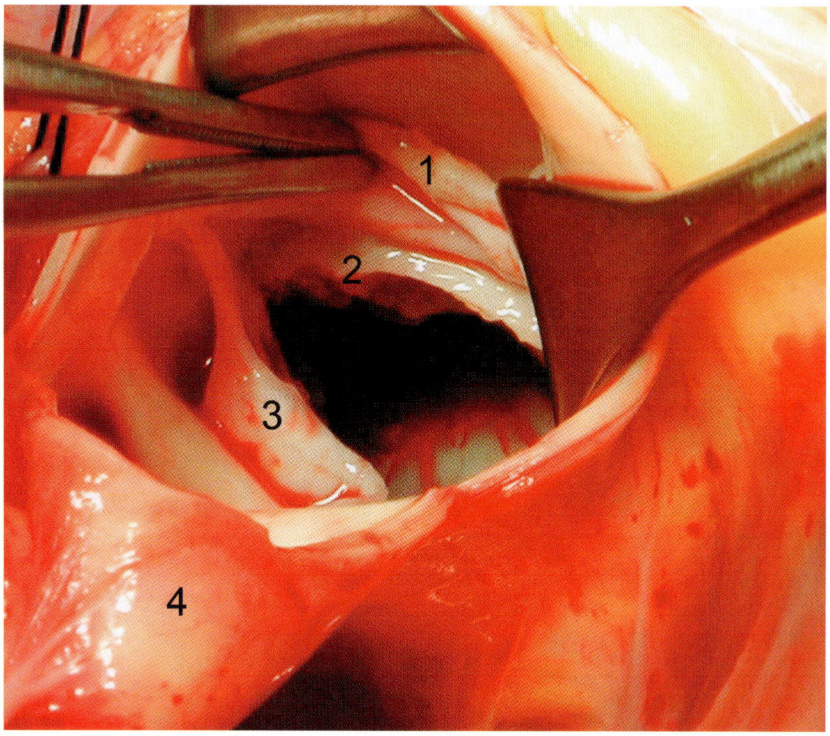

Figure 19.16. Operative view through an aortotomy after wedge resection of septal muscle in a patient with hypertrophic cardiomyopathy.

1. Wedge myectomy
2. Left coronary leaflet
3. Aortotomy incision

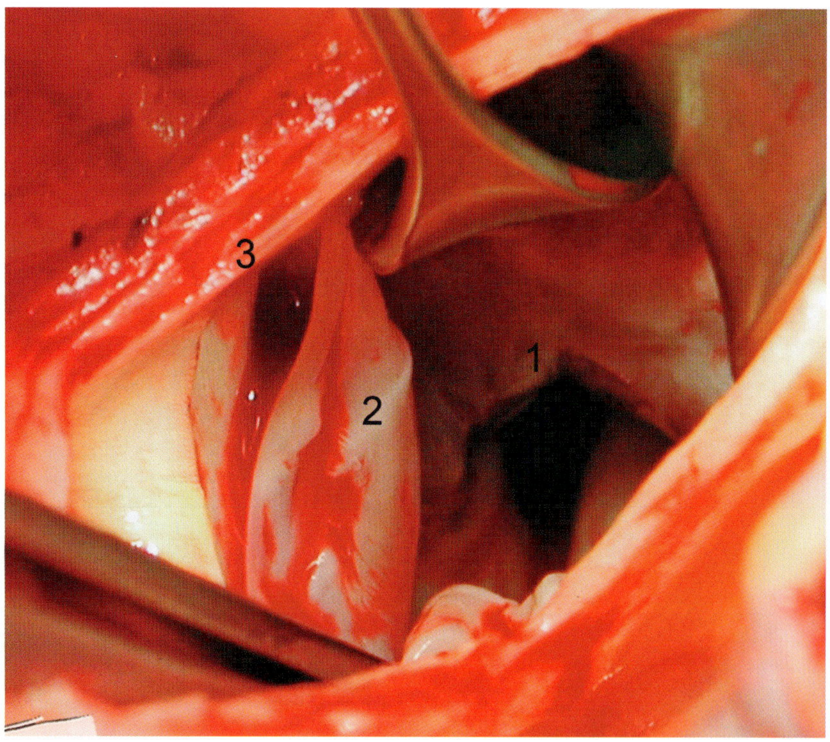

carrying out resections or myectomy. VSD-associated subaortic membrane has the tendency to recur, even long after VSD closure[2] (Figure 19.17). In the patient shown in Figures 19.18 to 19.20, there was prolapse of the aortic valve leaflets. Resection of the membrane and suspension valvuloplasty was performed.

VALVAR AORTIC STENOSIS/REGURGITATION

The most common cause for congenital aortic valvar stenosis is bicuspid aortic valve. This is a common anomaly, affecting up to 2% of the population.[3] The majority do not cause symptoms during childhood. Aortic stenosis and regurgitation are the main consequences, as well as dilatation of the aortic root.[4] Figures 19.21 and 19.22 are 2 examples of bicuspid aortic valve.

Figures 19.23 to 19.25 are from a 3-year-old child who has aortic stenosis and fusion of the aortic leaflets to the aortic wall, leaving only small openings to the aortic sinuses and coronary arteries.

When valvuloplasty is not possible, valve replacement is carried out. There are many options for bioprosthetic and artificial valves. Figures 19.26 to 19.33 show the technique of pulmonary autograft (the Ross procedure with root replacement). The pulmonary valve is harvested carefully along with a cuff of right ventricular (RV) outflow muscle, avoiding trauma to the first septal perforator artery. The aortic valve is excised, and the pulmonary valve is implanted into the aortic position. The autograft is oriented so that the left and right coronary arteries each face a sinus. The coronary artery buttons are implanted into the neoaortic root. Repair is completed by reconstructing the right ventricular outflow tract (RVOT) with a homograft. Neoaortic root dilatation is a common late complication.[5] This may be mitigated by wrapping a Dacron graft around the neoartic root.

Figures 19.34 to 19.42 are from a 10-year-old child with Loeys–Dietz syndrome. This disease shares many of the features of Marfan syndrome but is caused by a different genetic mutation.[6] In this patient, there was a dilated aortic root and aortic regurgitation. Aortic root replacement using the modified Bentall procedure was performed. A 21 mm St. Jude composite graft was implanted.

SUPRAVALVAR AORTIC STENOSIS

This is the least common type of aortic stenosis, and it is often associated with Williams syndrome[7] (Figure 19.43). Catheter-based interventions have a

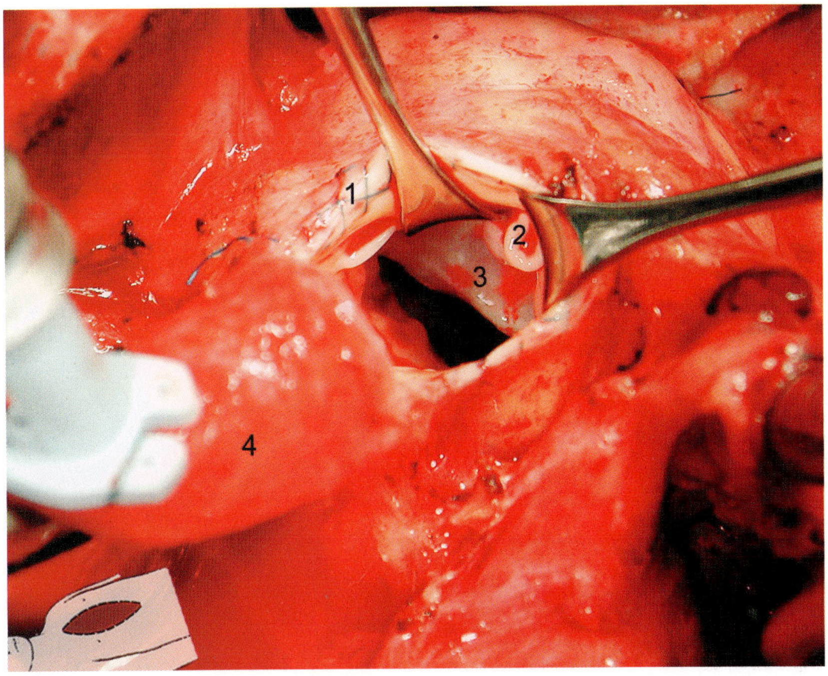

Figure 19.17. Redo aortotomy in a 3-year-old child who had previously undergone VSD closure and subaortic membrane resection. The membrane recurred and necessitated reoperation.

1. Aortotomy incision
2. Right coronary leaflet
3. Subaortic membrane
4. Ascending aorta

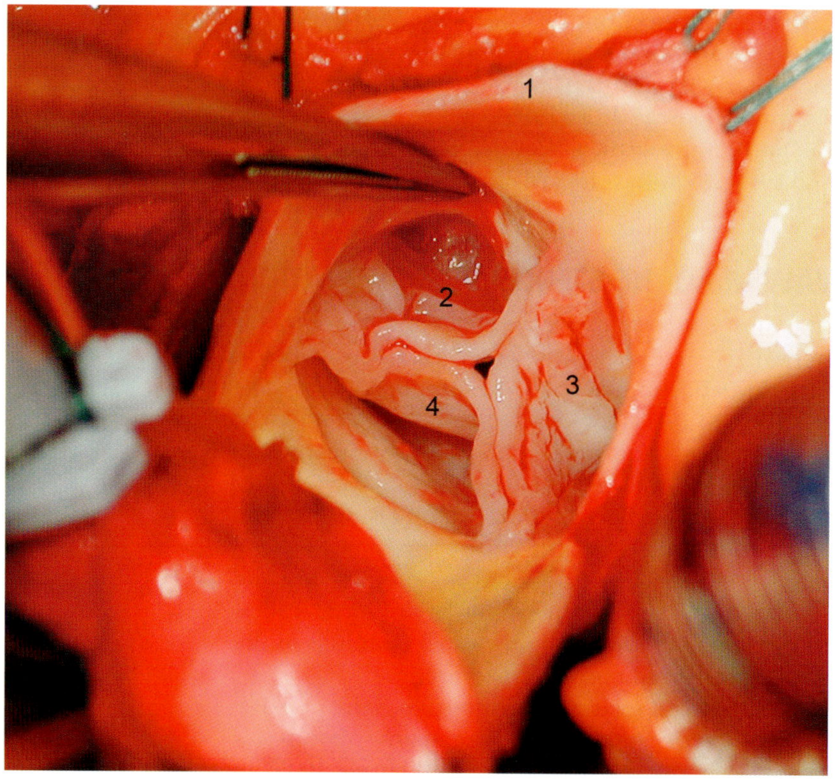

Figure 19.18. Aortic valve as seen through an aortotomy in a 14-year-old child. Note redundancy and prolapse of the left and right coronary leaflets. The patient also had a subaortic membrane (not shown).

1. Aortotomy incision
2. Right coronary leaflet
3. Noncoronary leaflet
4. Left coronary leaflet

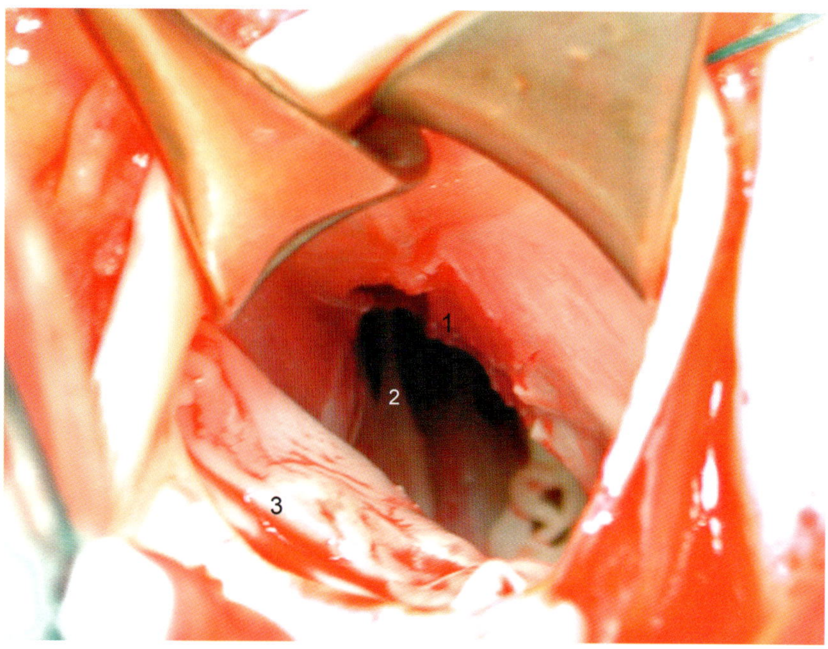

Figure 19.19. The same patient as in Figure 19.18 after resection of the subaortic membrane and myectomy.

1. Edge of myectomy
2. Mitral valve apparatus
3. Aortic valve

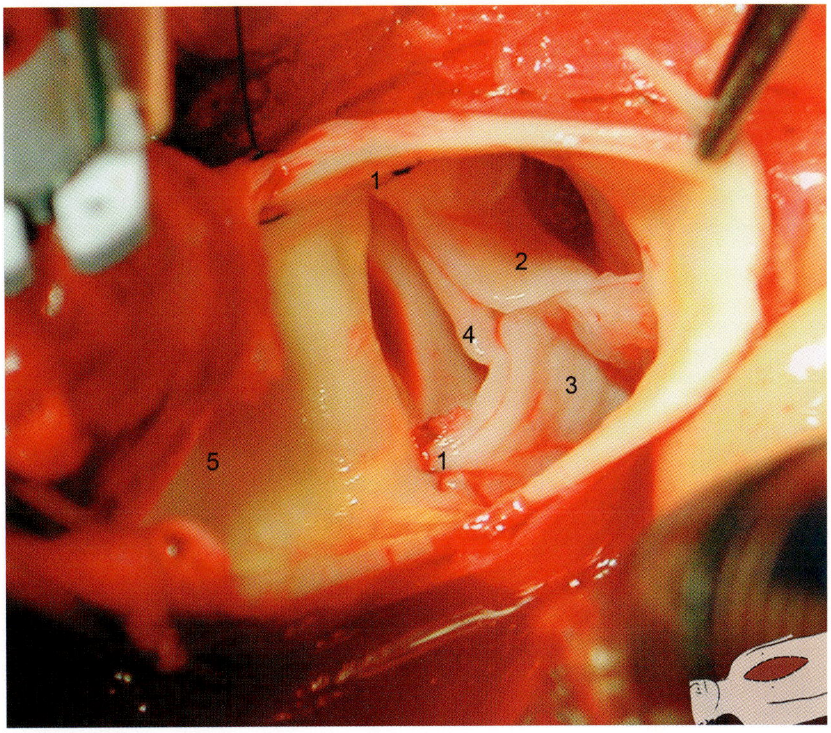

Figure 19.20. The same patient as in Figures 19.18 and 19.19 after valve repair. Suspension valvuloplasty was performed at 2 commissures: between the left and right leaflets, and between the left and noncoronary leaflets.

1. Sites of suspension valvuloplasty
2. Right coronary leaflet
3. Noncoronary leaflet
4. Left coronary leaflet
5. Ascending aorta

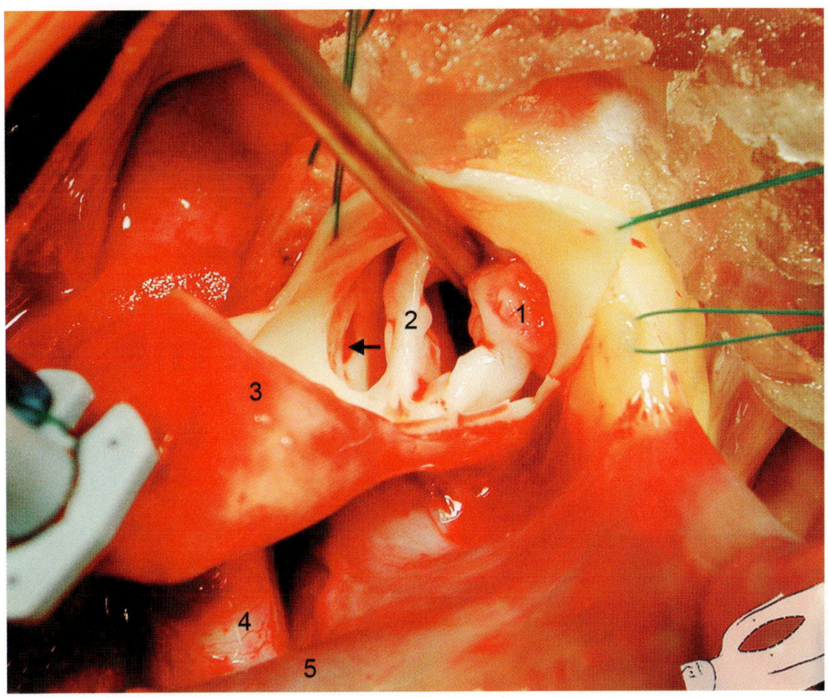

Figure 19.21. Bicuspid aortic valve in a 3-year-old child as seen through an aortotomy. The left and right coronary leaflets are conjoined, forming one large leaflet. Note the small, effective valve orifice. The arrow points to left coronary artery ostium. Surgery was indicated to relieve the stenosis and was achieved by commissurotomy between the left- and noncoronary leaflets and between the right- and noncoronary leaflets. Some shaving was also done to the valve tissue (not shown).

1. Right coronary leaflet
2. Left coronary leaflet
3. Ascending aorta
4. Right pulmonary artery (PA)
5. SVC

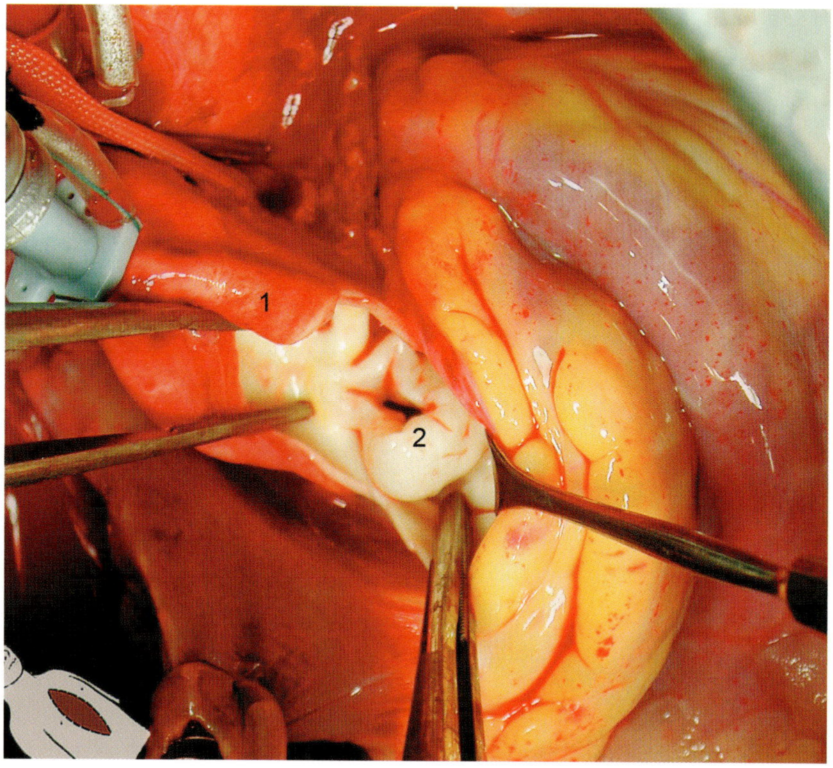

Figure 19.22. Bicuspid aortic valve in a 7-year-old child. Note the small valvar orifice and thickened valve leaflets.

1. Ascending aorta
2. Bicuspid aortic valve

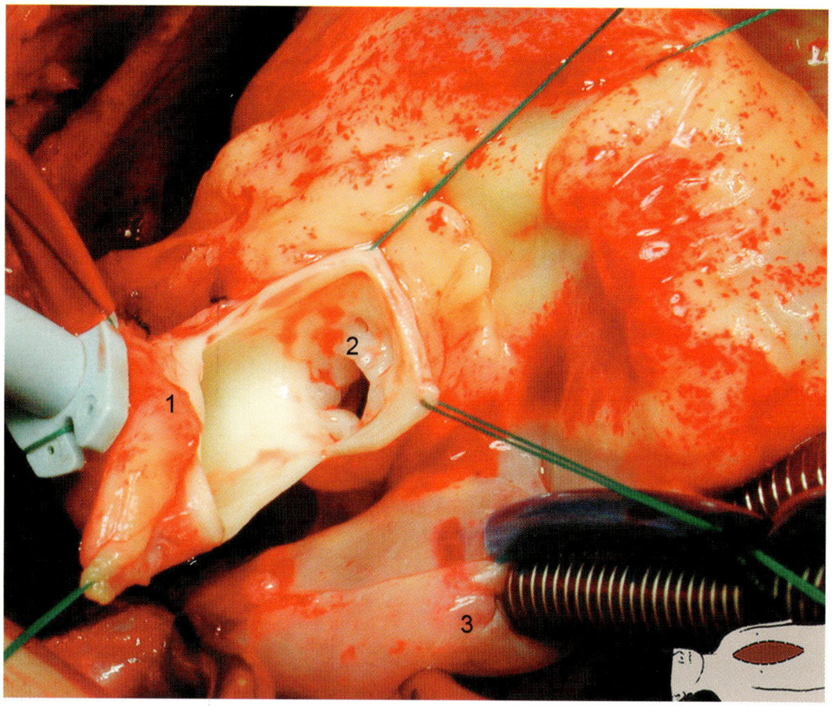

Figure 19.23. Aortotomy view in a 3-year-old child with valvar aortic stenosis. Both right and left coronary leaflets were fused to the aortic wall; the noncoronary leaflet was the only functional leaflet.

1. Ascending aorta
2. Right coronary leaflet
3. RAA

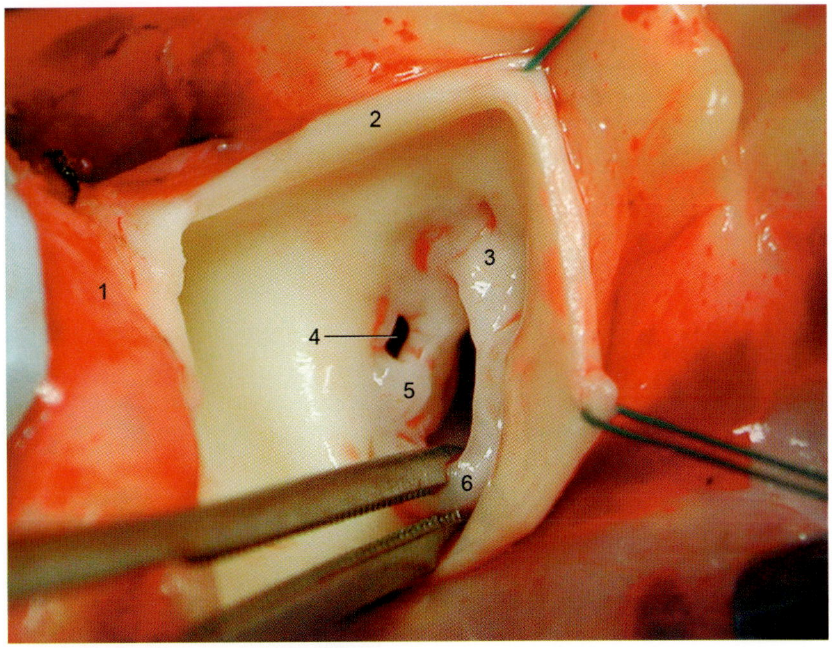

Figure 19.24. The same patient as in Figure 19.23. The left coronary leaflet is fused to the aortic wall, leaving a small opening, which is the only passage to the left aortic sinus and left coronary artery.

1. Ascending aorta
2. Aortotomy incision
3. Right coronary leaflet
4. Opening to left aortic sinus
5. Left coronary leaflet
6. Noncoronary leaflet

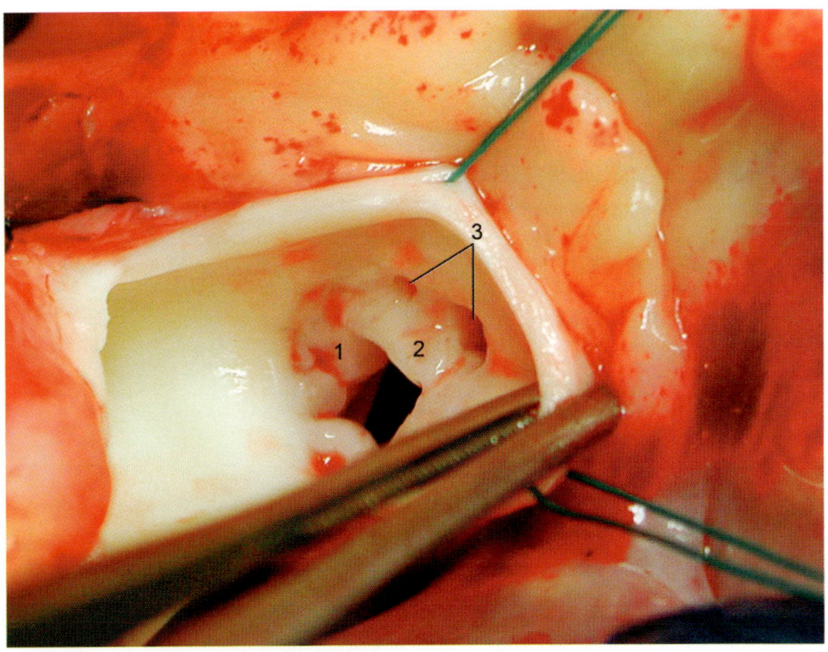

Figure 19.25. The same patient as in Figures 19.23 and 19.24. Similarly, the right coronary leaflet is also fused to the aortic wall, leaving 2 small openings as the only passage to the right aortic sinus and the right coronary artery. Treatment was achieved by freeing the leaflets and performing a commissurotomy (not shown).

1. Left coronary leaflet
2. Right coronary leaflet
3. Openings to right aortic sinus

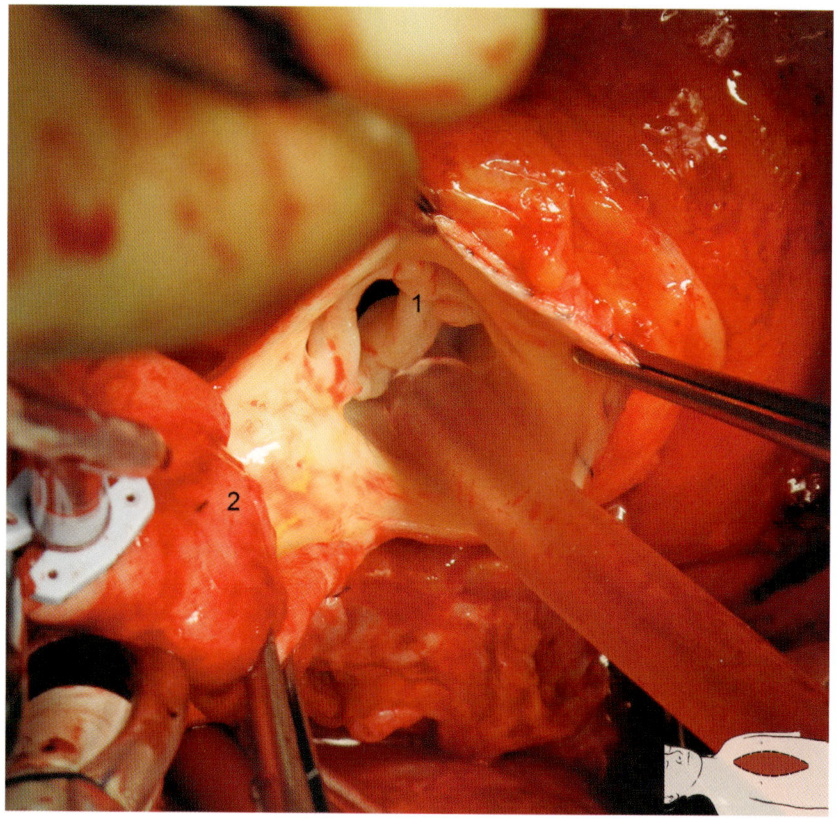

Figure 19.26. A redo aortotomy in a patient who had aortic valvotomy 10 years ago. The valve was not suitable for further repair, so a decision was made to replace it with the patient's own pulmonary valve (Ross procedure).

1. Aortic valve
2. Ascending aorta

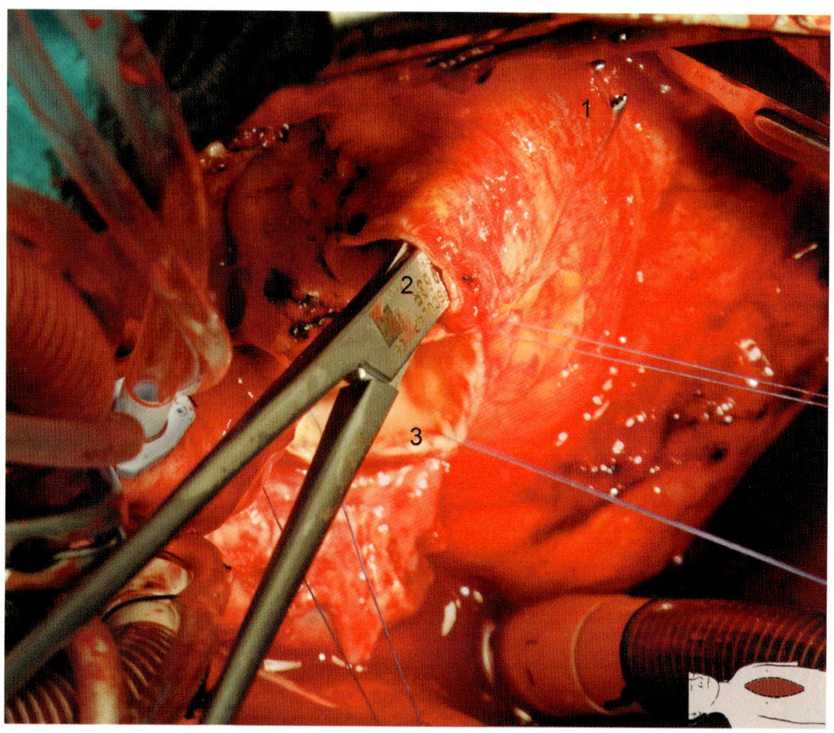

Figure 19.27. The same patient as in Figure 19.26. The pulmonary valve is being harvested. A pulmonary arteriotomy has been made. A curved clamp is passed through the pulmonary valve as a guide to locate the incision on the anterior aspect of the RV outflow.

1. RVOT
2. Forceps passed through pulmonary valve
3. Aortotomy incision

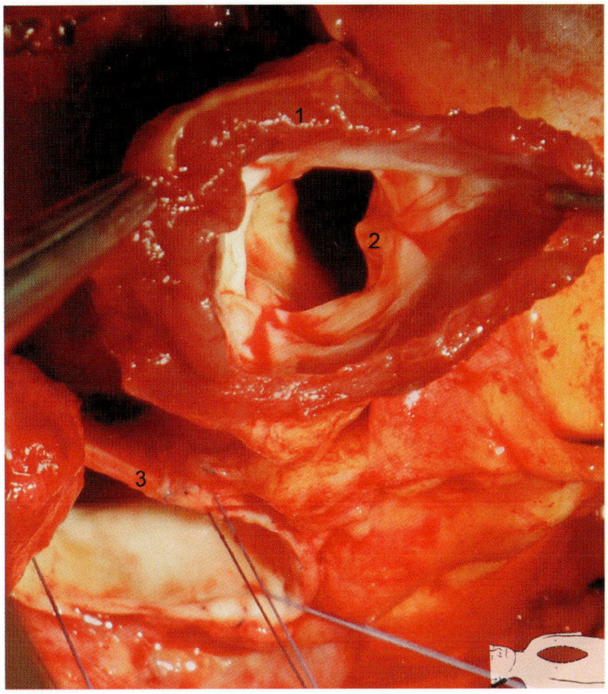

Figure 19.28. The same patient as in Figures 19.26 and 19.27 showing the harvested pulmonary valve with a portion of the RV infundibulum. The valve is shown here from the RV aspect.

1. RV outflow muscle
2. Pulmonary valve
3. Aortotomy incision

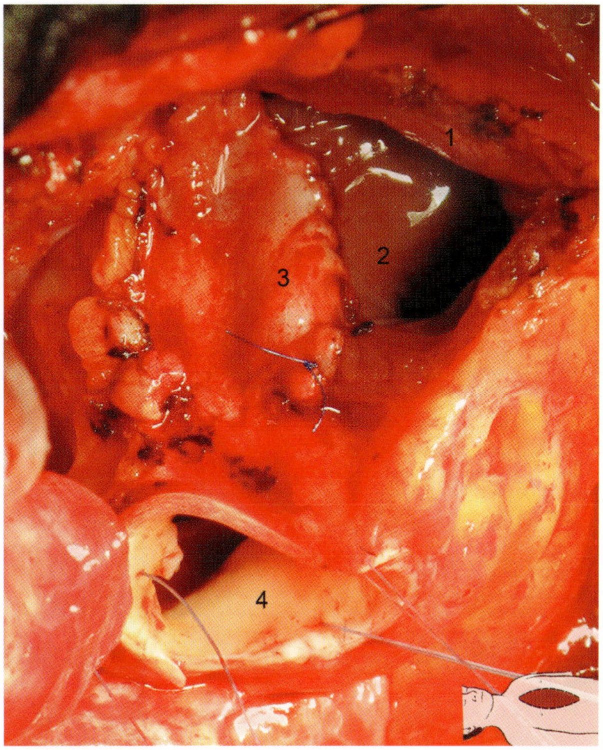

Figure 19.29. The same patient as in Figures 19.26 to 19.28 after removal of the pulmonary valve. A pericardial patch has been sutured to the superior part of the septum to support the anastomosis.

1. Site of explant in the RV outflow
2. Interventricular septum
3. Pericardial patch
4. Aorta

Figure 19.30. The same patient as in Figures 19.26 to 19.29. The coronary arteries have been detached from the aorta. The autograft (5) is being sutured to the aortic wall.

1. Site of explant in the RV outflow
2. Right coronary artery button
3. Left coronary artery button
4. Aortotomy incision
5. Autograft (patient's pulmonary valve)

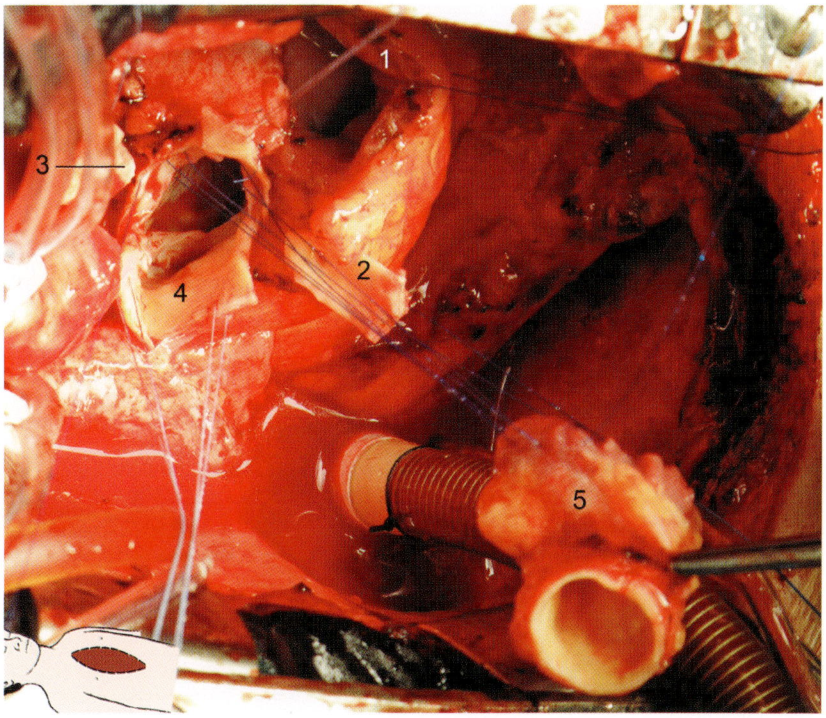

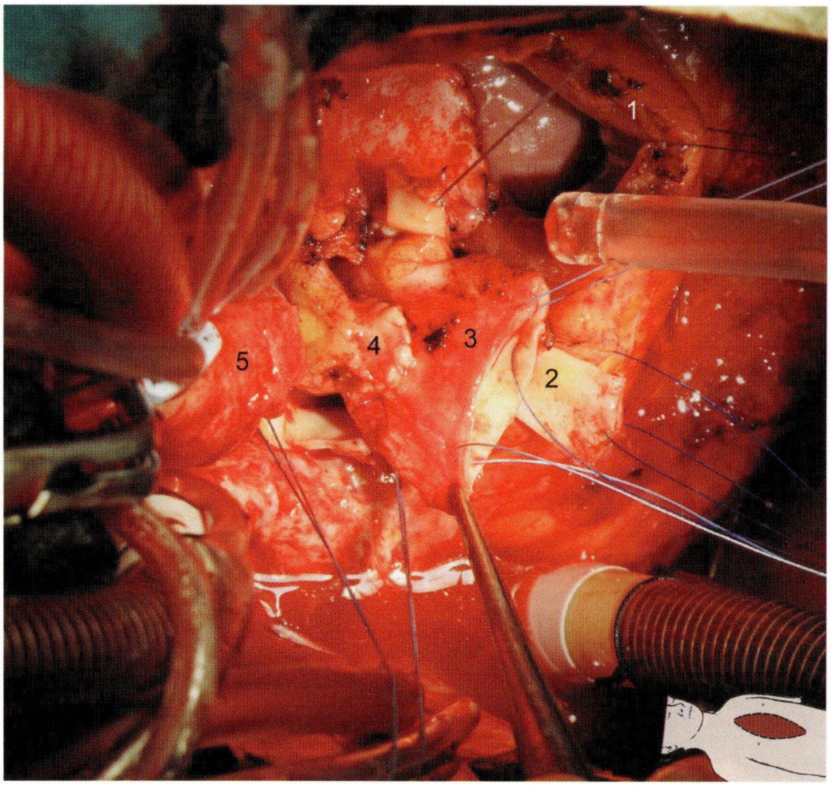

Figure 19.31. The same patient as in Figures 19.26 to 19.30 after suturing the autograft to the aortic position. The left coronary artery (4) has been sutured to the graft.

1. Site of explant in the RV outflow
2. Right coronary artery button
3. Autograft in aortic position
4. Left coronary button
5. Ascending aorta

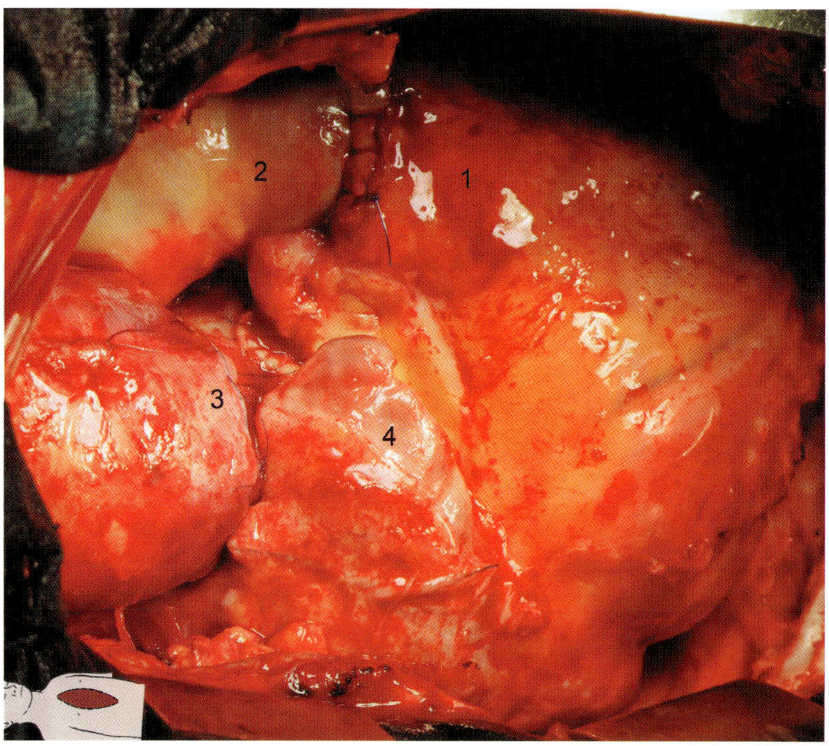

Figure 19.32. The same patient as in Figures 19.26 to 19.31. Both coronary arteries have been transferred, the distal ascending aorta has been anastomosed to the autograft, and a homograft has been implanted in the pulmonary valve position.

1. RV outflow
2. Pulmonary homograft
3. Ascending aorta
4. RAA

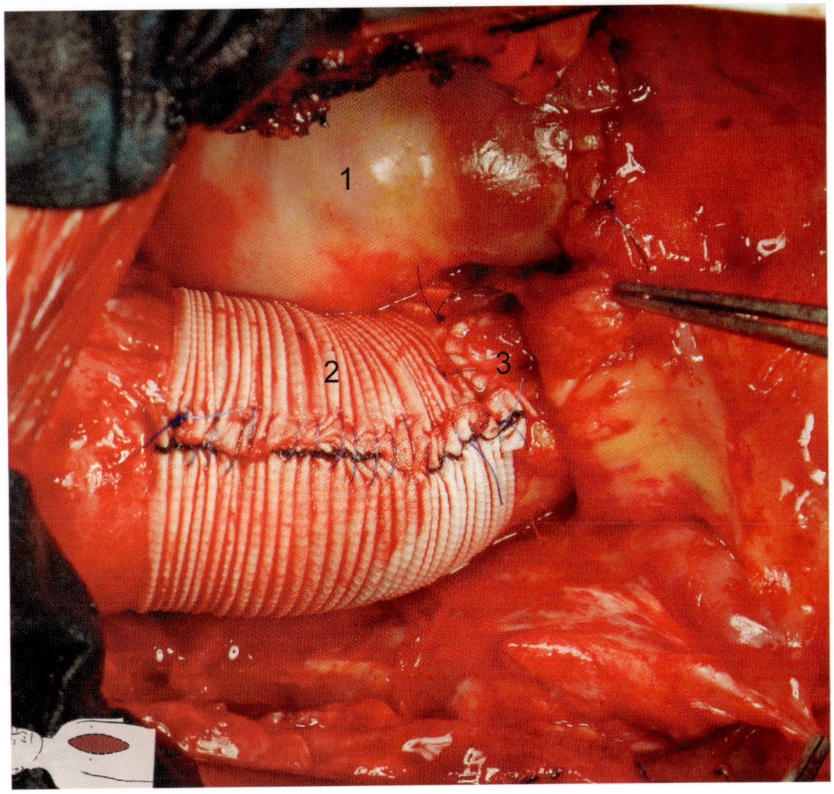

Figure 19.33. The same patient as in Figures 19.26 to 19.32. To prevent future dilatation, the ascending aorta is reinforced with a Hemashield graft.

1. Pulmonary homograft
2. Hemashield graft around ascending aorta
3. Right coronary artery button

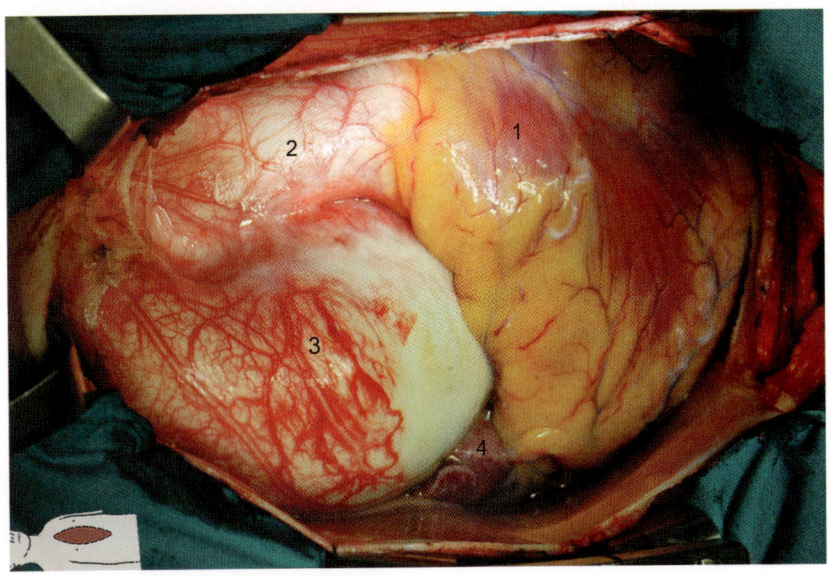

Figure 19.34. Median sternotomy view of a 10-year-old child with Loeys–Dietz syndrome. The ascending aorta is massively dilated (5 cm).

1. Outflow part of RV
2. MPA
3. Dilated ascending aorta
4. RAA

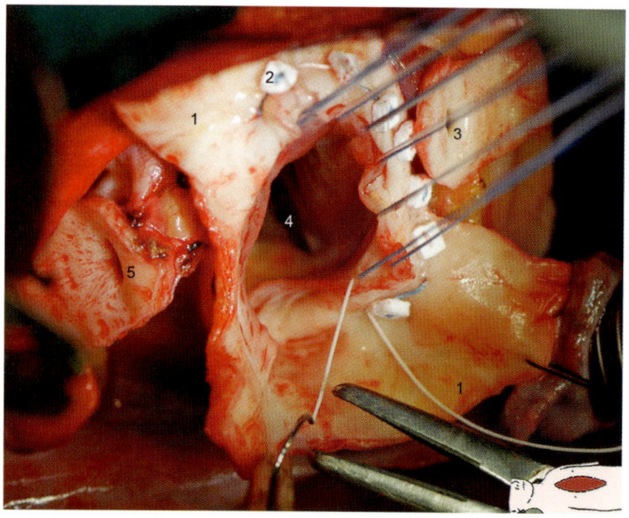

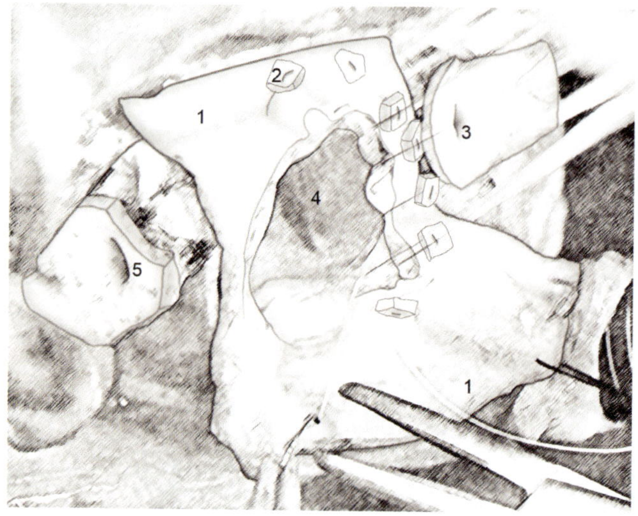

Figure 19.35 **Figure 19.36**

The same patient as in Figure 19.34. An aortotomy has been performed, and the aortic valve has been excised. The 2 coronary arteries have been detached from the aorta. Pledget-supported interrupted sutures are being placed circumferentially at the aortic root.

1. Wall of opened ascending aorta
2. Teflon pledget
3. Right coronary button
4. LV cavity
5. Left coronary button

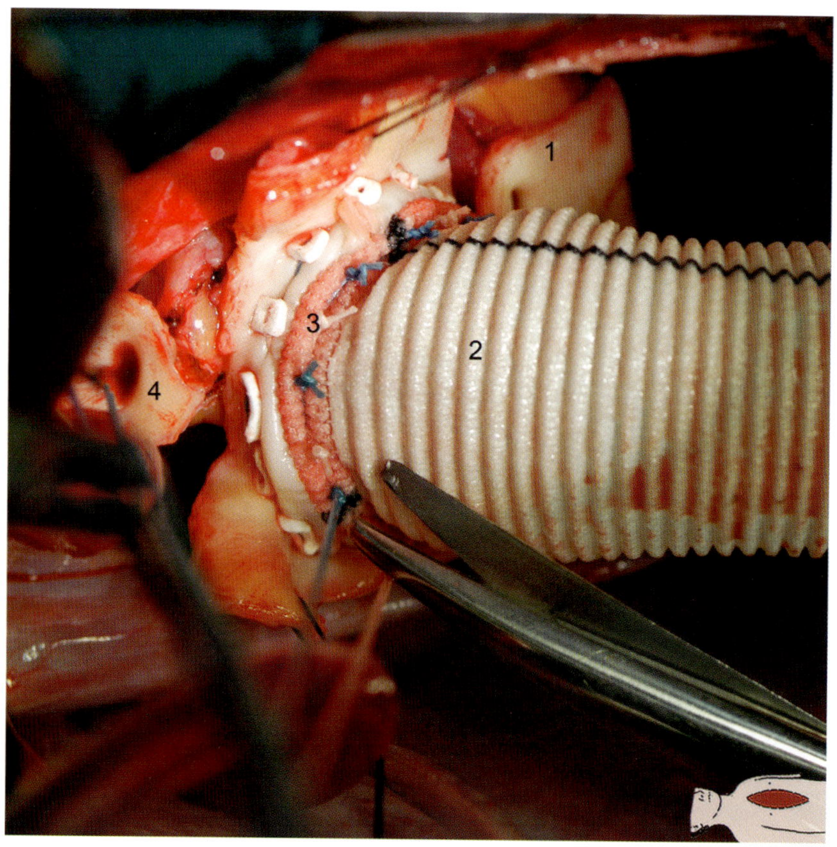

Figure 19.37. The same patient as in Figures 19.34 to 19.36. A modified Bentall procedure is performed using a 21 mm St. Jude composite graft. The valve end of the graft has been sutured in place using pledget-supported interrupted sutures. Note that the head of the patient is to the left of the picture, but the tube graft is turned down to show the left coronary artery behind it.

1. Right coronary artery button
2. St. Jude composite graft
3. Site of the graft valve
4. Left coronary artery button

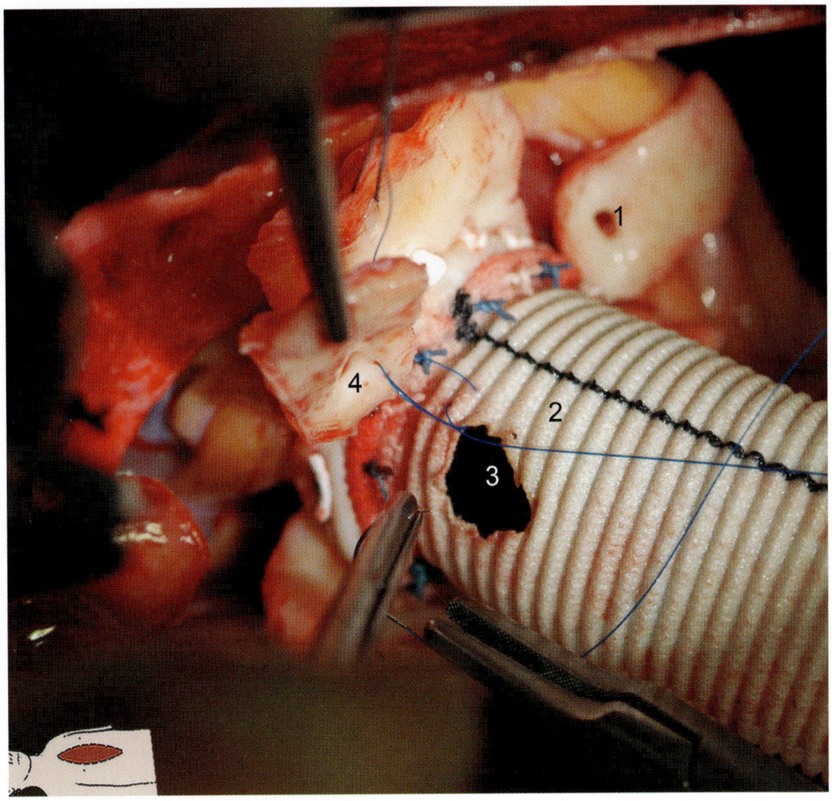

Figure 19.38. The same patient as in Figures 19.34 to 19.37. A hole has been made in the graft at the site that will receive the coronary artery.

1. Right coronary artery button
2. St. Jude composite graft
3. Hole at target site of left coronary artery
4. Left coronary artery button

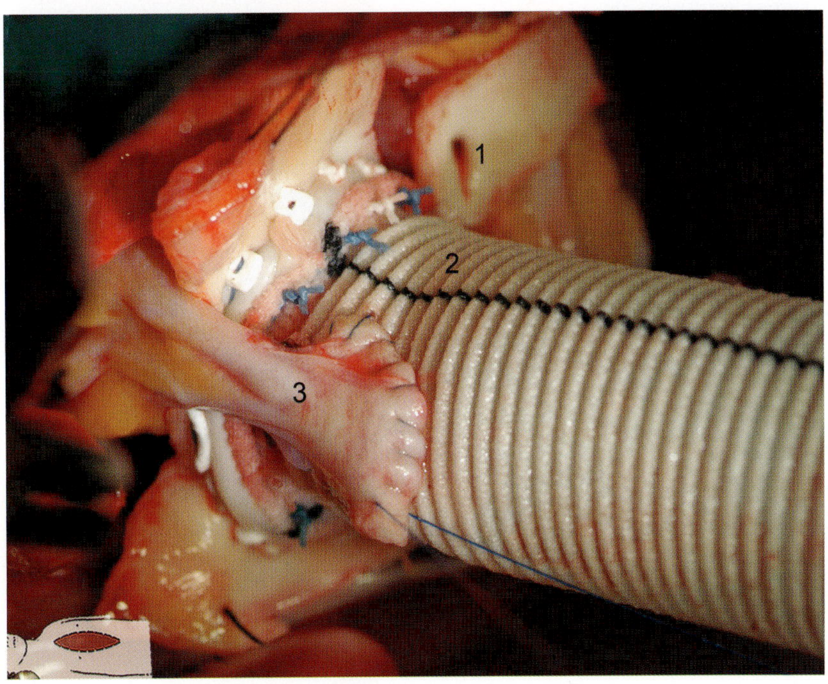

Figure 19.39. The same patient as in Figures 19.34 to 19.38 after suturing the left coronary artery to the graft.

1. Right coronary button
2. St. Jude composite graft
3. Left coronary artery

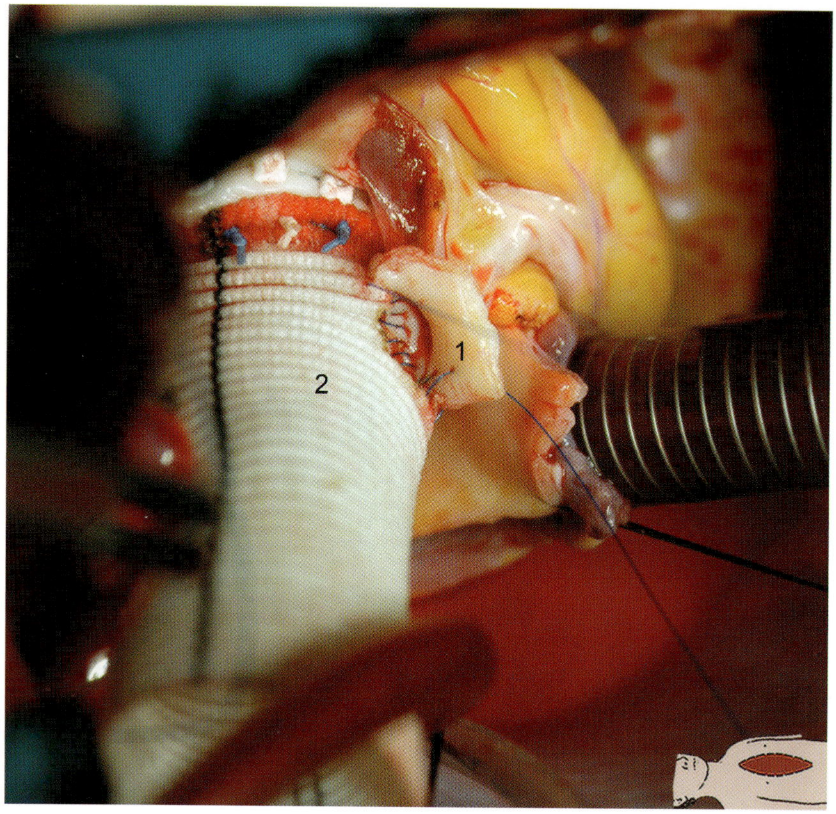

Figure 19.40. The same patient as in Figures 19.34 to 19.39. The right coronary artery button is being sutured to the graft, just above the valve.

1. Right coronary artery button
2. St. Jude composite graft

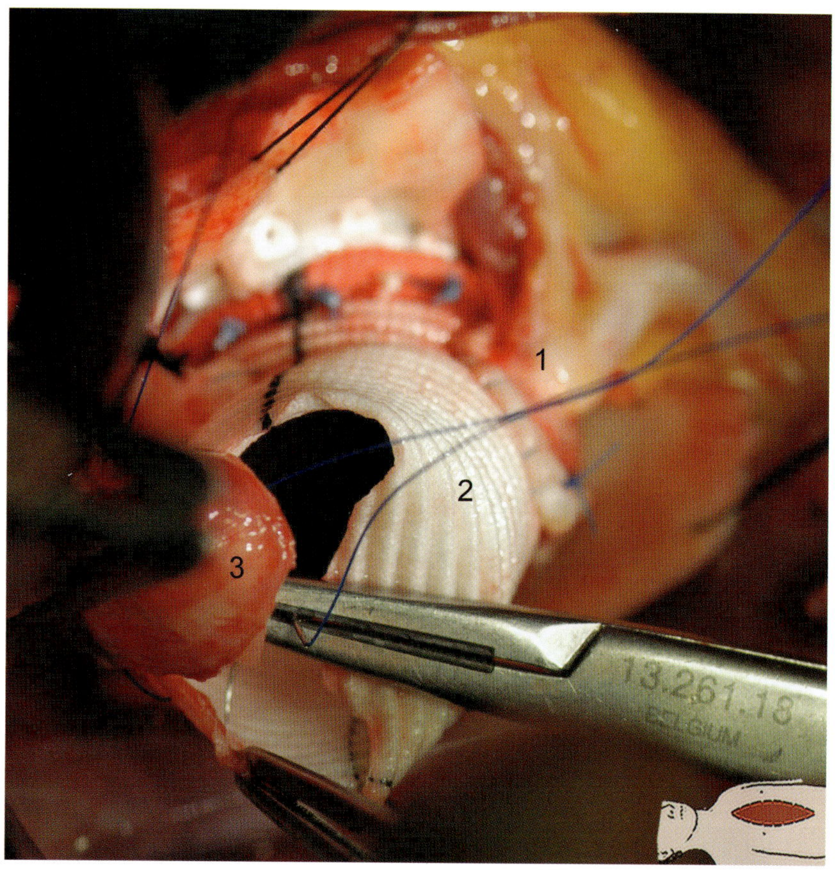

Figure 19.41. The same patient as in Figures 19.34 to 19.40. The distal end of the graft is being sutured to the distal part of the ascending aorta.

1. Right coronary artery
2. St. Jude composite graft
3. Transected distal ascending aorta

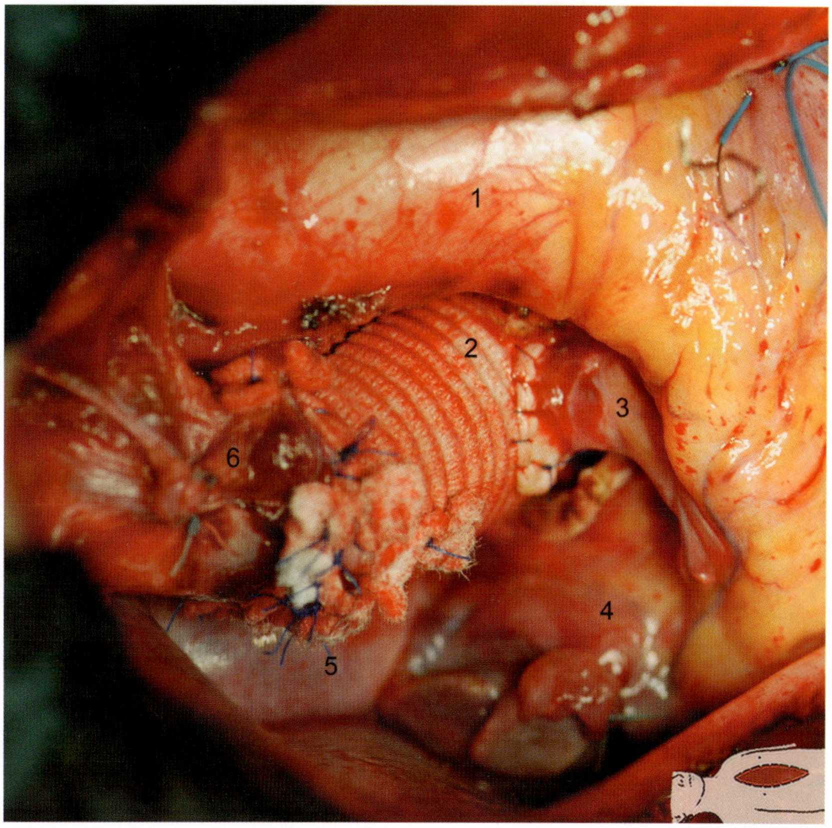

Figure 19.42. The same patient as in Figures 19.34 to 19.41 after completion of the aortic root replacement.

1. Main pulmonary artery (MPA)
2. St. Jude composite graft
3. Right coronary artery
4. Right atrium
5. SVC
6. Distal ascending aorta

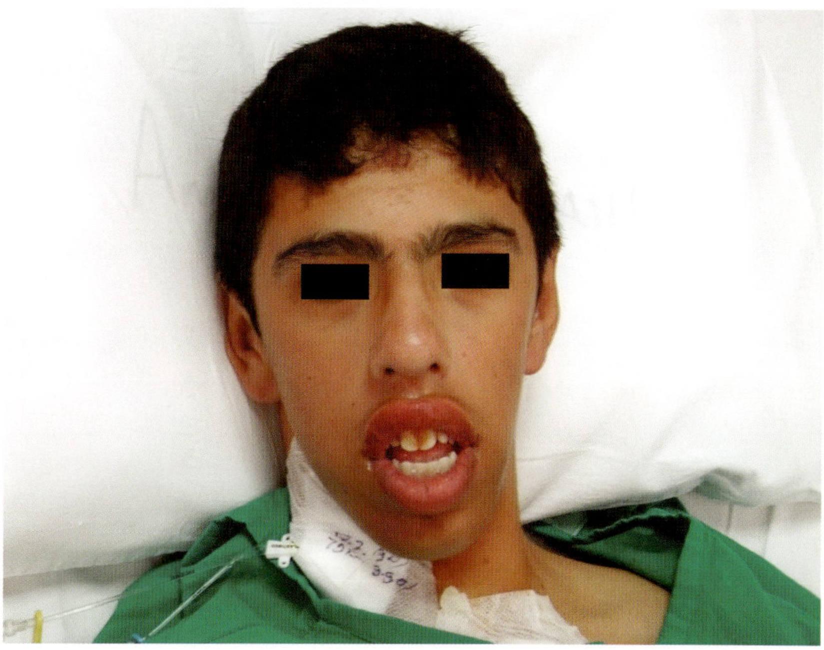

Figure 19.43. A patient with Williams syndrome in the intensive care unit after surgery for supravalvar aortic stenosis. Some of the typical facial features are shown. Note the medial eyebrow flare, periorbital fullness, and prominent lips with open mouth.

limited role because of the proximity to the aortic valve leaflets and coronary orifices; the narrowing affects the sinotubular junction of the aortic root and can extend to uniform hypoplasia of the lumen of the ascending aorta. Treatment is mainly surgical and involves placement of a patch in the supravalvar area using a variety of techniques. Figures 19.44 to 19.49 are intraoperative views from a 7-year-old child with Williams syndrome and supravalvar aortic stenosis.

Figures 19.50 to 19.52 are 2 examples of repair of supravalvar aortic stenosis. An inverted Y-shaped incision is made in the proximal aorta, extending the 2 arms of the Y down to the aortic "annulus." Then a pantaloon-shaped patch is sutured to the aortic root to augment the supravalvar area and relieve the stenosis.

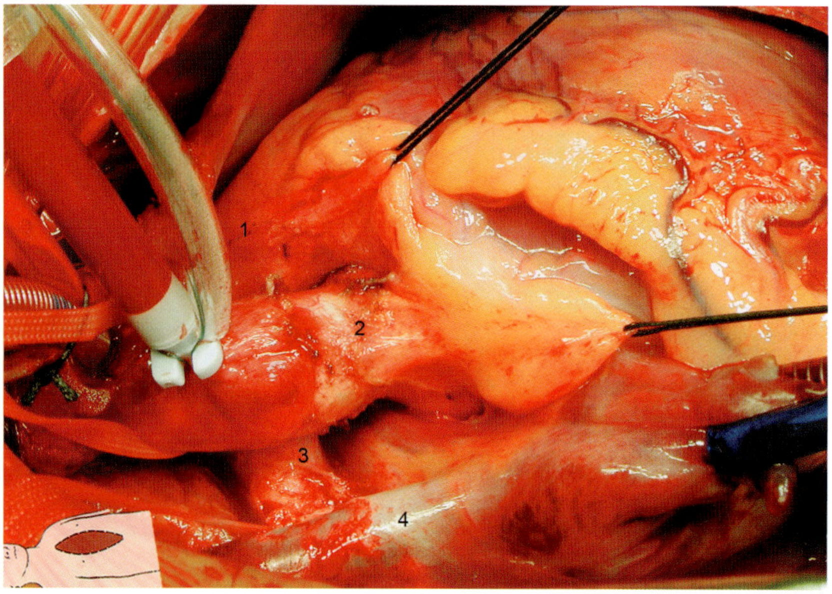

Figure 19.44. Median sternotomy view of a 7-year-old child with Williams syndrome. The site of supravalvar stenosis is evident externally as a circumferential constriction in the proximal ascending aorta.

1. MPA
2. Site of supravalvar stenosis
3. Right PA
4. SVC

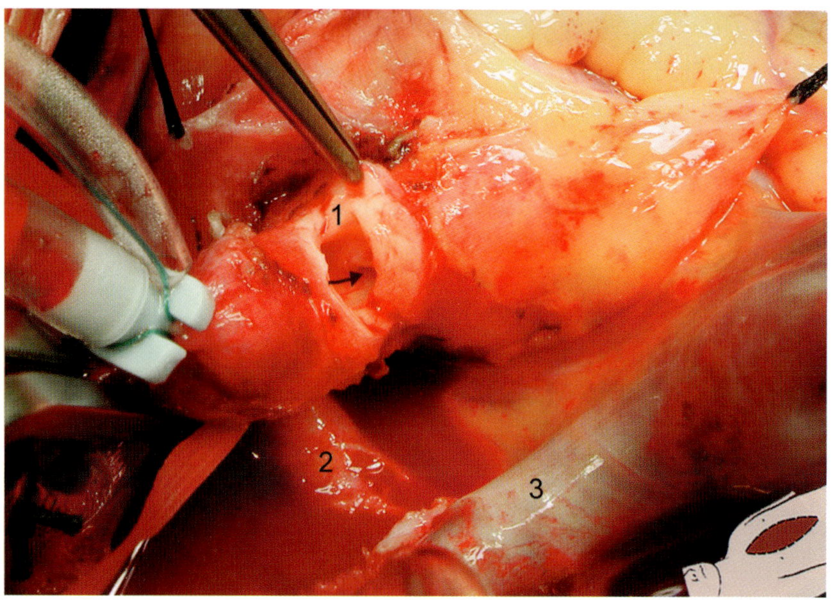

Figure 19.45. Transverse aortotomy is being performed on the same patient as shown in Figure 19.44. The aortic wall is extremely thick. The arrow points to the narrow lumen in the supravalvar area.

1. Aortic wall
2. Right PA
3. SVC

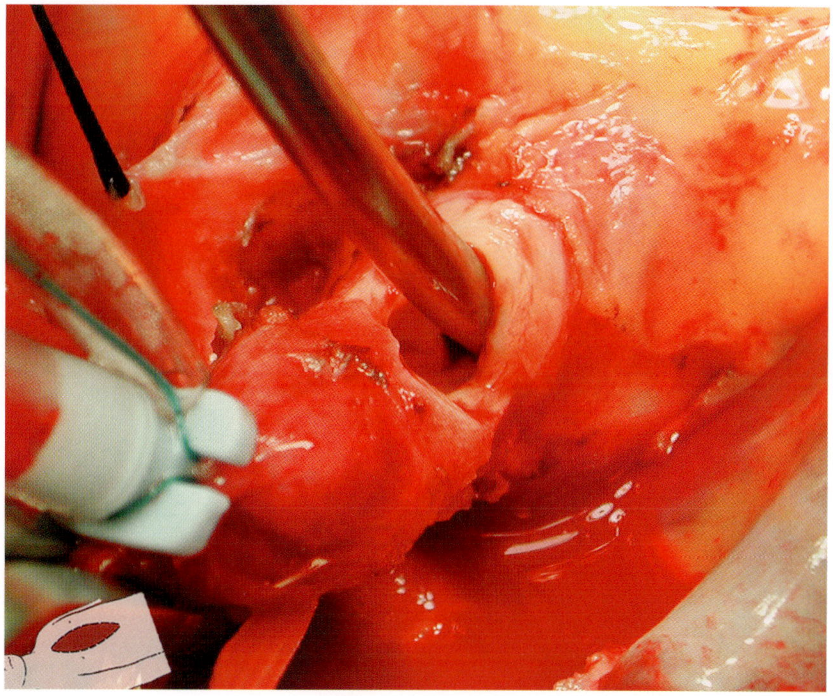

Figure 19.46. The same patient as in Figures 19.44 and 19.45. A suction catheter is passed through the narrowing in the supravalvar area.

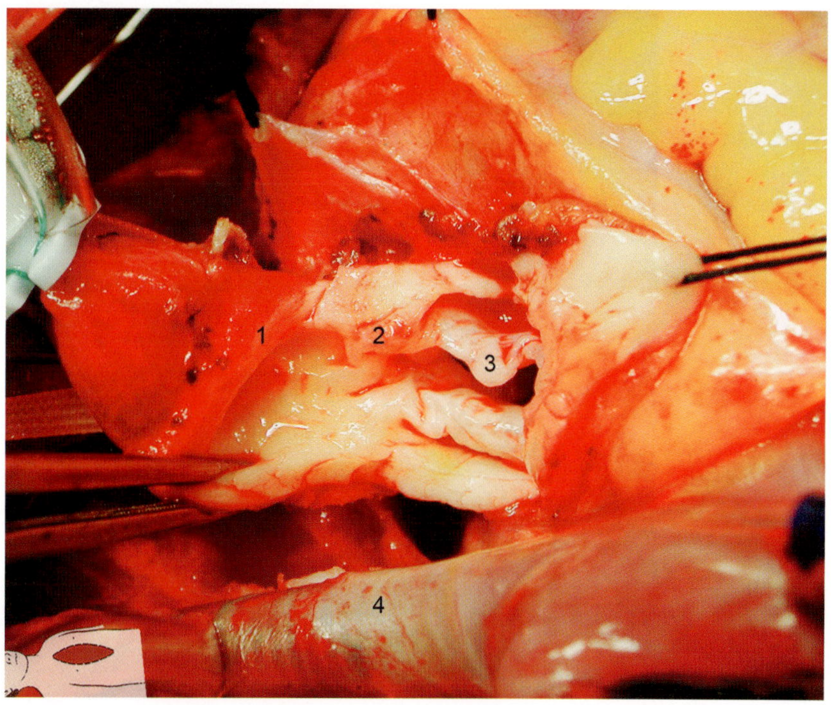

Figure 19.47. The same patient as in Figures 19.44 to 19.46. The incision is extended in both right and noncoronary aortic sinuses down to the attachment line of the valve leaflets ("annulus").

1. Aortotomy incision
2. Site of supravalvar narrowing
3. Right coronary leaflet
4. SVC

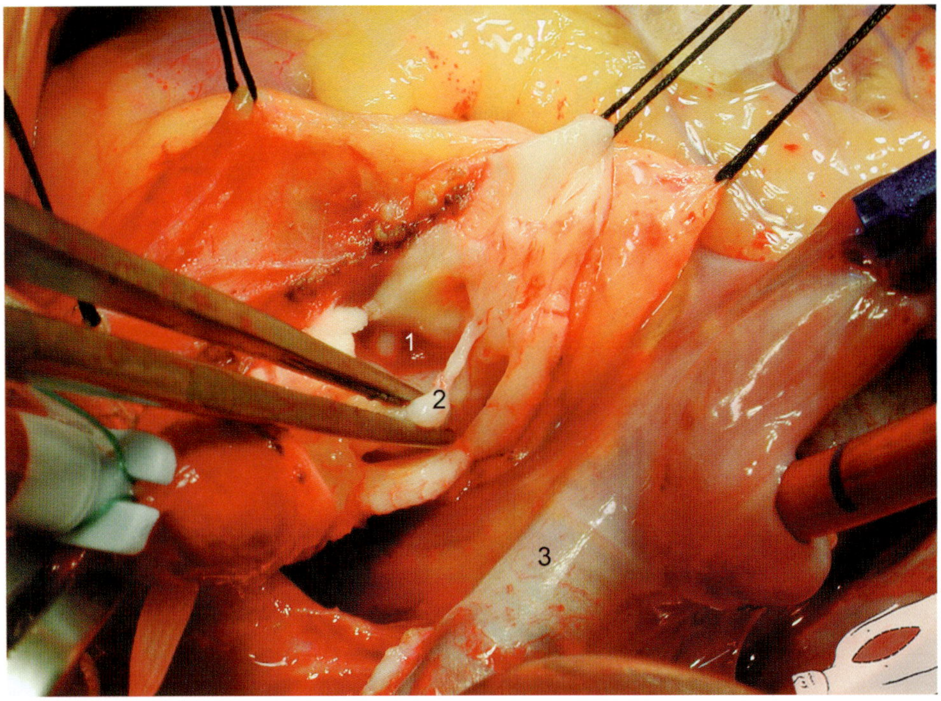

Figure 19.48. The same patient as in Figures 19.44 to 19.47. The right coronary cusp is pulled down to reveal the right coronary orifice.

1. Right coronary artery orifice
2. Right coronary leaflet
3. SVC

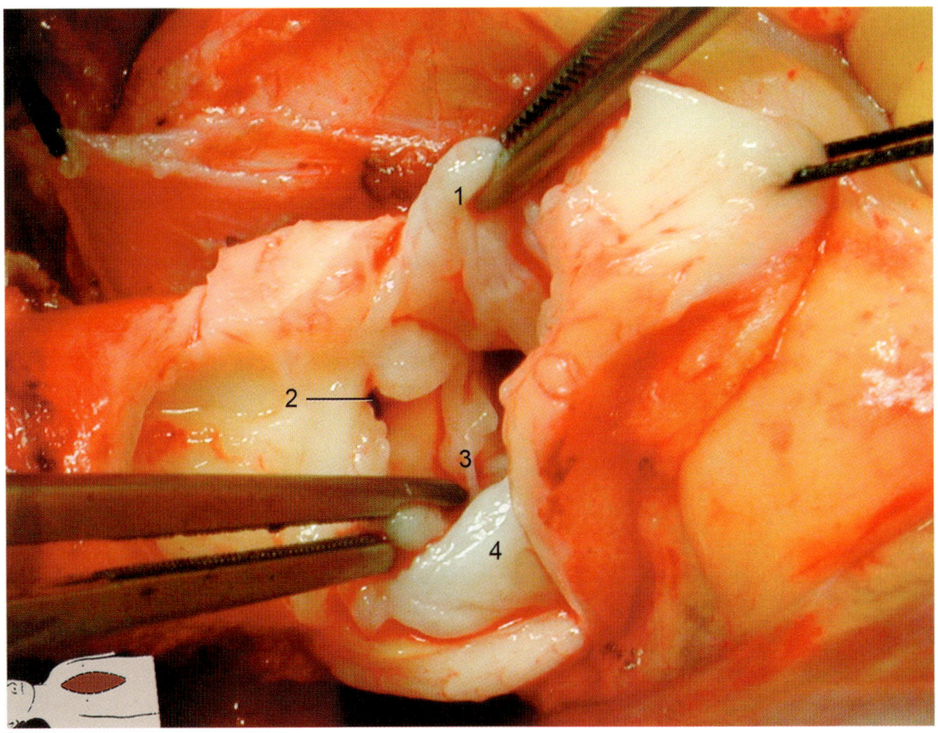

Figure 19.49. The same patient as in Figures 19.44 to 19.48. The right coronary cusp is pulled up, showing the left aortic sinus and orifice of left coronary artery.

1. Right coronary leaflet
2. Left coronary artery orifice
3. Left coronary leaflet
4. Noncoronary leaflet

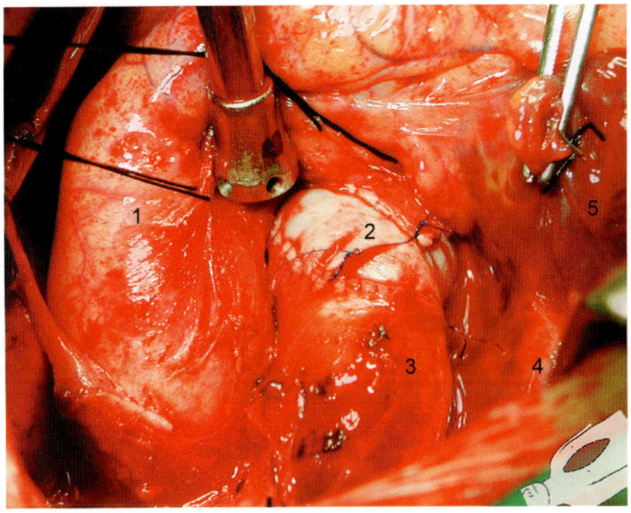

Figure 19.50

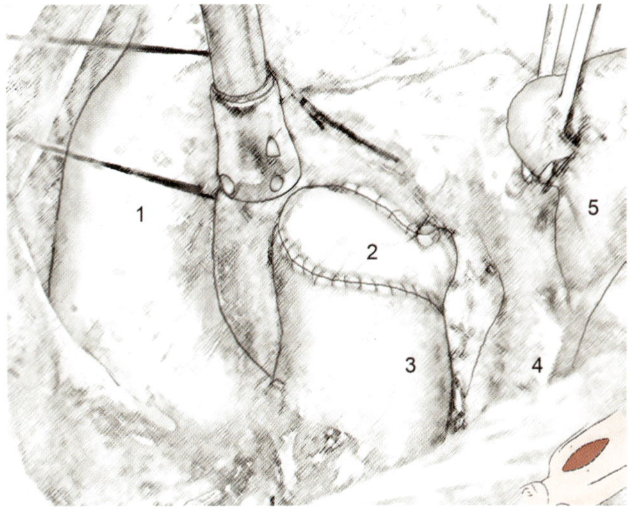

Figure 19.51

Median sternotomy view of an 8-year-old child with supravalvular aortic stenosis. Surgical repair has been performed using a pantaloon-shaped xenograft pericardium to augment the supravalvar area. One leg of the patch is sutured down in the noncoronary aortic sinus up to the valve "annulus"; the other leg is sutured similarly in the right aortic sinus.

1. MPA
2. Xenograft pericardial patch
3. Ascending aorta
4. SVC
5. RAA

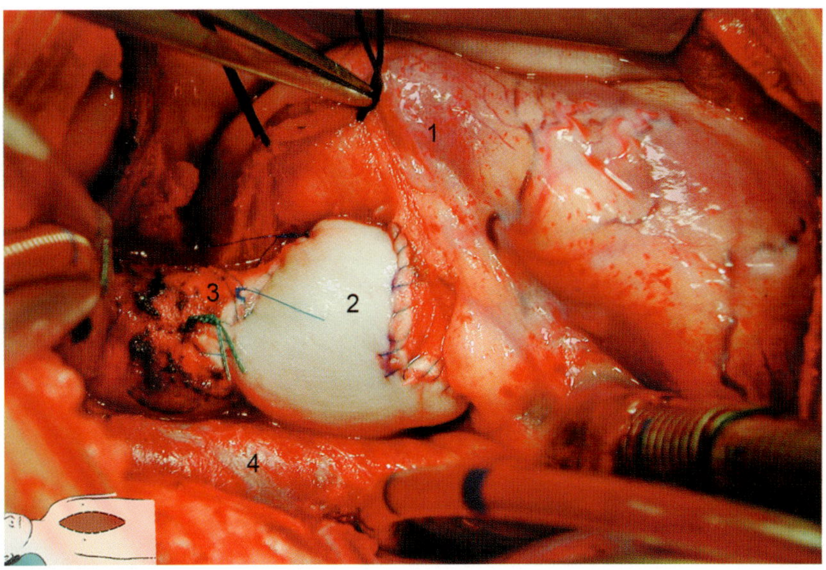

Figure 19.52. Median sternotomy view of a 3-year-old child with supravalvar aortic stenosis. Repair was performed using the same technique as that explained in Figure 19.50.

1. RV infundibulum
2. Xenograft pericardial patch
3. Ascending aorta
4. SVC

REFERENCES

1. Leichter DA, Sullivan I, Gersony WM. "Acquired" discrete subvalvular aortic stenosis: natural history and hemodynamics. *J Am Coll Cardiol.* 1989;14:1539.
2. Cicini MP, Giannico S, Marino B, et al. "Acquired" subvalvular aortic stenosis after repair of a ventricular septal defect. *Chest.* 1992;101:115.
3. Braverman AC, Güven H, Beardslee MA. The bicuspid aortic valve. *Curr Probl Cardiol.* 2005;30:470–522.
4. Lewin MB, Otto CM. The bicuspid aortic valve adverse outcomes from infancy to old age. *Circulation.* 2005;111:832–834.
5. Brown JW, Ruzmetov M, Rodefeld MD, et al. Incidence of and risk factors for pulmonary autograft dilation after Ross aortic valve replacement. *Ann Thorac Surg.* 2007;83:1781–1789.
6. Loeys BL, Schwarze U, Holm T, et al. Aneurysm syndromes caused by mutations in the TGF-β receptor. *N Engl J Med.* 2006;355:788–798.
7. Collins RT, Kaplan P, Somes GW, Rome JR. Cardiovascular abnormalities, interventions, and long-term outcomes in infantile Williams syndrome. *J Pediatr.* 2010;156:253–258.

CHAPTER 20

Valve Surgery

Aortic valve disease was discussed in chapter 19, and the pulmonary valve was discussed in chapters 13 and 14. In this chapter, we discuss examples of diseases or malformations of the mitral and tricuspid valves and also include examples of the left and right components of the valve in atrioventricular septal defect (AVSD).

MITRAL VALVE

A double orifice mitral valve is a rare anomaly, commonly found as an ancillary finding in the setting of a more complex congenital heart disease. The most common association of a double orifice left atrioventricular (AV) valve is with AVSD.[1] Figures 20.1 and 20.2 are from a 1-year-old child with partial AVSD and double orifice left valve, caused by a complete bridge of leaflet tissue.

Mitral valve cleft is another anomaly that may occur in isolation. It should be distinguished from the so-called "cleft" in hearts with AVSD, which is the space between the superior and inferior bridging leaflets of the left AV valve. Figure 20.3 is an example of mitral valve cleft in a patient with Down syndrome and ventricular septal defect (VSD) (not AVSD), whereas Figure 20.4 is from a patient who had partial AVSD. For more examples, refer to chapter 5. Leaflet prolapse may occur concomitantly with a mitral cleft, as shown in Figure 20.5.

A supravalvar mitral ring, or membrane, is a rare anomaly that functionally results in mitral stenosis (Figures 20.6–20.8). The ring is located just above the

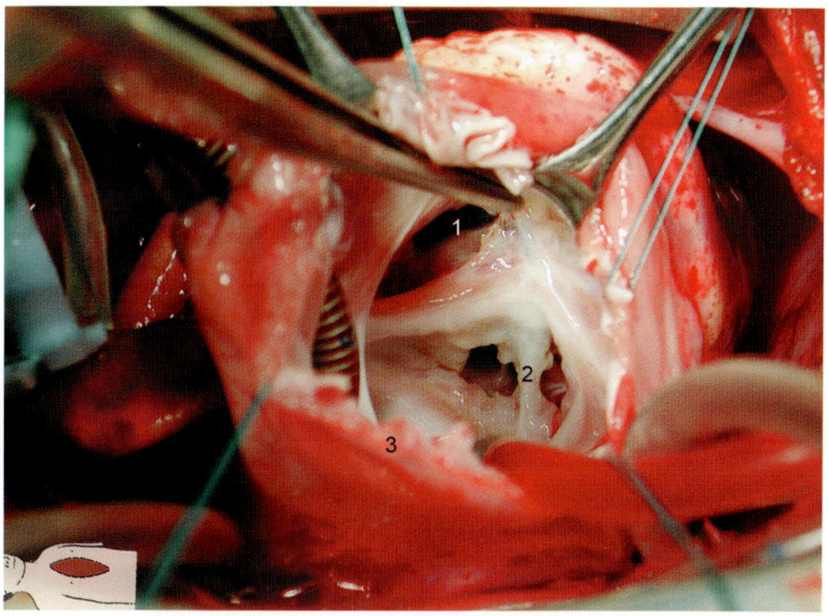

Figure 20.1. Double orifice left AV valve as seen through a median sternotomy and right atriotomy in a 1-year-old child. The patient also has a large primum AVSD. There was no valvar stenosis or regurgitation, so the valve was left untouched, and the atrial communication was repaired by the usual technique.

1. Right ventricular cavity
2. Left AV valve
3. Right atrial wall

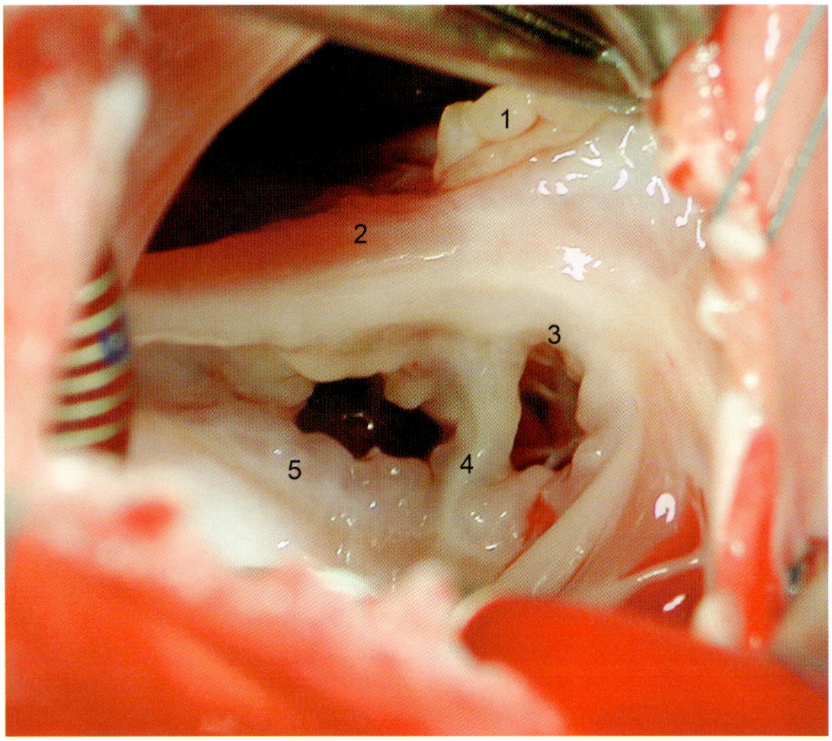

Figure 20.2. Close-up view of the left AV valve of the same patient as in Figure 20.1. Note the bridge of leaflet tissue (4) that divides the valve orifice into 2.

1. Right AV valve
2. Interventricular septum
3. Inferior bridging leaflet
4. Bridge of leaflet tissue
5. Superior bridging leaflet

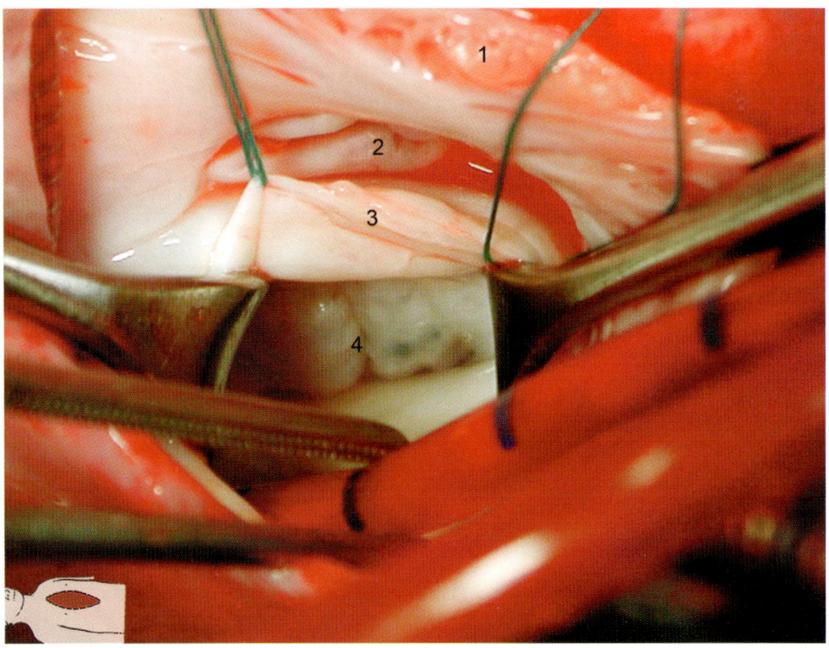

Figure 20.3. Right atriotomy view in a 9-month-old infant with Down syndrome, VSD, and mitral valve cleft. The mitral valve is seen through a transseptal approach. The cleft was treated by primary suturing (not shown).

1. Right atrial wall
2. Tricuspid valve
3. Flap of opened interatrial septum
4. Mitral valve cleft

Figure 20.4. The left AV valve as seen through a left atriotomy in a 20-year-old patient who previously had undergone partial AVSD repair. Note the "cleft" and poor coaptation of the valve. The median commissure was closed and an annuloplasty was performed by implanting a 33 mm St. Jude ring (not shown).

1. Right atrium
2. Interatrial septum
3. Left AV valve
4. Left atrial wall

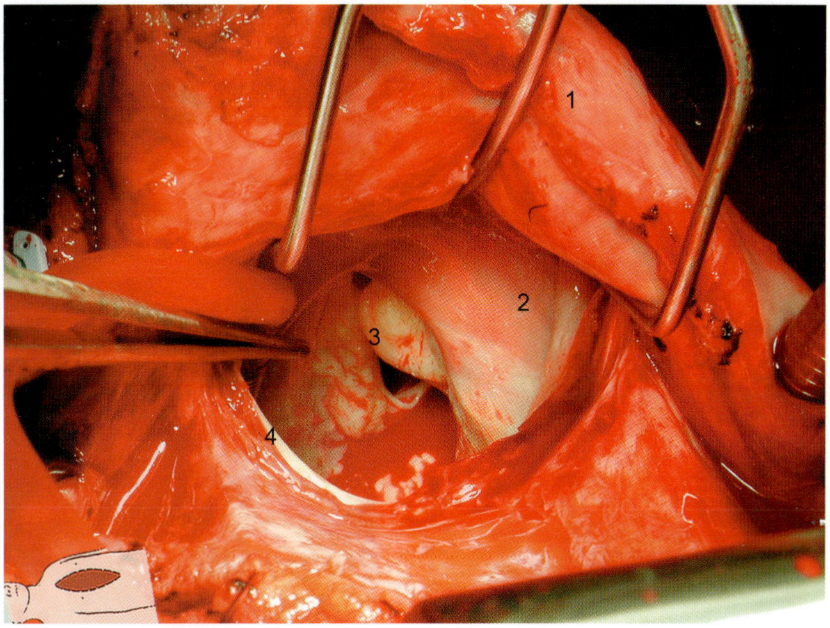

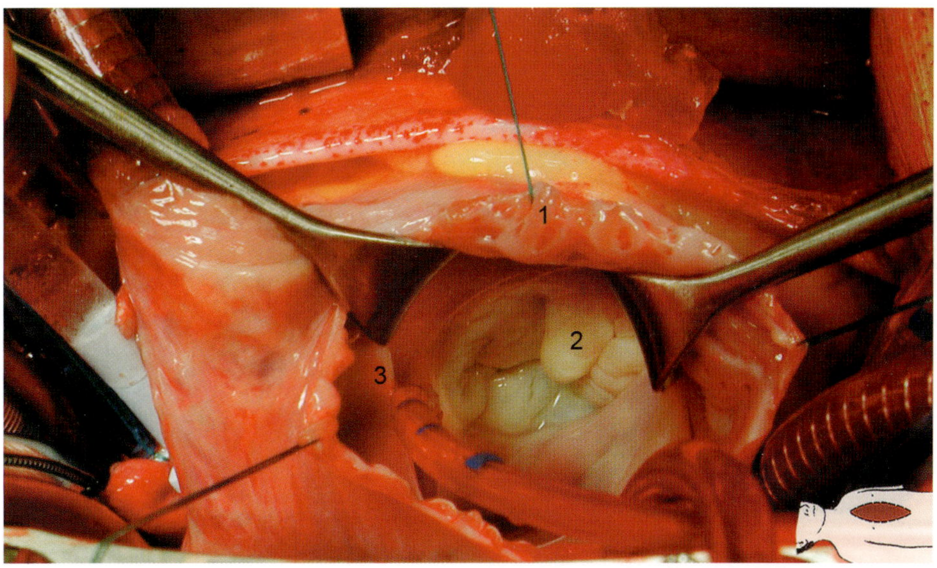

Figure 20.5. A median sternotomy and right atriotomy view in a 6-year-old child with a large secundum atrial septal defect (ASD). The mitral valve is examined through the ASD. Note the cleft and prolapse of the anterior leaflet.

1. Right atrium wall
2. Prolapsed portion of anterior leaflet
3. Edge of secundum ASD

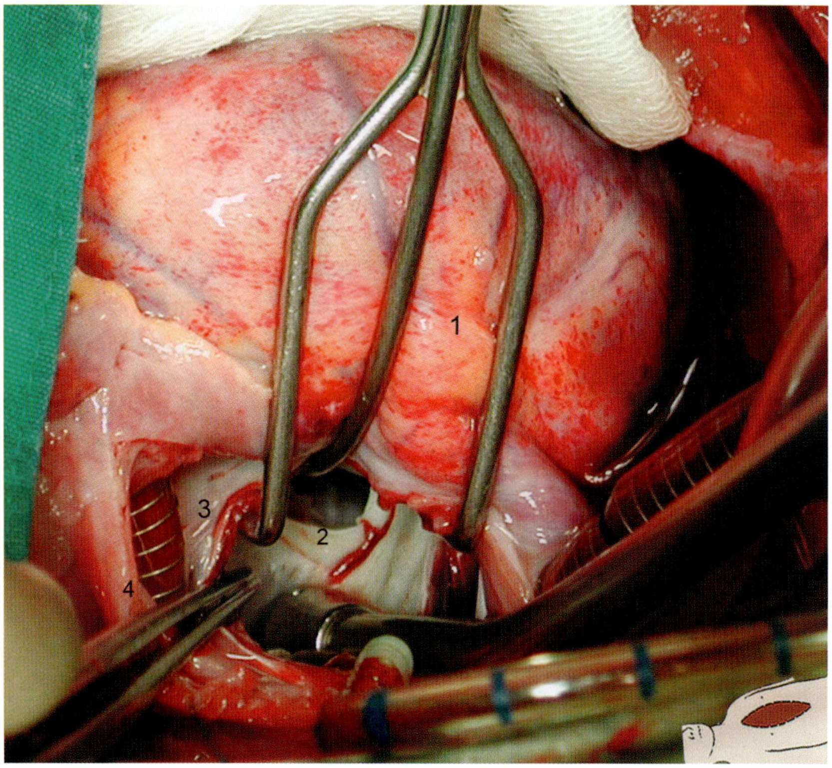

Figure 20.6. Right atriotomy view in an 11-year-old child with supravalvar mitral ring. The ring (2) is seen through a transseptal approach.

1. Right ventricle (RV)
2. Supravalvar mitral ring
3. Atrial septum
4. Right atriotomy incision

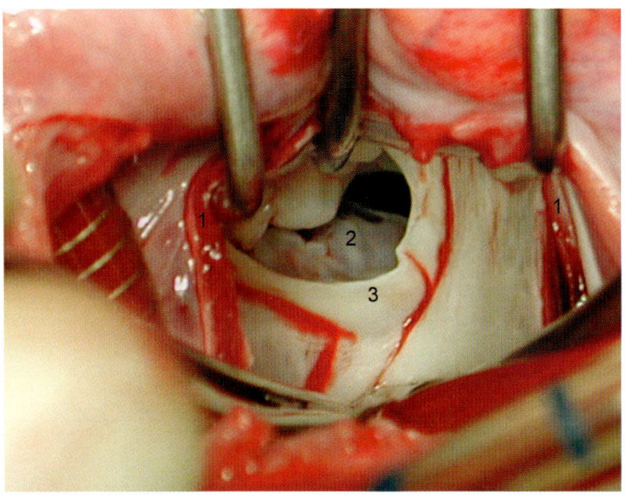

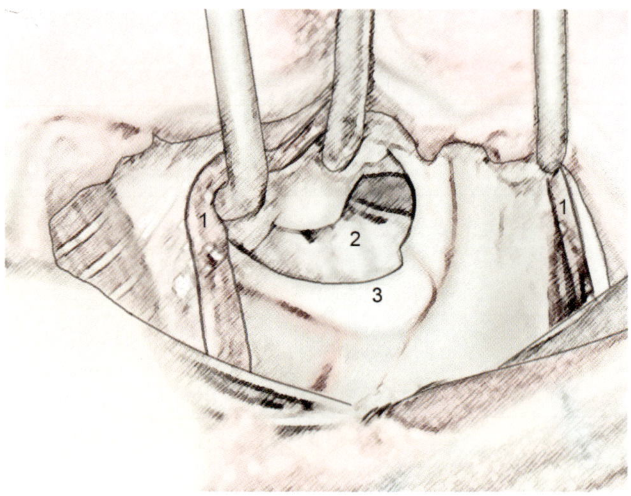

Figure 20.7 **Figure 20.8**

Close-up view of the same patient shown in Figure 20.6. The supravalvar mitral membrane is seen through a transseptal approach. Note the mitral valve immediately beneath the membrane.

1. Incision in atrial septum
2. Mitral valve
3. Supravalvar mitral ring

mitral valve orifice at a plane below the opening of the left atrial appendage (LAA).

Rheumatic heart disease used to be a common cause of valve disease, and it is still prevalent in many countries. The mitral and aortic valves are most commonly involved.[2] Figures 20.9 to 20.14 are from a 12-year-old child with rheumatic aortic and mitral valve disease. Both valves were replaced with mechanical valves.

Aortic-mitral double annulus enlargement procedure with attendant valve replacement[3] was performed on the patient shown in Figure 20.15 who had concomitant mitral and aortic valve disease. The procedure is shown diagrammatically in Figures 20.16 and 20.17.

Although mechanical valves have a good history of durability, valve dysfunction may result from thrombosis, endocarditis, or pannus formation. Figures 20.18 to 20.20 show an explanted valve that malfunctioned because of pannus that interfered with valve disk movement.

TRICUSPID VALVE

Some of the tricuspid valve anomalies have been discussed in other chapters. Figures 20.21 and 20.22 show a common AV valve from a 1-year-old child with partial AVSD who has so-called primum ASD and regurgitation of both right and left components of the AV valve that are neither tricuspid nor mitral. Nevertheless, inspection of the left valve reveals a commissural "cleft." The right valve, interestingly, has a "fenestration" or accessory orifice caused by a bridge of leaflet tissue connecting the inferior bridging and right inferior leaflets.

Ebstein anomaly of the tricuspid valve (Figure 20.23) is characterized by displacement of the tricuspid valve annulus into the RV, an enlarged right atrium, tricuspid regurgitation, and variable degrees of hypoplasia of the RV. A patent foramen ovale or ASD is invariably present. Figures 20.24 to 20.28 are from a 7-year-old child with Ebstein anomaly of the tricuspid valve. The anomaly was repaired using the modified Carpentier technique.[4] The atrialized portion of the RV was plicated, and the anterior leaflet was mobilized and repositioned superiorly to achieve better coaptation. A Glenn shunt may concomitantly be performed to partially volume-unload the RV.[5]

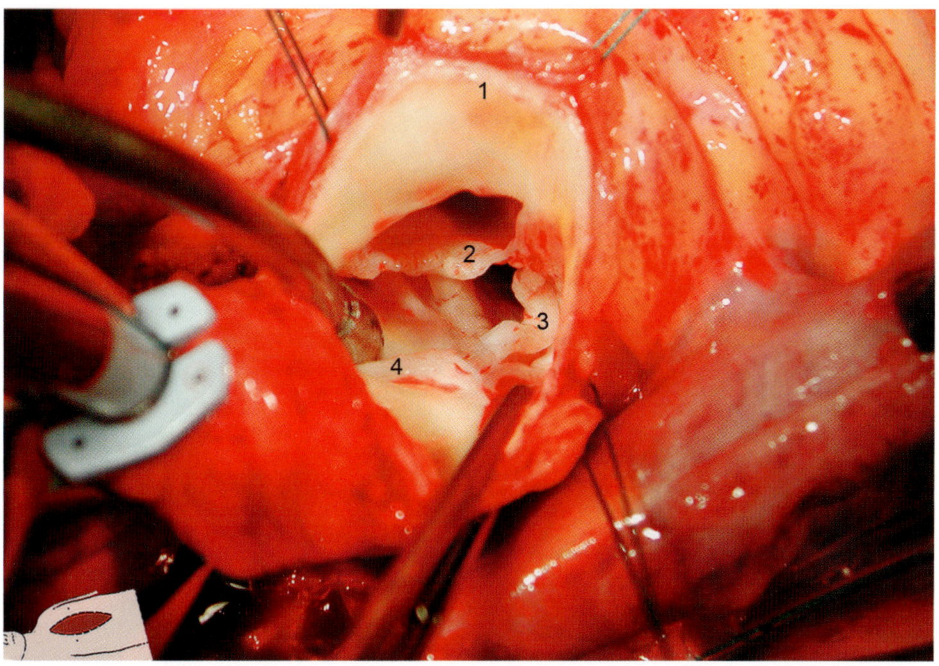

Figure 20.9. Rheumatic heart disease in a 12-year-old child. The aortic valve is seen through an aortotomy. The leaflets are thickened with poor excursion. The left coronary cusp is adherent to the aortic wall.

1. Aortotomy incision
2. Right coronary leaflet
3. Noncoronary leaflet
4. Left coronary leaflet

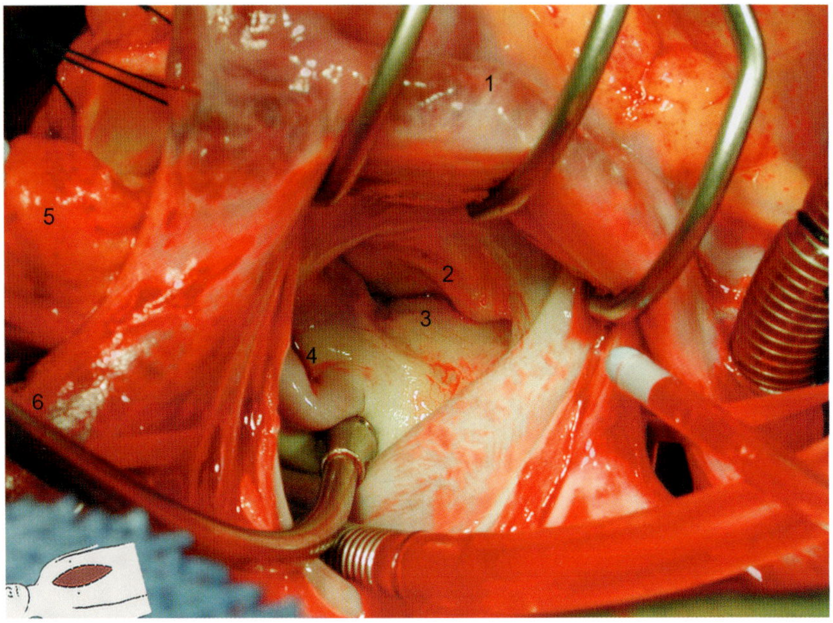

Figure 20.10. Left atriotomy of the same patient shown in Figure 20.9. The mitral valve is shown. It has relatively better coaptation than the aortic valve. The leaflets, however, are thickened and degenerated, as further shown in Figure 20.11.

1. Right atrium
2. Anterior leaflet of mitral valve
3. Posterior leaflet of mitral valve
4. Opening of LAA
5. Ascending aorta
6. Superior vena cava (SVC)

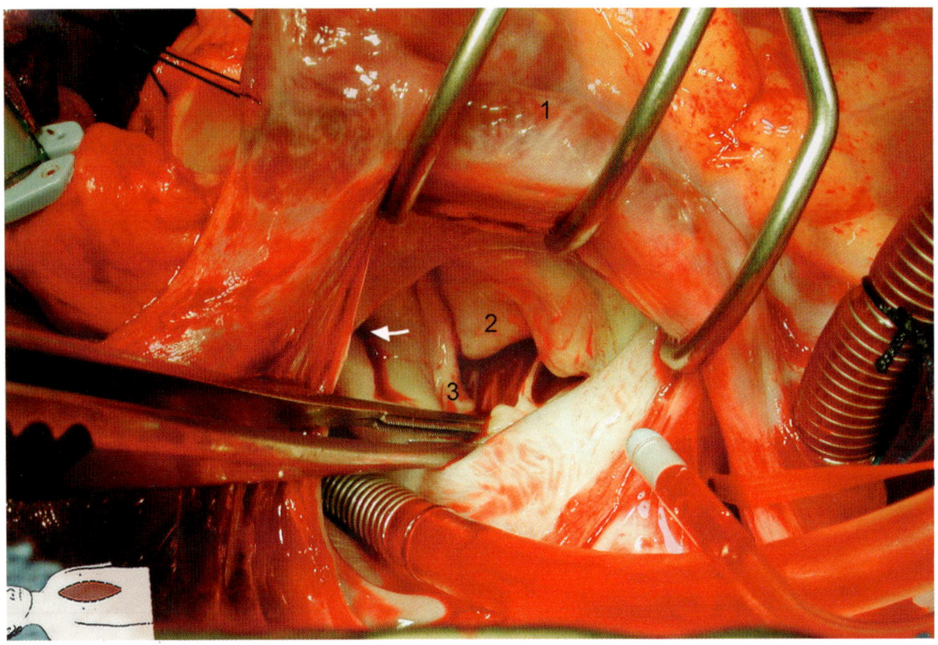

Figure 20.11. The same patient as in Figures 20.9 and 20.10. Note the thickened, degenerated mitral valve leaflets. The arrow points to the opening of the LAA.

1. Right atrium
2. Anterior leaflet of mitral valve
3. Posterior leaflet of mitral valve

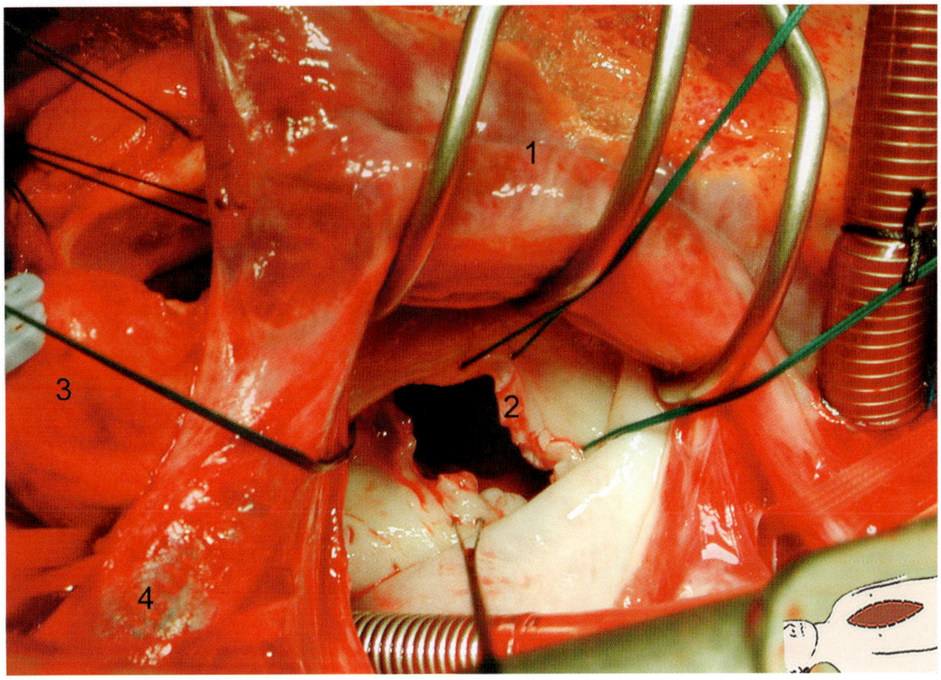

Figure 20.12. The same patient as in Figures 20.9 to 20.11 after resection of the mitral valve.

1. Right atrium
2. Remnants of mitral valve
3. Ascending aorta
4. SVC

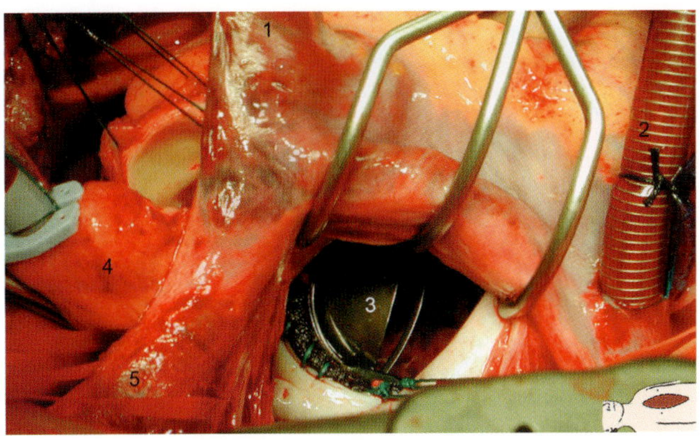

Figure 20.13

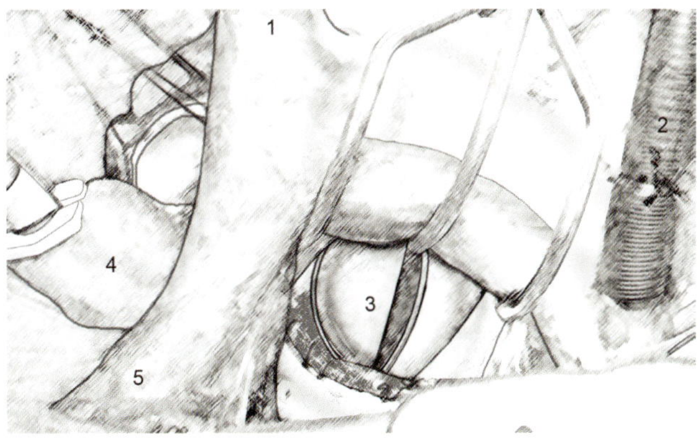

Figure 20.14

The same patient as in Figures 20.9 to 20.12. A mechanical valve (Sorin Bicarbon Fitline, 25 mm) has been implanted in the mitral valve position.

1. Right atrium
2. Inferior vena cava cannula
3. Mechanical mitral valve (Sorin Bicarbon Fitline, 25 mm)
4. Ascending aorta
5. SVC

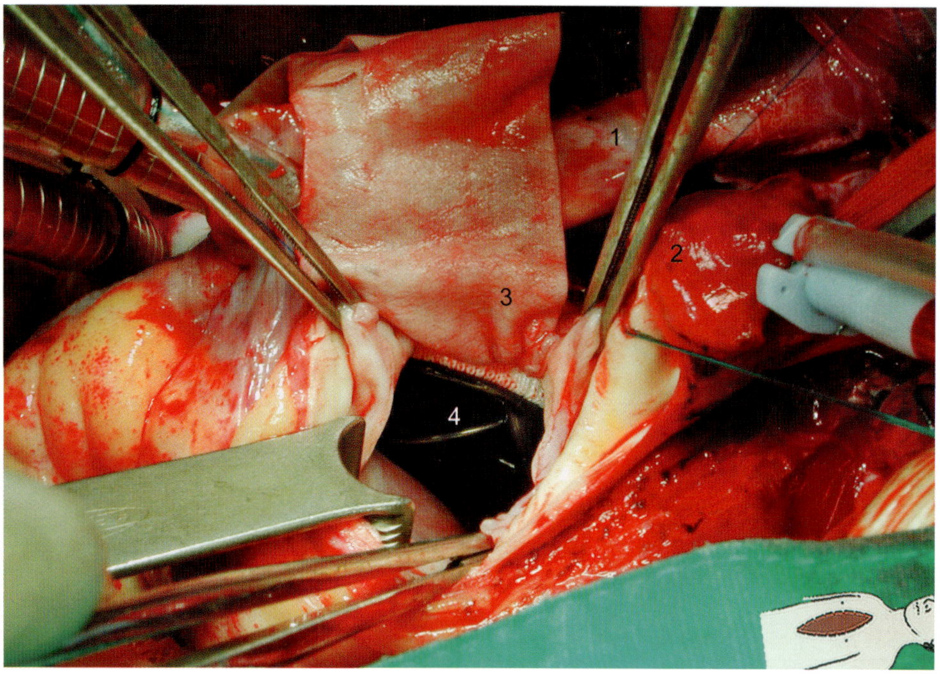

Figure 20.15. Median sternotomy view of a 9-year-old child, shown from the left side of the patient. An aortotomy incision was made, and an incision was made between the left and noncoronary sinuses and extended through the area of fibrous continuity between the aortic and mitral valves and the anterior leaflet of the mitral valve. A xenograft pericardial patch was then inserted to enlarge both annuli. A mechanical mitral valve has been inserted as shown, and an aortic valve will also be inserted to complete the procedure. See Figures 20.16 and 20.17 for diagrammatic illustrations.

1. SVC
2. Ascending aorta
3. Xenograft pericardial patch
4. Mechanical mitral valve

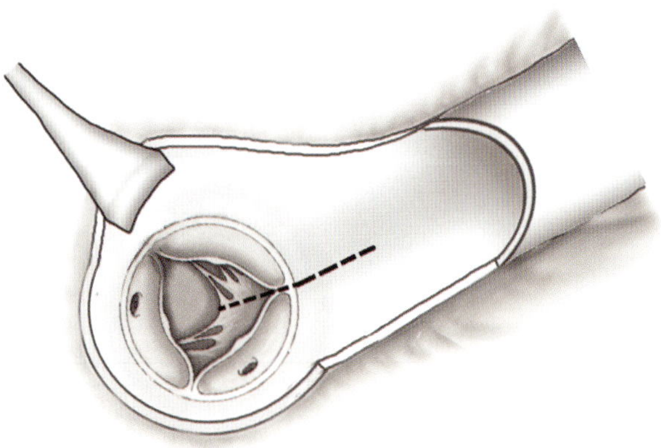

Figure 20.16

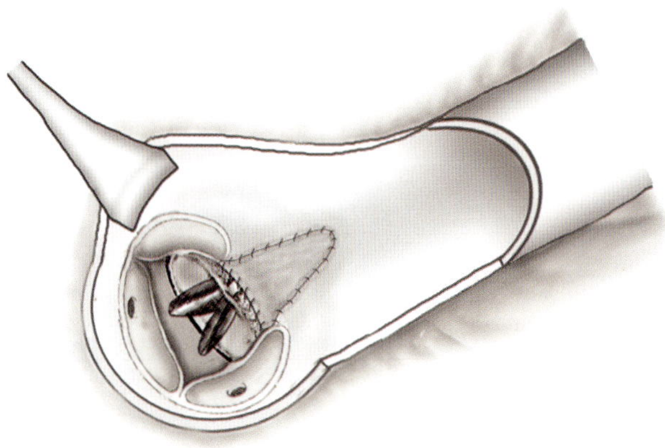

Figure 20.17

Aortic-mitral double annulus enlargement procedure with attendant valve replacement. An incision is made in the aortic annulus and extended through the area of fibrous continuity between the aortic and mitral valves into the anterior leaflet of the mitral valve. A xenograft pericardial patch is then inserted to enlarge both annuli. A mechanical mitral valve is inserted as shown, and an aortic valve will also be inserted to complete the procedure.

Figure 20.18. An explanted mechanical valve from a 6-year-old child who had mechanical valve dysfunction. This is a tilting single-disk valve (Bjork Shiley). The picture shows a fairly normal-looking valve when viewed from the left ventricular aspect.

1. Valve ring
2. Tilting disk
3. Teflon pledget
4. Strut holding the disk

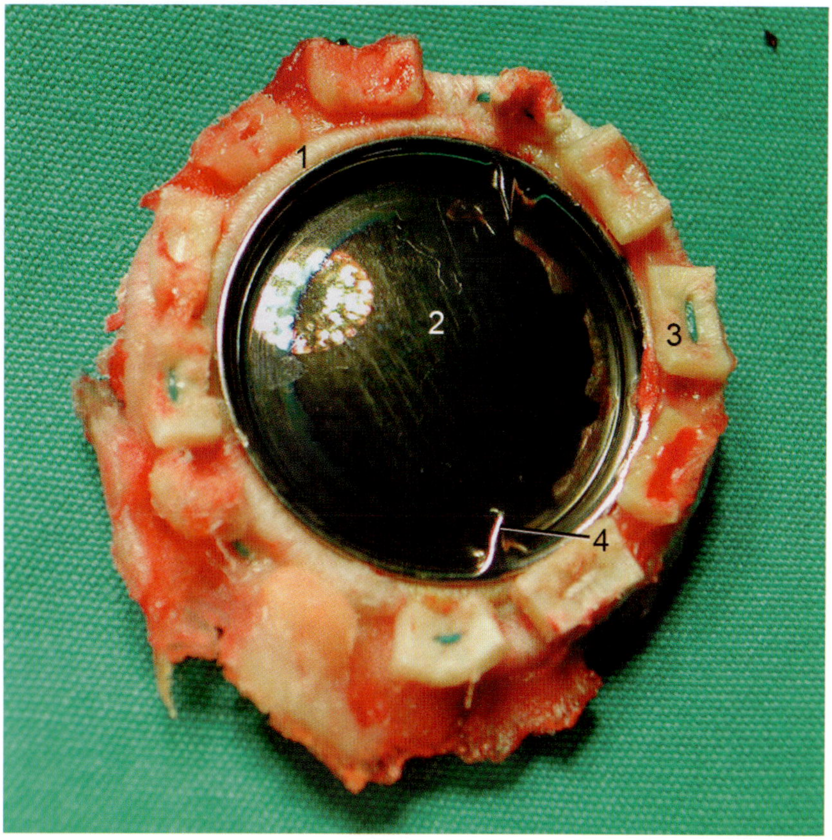

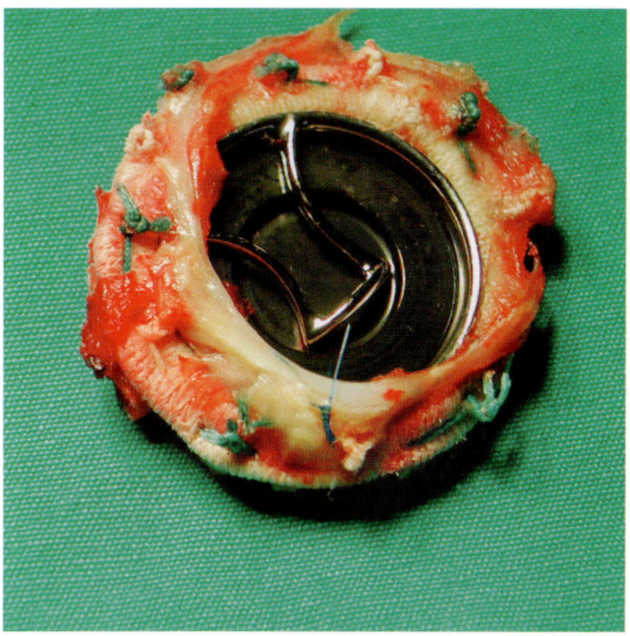

Figure 20.19

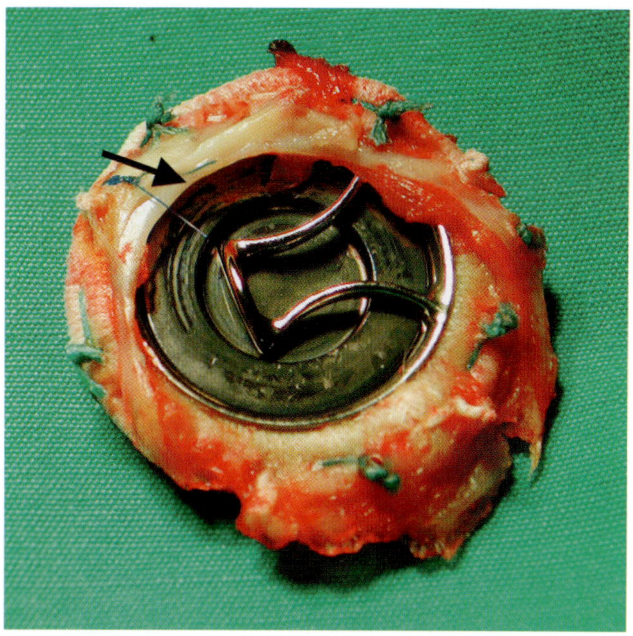

Figure 20.20

The atrial aspect of the same valve as shown in Figure 20.18. The arrow in Figure 20.20 points to the abnormal tissue formation (pannus) that caused valve dysfunction by impeding the movement of the disk. This resulted in mitral stenosis.

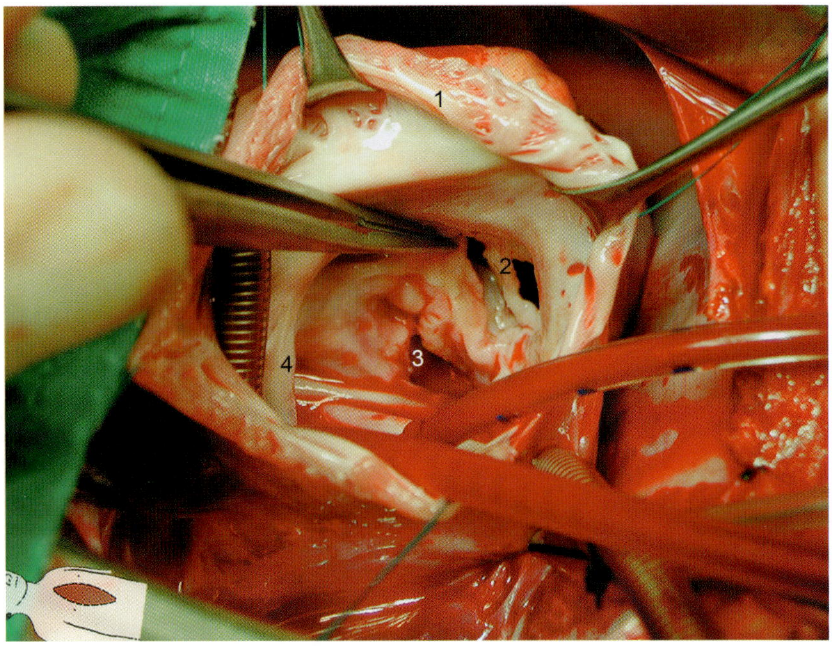

Figure 20.21. Right atriotomy view of a 1-year-old child with partial AVSD. The left AV valve is seen through the primum ASD. Note the "cleft" in the left valve. The right AV valve is also abnormal and is further shown in Figure 20.22.

1. Right atrial wall
2. Right AV valve
3. Left AV valve
4. Edge of primum ASD

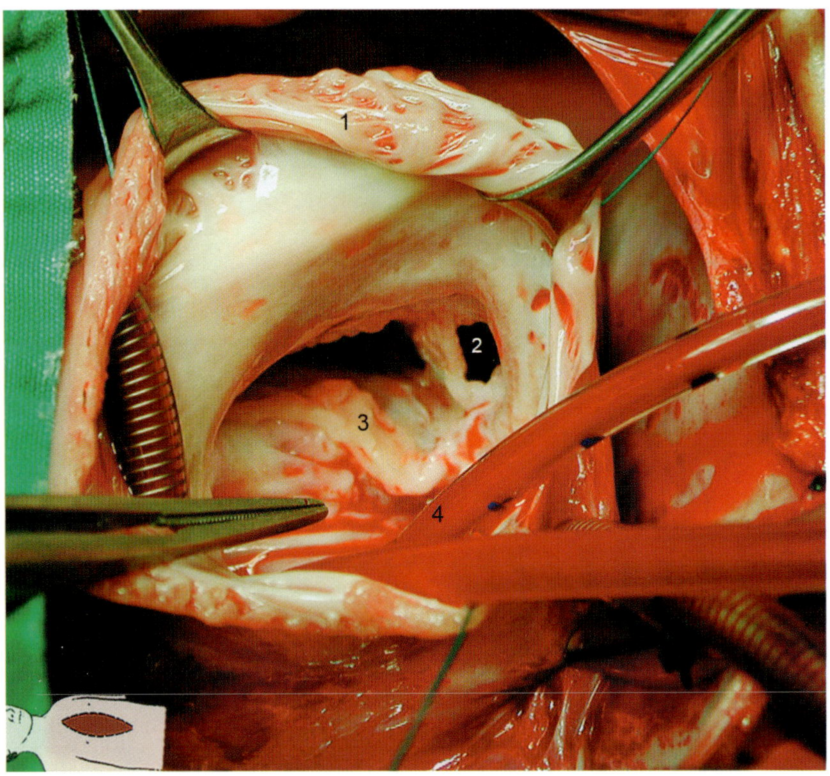

Figure 20.22. The same patient as in Figure 20.21. Note the accessory orifice in the right component of the AV valve caused by a bridge of tissue between adjacent leaflets.

1. Right atrial wall
2. "Fenestration" between inferior bridging and right inferior leaflets of right AV valve
3. Fused superior and inferior bridging leaflets of right AV valve
4. Suction catheter in left atrium

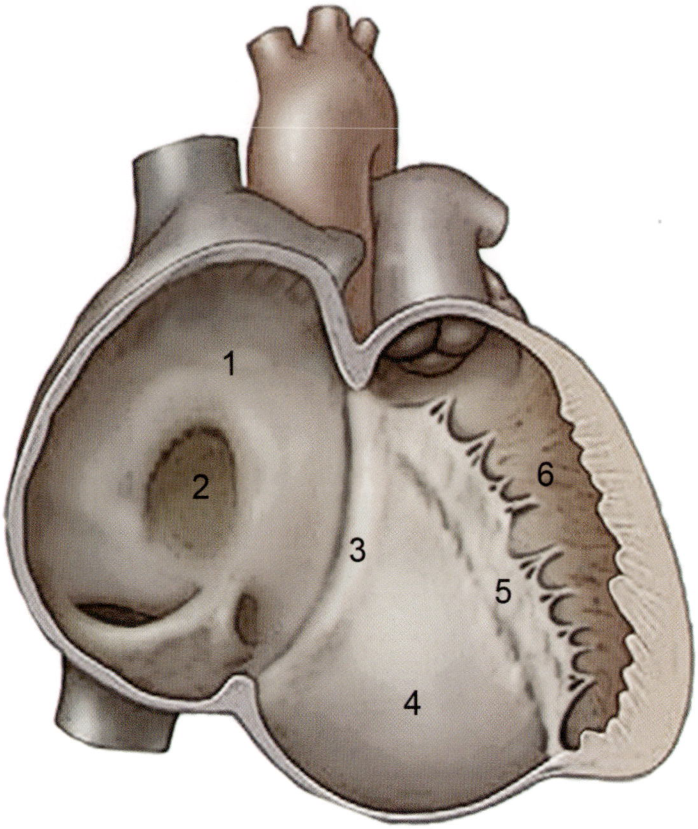

Figure 20.23. Diagrammatic illustration of Ebstein anomaly of the tricuspid valve. The septal and posterior leaflets are displaced into the RV, resulting in a small functional RV. The tricuspid valve is usually incompetent, and the right atrium is massively dilated.

1. Right atrium
2. ASD
3. Level of right AV junction where the tricuspid annulus normally inserts
4. "Atrialized portion" of RV
5. Displaced tricuspid valve leaflet
6. Functional RV

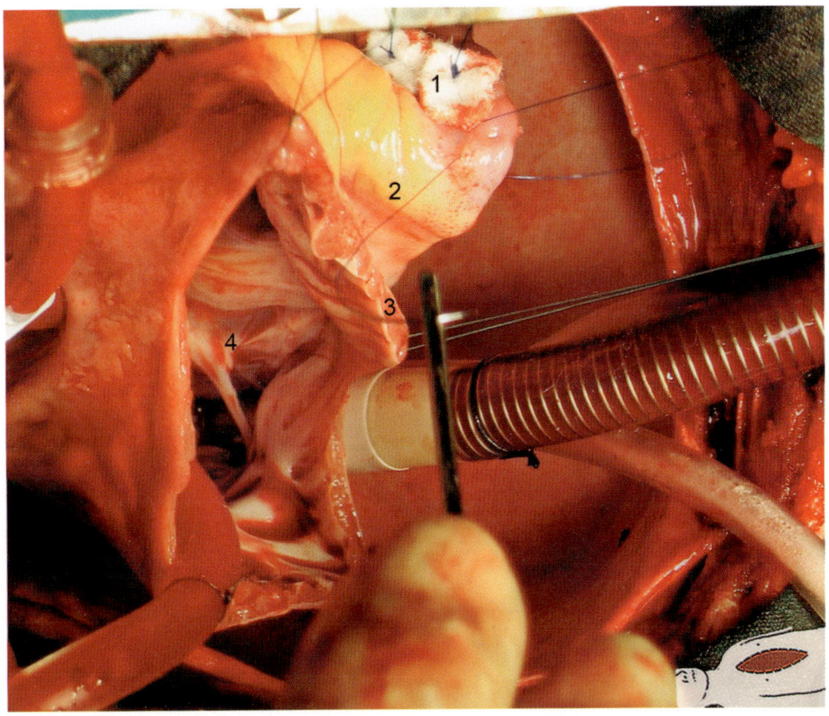

Figure 20.24. Median sternotomy view of a 7-year-old child with Ebstein anomaly of the tricuspid valve. The atrialized portion of the RV has been plicated with pledget-supported sutures, visible here on the external aspect of the heart.

1. Teflon pledgets supporting the sutures used in plication
2. Atrialized RV
3. Right atriotomy
4. Tricuspid valve

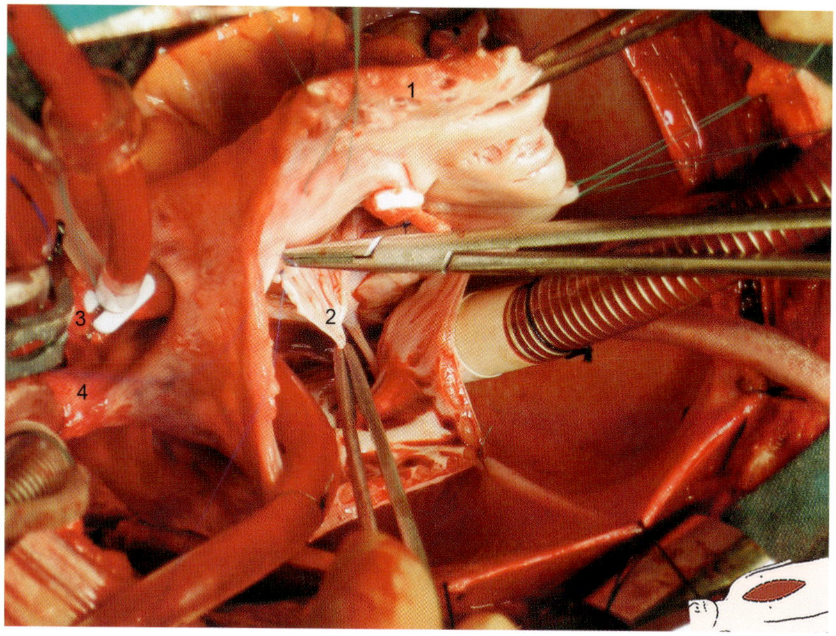

Figure 20.25. The same patient as in Figure 20.24. The internal aspect of the atrialized RV is seen. The tricuspid valve is displaced toward the apex of the RV.

1. Right atriotomy
2. Anterior leaflet of tricuspid valve
3. Ascending aorta
4. SVC

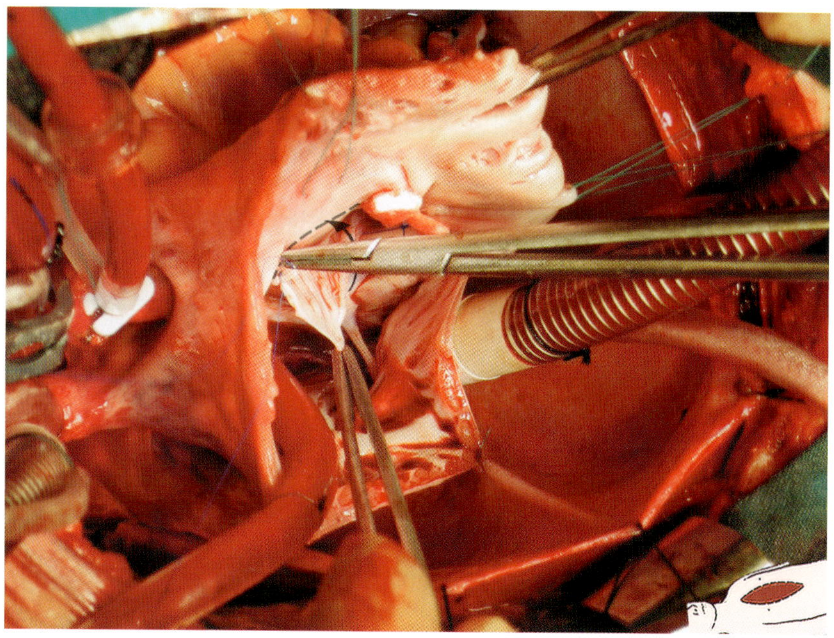

Figure 20.26. The same photo as in Figure 20.25, marked with the target site to which the anterior leaflet will be transferred.

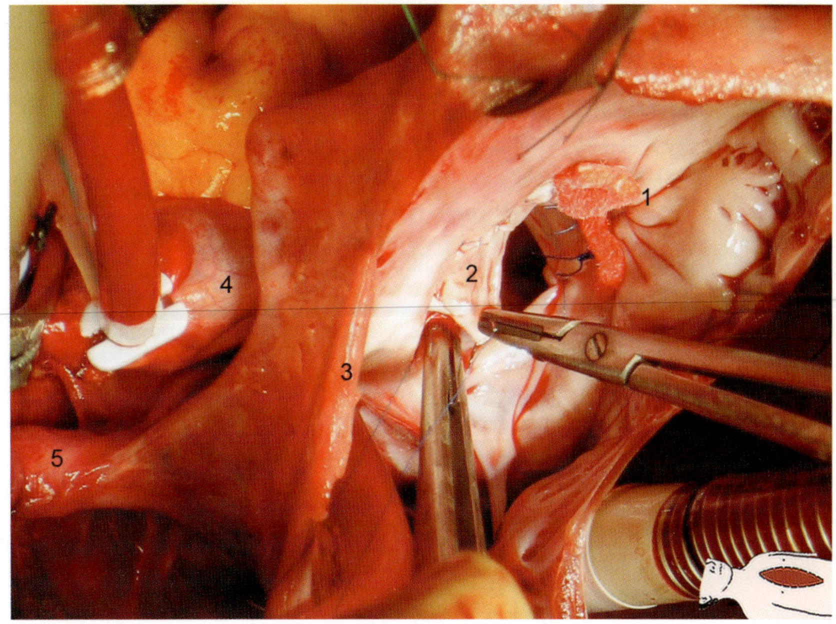

Figure 20.27. The same patient as in Figures 20.24 to 20.26 after transferring the anterior leaflet to its new location.

1. Corrugation at site of plication of atrialized RV
2. Relocated anterior leaflet of tricuspid valve
3. Right atrium wall
4. Ascending aorta
5. SVC

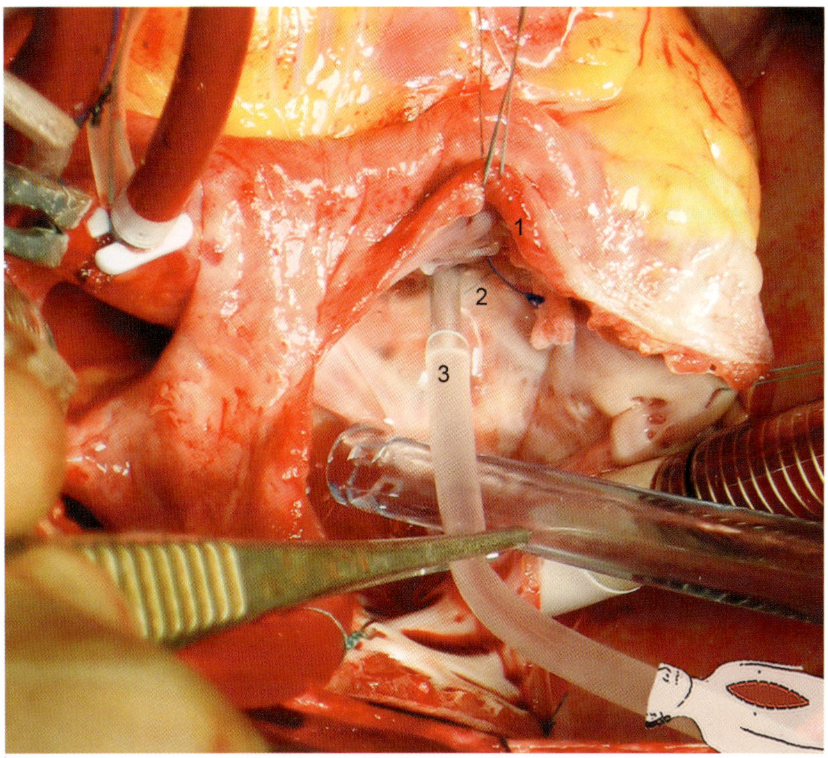

Figure 20.28. The same patient as in Figures 20.24 to 20.27. Competence of the repaired tricuspid valve is being tested by injecting saline solution in the RV.

1. Right atriotomy incision
2. Tricuspid valve
3. Catheter injecting saline into the RV

REFERENCES

1. Zalzstein E, Hamilton R, Zucker N, Levitas A, Gross G. Presentation, natural history, and outcome in children and adolescents with double orifice mitral valve. *Am J Cardiol.* 2004;93:1067–1069.
2. Caldas I, Terreri M, Moises V, et al. What is the true frequency of carditis in acute rheumatic fever? A prospective clinical and Doppler blind study of 56 children with up to 60 months of follow-up evaluation. *Pediatr Cardiol.* 2008;29:1048–1053.
3. Manouguian S, Kirchhoff P. Patch enlargement of the aortic and the mitral valve rings with aortic-mitral double-valve replacement. *Ann Thorac Surg.* 1980;30:396–399.
4. Carpentier A, Chauvaud S, Mace L, et al. A new reconstructive operation for Ebstein's anomaly of the tricuspid valve. *Thorac Cardiovasc Surg.* 1988;96:92–101.
5. Al-Najashi KS, Balint OH, Oechslin E. Mid-term outcomes in adults with Ebstein anomaly and cavopulmonary shunts. *Ann Thorac Surg.* 2009;88:131–136.

CHAPTER 21

Coronary Artery Abnormalities

CORONARY ARTERY FISTULA

Coronary artery fistula is an abnormal communication between the coronary artery system and one of the cardiac chambers or the large vessels close to the heart. Because of the multitude of possible connections, the anatomy can vary considerably. Most commonly, the right coronary artery is involved and the communication is with right-sided cardiac structures.[1]

Symptoms most commonly arise from volume overload, usually on the left ventricle (LV), and myocardial ischemia from coronary artery steal.[2]

Most fistulas are amenable to catheter-based coil occlusion.[3] The other option is surgical closure. Figure 21.1 shows a fistulous communication between the right coronary artery and the pulmonary artery (PA). Interestingly, this heart has a rather deep interventricular groove, creating a bifid apex (Figure 21.2). Fistulas tend to enlarge with time and may become quite dilated and tortuous, as shown in Figures 21.3 to 21.5 in an adult patient who presented with chest pain. The distal end of the fistula opened into the coronary sinus (CS): a coronary arteriovenous fistula. The opening was closed and the fistula was ligated at multiple sites.

MISCELLANEOUS CORONARY ARTERY ABNORMALITIES

Various coronary artery abnormalities are encountered in the field of pediatric cardiology, often in association with congenital heart disease. Some of these abnormalities, as well as variations in normal anatomy, have been discussed in chapters 13 and 15. We will present here some other examples.

Figures 21.6 to 21.13 show a ventricular septal aneurysm arising from a perforating branch of the left anterior descending (LAD) coronary artery. The LAD itself is massively enlarged. The cavity of the aneurysm was obliterated by suturing together its walls. Figure 21.14 shows a small aneurysm at the origin of the right coronary artery, found incidentally during surgery for ventricular septal defect (VSD).

An aortic-ventricular tunnel is an abnormal communication between the aorta and one of the ventricles, usually the left. While it is not a coronary artery abnormality, an aortoventricular tunnel is closely related to the coronary arteries as it originates just above the aortic sinus of Valsalva and may run along the course of a coronary artery, as shown in Figures 21.15 and 21.16.

An intramural coronary artery runs within the wall of the aorta for a distance before exiting the aorta. It is prone to compression and can lead to myocardial ischemia.[4] An example is shown in Figures 21.17 and 21.18. This patient was treated by unroofing the intramural segment of the coronary artery.

ANOMALOUS LEFT CORONARY ARTERY FROM THE PULMONARY ARTERY (ALCAPA)

This is an uncommon congenital anomaly that compromises the left coronary artery system, resulting in left ventricular ischemia, myocardial infarction, mitral regurgitation, and dilated poorly contractile LV. Symptoms usually appear at about 2 to 3 months of age after PA pressure drops. Surgery is indicated once the diagnosis is made. Many surgical techniques can

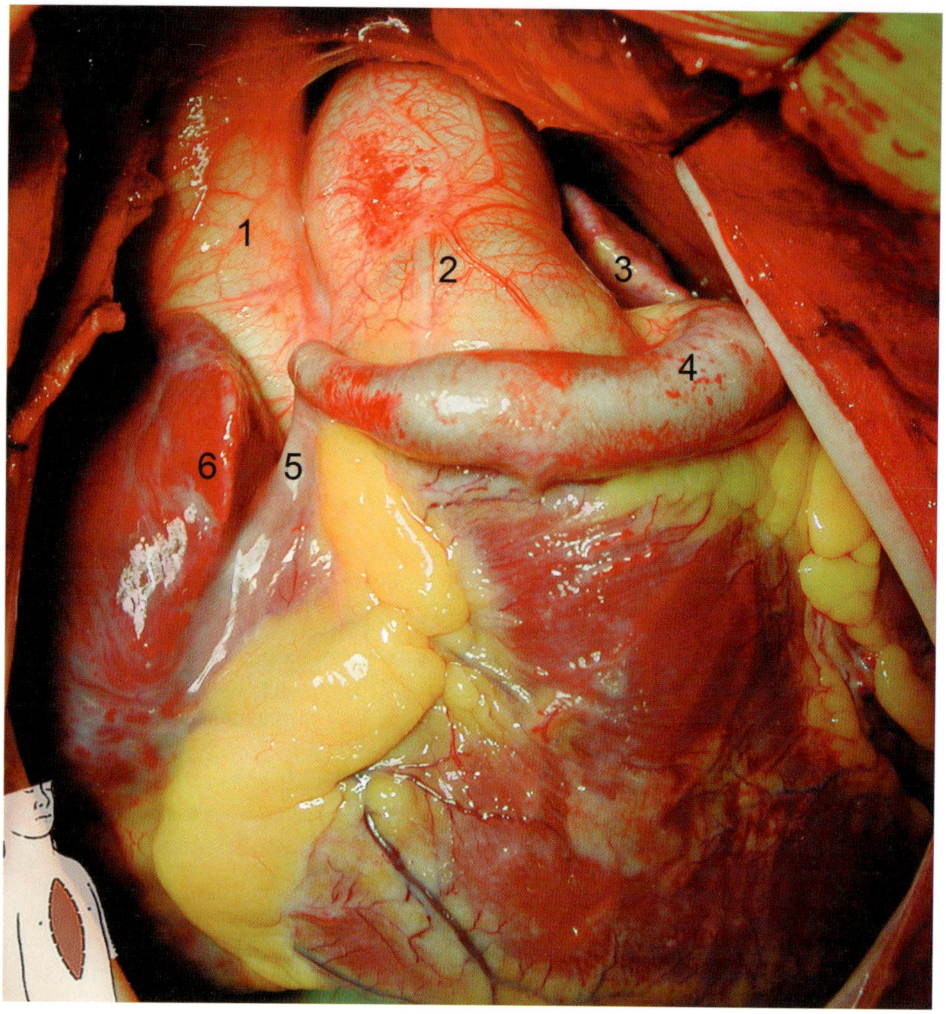

Figure 21.1. Median sternotomy view of a 5-year-old child with coronary artery fistula. The right coronary artery communicates with the PA.

1. Ascending aorta
2. Main pulmonary artery (MPA)
3. Left atrial appendage (LAA)
4. Fistula between right coronary artery and PA
5. Right coronary artery
6. Right atrial appendage (RAA)

be used to repair this anomaly, including coronary artery transfer, bypass grafting, and intrapulmonary tunneling.[5]

Figures 21.19 to 21.28 are intraoperative pictures of an infant who has ALCAPA. The anomalous left coronary artery arises from the posterior-facing sinus of the pulmonary valve. The coronary artery was transferred with a button of pulmonary wall to its new location on the aorta. This is similar to the technique used during coronary artery transfer for transposition of the great arteries.

An intrapulmonary tunnel is another procedure used to treat ALCAPA that was initially described by Takeuchi et al.[6] It may be preferable when coronary artery transfer is not easy, for example, when the left coronary artery arises from the PA at its farthest point from the aorta. Figure 21.29 is a diagrammatic illustration of this technique. Figure 21.30 is from a 1-year-old infant who presented with mitral valve regurgitation and was found to have ALCAPA. She was treated with an intrapulmonary tunnel, as shown in Figures 21.31 to 21.38.

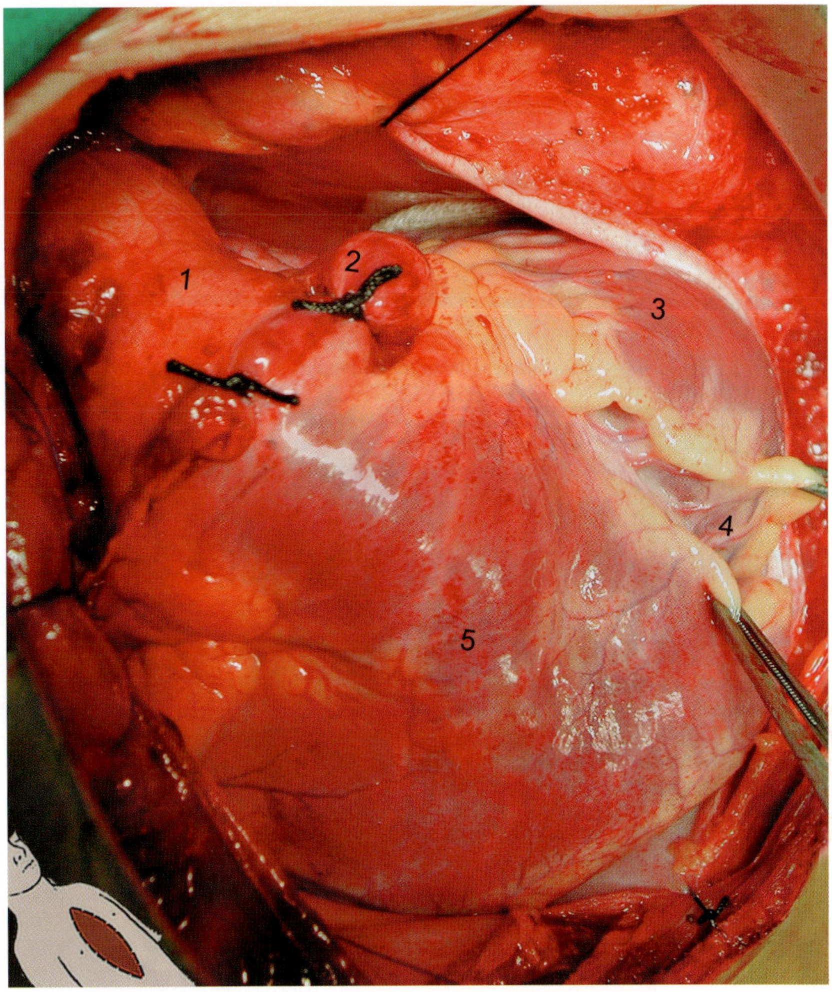

Figure 21.2. The same patient as in Figure 21.1 after ligation of the fistula between the right coronary artery and the PA. Note the deep groove between the ventricles, creating a bifid apex.

1. MPA
2. Ligated fistula
3. LV
4. Deep groove between LV and right ventricle (RV)
5. RV

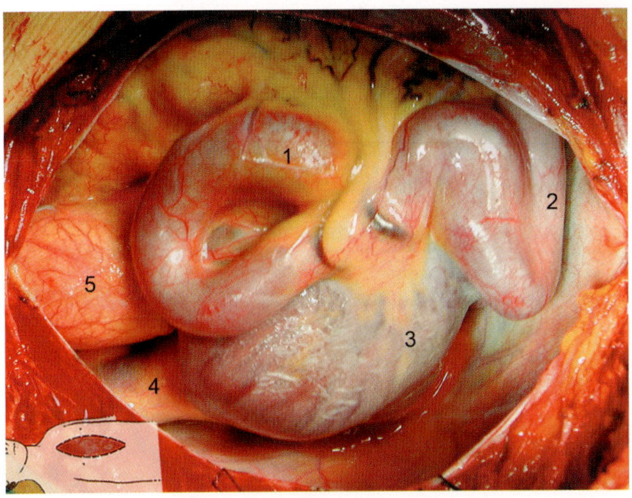

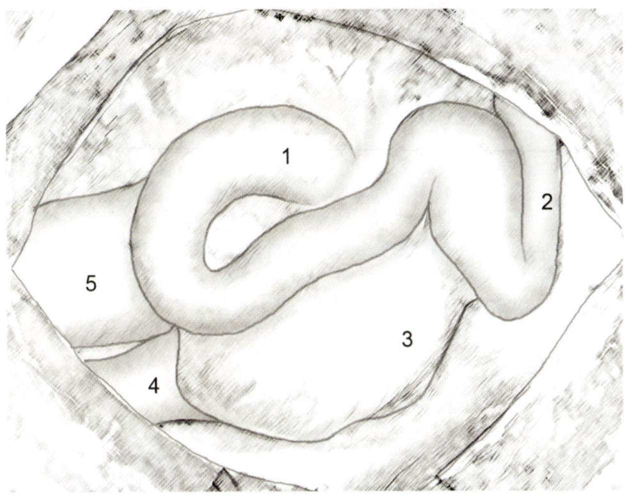

Figure 21.3 **Figure 21.4**

A median sternotomy view of a 30-year-old patient with a large right coronary artery fistula that drains into the CS. Note the massively dilated, tortuous coronary artery.

1. Right coronary artery
2. Distal end of artery (eventually drains to CS)
3. Right atrium
4. Superior vena cava (SVC)
5. Ascending aorta

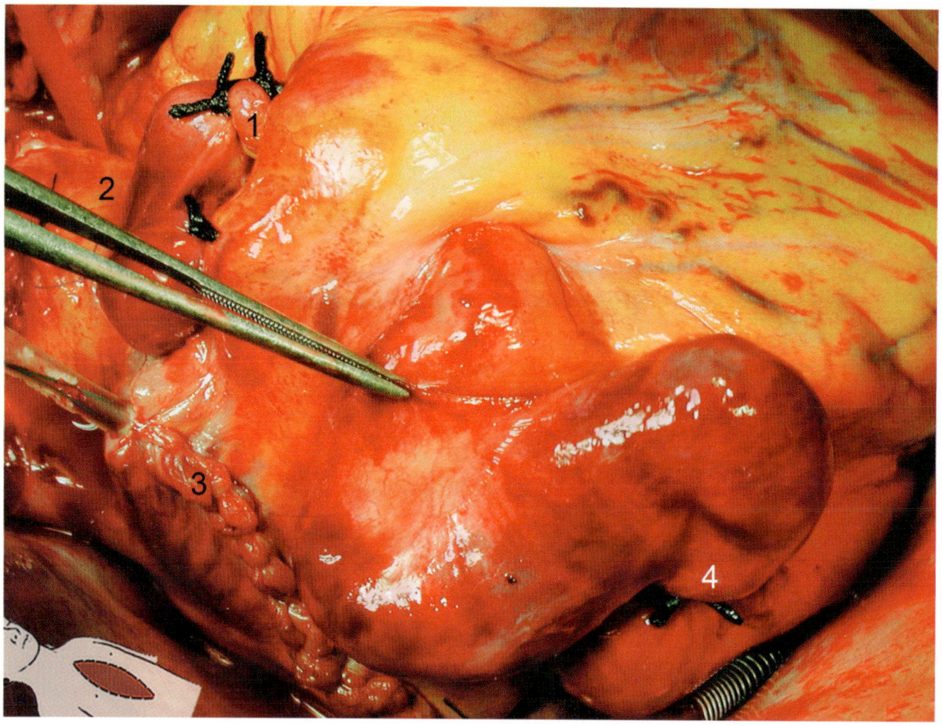

Figure 21.5. The same patient as in Figure 21.3 after ligation of the fistula. The opening into the CS was closed via right atriotomy.

1. Right coronary artery
2. Ascending aorta
3. Right atriotomy
4. Dilated tortuous right coronary artery

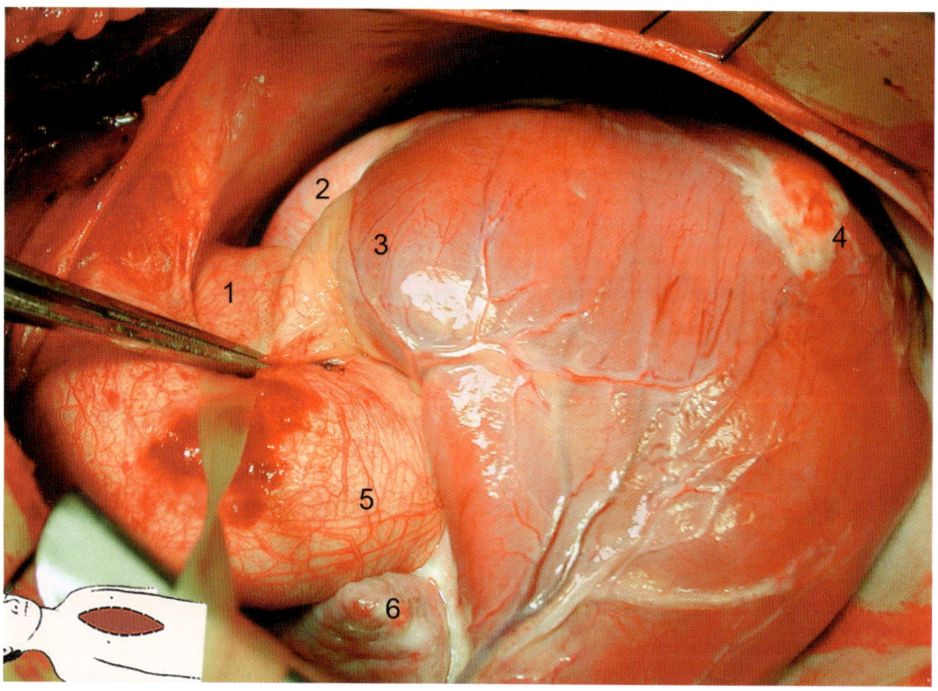

Figure 21.6. Median sternotomy view of a 5-year-old infant with a coronary artery aneurysm arising from a septal branch of the LAD. The LAD is dilated and the aneurysm itself (4) is seen making a bulge close to the apex.

1. MPA
2. LAD coronary artery
3. RV outflow
4. Bulge made by underlying aneurysm
5. Ascending aorta
6. RAA

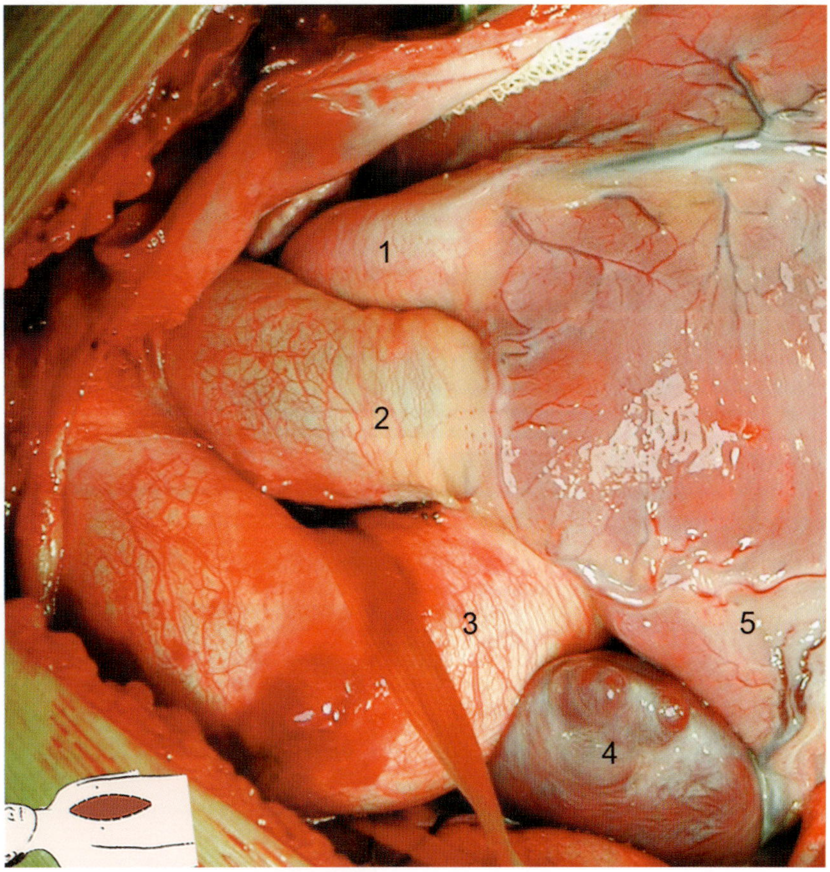

Figure 21.7. The same patient as in Figure 21.6. Note the massively dilated proximal part of the LAD.

1. LAD coronary artery
2. MPA
3. Ascending aorta
4. RAA
5. RV

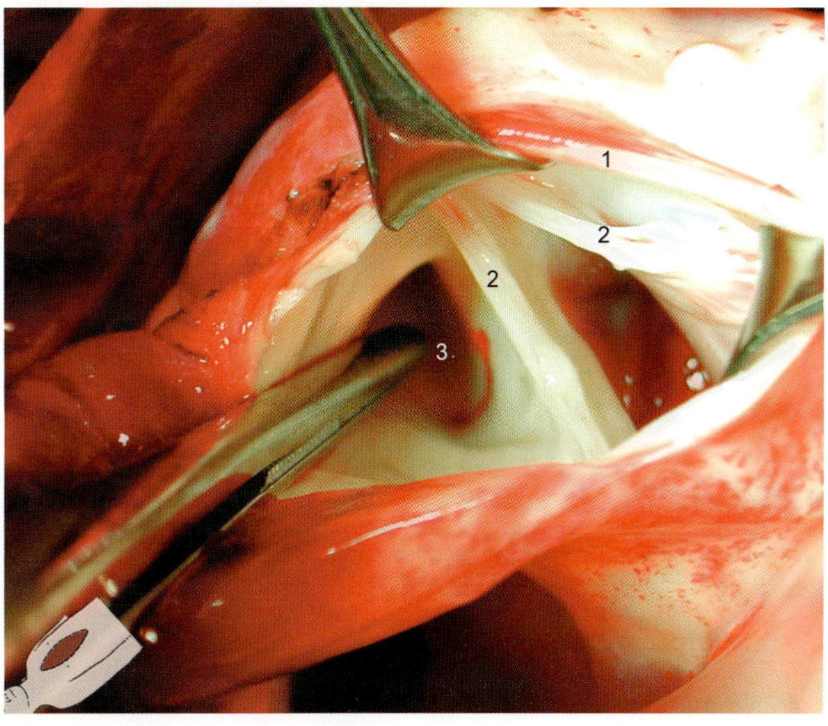

Figure 21.8. An aortotomy view of the same patient shown in Figures 21.6 and 21.7. The orifice of the left coronary artery is dilated.

1. Aortotomy incision
2. Aortic valve leaflets
3. Orifice of left coronary artery

Figure 21.9. The same patient as in Figures 21.6 to 21.8. The aneurysm in the interventricular septum has been opened.

1. Apex
2. LAD coronary artery
3. Proximal part of LAD
4. Interventricular septal aneurysm
5. RV
6. RAA
7. Aortotomy incision

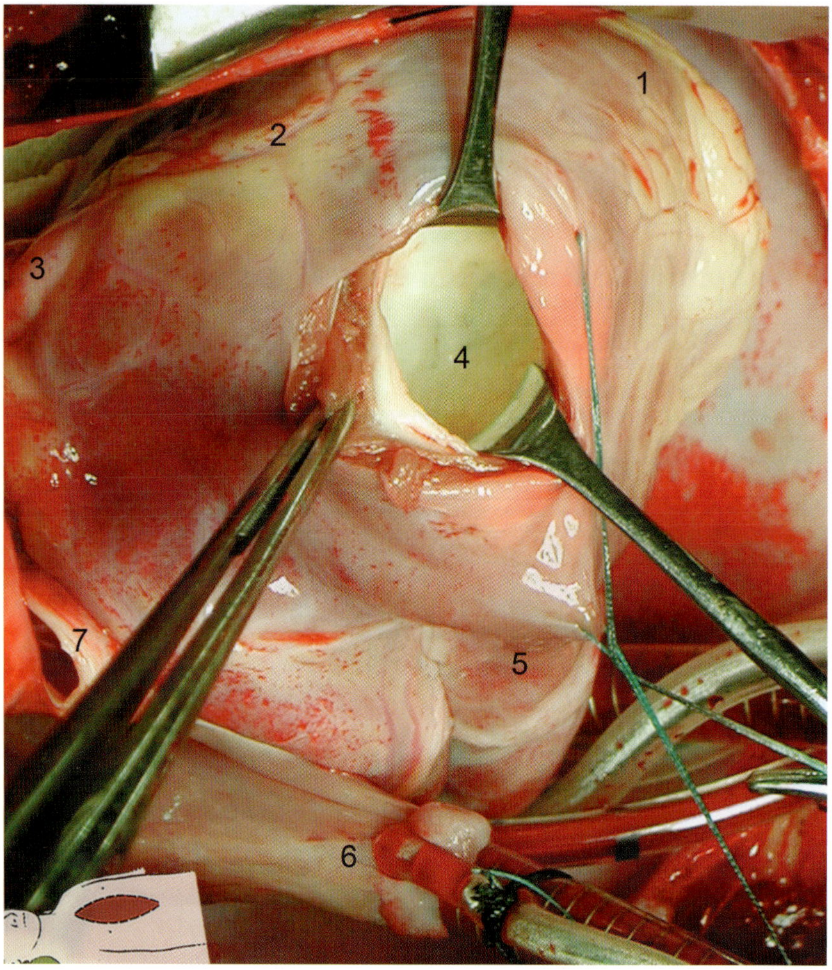

Figure 21.10. The same patient as in Figures 21.6 to 21.9. The camera is oriented superiorly to show the upper part of the aneurysm. The arrow points to the orifice of the artery feeding the aneurysm.

1. Wall of the aneurysm
2. Aortotomy incision

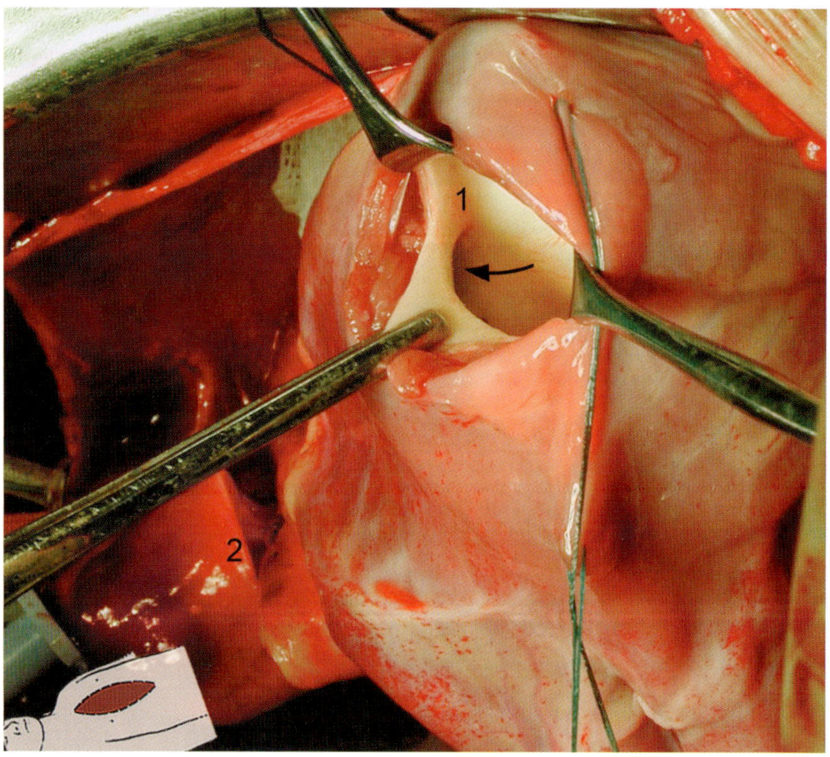

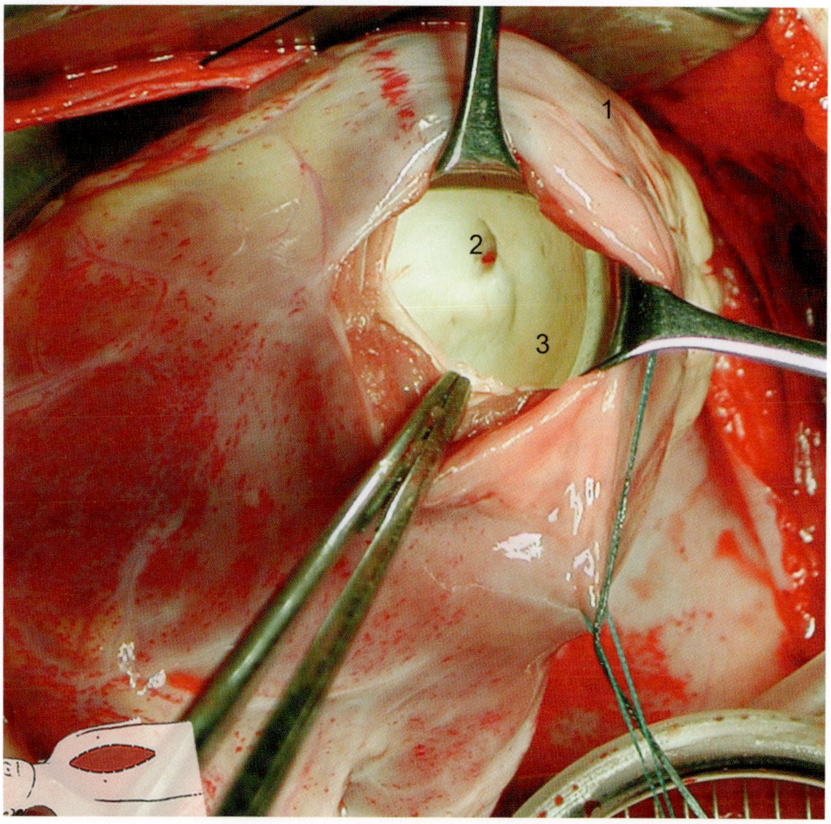

Figure 21.11. The same patient as in Figures 21.6 to 21.10. The camera is oriented inferiorly to show the caudal part of the aneurysm.

1. Apex
2. A coronary artery branch
3. Body of the aneurysm

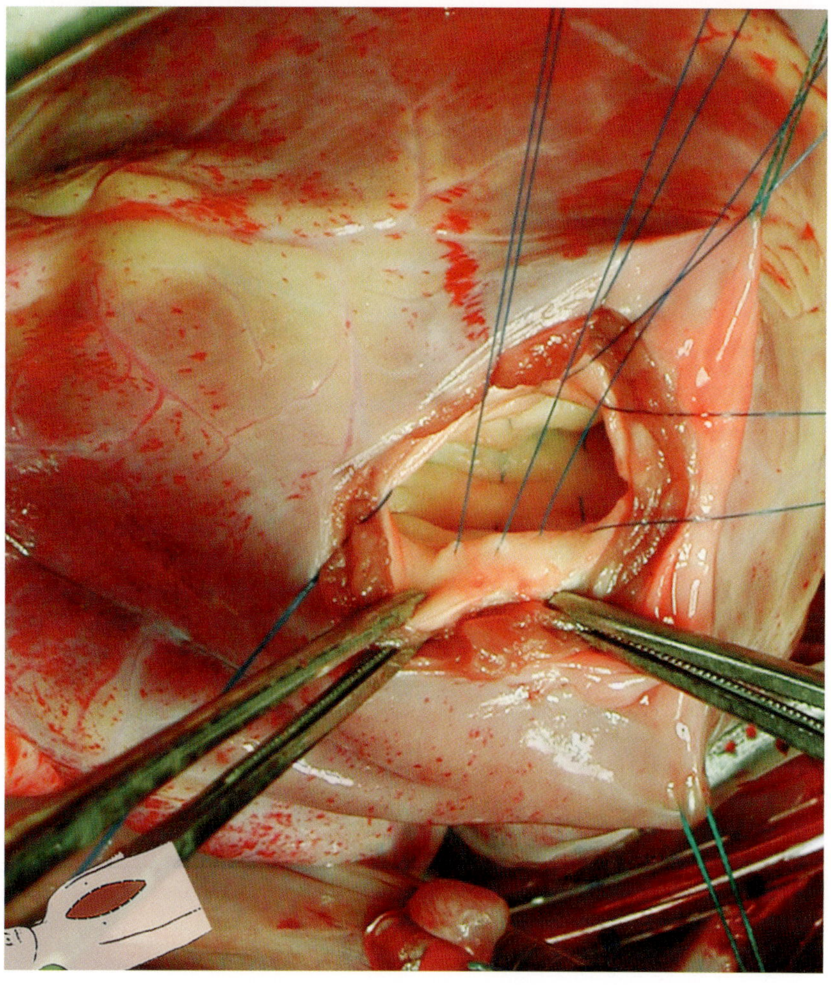

Figure 21.12. The same patient as in Figures 21.6 to 21.11. Sutures have been placed in the walls of the aneurysm.

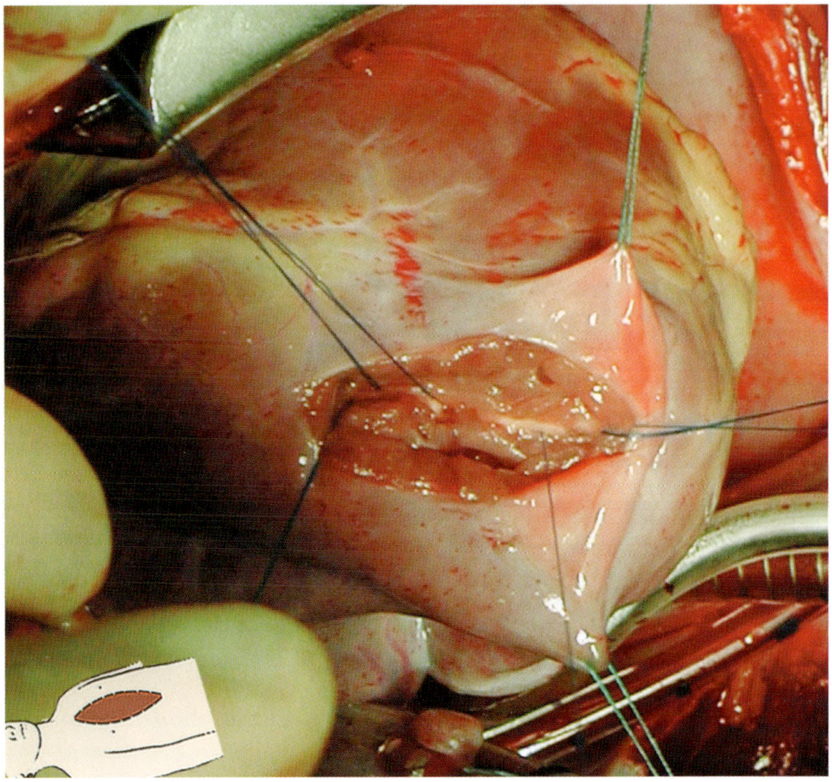

Figure 21.13. The same patient as in Figures 21.6 to 21.12. The sutures have been tightened, thus obliterating the cavity of the aneurysm.

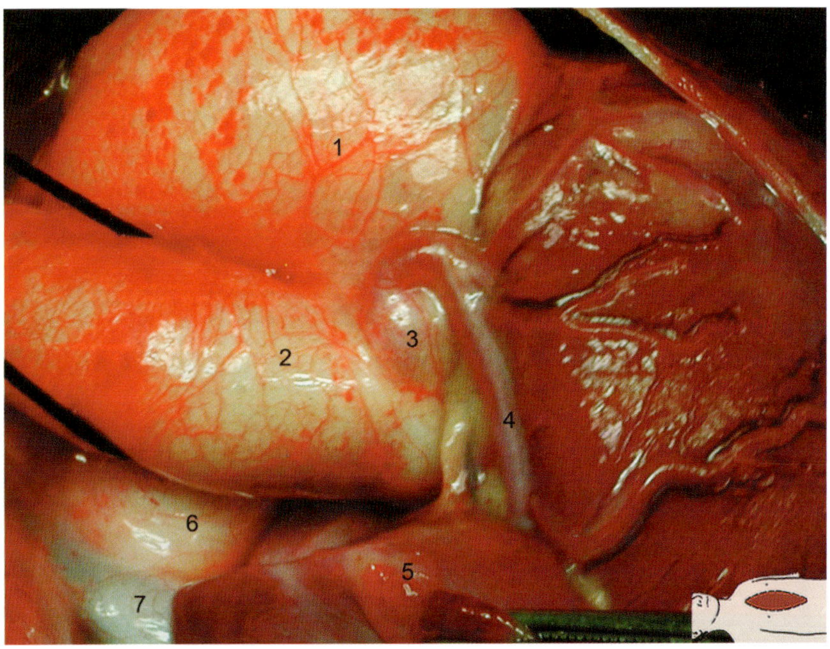

Figure 21.14. Median sternotomy view of a 4-month-old infant, operated on for closure of 2 VSDs. Incidentally, the right coronary artery is found to have an aneurysm at its origin. Note the dilated main (1) and right (6) pulmonary arteries as a result of left-to-right shunting across the VSD.

1. MPA
2. Ascending aorta
3. Right coronary artery aneurysm
4. Right coronary artery
5. RAA
6. Right PA
7. SVC

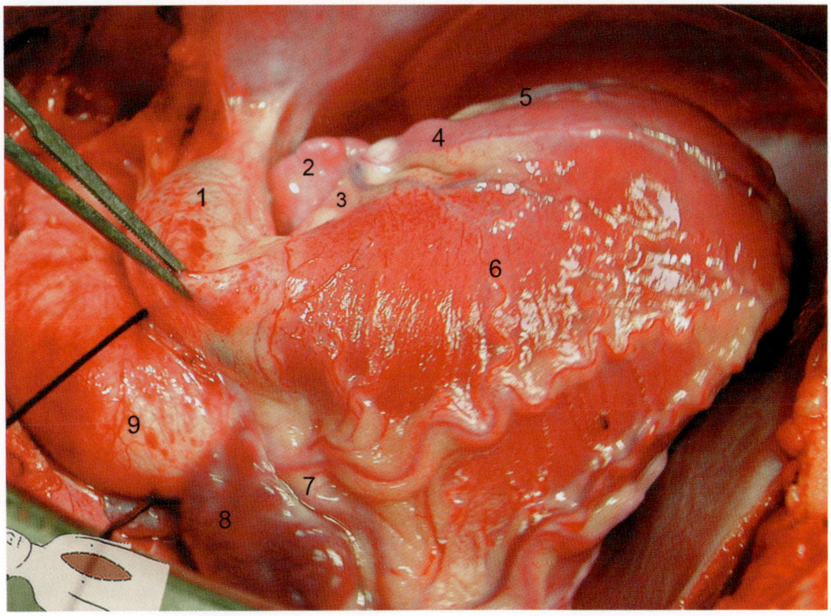

Figure 21.15. Median sternotomy view of a 10-month-old infant with an aorta-to-RV tunnel. It originates from the left sinus of Valsalva and runs alongside the LAD.

1. MPA
2. LAA
3. Left coronary artery
4. Bulge overlying the tunnel
5. LAD coronary artery
6. RV
7. Right coronary artery
8. RAA
9. Ascending aorta

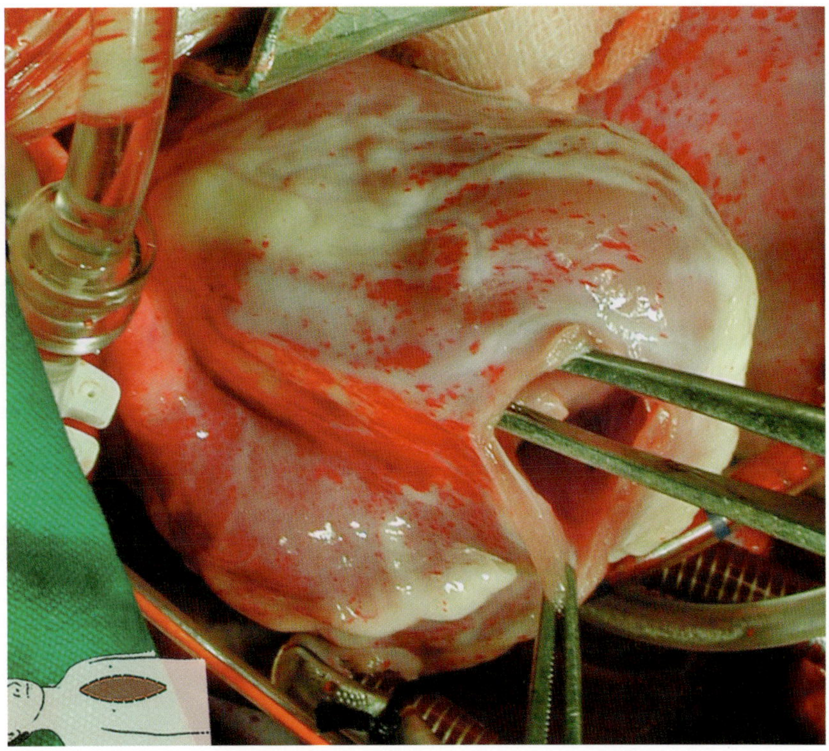

Figure 21.16. The same patient as in Figure 21.15. A right ventriculotomy has been performed to close the tunnel from within the RV cavity.

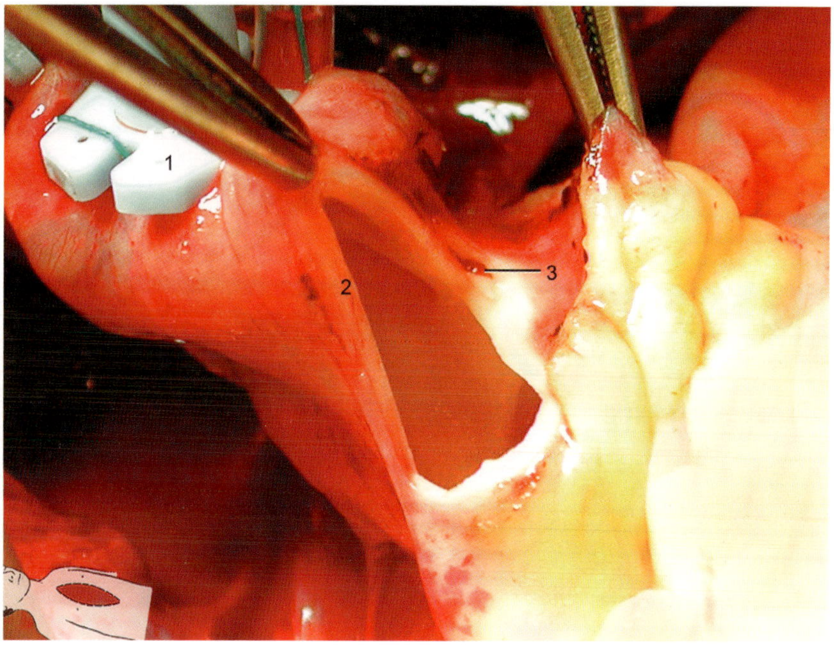

Figure 21.17. Median sternotomy view of a 9-year-old child with subaortic stenosis. The right coronary artery was intramural. It has an unusually high take-off from the ascending aorta, well above the sinus of Valsalva and above the sinotubular junction, so it was accidentally cut during aortotomy.

1. Cardioplegia catheter
2. Aortotomy incision
3. Intramural right coronary artery

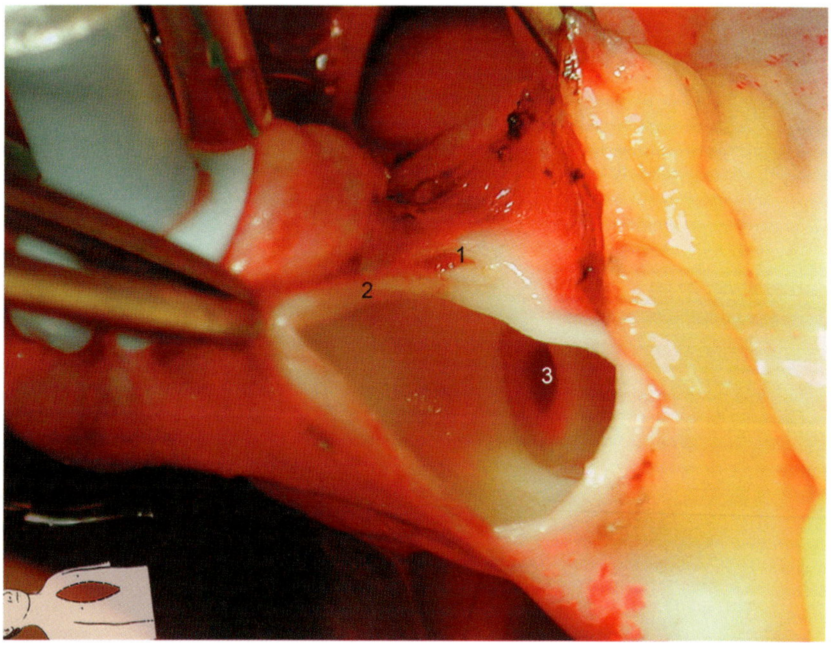

Figure 21.18. Another view of the same patient shown in Figure 21.17. The left coronary artery orifice is seen in the normal place, below the sinotubular junction. The intramural portion of the right coronary artery was unroofed by resecting its inner wall.

1. Intramural right coronary artery
2. Aortotomy incision
3. Orifice of left coronary artery

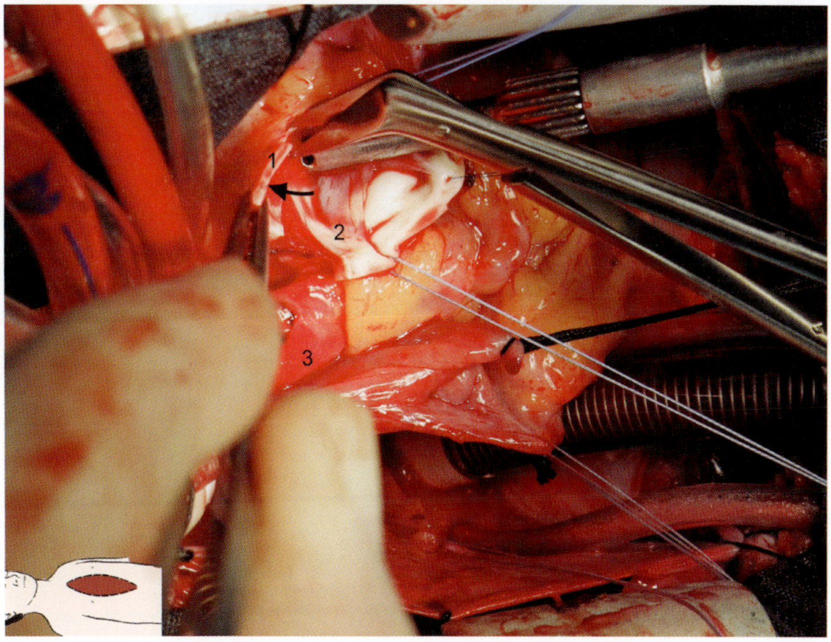

Figure 21.19. ALCAPA as seen through a median sternotomy. Pulmonary arteriotomy has been performed. The arrow points to the site of orifice of the coronary artery from posterior sinus.

1. Wall of MPA
2. Pulmonary valve
3. Ascending aorta

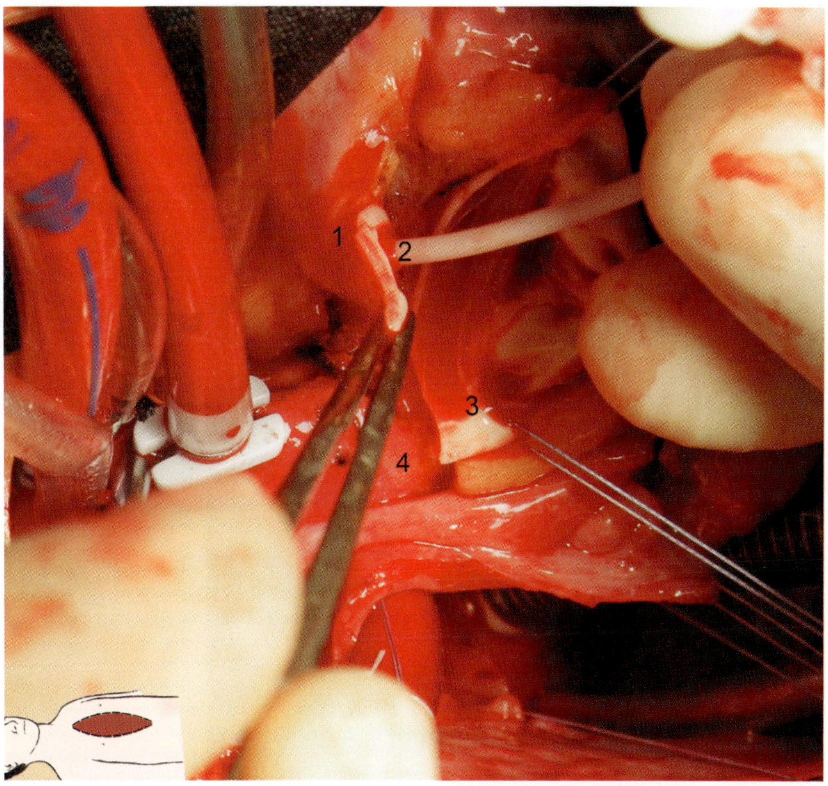

Figure 21.20. The same patient as in Figure 21.19. A coronary perfusion catheter is placed in the orifice of the left coronary artery.

1. Left coronary artery
2. Catheter inside orifice of coronary artery
3. Pulmonary valve
4. Ascending aorta

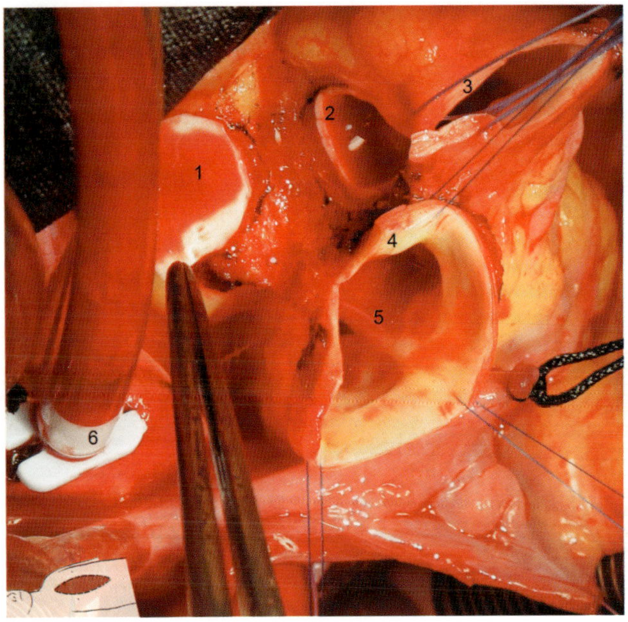

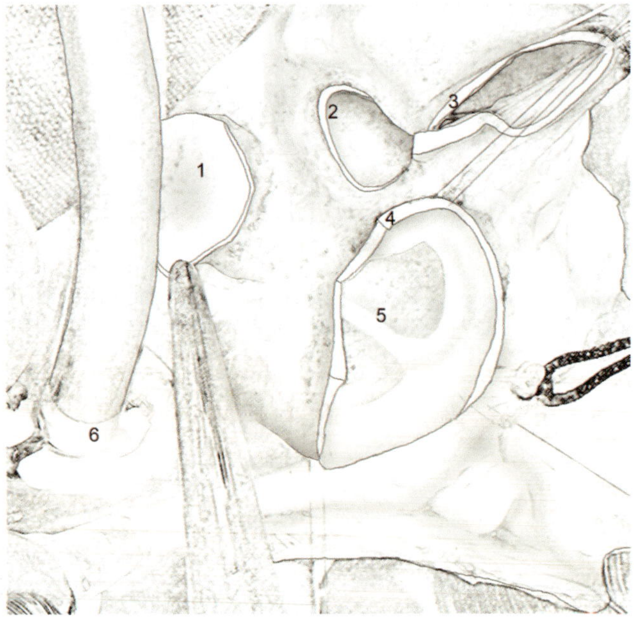

Figure 21.21 **Figure 21.22**

The same patient as in Figures 21.19 and 21.20. The coronary artery has been detached from the MPA with a cuff of PA wall (1). The target site on the aorta has been incised vertically.

1. Left coronary artery with a button of PA wall
2. Original site of coronary artery
3. MPA
4. Ascending aorta
5. Aortic valve
6. Cardioplegia catheter

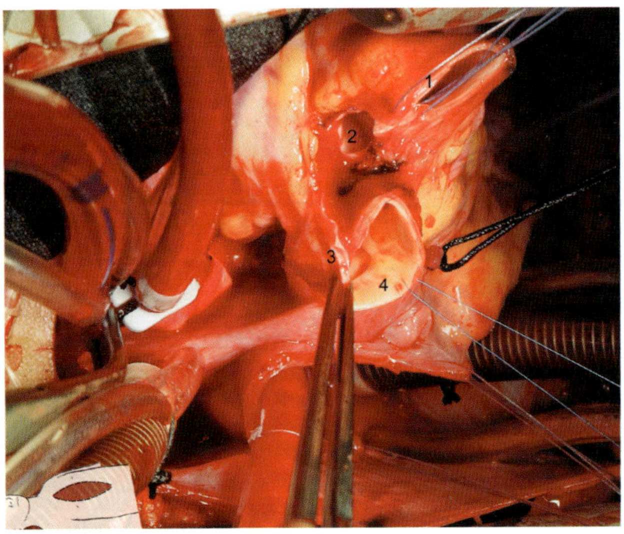

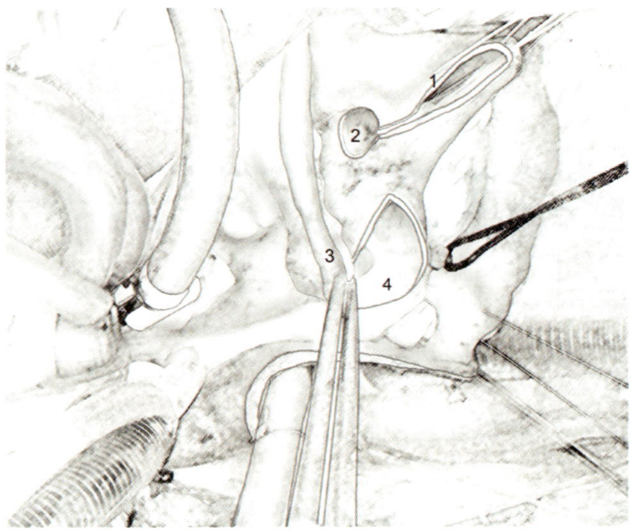

Figure 21.23 **Figure 21.24**

The same patient as in Figures 21.19 to 21.22. The coronary artery is mobilized and is pulled to its target location on the aortic wall.

1. MPA
2. Original site of coronary artery
3. Left coronary artery
4. Ascending aorta

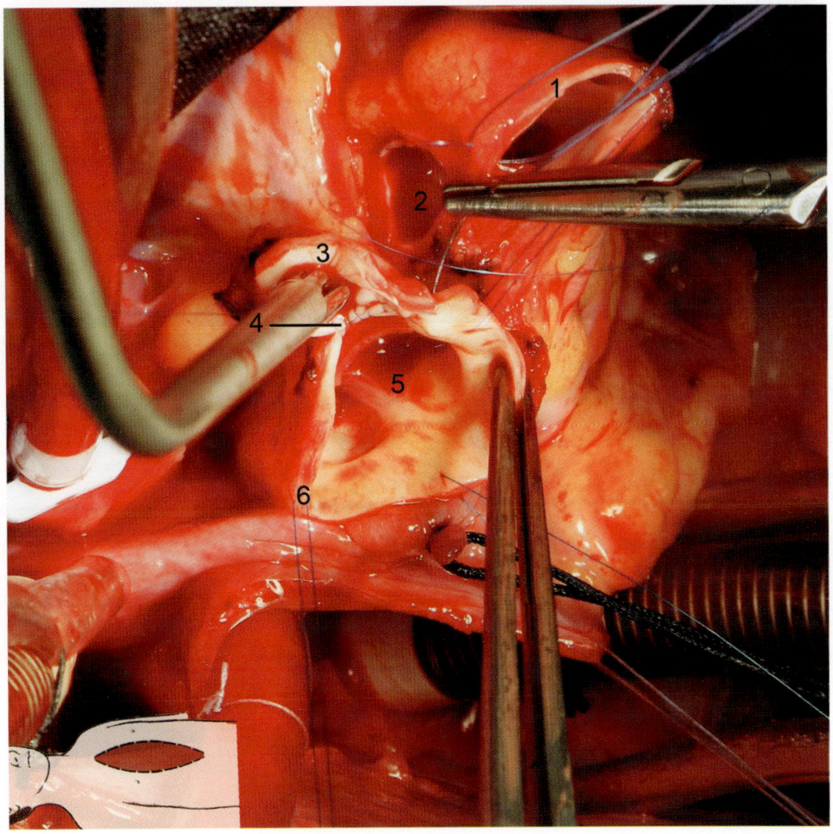

Figure 21.25. The same patient as in Figures 21.19 to 21.24. The left coronary artery has been transferred to its new location and is being anastomosed to the aortic wall.

1. MPA
2. Original site of coronary artery
3. Left coronary artery button
4. Anastomosis of coronary artery to aorta
5. Aortic valve
6. Wall of ascending aorta

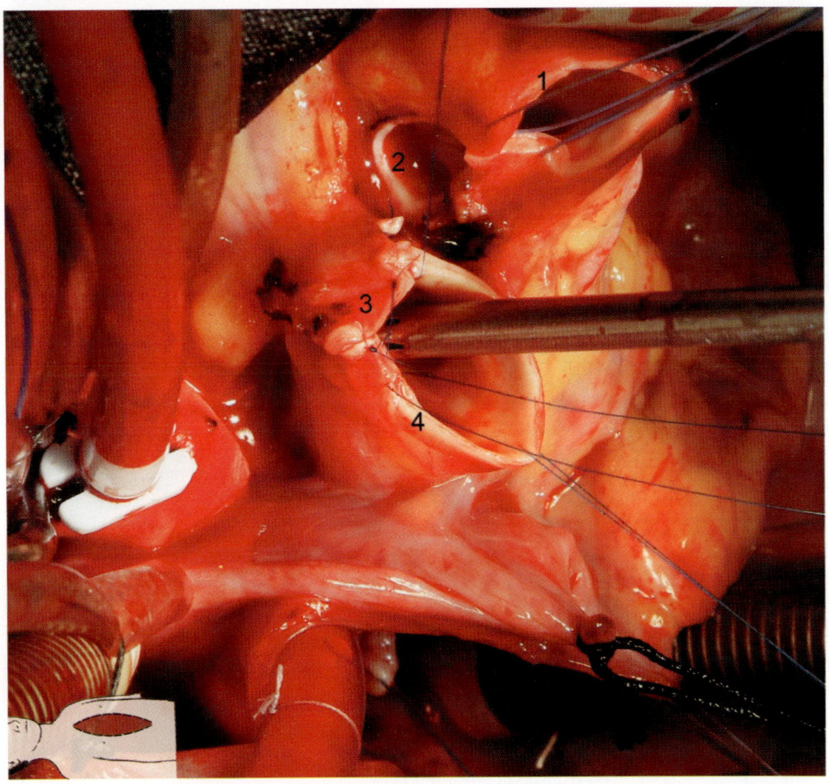

Figure 21.26. The same patient as in Figures 21.19 to 21.25 after transfer of the left coronary artery to its new location on the aortic wall.

1. MPA
2. Original site of coronary artery
3. Left coronary artery
4. Ascending aorta

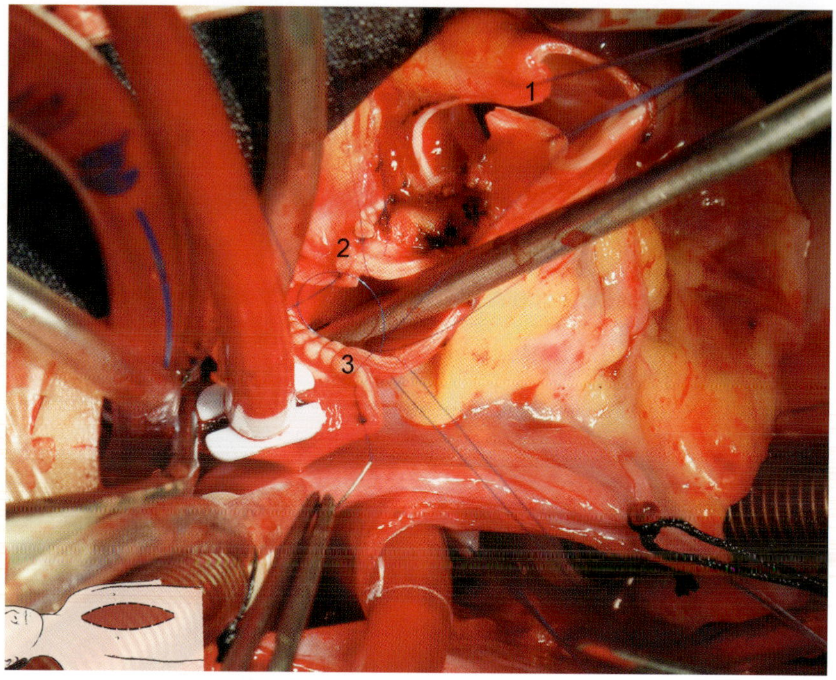

Figure 21.27. The same patient as in Figures 21.19 to 21.26. The anastomosis of the left coronary artery to the aorta has been completed. The proximal and distal ends of the aorta are now being anastomosed together.

1. MPA
2. Left coronary artery
3. Aortic anastomosis

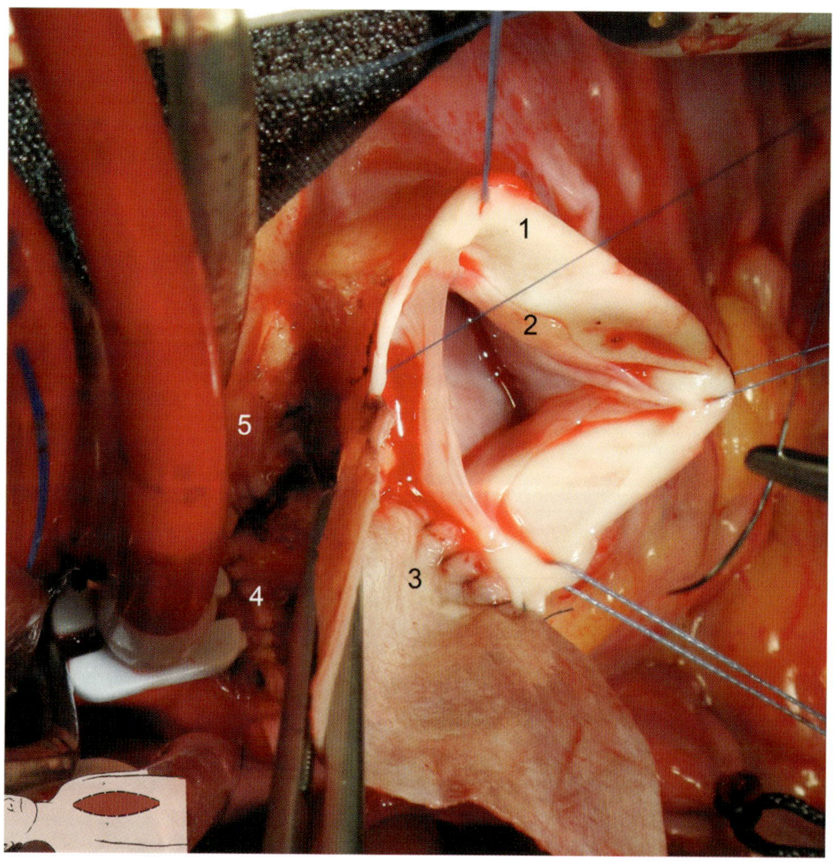

Figure 21.28. The same patient as in Figures 21.19 to 21.27. A pericardial patch is being sutured to close the defect in the PA where the coronary button was removed.

1. MPA
2. Pulmonary valve
3. Pericardial patch
4. Aortic anastomosis
5. Left coronary artery

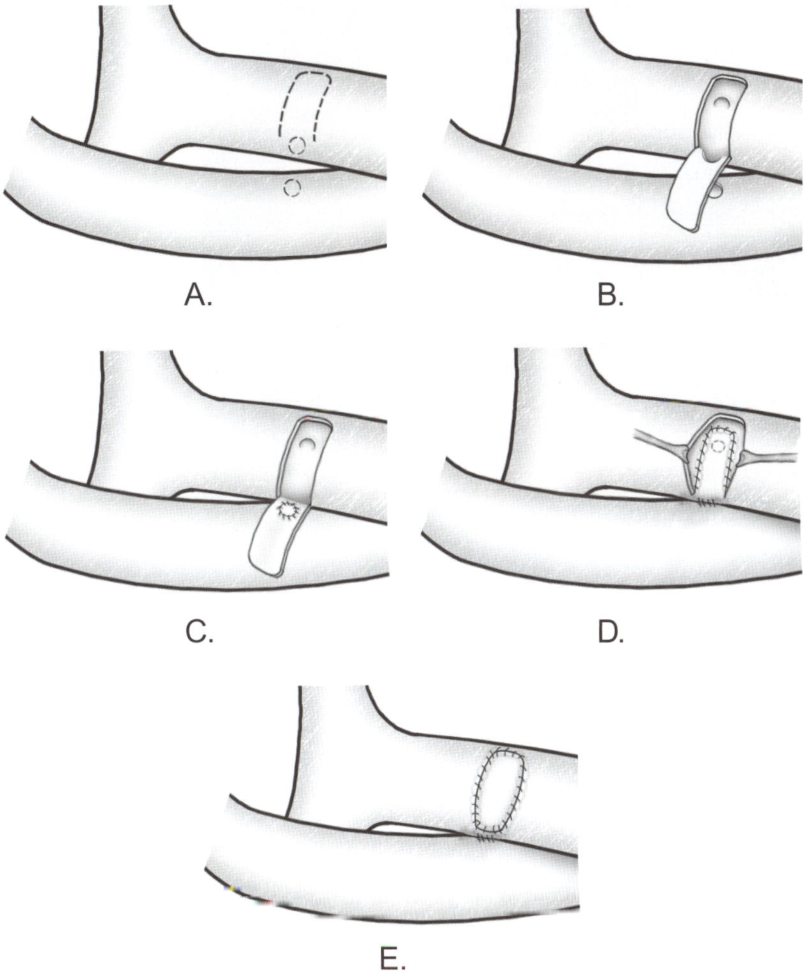

Figure 21.29. Schematic illustration of the Takeuchi (intrapulmonary tunnel) procedure used to treat ALCAPA. (**A**) The interrupted line marks the site of the aortopulmonary window (APW) and the PA flap. (**B**) A PA flap has been made. Two punch holes are made in adjacent opposing walls of the PA and the aorta. The orifice of the anomalous left coronary artery is seen on the posterior wall of the PA. (**C**) The 2 punch holes are stitched together to create an APW. (**D**) The flap is stitched to the posterior wall of the PA, thus creating a tunnel from the coronary artery to the aorta. (**E**) A pericardial flap is used to close the defect in the anterior pulmonary wall.

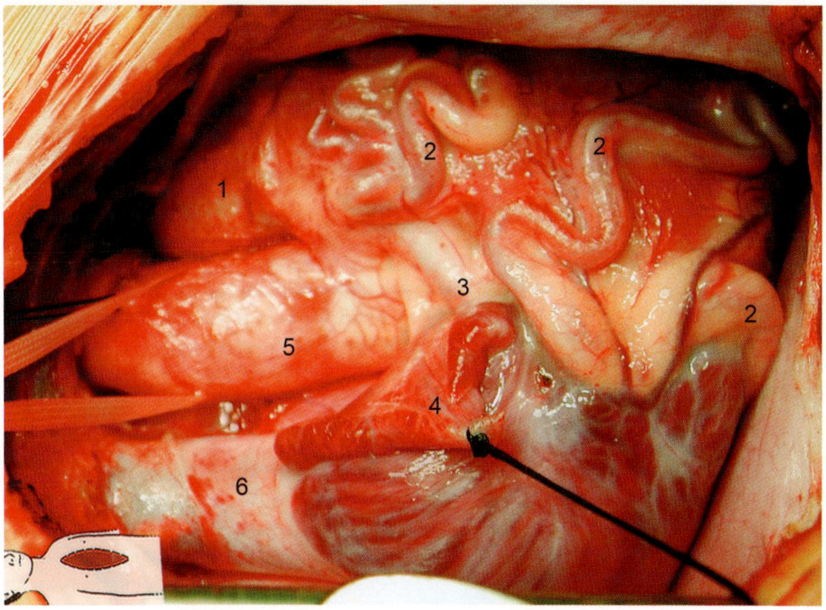

Figure 21.30. ALCAPA as seen through a median sternotomy in a 1-year-old child who presented with mitral regurgitation. Note the dilated coronary arteries.

1. MPA
2. Dilated coronary arteries
3. Right coronary artery
4. RAA
5. Ascending aorta
6. SVC

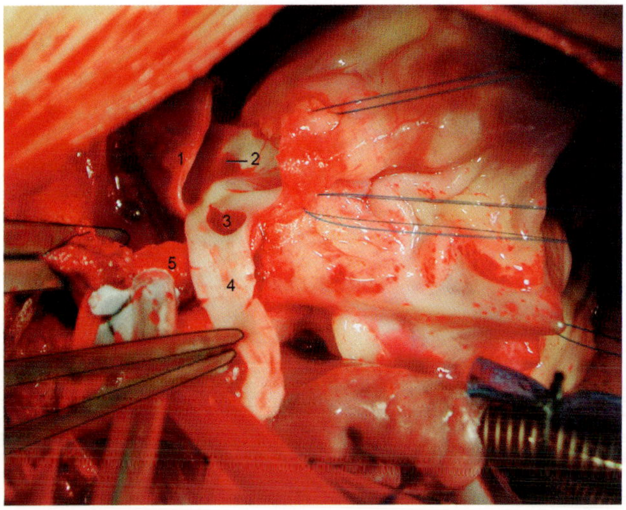

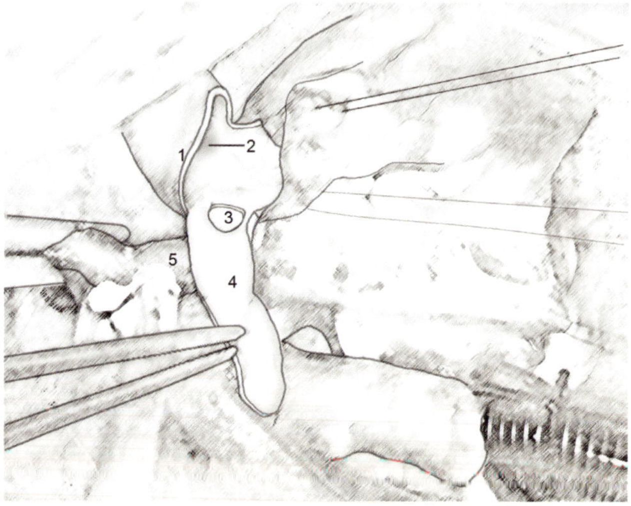

Figure 21.31 **Figure 21.32**

The same patient as in Figure 21.30, now on cardiopulmonary bypass. The anterior wall of the pulmonary artery has been opened in a manner that makes a flap. A punch hole (3) has been made in its wall; the hole will be used to create an APW. The internal orifice of the anomalous coronary artery is on the postero-lateral wall (2) and is covered with pooled blood.

1. MPA
2. Coronary artery orifice
3. Punch hole in pulmonary wall
4. PA flap
5. Ascending aorta

Figure 21.33. The same patient as in Figures 21.30 to 21.32. A counter-punch hole (4) has been made in the aortic wall. This is further shown in Figure 21.34.

1. MPA
2. Site of orifice of anomalous coronary artery
3. Punch hole in PA wall
4. Counter-punch hole in ascending aorta
5. Ascending aorta

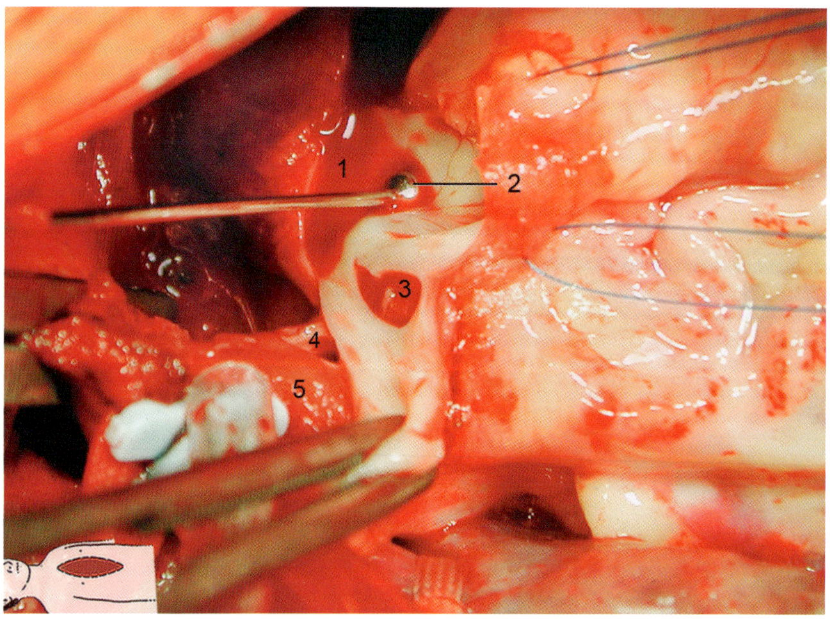

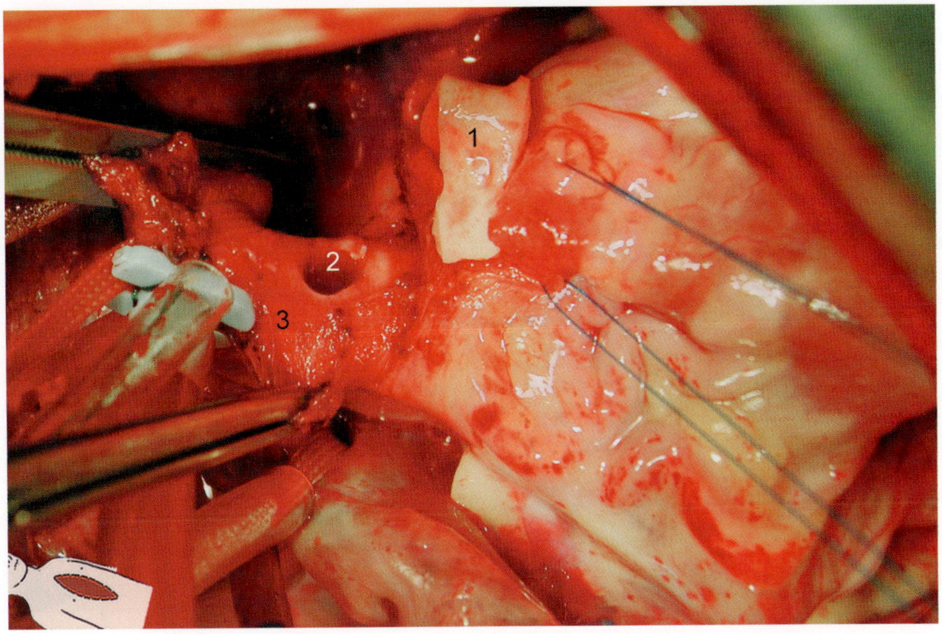

Figure 21.34. The same patient as in Figures 21.30 to 21.33 showing the aortic part of the APW.

1. PA flap
2. Counter-punch hole in ascending aorta
3. Ascending aorta

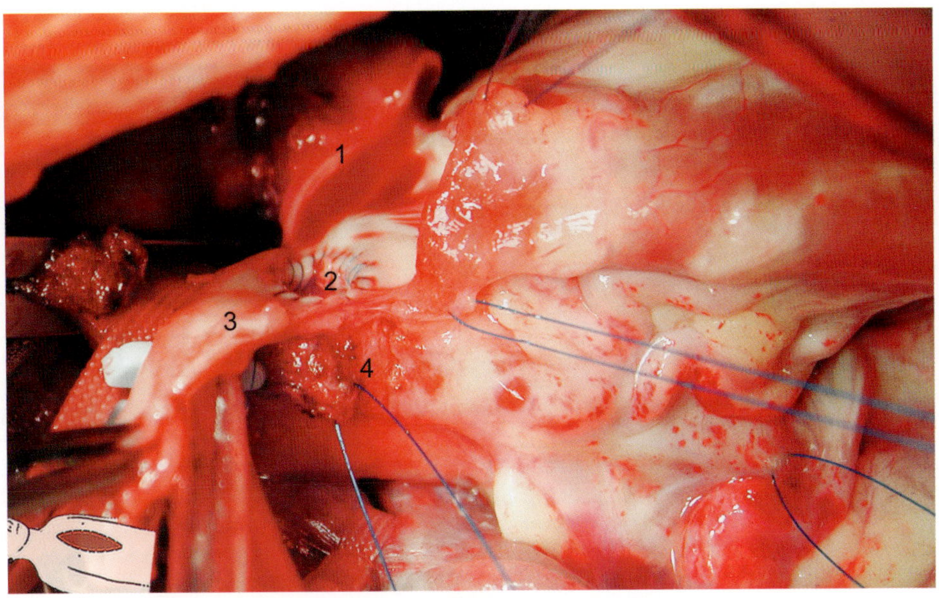

Figure 21.35. The same patient as in Figures 21.30 to 21.34. The 2 holes are stitched together to create an APW.

1. MPA
2. APW
3. PA flap
4. Ascending aorta

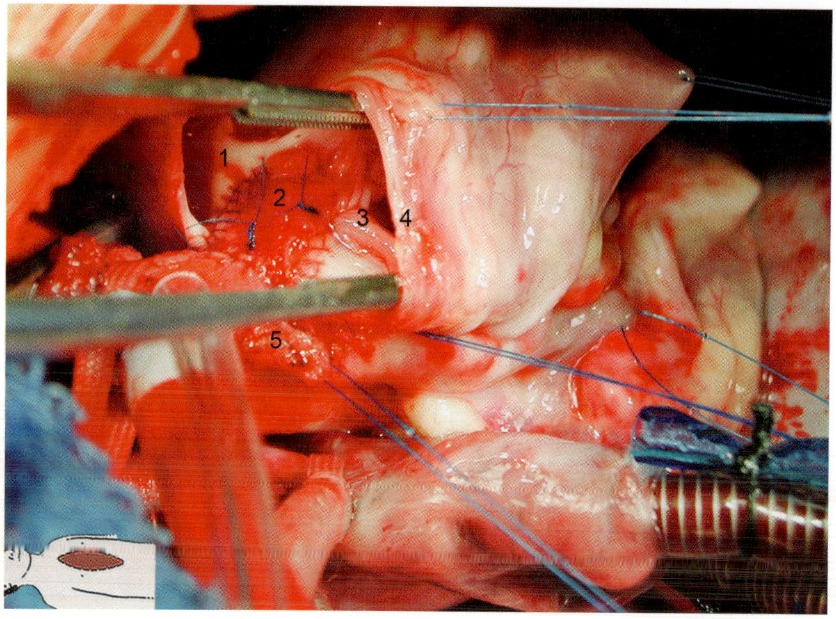

Figure 21.36. The same patient as in Figures 21.30 to 21.35. The flap has been stitched to the posterior wall of the MPA, creating a tunnel. The coronary artery now has direct communication with the aorta through the APW.

1. Lumen of MPA
2. Tunnel made of PA flap
3. Pulmonary valve
4. Wall of MPA
5. Ascending aorta

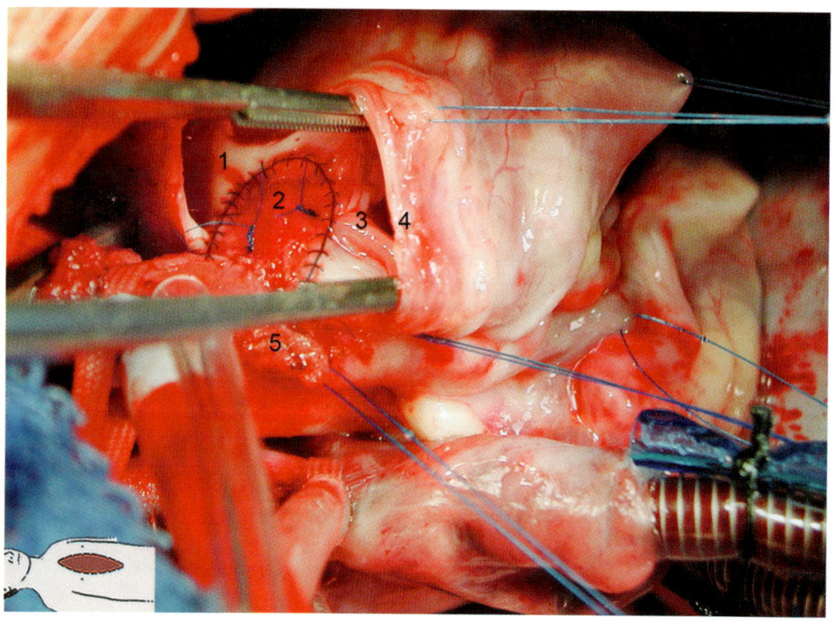

Figure 21.37. The same photo as Figure 21.36, with the intrapulmonary tunnel outlined.

1. Lumen of MPA
2. Tunnel made of PA flap
3. Pulmonary valve
4. Wall of PA
5. Ascending aorta

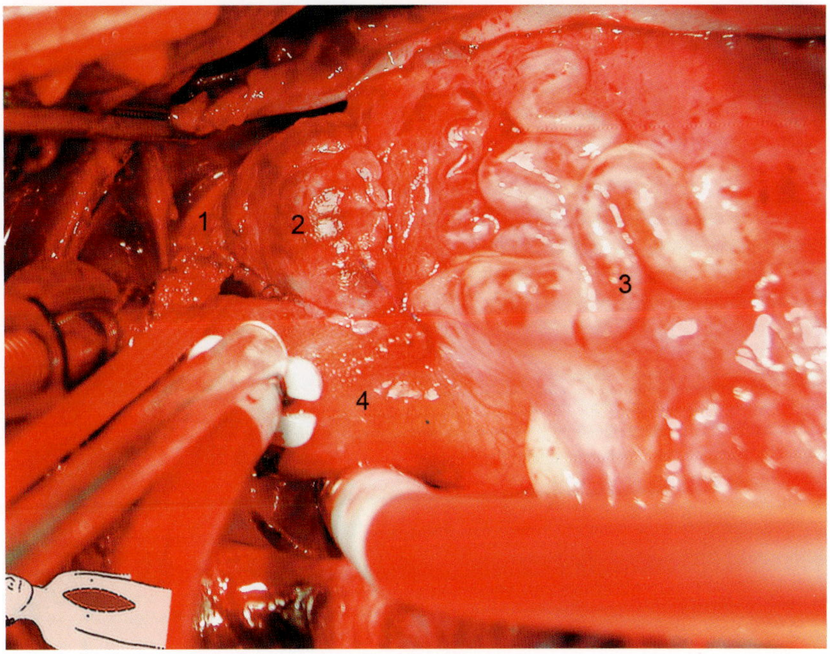

Figure 21.38. The same patient as in Figures 21.30 to 21.37 after completion of repair. The defect in the anterior wall of the MPA has been closed by a pericardial patch.

1. MPA
2. Pericardial patch
3. Dilated coronary artery
4. Ascending aorta

REFERENCES

1. Ceresnak S, Gray RG, Altmann K, et al. Coronary artery fistulas: a review of the literature and presentation of two cases of coronary fistulas with drainage into the left atrium. *Congenit Heart Dis.* 2007;2:208–213.
2. Gowda RM, Vasavada BC, Khan IA. Coronary artery fistulas: clinical and therapeutic considerations. *Int J Cardiol.* 2006;107:7–10.
3. Xu L, Xu Z, Jiang S, et al. Transcatheter closure of coronary artery fistula in children. *Chin Med J.* 2010;123(7):822–826.
4. Mumtaz MA, Lorber RE, Arruda J, et al. Surgery for anomalous aortic origin of the coronary artery. *Ann Thorac Surg.* 2011;91:811–815.
5. Amanullah MA, Rostron AJ, Hamilton J, Chaudhari MP, Hasan A. Towards an anatomically correct repair for anomalous left coronary artery arising from the pulmonary trunk. *Cardiol Young.* 2008;18:372–378.
6. Takeuchi S, Imamura H, Katsumoto K, et al. New surgical method for repair of anomalous left coronary artery from pulmonary artery. *J Thorac Cardiovasc Surg.* 1979;78:7–11.

CHAPTER 22

Cardiac Tumors

Cardiac tumors, primary or secondary, are rare. In children, the most common primary cardiac tumors are rhabdomyoma, fibroma, and myxoma. Teratoma is also encountered, especially in fetuses and neonates.[1] Symptoms are nonspecific and may be related to obstruction of blood flow across the valves, or arrhythmia. Diagnosis often comes as a surprise during echocardiography.

When treatment is indicated for cardiac tumors, surgery is currently the only option available.[2]

Rhabdomyoma is the most common cardiac tumor in the pediatric age group. It is associated with tuberous sclerosis (a genetic disorder characterized by epilepsy, mental retardation, and cardiac and cutaneous angiofibroma). Rhabdomyoma often regresses spontaneously and may not require intervention.[3] Figures 22.1 and 22.2 are intraoperative views from a 2-month-old infant with multiple rhabdomyomas in the left and right ventricles (LVs and RVs). Surgery was performed to relieve LV outflow obstruction. The excised tumors are shown in Figure 22.3. Another example of rhabdomyoma is shown in Figures 22.4 and 22.5.

Fibroma is often solitary, but it may blend imperceptibly with adjacent myocardium.[1] Figure 22.6 shows the heart of a 2-month-old infant with cardiac fibroma. The tumor extensively infiltrates the LV myocardium, rendering surgical excision infeasible.

Myxoma is the most common primary tumor of the heart in adults, but is rare in children. The most common site is the left atrium. It has a finely lobulated, mucoid, gelatinous appearance.[4] Symptoms arise from mitral inflow obstruction, heart failure, and embolic phenomena. Figures 22.7 and 22.8 are from a 30-month-old child with left atrial myxoma. The excised tumor is shown in Figure 22.9.

Secondary cardiac tumors are also rare. Direct extension from the inferior vena cava (IVC) to the right atrium can occur in a Wilms tumor, renal myosarcoma, and leiomyosarcoma.[5] An example of a child with a Wilms tumor and secondary extension to the IVC and the heart is shown in Figures 22.10 and 22.11. Nephrectomy was done, and the tumor extensions were excised from the IVC and the right atrium (not shown).

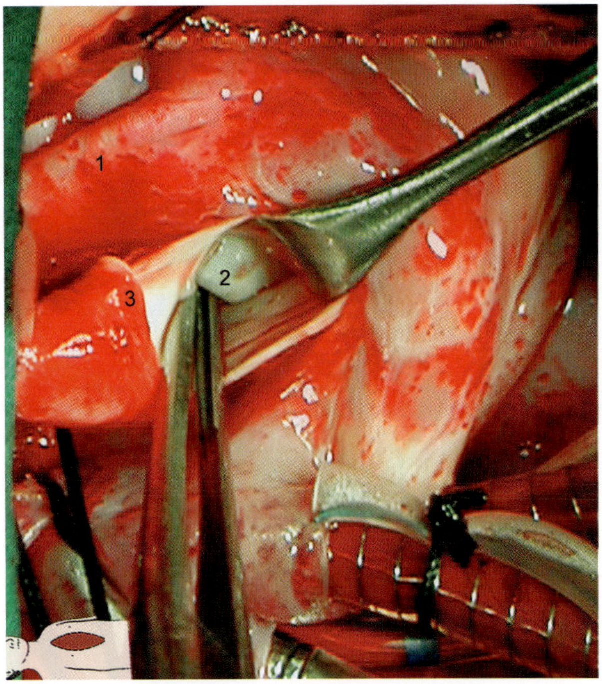

Figure 22.1. Median sternotomy view of a 2-month-old infant with rhabdomyoma. There were multiple tumor masses, one of which was obstructing the LV outflow tract and is shown here through an aortotomy incision.

1. MPA
2. Rhabdomyoma
3. Ascending aorta

Figure 22.2. A right atriotomy view of the same patient as in Figure 22.1 revealing another large tumor in the RV.

1. Rhabdomyoma
2. Tricuspid valve
3. Right atrium

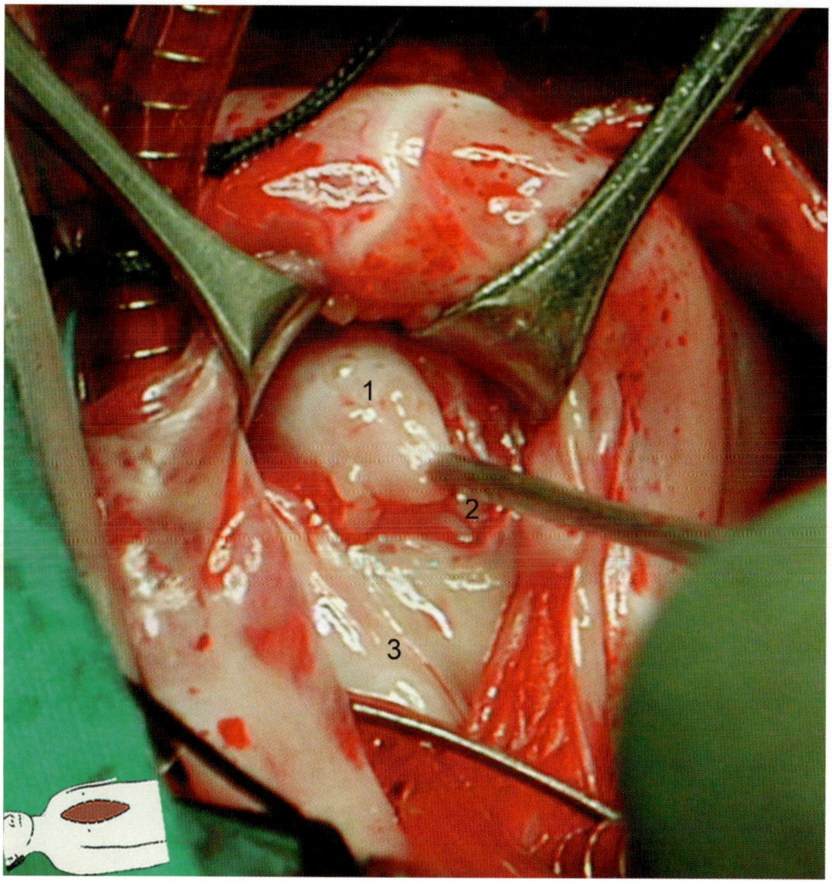

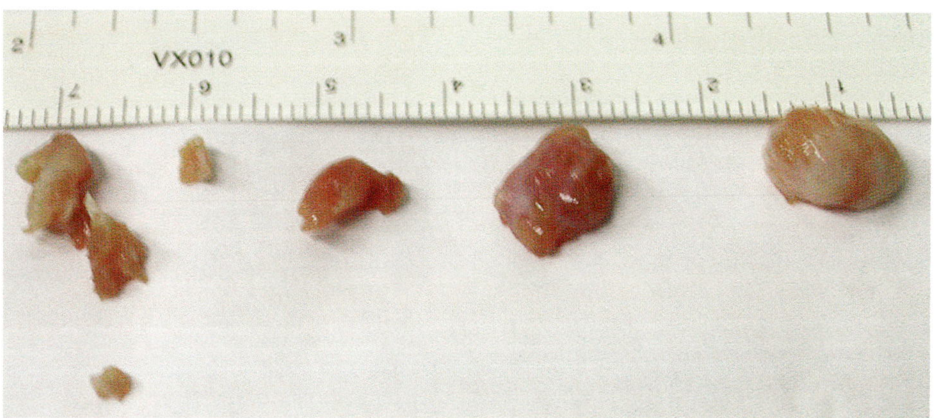

Figure 22.3. The tumor masses that were resected from the patient shown in Figures 22.1 and 22.2. Histopathologic examination confirmed rhabdomyoma.

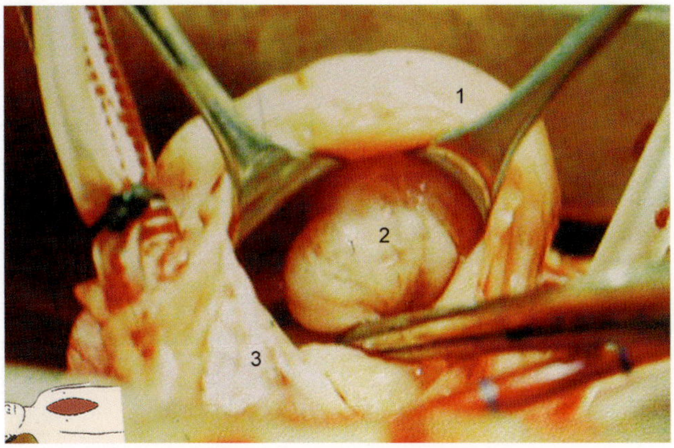

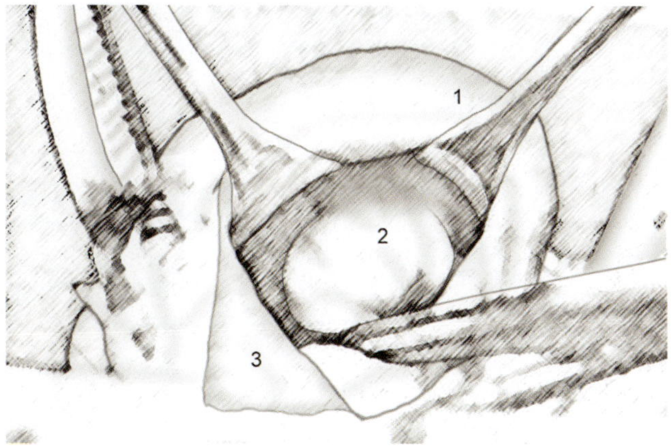

Figure 22.4 **Figure 22.5**

A right atriotomy view of a 2-month-old infant with rhabdomyoma. A large tumor is attached to the RV free wall and tricuspid valve, impeding inflow to the RV. The tumor was excised and a tricuspid valvuloplasty was performed (not shown).

1. RV
2. Rhabdomyoma
3. Right atrial wall

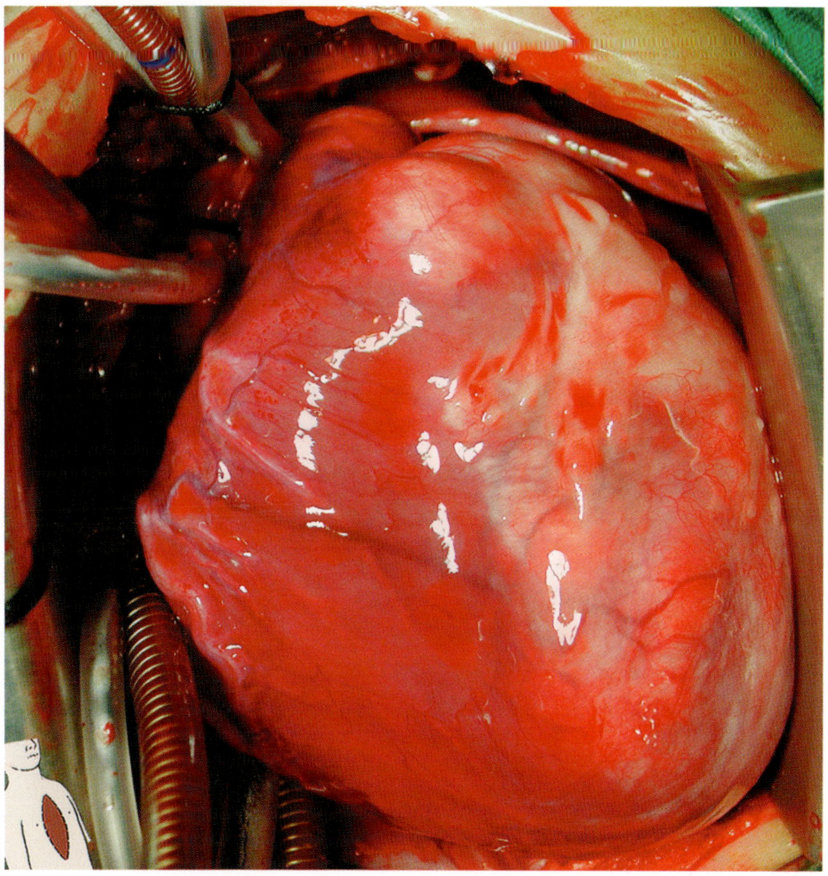

Figure 22.6. Median sternotomy view of a 2-month-old infant with a cardiac tumor. Note the extensive infiltration of the LV free wall. Surgical excision was not possible. A biopsy was taken, and histopathologic examination of the specimen revealed fibroma.

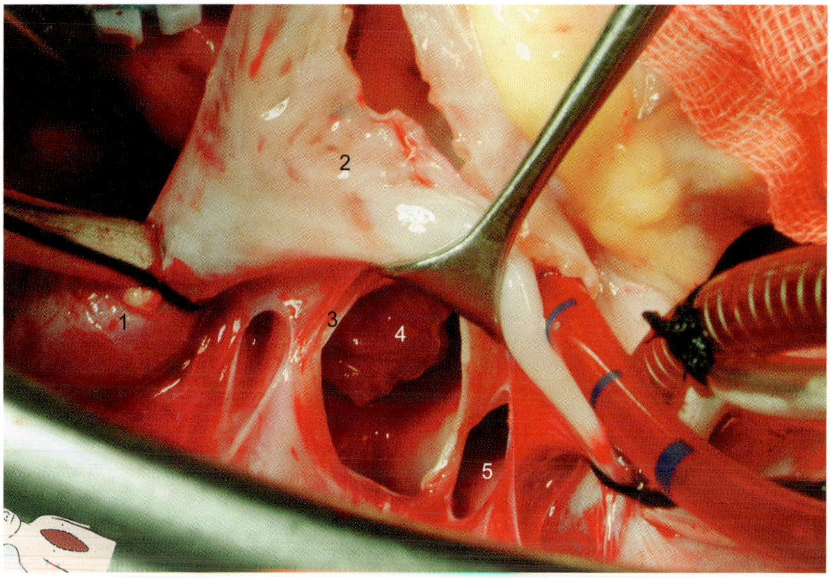

Figure 22.7. A left atrial myxoma in a 30-month-old child. The tumor is seen through a left atriotomy incision. The myxoma is attached to the posterosuperior wall of the left atrium.

1. Superior vena cava (SVC)
2. Right atrium
3. Left atrial wall
4. Myxoma
5. Oblique pericardial sinus

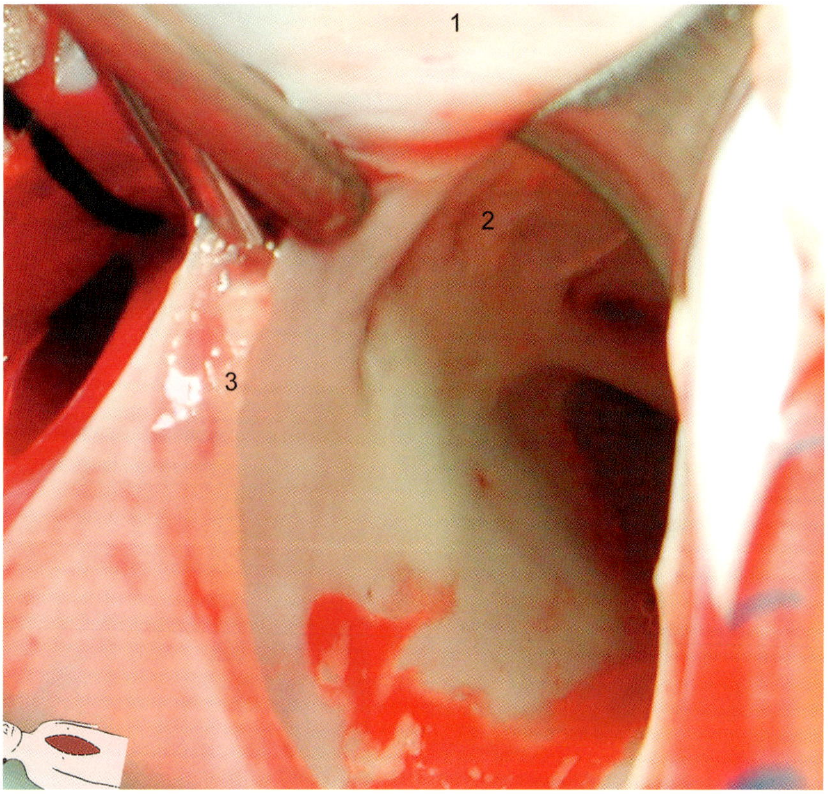

Figure 22.8. The left atrium after excision of the myxoma. The tumor bed in the left atrium superior wall is shown.

1. Right atrium
2. Tumor bed
3. Left atrial wall

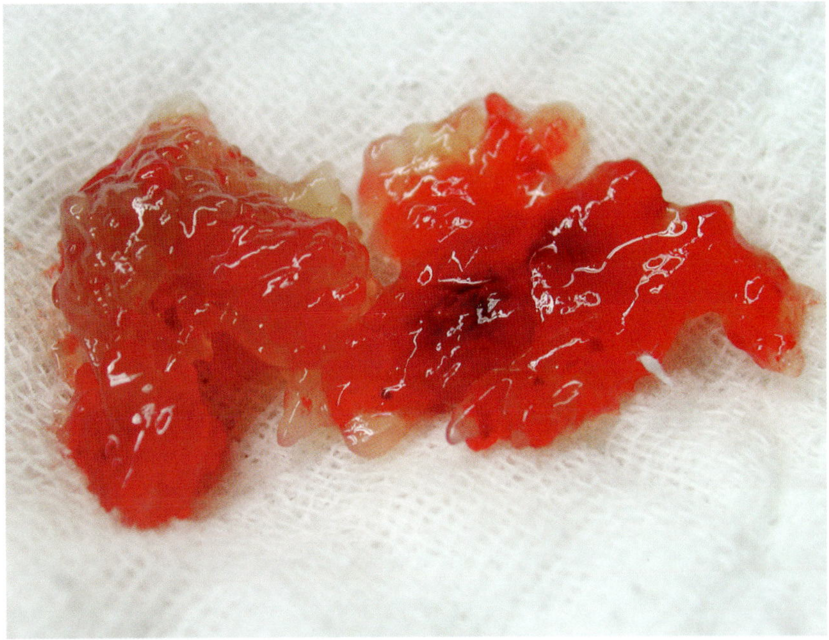

Figure 22.9. The myxoma that was excised from the patient in Figures 22.7 and 22.8. Note the polypoid, gelatinous appearance of the mass with areas of hemorrhage.

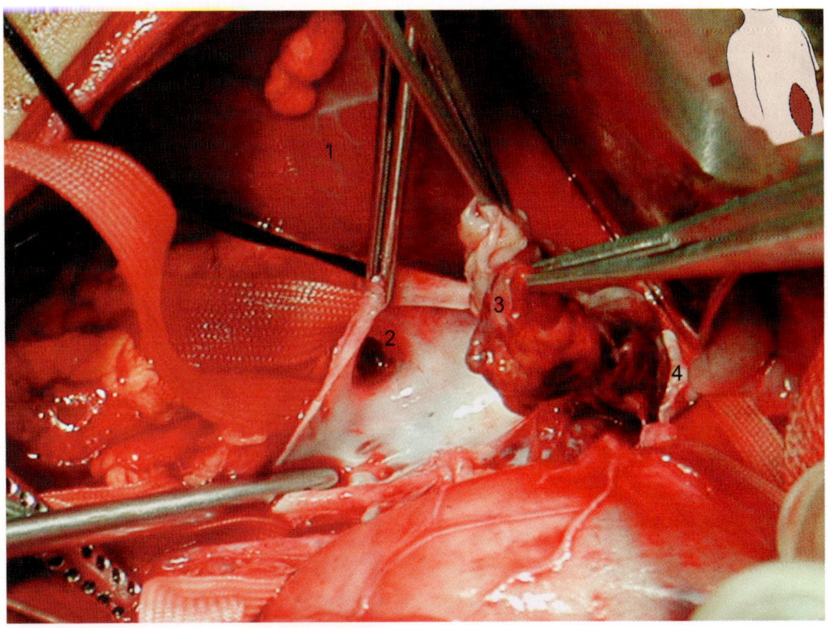

Figure 22.10. A laparotomy view of a 6-year-old child with a Wilms tumor. The child is on deep hypothermic circulatory arrest. The tumor arises from the left kidney and extends through the renal vein to the IVC and cephalad to the right atrium. In this picture, the mass is seen coming off the left renal vein.

1. Liver
2. IVC
3. Tumor
4. Left renal vein

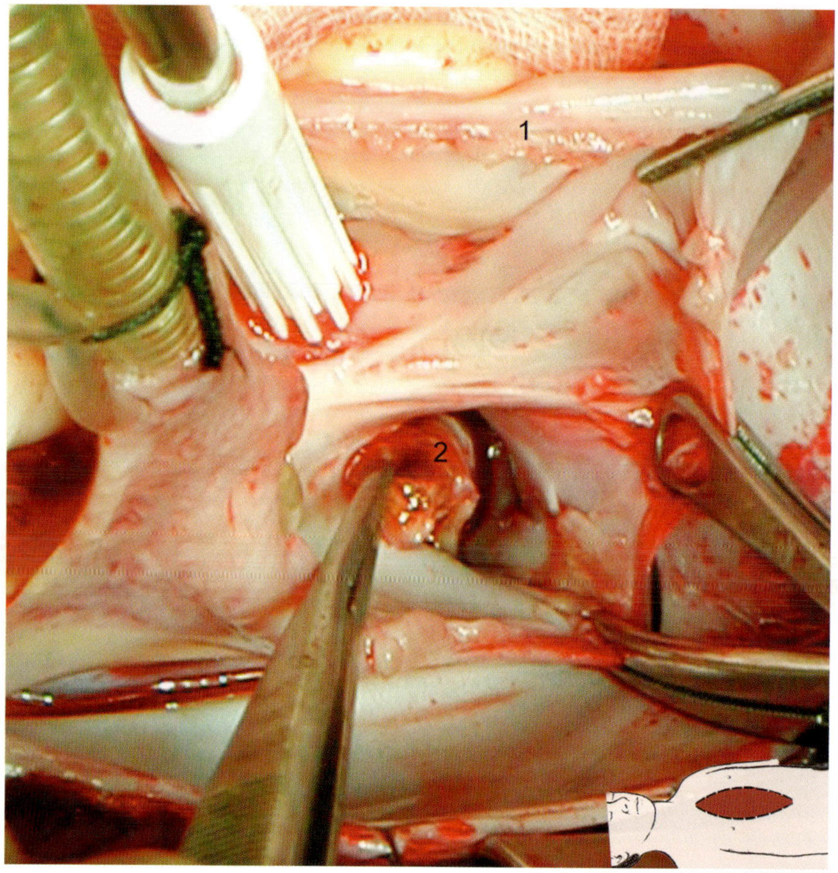

Figure 22.11. The same patient as in Figure 22.10. A median sternotomy was performed; the right atrium was opened with the child still on deep hypothermic circulatory arrest. The tumor mass is seen protruding from the IVC into the right atrium.

1. Right atrial wall
2. Tumor

A blood cyst is a curious lesion often found incidentally during echocardiography or intraoperatively during surgery for other reasons. It is thought to arise from infolding of the endothelium into atrioventricular or semilunar valves. Most are asymptomatic.[6]

Figures 22.12 and 22.13 are from a 4-year-old child with transposition of the great arteries (TGA), ventricular septal defect (VSD), and pulmonary stenosis. A blood cyst is seen on the pulmonary valve.

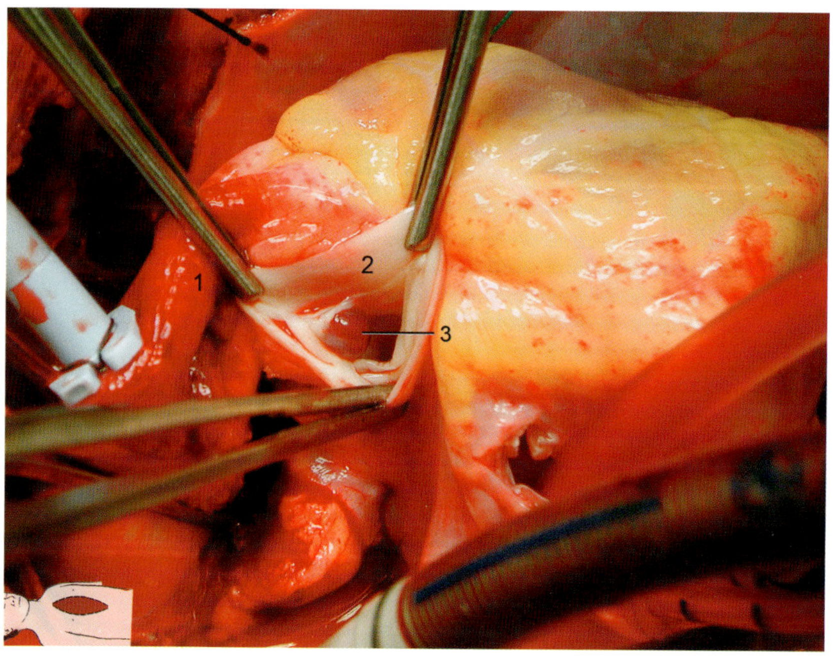

Figure 22.12. Median sternotomy view of a 4-year-old child with TGA, VSD, and pulmonary stenosis. The pulmonary valve is exposed through an arteriotomy. A blood cyst is visible on the undersurface of the pulmonary valve leaflet.

1. Ascending aorta
2. Proximal main PA
3. Blood cyst

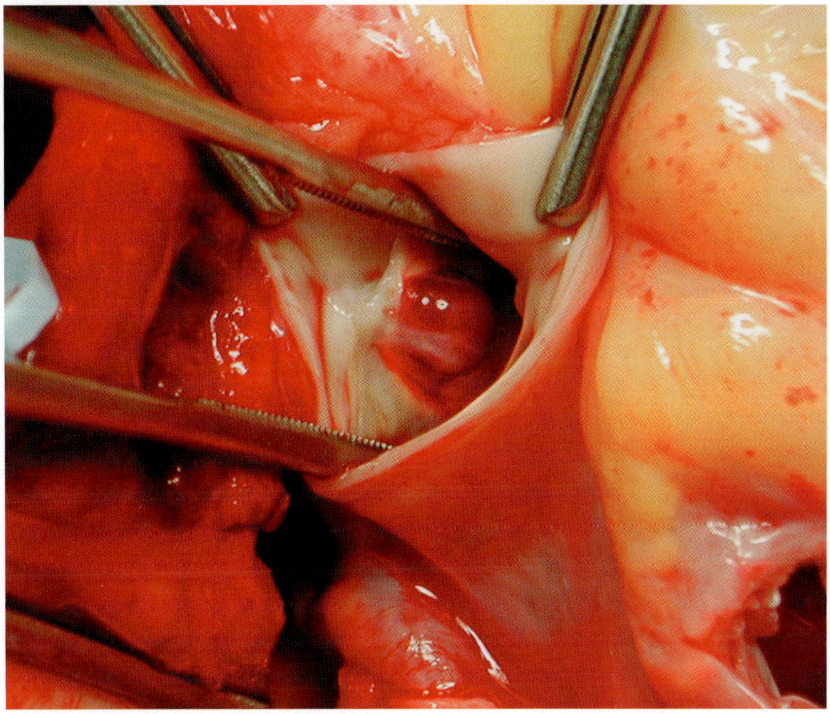

Figure 22.13. Close-up view of the same patient shown in Figure 22.12. The blood cyst arises from the undersurface of the pulmonary valve leaflet.

REFERENCES

1. Isaacs H. Fetal and neonatal cardiac tumors. *Pediatr Cardiol.* 2004;25:252–273.
2. Günther T, Schreiber C, Noebauer C, et al. Treatment strategies for pediatric patients with primary cardiac and pericardial tumors: a 30-year review. *Pediatr Cardiol.* 2008;29:1071–1076.
3. Józwiak S, Kotulska K, Kasprzyk-Obara J, et al. Clinical and genotype studies of cardiac tumors in 154 patients with tuberous sclerosis complex. *Pediatrics.* 2006; 118:1146–1151.
4. Nomura K, Nakamura Y, Uno Y, Yamashiro M. Pediatric left atrial myxoma: surgical excision and mitral valve plasty. *Ann Thorac Cardiovasc Surg.* 2007;13:65–67.
5. Marx GR, Moran AM. Cardiac tumors. In: Allen HD, Driscoll DJ, Shaddy RE, Feltes TF, eds. *Moss and Adams' Heart Disease in Infants, Children, and Adolescents: Including the Fetus and Young Adults.* 7th ed. Philadelphia, PA: Lippincott Williams & Wilkins; 2008:1479–1495.
6. Agac MT, Acar Z, Turan T, Karadag B, et al. Blood cyst of tricuspid valve: an incidental finding in a patient with ventricular septal defect. *Eur J Echocardiogr.* 2009;10(4):588–589.

CHAPTER 23

Infective Endocarditis

Infective endocarditis is a dreaded complication of congenital and acquired structural heart disease. Despite medical and surgical advances, it continues to have substantial morbidity and mortality. High-risk lesions include complex and cyanotic heart disease, ventricular septal defect (VSD), patent ductus arteriosus, valvular heart disease, and the presence of prosthetic materials such as shunts, grafts, and artificial valves.[1]

Common causative organisms include streptococci, staphylococci, the HACEK group (*Haemophilus parainfluenza, Actinobacillus, Cardiobacterium, Ekinella, Kingella*), and fungi.[2]

The mainstay of treatment is parenteral antibiotics, but surgery may be necessary in certain situations.[3] Surgical procedures in the setting of endocarditis include the removal of vegetations, drainage of abscesses, repair/replacement of damaged valves, and repair of underlying structural disease.

An abnormal mitral or aortic valve is a common predisposing factor in both adults and children. Figure 23.1 shows large aortic valve vegetations in an 8-year-old child. The valve was replaced with a pulmonary autograft (Ross procedure). Figure 23.2 shows a bicuspid aortic valve that was damaged by infective endocarditis. Aortic root dilatation is seen in infective endocarditis as well as in many other conditions, including bicuspid aortic valve. An example is shown in Figures 23.3 and 23.4.

Mycotic aneurysms are uncommon complications of infective endocarditis. They result from septic embolization of vegetations to the arterial vasa vasorum, or from intraluminal spread of infection through the endothelium outward through the arterial wall.[3] Figures 23.5 to 23.7, from a 10-year-old child, show the gross appearance of a pulmonary artery (PA) mycotic aneurysm. The underlying structural disease was VSD and pulmonary stenosis. There were vegetations on the tricuspid and pulmonary valves (Figures 23.8–23.10). These are usual sites for vegetations because they tend to develop at sites of turbulent blood flow, adjacent to septal defects or stenotic valves.[4] This is further

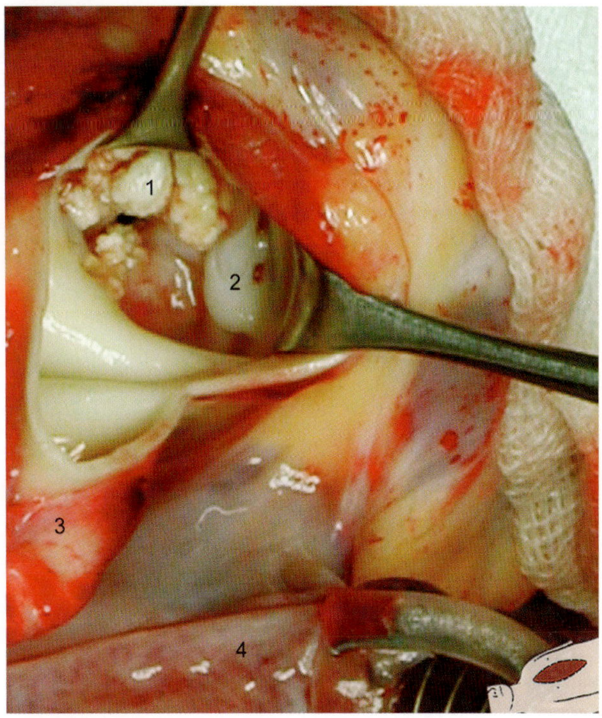

Figure 23.1. An intraoperative view of the aortic valve via median sternotomy and aortotomy in an 8-year-old child. Large vegetations are seen on the left and noncoronary cusps. The valve was severely damaged beyond repair. A Ross procedure was performed (not shown).

1. Vegetation on left coronary cusp
2. Right coronary cusp
3. Ascending aorta
4. Right atrial appendage (RAA)

Congenital Heart Disease: A Surgical Color Atlas © 2015 A. Sukru Mercan, Zakariya Hubail, S. Yen Ho.
Cardiotext Publishing, ISBN: 978-1-935395-90-4.

illustrated by the patients shown in Figures 23.11 to 23.16.

Occasionally, a calcified old vegetation, reminiscent of a previous infective endocarditis, may be encountered during repair of congenital heart defects (Figure 23.17).

In many series, tetralogy of Fallot (TOF) is responsible for a significant number of infective endocarditis cases.[1] Figures 23.18 and 23.19 are from a 2-year-old child with TOF who developed infective endocarditis. Two vegetations are seen in the right ventricle (RV) outflow tract. Figures 23.20 to 23.24 are from 2 other patients who underwent RV-to-PA conduit replacement because of the infective endocarditis/endarteritis.

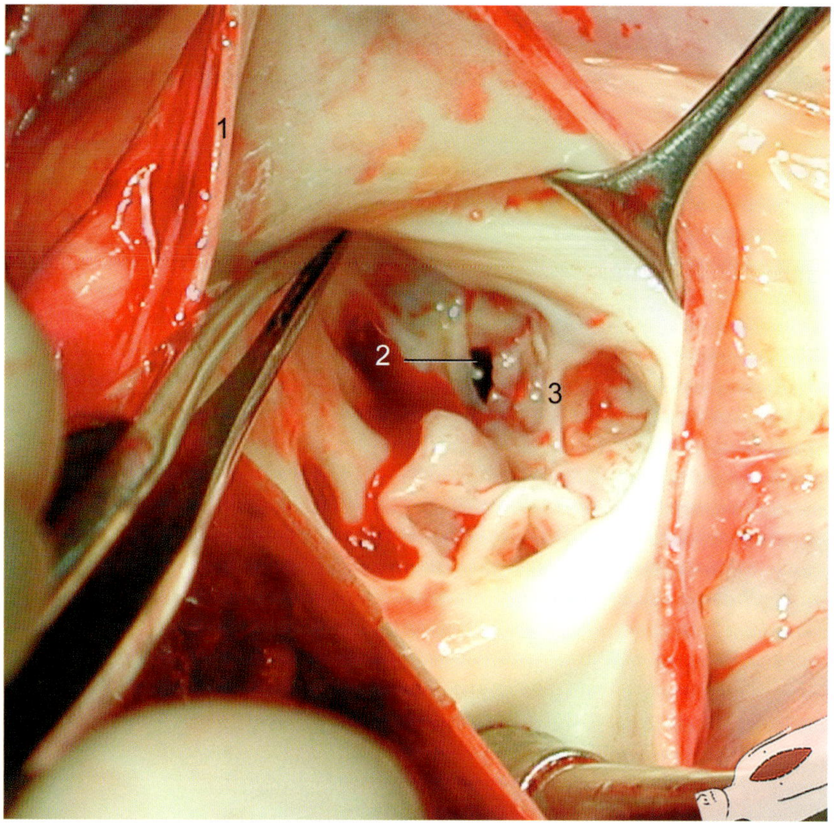

Figure 23.2. An aortotomy view of a 13-year-old child with a bicuspid aortic valve and VSD. Shown here is the bicuspid aortic valve. The left and right coronary cusps were fused with a prominent raphe between them. A perforation, caused by endocarditis, is seen in the left coronary cusps.

1. Oblique aortotomy incision
2. Perforation in left coronary cusp
3. Raphe

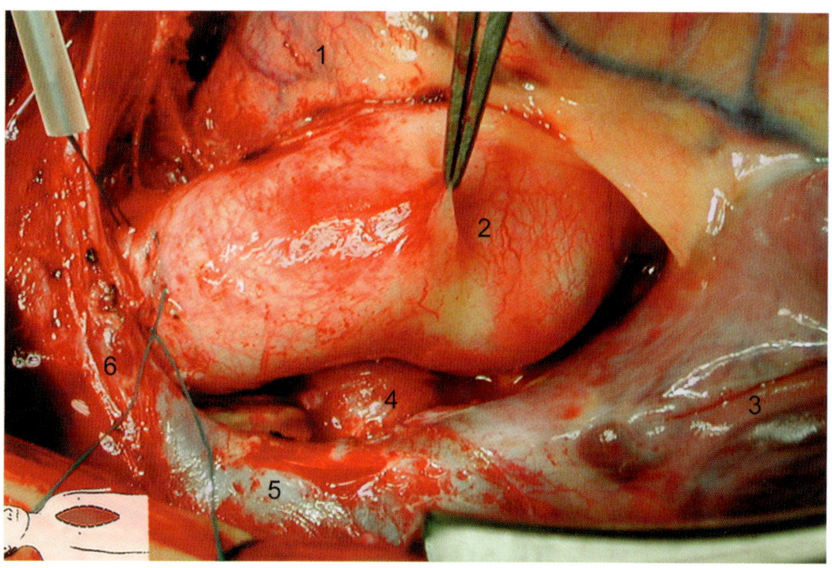

Figure 23.3. Median sternotomy view of an 11-year-old child with subaortic membrane complicated by infective endocarditis. Note the dilated ascending aorta.

1. Main pulmonary artery (MPA)
2. Ascending aorta
3. Right atrium
4. Right PA
5. Superior vena cava (SVC)
6. Innominate vein

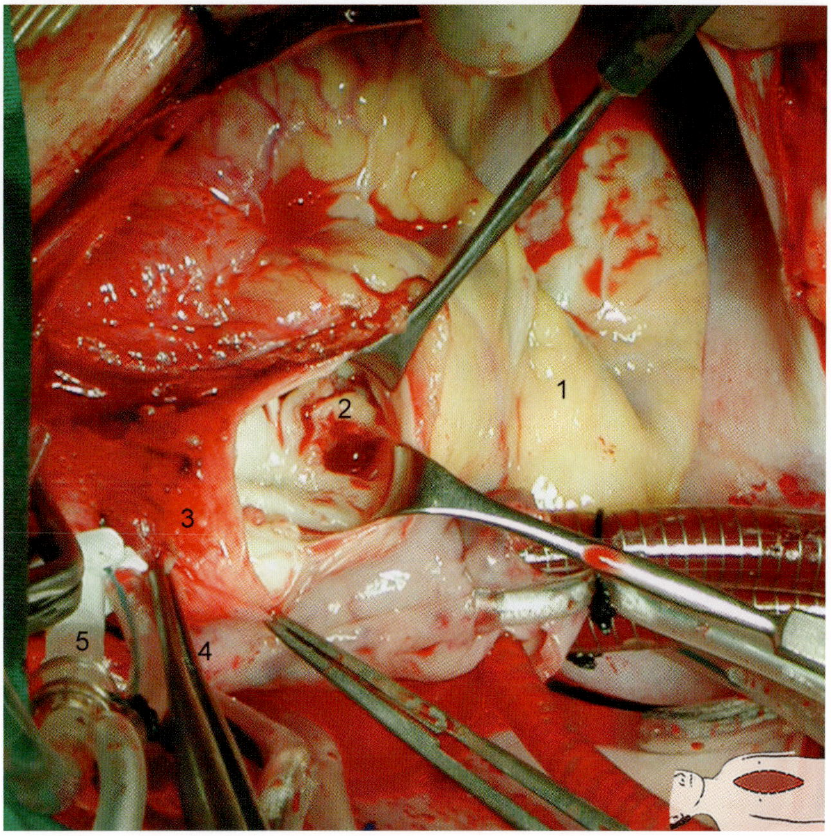

Figure 23.4. Aortotomy view of the same patient shown in Figure 23.3. The valve is bicuspid, and the left coronary cusp is damaged.

1. RV
2. Aortic valve
3. Ascending aorta
4. SVC
5. Cardioplegia catheter

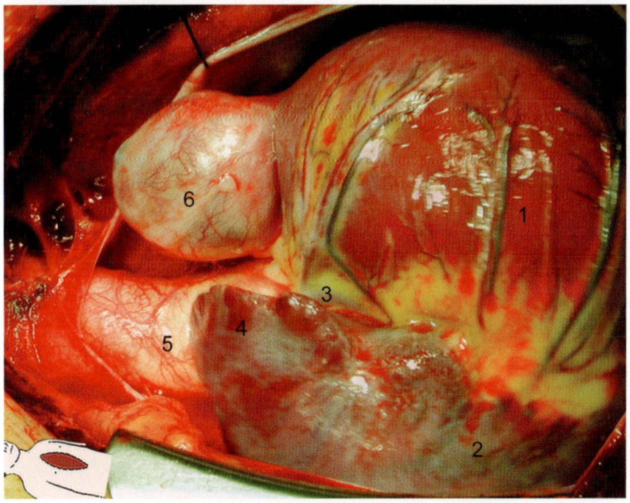

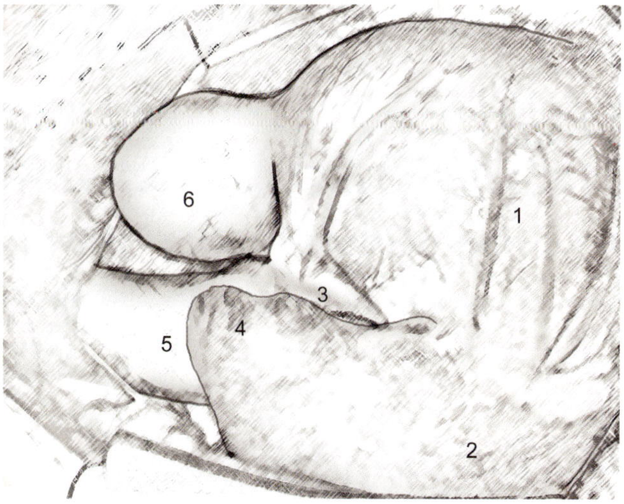

Figure 23.5 **Figure 23.6**

A mycotic aneurysm of the MPA in a 10-year-old child, as seen through a median sternotomy. This child's underlying diseases were VSD and pulmonary stenosis. There were vegetations on the tricuspid and pulmonary valves (Figures 23.8 to 23.10).

1. RV
2. Right atrium
3. Right coronary artery
4. RAA
5. Ascending aorta
6. MPA aneurysm

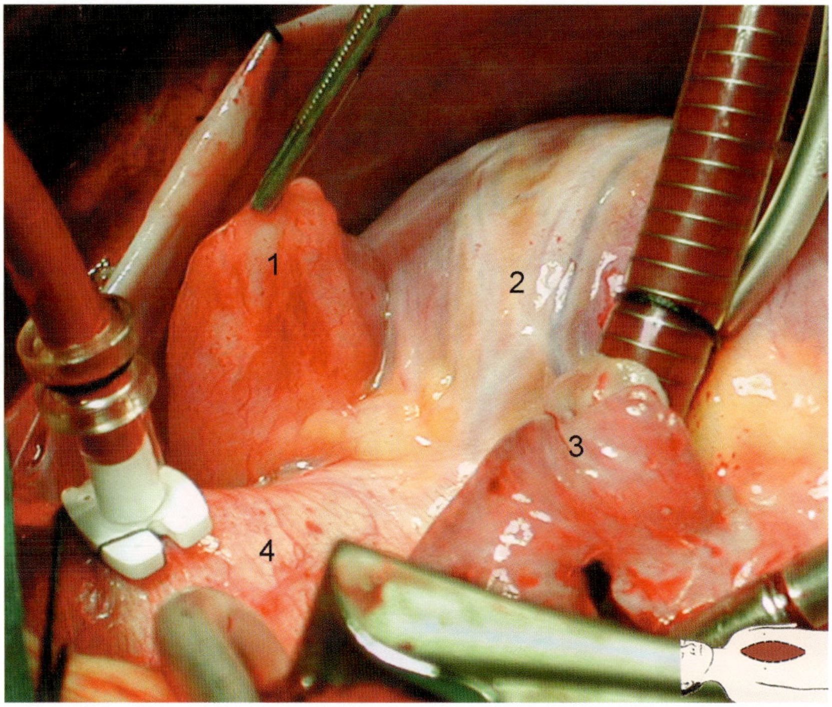

Figure 23.7. The same patient as in Figure 23.5, now on cardiopulmonary bypass. The MPA is empty, and the redundant wall of the aneurysm is clearly seen.

1. PA aneurysm
2. RV
3. RAA
4. Ascending aorta

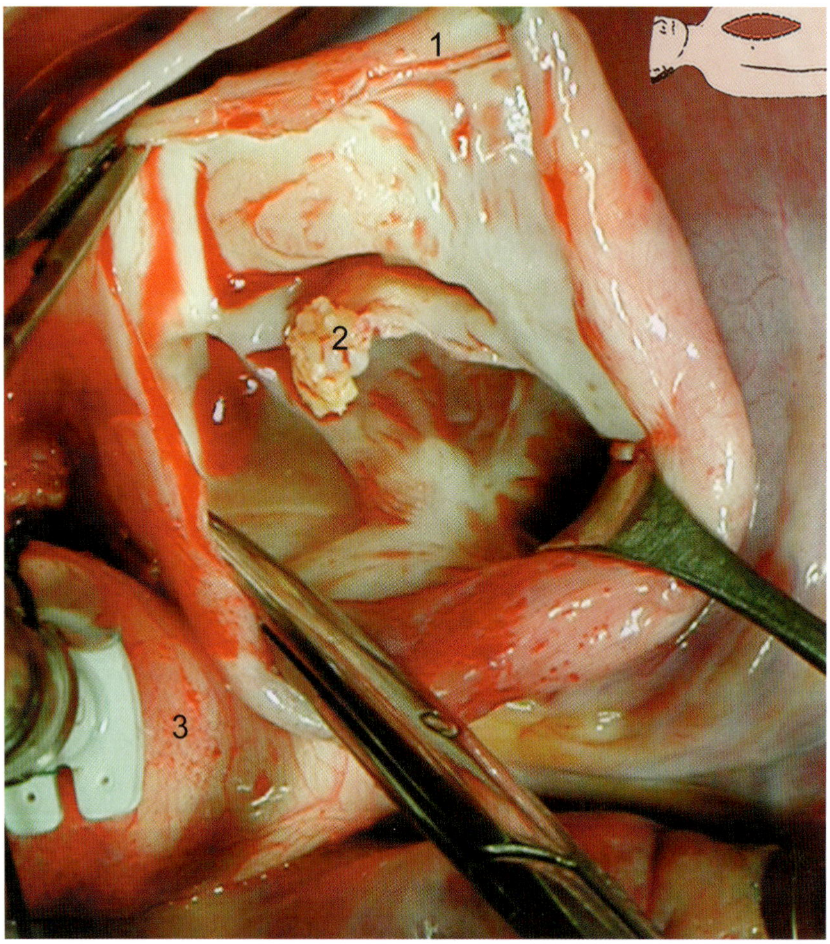

Figure 23.8. The pulmonary valve of the same patient shown in Figures 23.5 to 23.7, seen through a pulmonary arteriotomy. A sizable vegetation is loosely attached to the valve leaflet.

1. Pulmonary arteriotomy incision
2. Vegetation
3. Ascending aorta

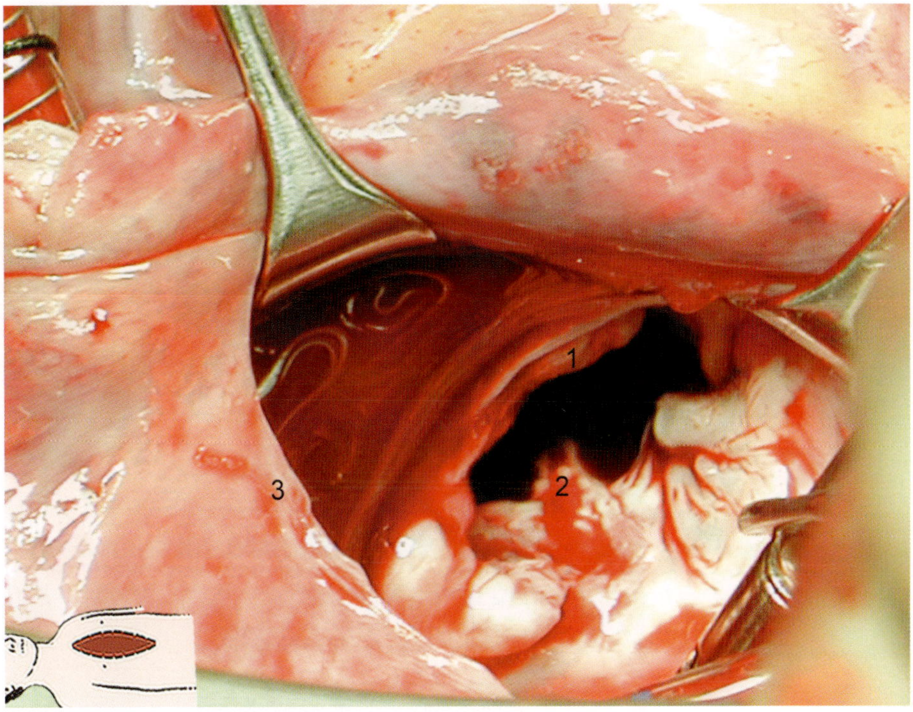

Figure 23.9. The same patient as in Figures 23.5 to 23.8. A right atriotomy reveals a vegetation on the septal leaflet of the tricuspid valve.

1. Anterior leaflet of tricuspid valve
2. Vegetation on the septal leaflet of the tricuspid valve
3. Right atrial wall

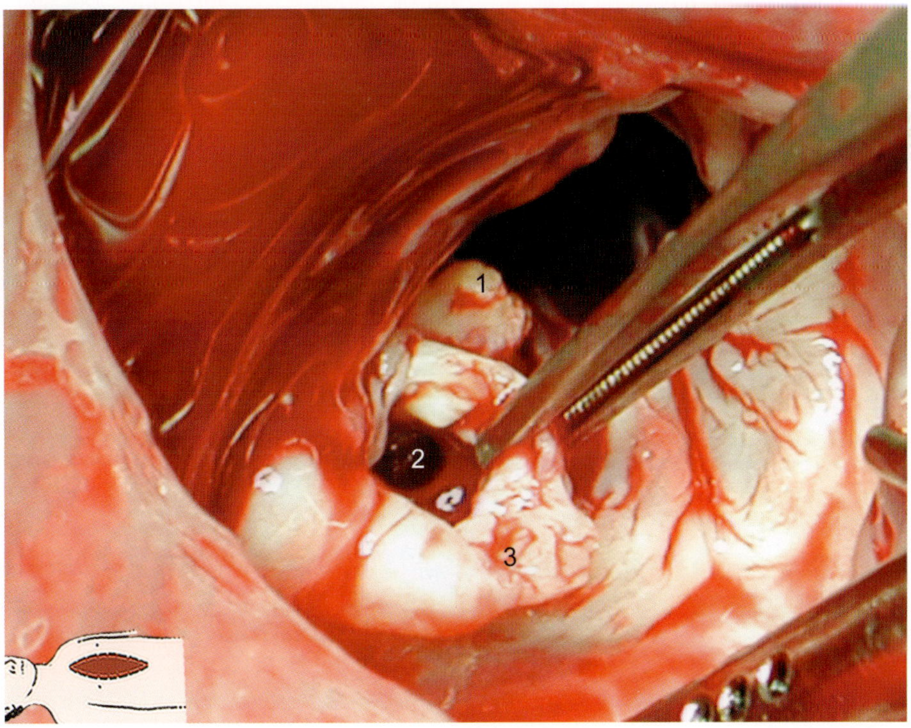

Figure 23.10. The same patient as in Figures 23.5 to 23.9. The tricuspid valve is retracted to show the VSD.

1. Vegetation
2. VSD
3. Tricuspid valve

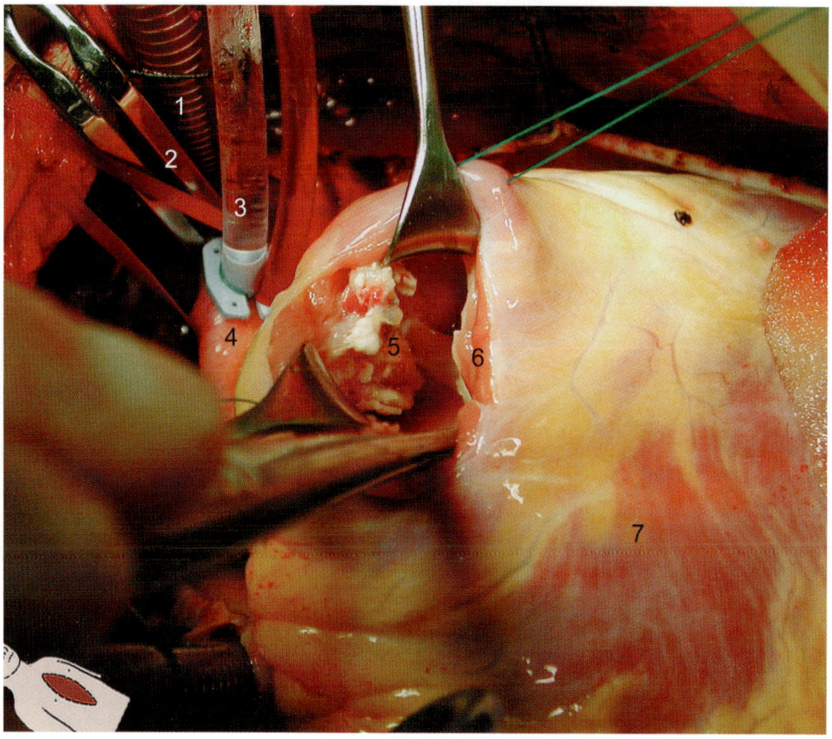

Figure 23.11. A right ventriculotomy view of a 14-year-old child with VSD and double-chambered RV. A vegetation is seen on the RV free wall opposite the site of VSD and anomalous muscle bundle.

1. Aortic cannula
2. Aortic cross-clamp
3. Cardioplegia catheter
4. Ascending aorta
5. Vegetation
6. Right ventriculotomy incision
7. RV

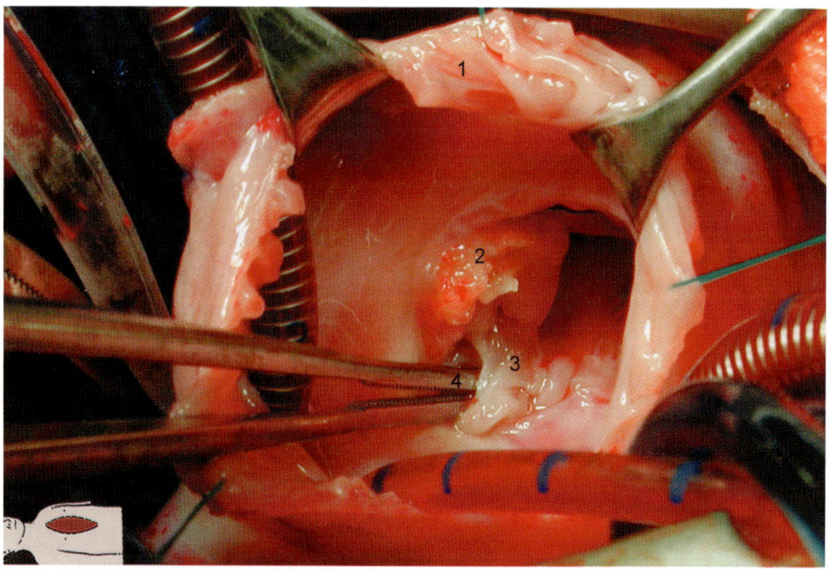

Figure 23.12. A right atriotomy view of a 6-year-old child with VSD and infective endocarditis. A vegetation is seen on the anterior leaflet of the tricuspid valve. The tip of the forceps in the VSD.

1. Right atrial wall
2. Vegetation
3. Septal leaflet of tricuspid valve
4. Forceps in the VSD

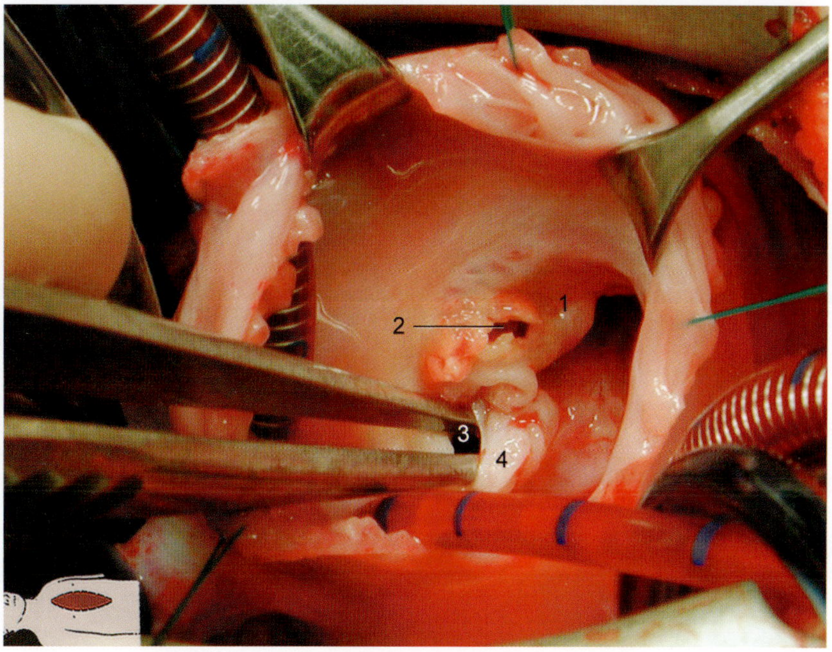

Figure 23.13. The same patient as in Figure 23.12. A defect is seen in the anterior leaflet of the tricuspid valve caused by infective endocarditis.

1. Anterior leaflet of the tricuspid valve
2. Defect in anterior leaflet
3. VSD
4. Septal leaflet of the tricuspid valve

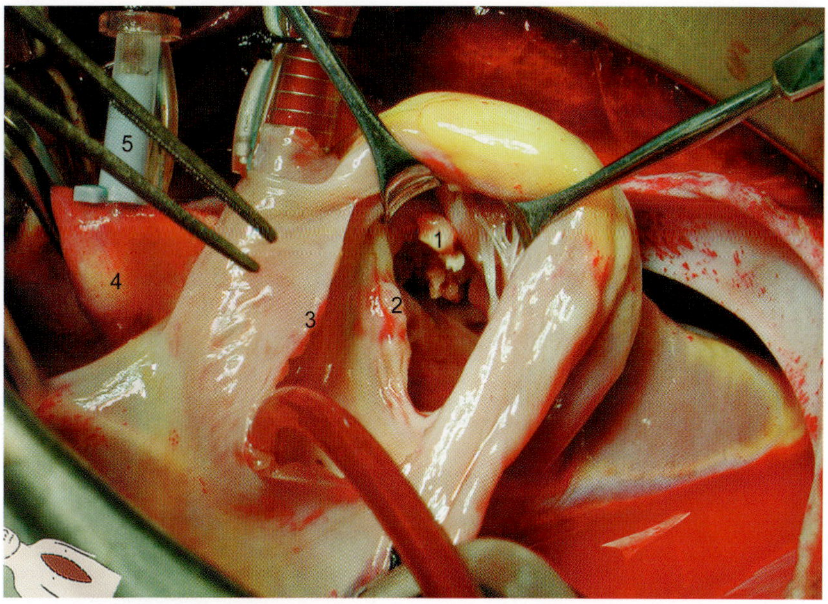

Figure 23.14. Median sternotomy/right atriotomy view of a child with VSD and infective endocarditis. The vegetation is attached to the anterior leaflet of the tricuspid valve.

1. Vegetation
2. Septal leaflet
3. Right atriotomy incision
4. Ascending aorta
5. Cardioplegia catheter

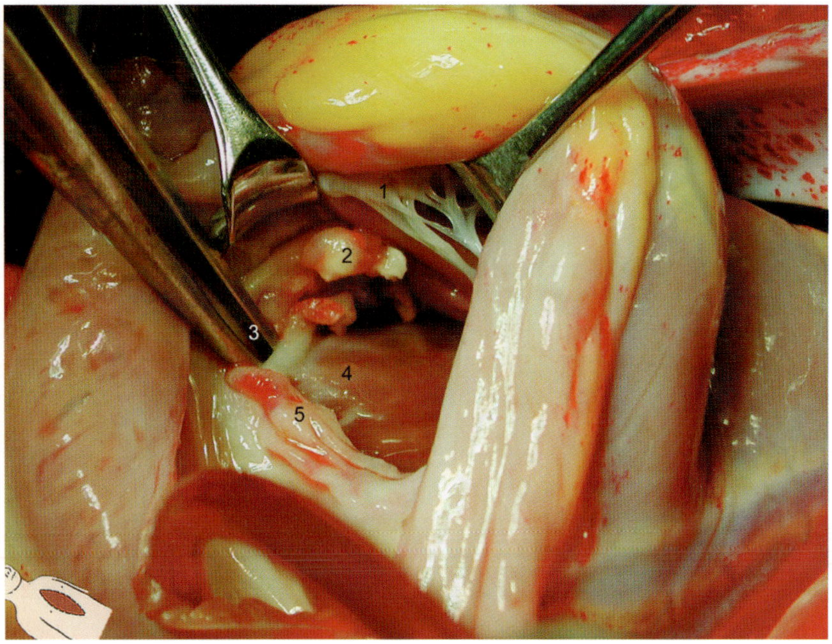

Figure 23.15. The same patient as in Figure 23.14. A pair of forceps is passed through the VSD.

1. Tricuspid valve
2. Vegetation
3. VSD
4. Interventricular septum
5. Septal leaflet

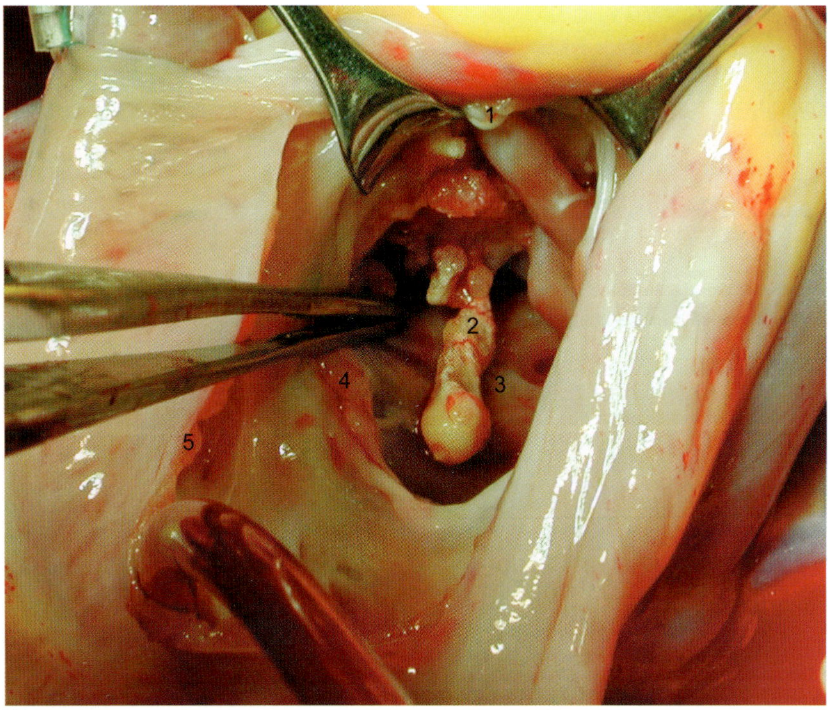

Figure 23.16. The same patient as in Figures 23.14 and 23.15, showing the extent and size of the vegetation.

1. Anterior leaflet
2. Vegetation
3. Interventricular septum
4. Septal leaflet
5. Right atriotomy incision

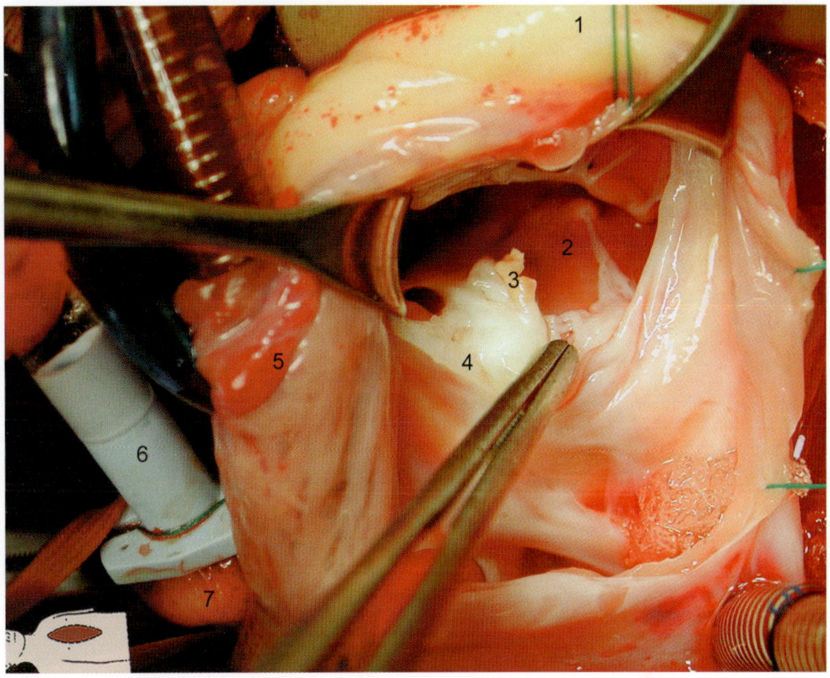

Figure 23.17. Median sternotomy/right atriotomy view of a 30-month-old child during surgery to close a VSD. A calcified old vegetation is seen on the septal leaflet of the tricuspid valve, caused by a previous endocarditis.

1. RV
2. Interventricular septum
3. Vegetation
4. Septal leaflet
5. RAA
6. Cardioplegia catheter
7. Ascending aorta

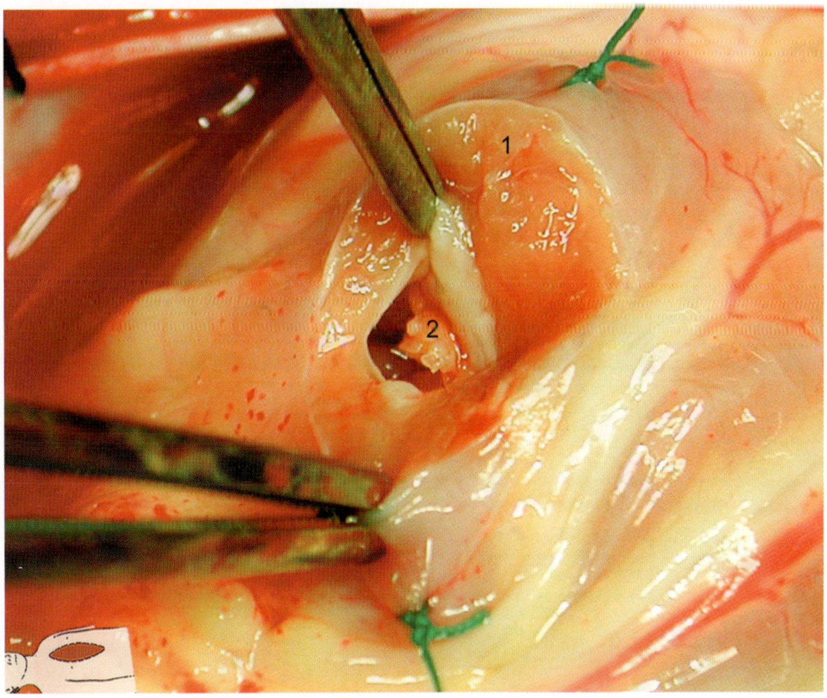

Figure 23.18. Right ventriculotomy view of a 2-year-old child with TOF. A vegetation is encountered on the free wall of the RV. Note the hypertrophied ventricular muscle characteristic of TOF.

1. RV wall
2. Vegetation

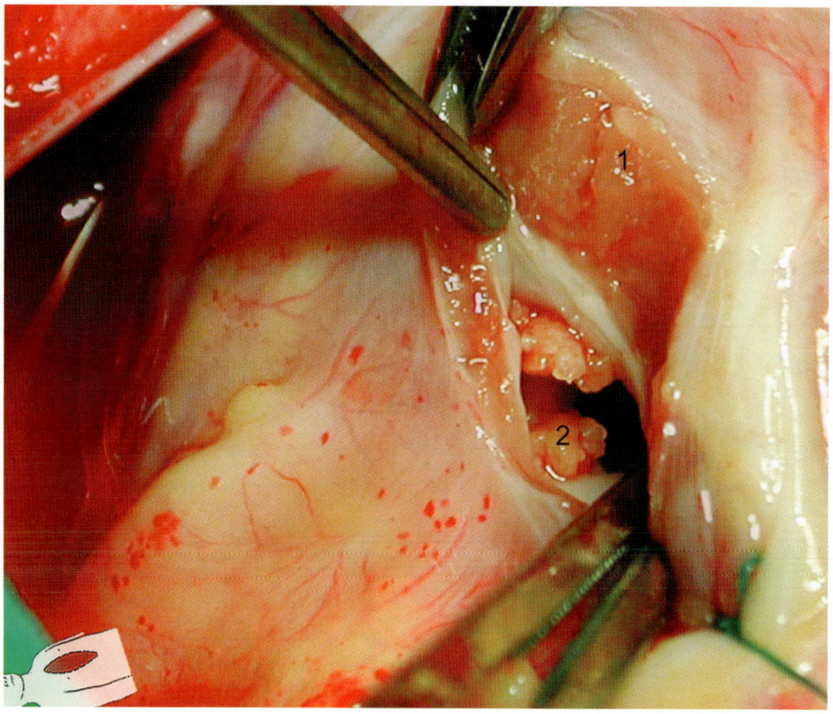

Figure 23.19. The same patient as in Figure 23.18. Another vegetation is seen facing the one on the free wall.

1. RV wall
2. Vegetation

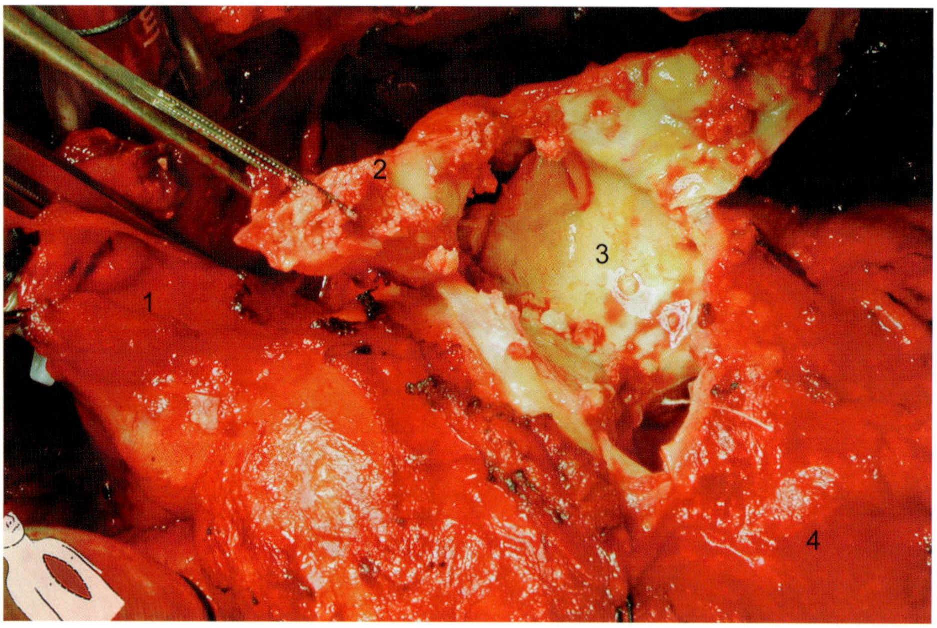

Figure 23.20. Median sternotomy view of a 23-year-old patient with pulmonary atresia during reoperation for conduit replacement. The incision was started at the RV outflow and extended up to the distal part of the conduit. Multiple vegetations are visible.

1. Ascending aorta
2. Vegetation on the conduit
3. Opened conduit
4. RV

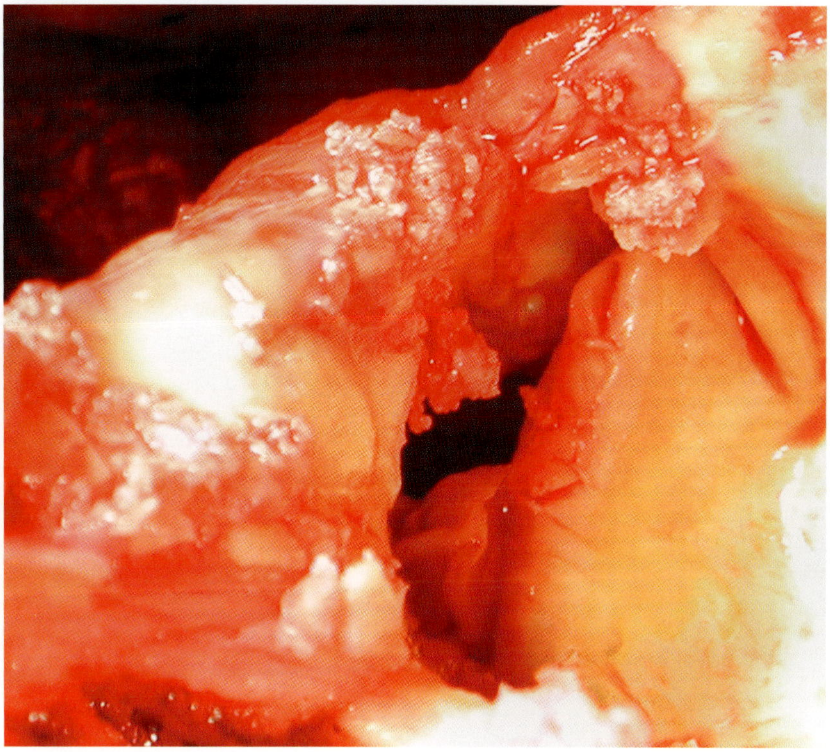

Figure 23.21. A close-up view of the conduit of the same patient as in Figure 23.20. Note the extensive vegetations lining the inside of the conduit.

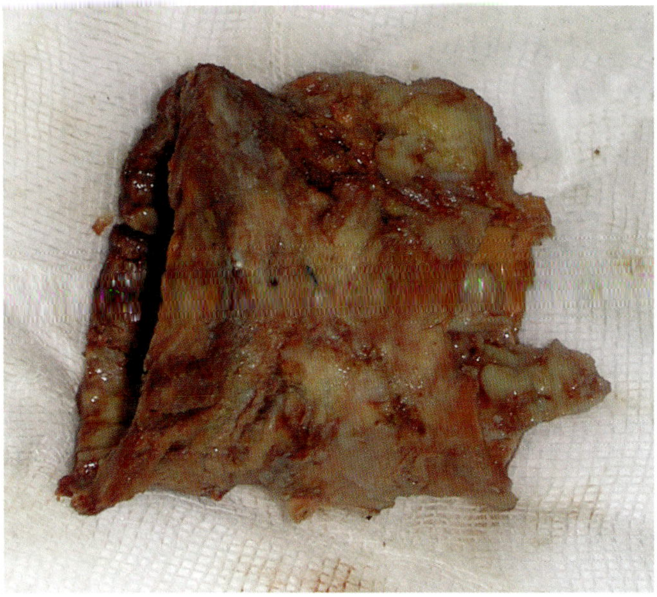

Figure 23.22

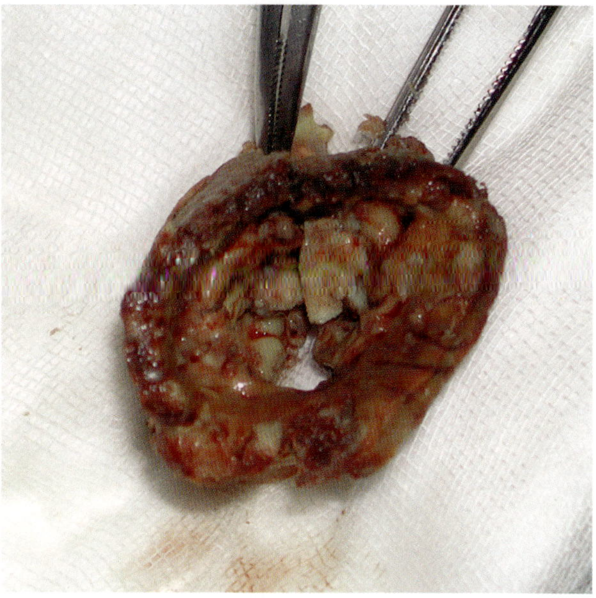

Figure 23.23

An excised conduit from a 12-year-old child with TOF who developed infective endocarditis. Multiple vegetations are seen on the valve and inner walls of the conduit.

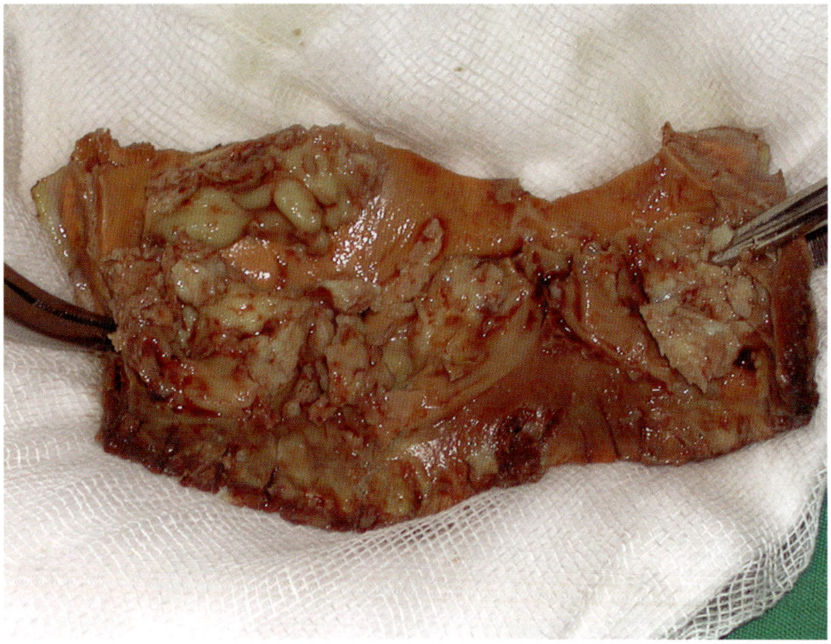

Figure 23.24. The same conduit as that shown in Figures 23.22 and 23.23. The conduit has been opened to show the extent of the vegetations and the severely damaged conduit valve.

REFERENCES

1. Day M, Gauvreau K, Shulman S, Newburger J. Characteristics of children hospitalized with infective endocarditis. *Circulation*. 2009;119:865–870.
2. Ferrieri P, Gewitz M, Gerber M, et al. Unique features of infective endocarditis in childhood. *Pediatrics*. 2002;109:931–943.
3. Baddour L, Wilson W, Bayer A, et al. Infective endocarditis diagnosis, antimicrobial therapy, and management of complications. *Circulation*. 2005; 111:e394–e433.
4. Mauri L, de Lemos J, O'Gara P. Infective endocarditis. *Curr Probl Cardiol*. 2001;9:562–610.

CHAPTER 24

Miscellaneous Conditions

In this chapter, we present some miscellaneous congenital cardiac conditions that are not covered in the preceding chapters.

Normally, the heart lies in the mediastinum with its apex pointing toward the left. Rarely, the heart may be bifid and thus has 2 apices as shown in Figure 24.1 from a 5-year-old child with tetralogy of Fallot (TOF). Another less dramatic example of a bifid heart was presented in Figure 21.2.

Arterial tortuosity is seen in many conditions, including cutis laxa, Ehlers–Danlos syndrome, and the so-called arterial tortuosity syndrome.[1] It may lead to arterial stenosis caused by kinking and twisting of the arteries. Two cases are presented; the first (Figures 24.2 to 24.8) has crossed pulmonary arteries (PAs) resulting in stenosis, and the second (Figures 24.9–24.11) is an incidental finding with no hemodynamic consequences in a child who had a ventricular septal defect (VSD).

A double-orifice tricuspid valve is a very rare condition. Figures 24.12 to 24.15 are from an 8-year-old child who also had a VSD, atrial septal defect (ASD), and pulmonary stenosis. The accessory valve orifice has rudimentary leaflets and papillary muscle of its own. Interestingly, a diverticulum was found on the inferolateral wall of the right ventricle (RV) of the same patient (see Figure 24.12). See Figures 20.1 and 20.2 for a double orifice mitral valve.

Budd–Chiari syndrome is characterized by hepatic venous outflow obstruction, resulting from a variety

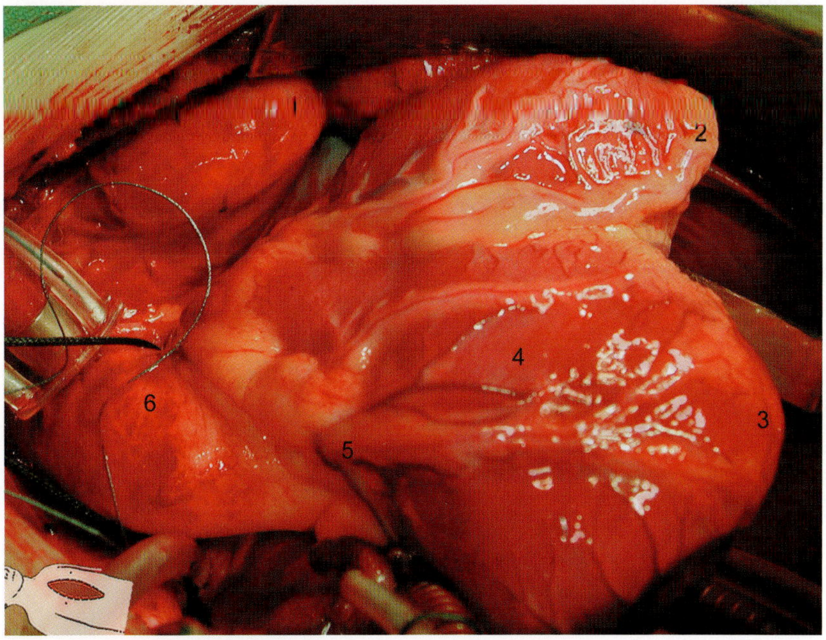

Figure 24.1. Bifid heart in a 5-year-old child with TOF, seen through a median sternotomy. The heart has 2 apices. Note the inconspicuous main pulmonary artery (MPA).

1. Left lung
2. Left apex
3. Right apex
4. RV
5. Right coronary artery
6. Ascending aorta

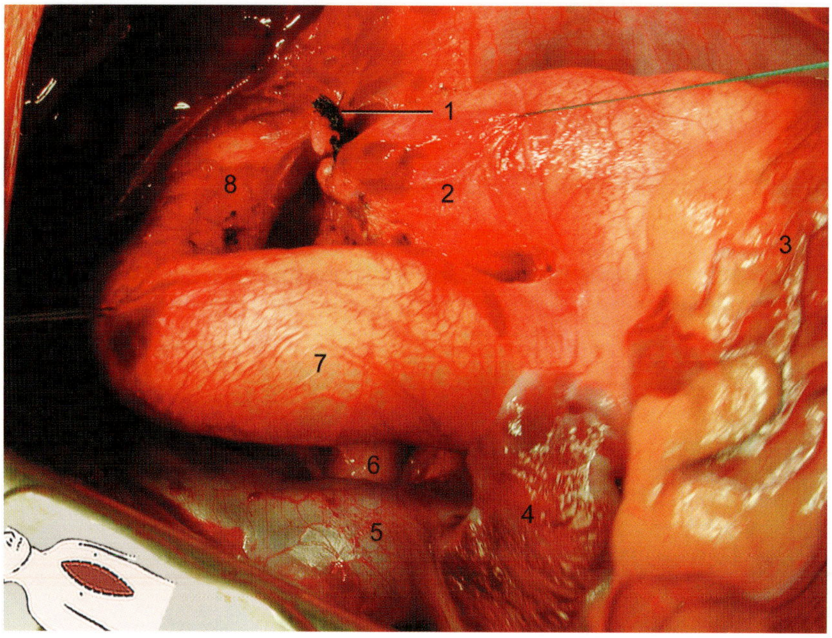

Figure 24.2. Median sternotomy view of a 3-year-old child with branch pulmonary stenosis caused by crossed PAs. Also note the elongated aorta.

1. Ligamentum arteriosum (ligated)
2. MPA
3. RV
4. Right atrial appendage (RAA)
5. Superior vena cava (SVC)
6. Right PA
7. Ascending aorta
8. Transverse aortic arch

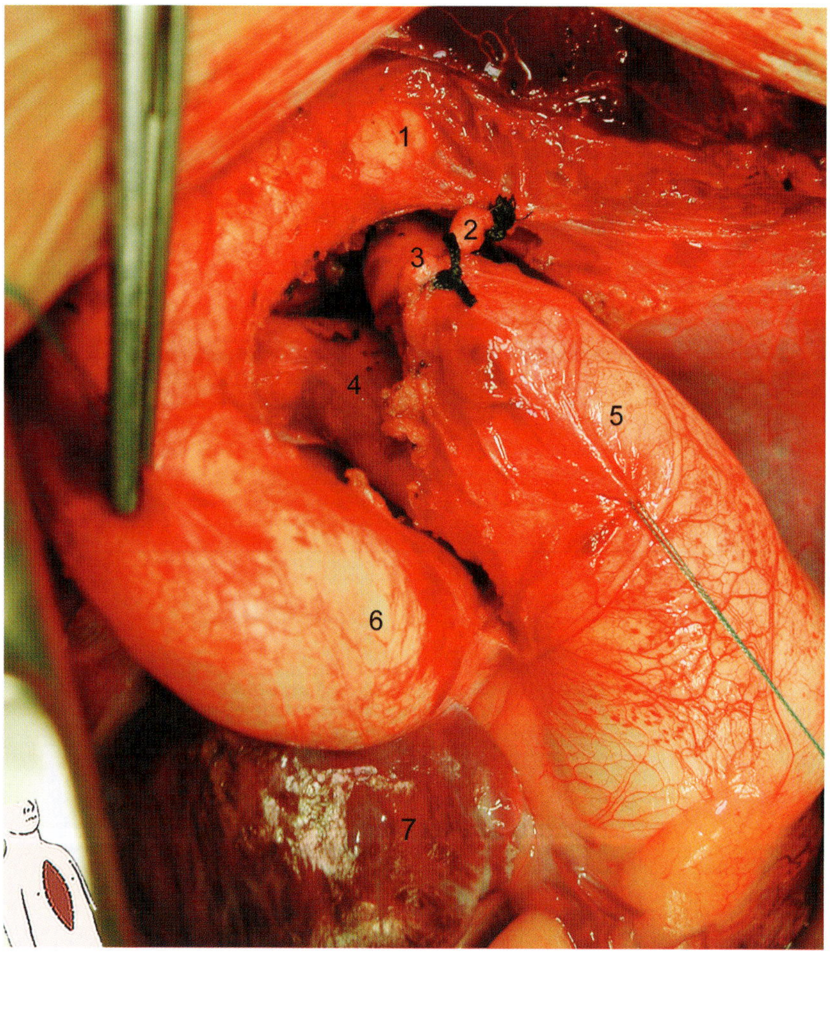

Figure 24.3. The same patient as in Figure 24.2 with the aorta retracted to the right to show the bifurcation of the MPA. The PA is twisted counterclockwise; the right branch arises from a leftward posterior location, whereas the left branch arises from a rightward anterior location, resulting in kinking.

1. Transverse aorta
2. Ligamentum arteriosum (ligated)
3. Left PA
4. Right PA
5. MPA
6. Ascending aorta
7. RAA

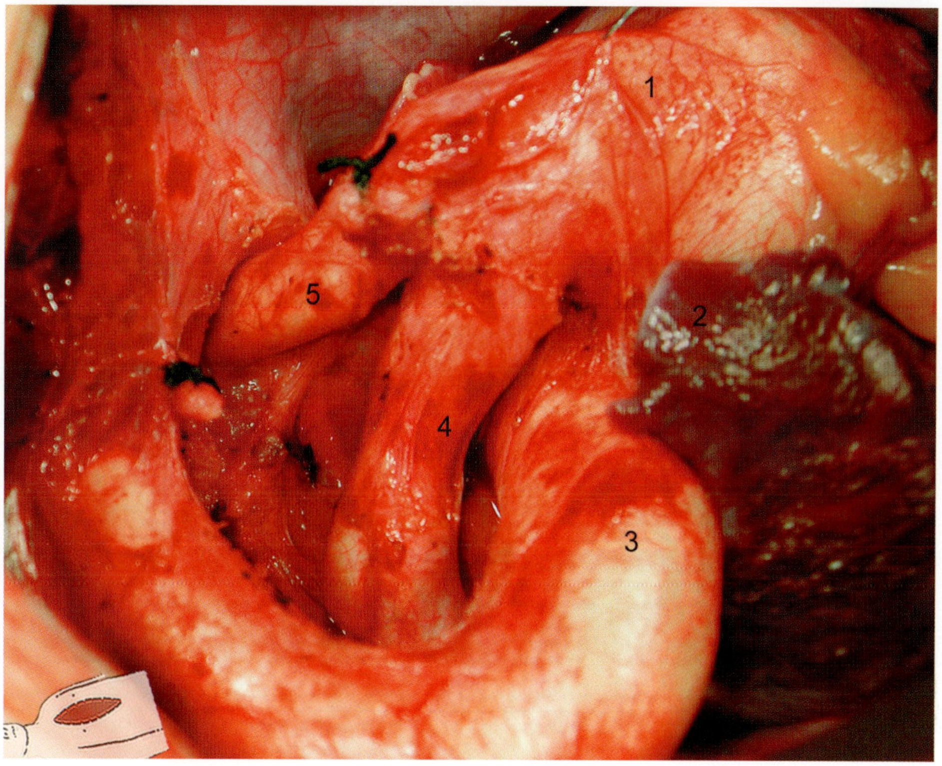

Figure 24.4. The same patient as in Figures 24.2 and 24.3 with the aorta and the PA retracted to better show the bifurcation of the MPA.

1. MPA
2. RAA
3. Ascending aorta
4. Right PA
5. Left PA

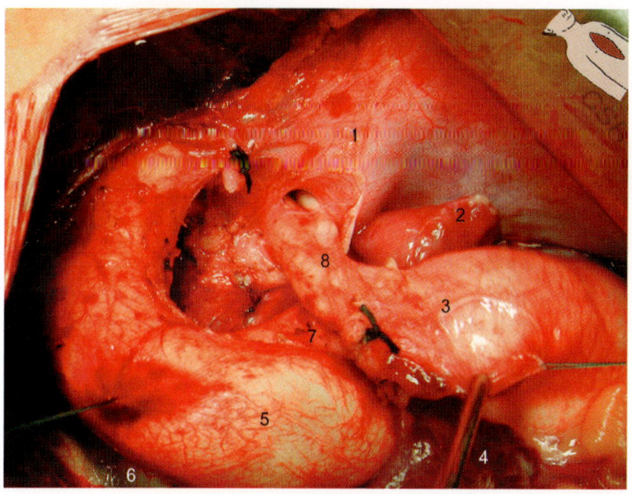

Figure 24.5

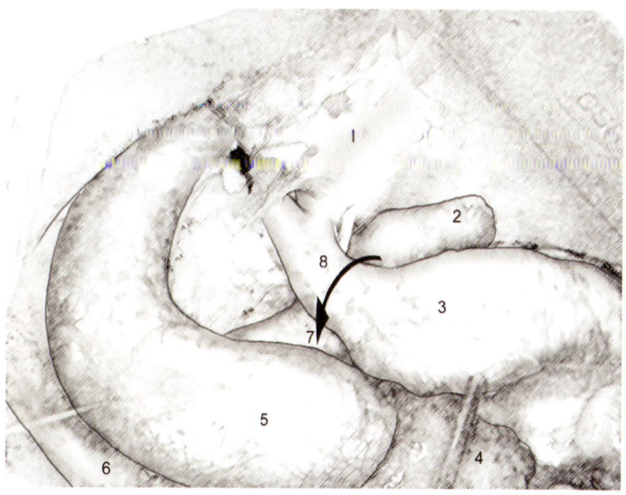

Figure 24.6

The same patient as in Figures 24.2 to 24.4. There is counterclockwise rotation of the MPA around itself, resulting in kinking of the PAs, especially the left.

1. Left lung
2. Left atrial appendage (LAA)
3. MPA
4. RAA
5. Ascending aorta
6. SVC
7. Right PA
8. Left PA

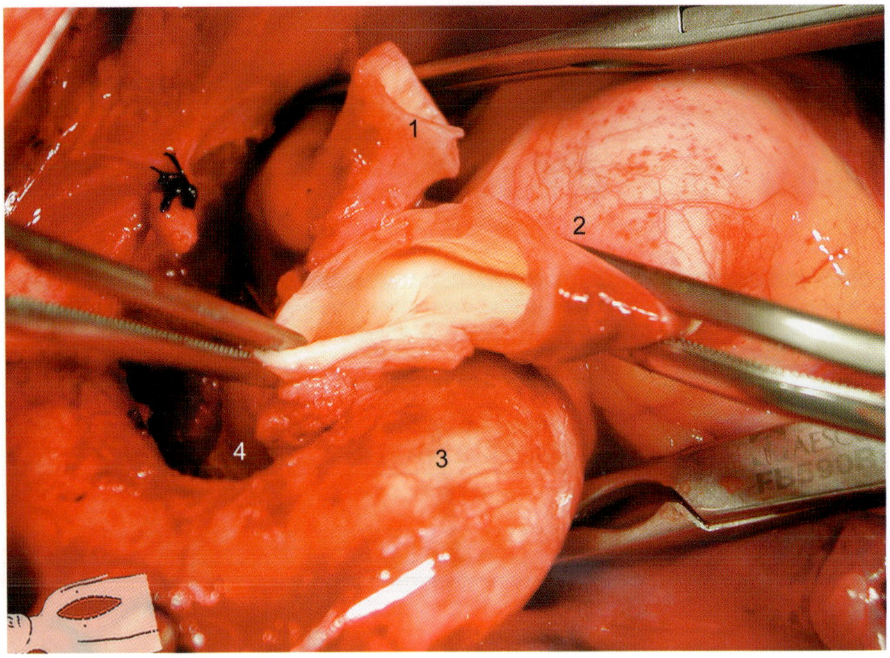

Figure 24.7. The same patient as in Figures 24.2 to 24.6 during repair. The left PA has been detached from its origin on the superior aspect of the MPA.

1. Left PA
2. MPA
3. Ascending aorta

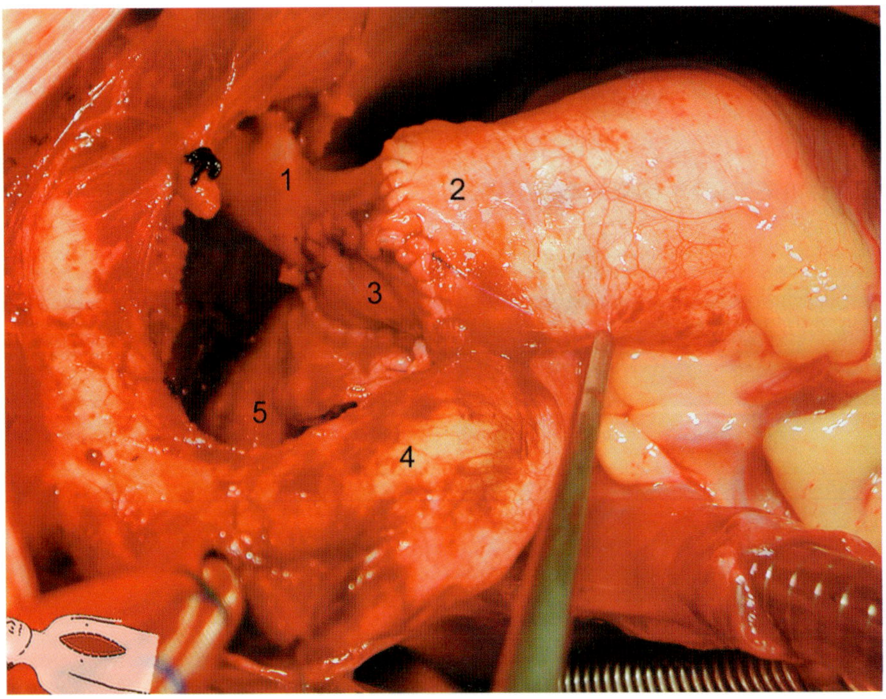

Figure 24.8. The same patient as in Figures 24.2 to 24.7 after repair. The left PA has been relocated to a more normal location on the left aspect of the MPA. Some resection in the PA wall was also done to achieve proper anatomic alignment. Its original site (3) has been covered by a patch of autologous pericardium.

1. Left PA
2. MPA
3. Autologous pericardial patch
4. Ascending aorta
5. Right PA

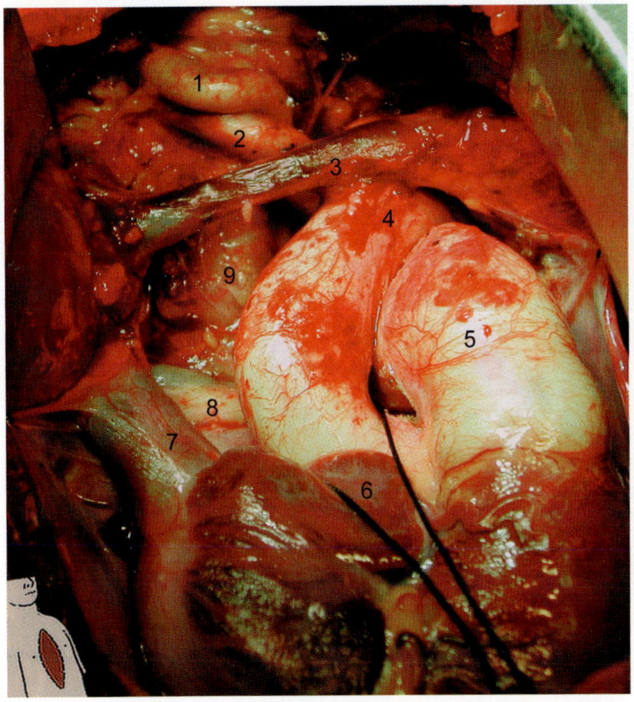

Figure 24.9

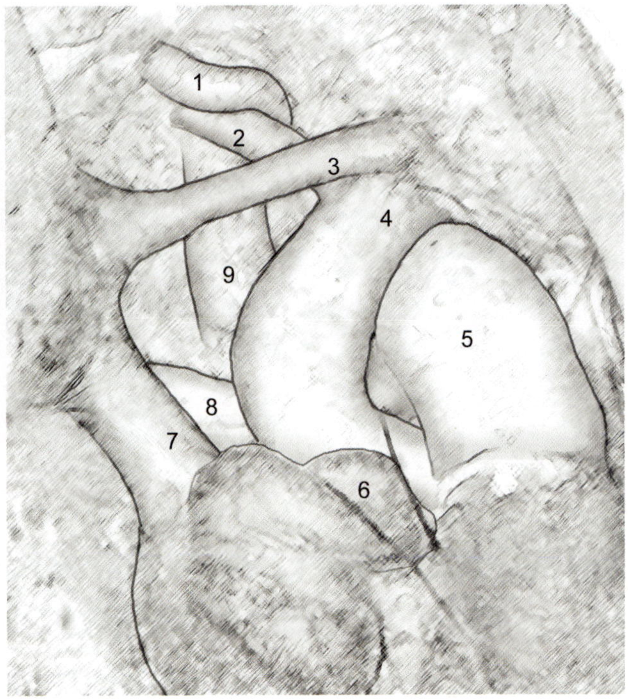

Figure 24.10

Intraoperative view of a child operated on for closure of VSD. The major arteries, including neck arteries, were elongated, tortuous, and twisted. The MPA is dilated secondary to left-to-right shunting across the VSD.

1. Right common carotid artery
2. Right subclavian artery
3. Innominate vein
4. Aortic arch
5. MPA
6. RAA
7. SVC
8. Right PA
9. Trachea

of causes. The large hepatic veins and inferior vena cava (IVC) are involved.[2] Figure 24.16 shows the very small orifice of the IVC as seen in the right atrium in a 13-year-old child with Budd–Chiari syndrome. This was treated by resection of obstructive tissue and enlargement of the IVC opening (not shown).

Figure 24.17 is a still frame from an echocardiogram done on the third postoperative day for a 1-month-old infant who has had an arterial switch operation. A mass was seen in the left atrium. The infant was reopened again, and the mass turned out to be an invaginated LAA (Figure 24.18).

Pulmonary vein (PV) stenosis is usually seen in the context of anomalous pulmonary venous connections or after surgery involving the PVs. Primary stenosis of the PVs is exceedingly rare.[3] If left untreated, diffuse hypoplasia of the veins may ensue and may culminate in death.[4] Figure 24.19 shows stenosis of the left PVs in an 11-month-old infant who also had a VSD. Figures 24.20 to 24.25 are from another child, 18 months old, who had subvalvar aortic stenosis in addition to the pulmonary venous abnormality. The left and right PVs were stenotic. In this patient, the PVs were patch-augmented with autologous pericardium.

An abnormally located and/or dilated vessel may occasionally compress the airways, leading to respiratory distress and tracheobronchomalacia. Figure 24.26 is a median sternotomy view of a 3 month-old infant with dextrocardia, double outlet right ventricle (DORV), and pulmonary stenosis. There was tracheal compression by a dilated, abnormally coursing aortic arch. Aortopexy was performed by suspending the aortic arch to the anterior chest wall using a piece of Dacron passed around the arch.

Anomalous origin of one of the PAs from the aorta is a rare abnormality that leads to left-to-right shunting and may cause congestive heart failure and pulmonary hypertension. The right PA is more commonly involved.[5] An example is shown in Figures 24.27 to 24.31. Figures 24.32 to 24.34 are from a 10-month-old infant with hypoplastic right PA that needed patch angioplasty.

Unilateral absence of one of the branch PAs is another rare abnormality. It is usually associated with

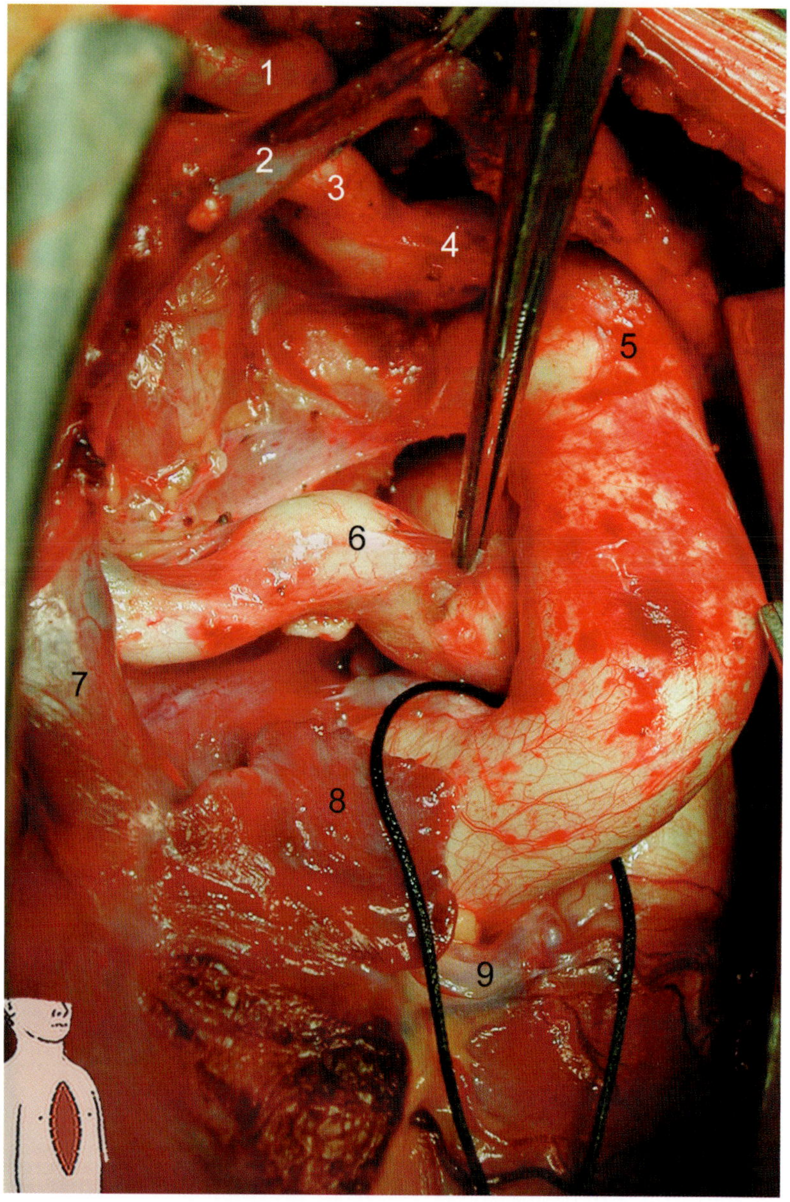

Figure 24.11. The same patient as in Figure 24.9. The aorta is retracted leftward to reveal the elongated, tortuous right PA. Even the coronary artery looked abnormal.

1. Right common carotid artery
2. Innominate vein
3. Right subclavian artery
4. Innominate artery
5. Aortic arch
6. Right PA
7. SVC
8. RAA
9. Right coronary artery

a ductus arteriosus feeding an intrapulmonary PA, or the involved lung may be supplied by aortopulmonary collateral arteries.[6] In the patient shown in Figures 24.35 and 24.36, the right PA is absent, the right lung is hypoplastic, and the lung is supplied by aortopulmonary collateral arteries. The mediastinal structures are shifted to the right, altering their spatial orientation. Right pneumonectomy was performed because the right lung was nonfunctional and acted as focus of infection.

Double outlet left ventricle (DOLV) is an exceedingly rare condition in which both great arteries originate from the morphologic LV. The patients usually have normal visceral and atrial situs. The most common associated anomalies are VSDs and pulmonary stenosis.[7] Figures 24.37 to 24.43 are from a 4-month-old infant with DOLV and VSD. The PA was oversewn, the VSD was closed by a Dacron patch in a way that commits the aorta to the LV, and a xenograft conduit was placed between the RV and the PAs.

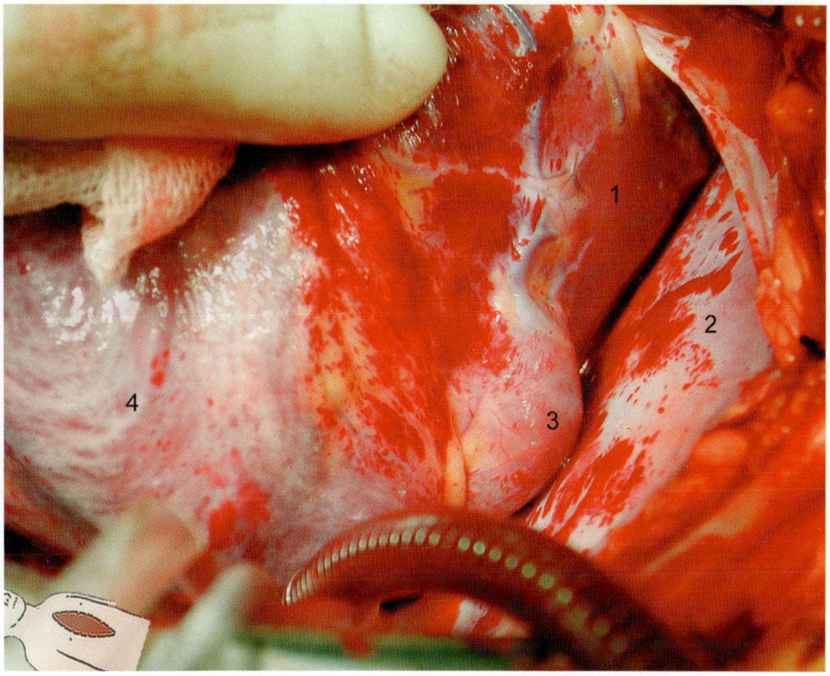

Figure 24.12. The right aspect of the heart as seen through a median sternotomy in an 8-year-old child during surgery for repair of VSD, ASD, and pulmonary stenosis. A small diverticulum is seen on the inferolateral side of the RV adjacent to the atrioventricular groove.

1. RV
2. Diaphragmatic side of pericardial sac
3. Diverticulum
4. Right atrium

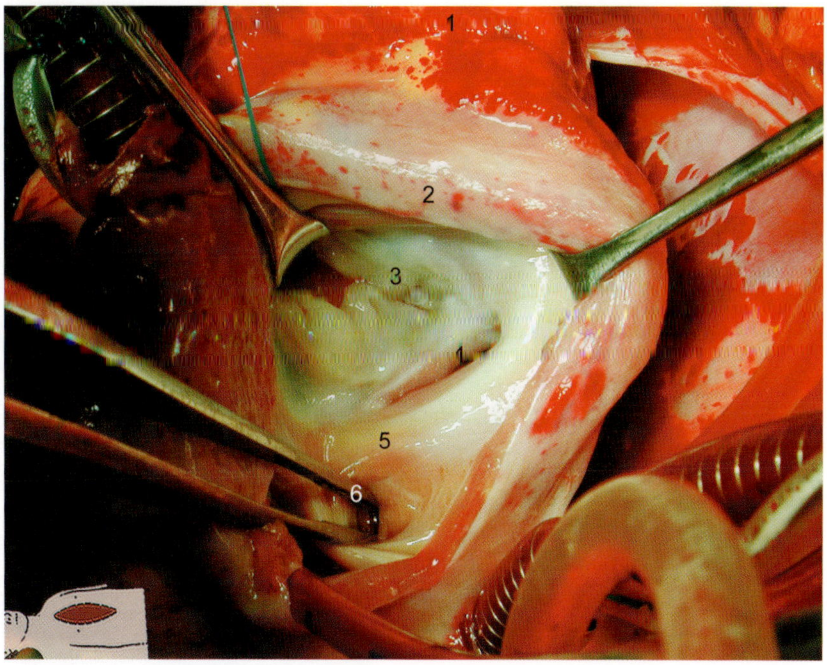

Figure 24.13. Right atriotomy view of the same patient as in Figure 24.12. An accessory tricuspid valve opening is seen to the right of the main tricuspid valve orifice.

1. RV
2. Right atrial wall
3. Tricuspid valve
4. Accessory tricuspid valve orifice
5. Annulus of tricuspid valve
6. Forceps in coronary sinus (CS)

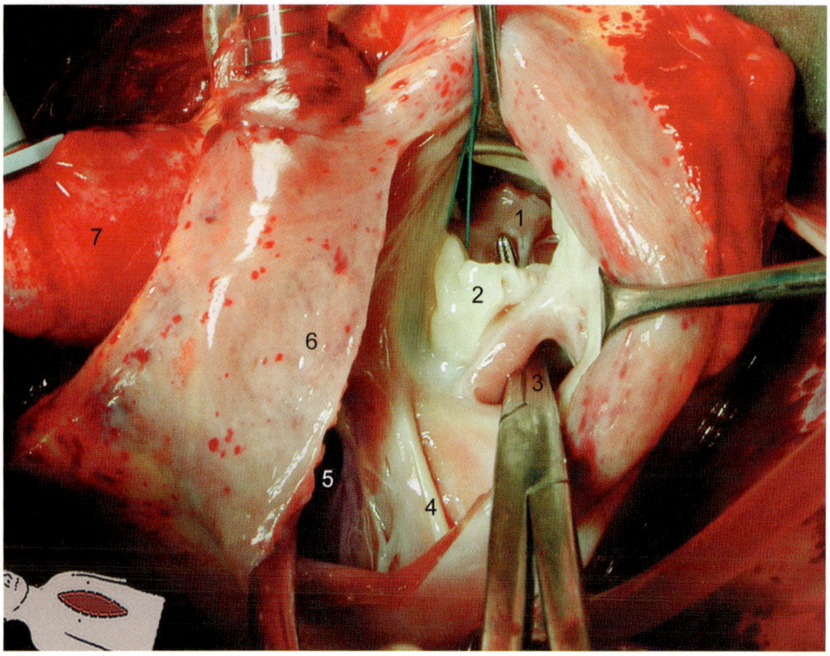

Figure 24.14. The same patient as in Figures 24.12 and 24.13. The forceps pass through the accessory valve orifice into the RV cavity.

1. RV cavity
2. Tricuspid valve
3. Forceps in accessory tricuspid valve orifice
4. Tendon of Todaro
5. ASD
6. Right atrial wall
7. Ascending aorta

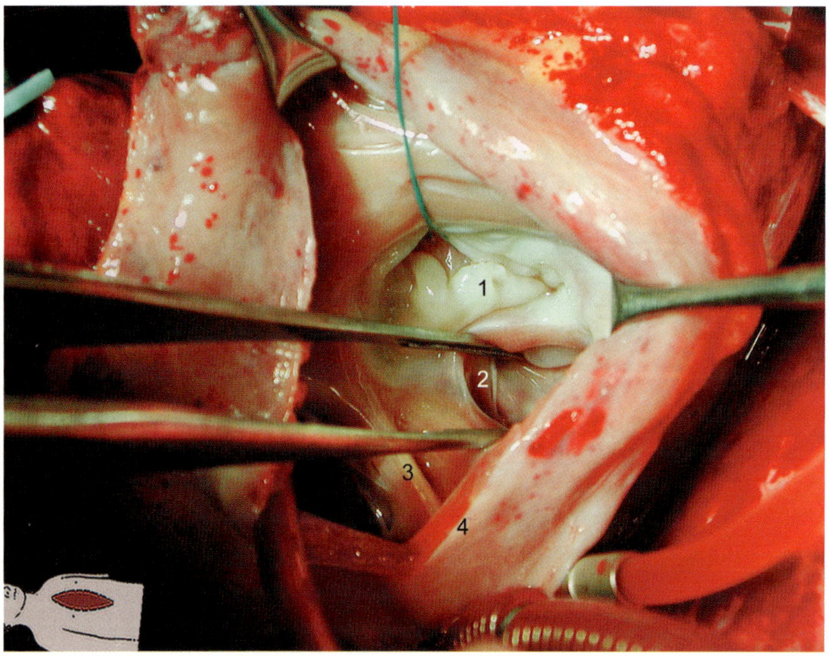

Figure 24.15. The same patient as in Figures 24.12 to 24.14. The accessory valve orifice has its own rudimentary leaflets and papillary muscles. It was closed with a Dacron patch (not shown).

1. Tricuspid valve
2. Accessory tricuspid valve
3. Tendon of Todaro
4. Right atrial wall

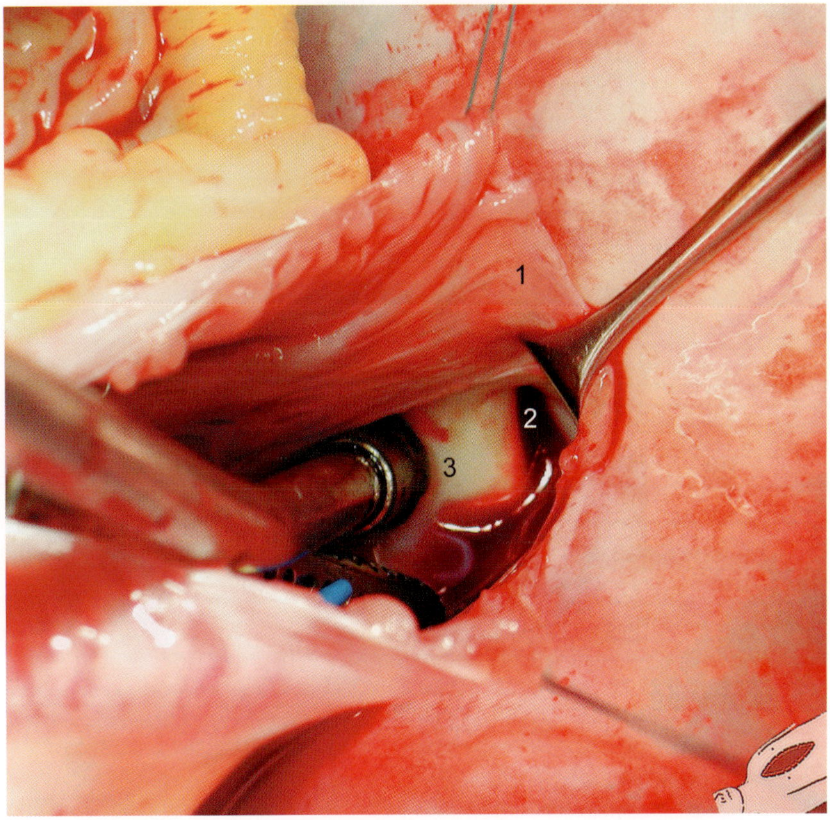

Figure 24.16. Right atriotomy view of a 13-year-old child with Budd–Chiari syndrome. There is near-complete obliteration of the IVC at its junction with the right atrium. Blood is seen oozing from the orifice of the IVC.

1. Right atrial wall
2. IVC orifice
3. Floor of right atrium

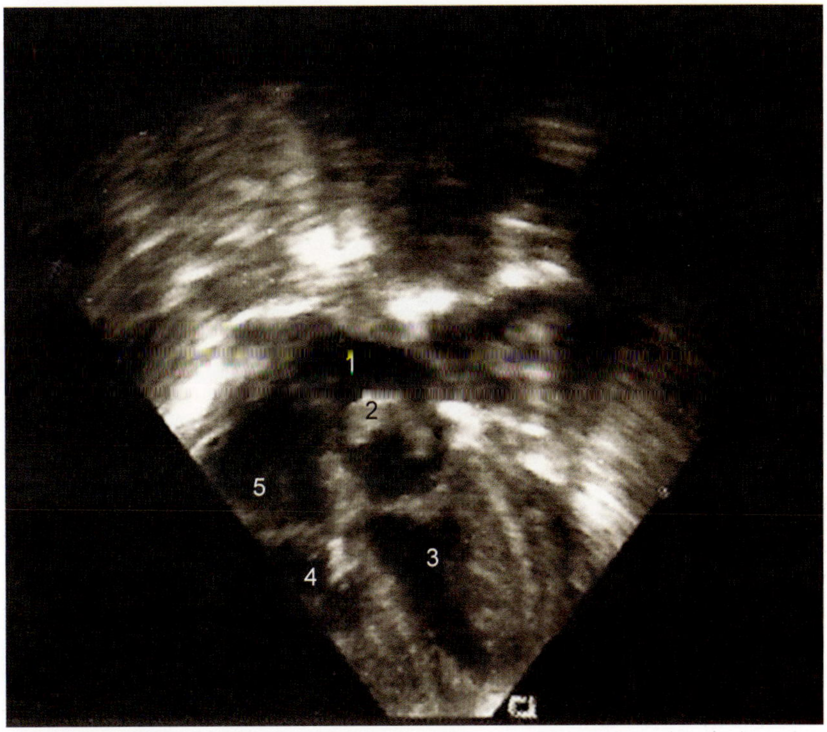

Figure 24.17. An echocardiogram still frame from a 1-month-old infant 3 days after an arterial switch operation. In this 4-chamber view, a mass is seen in the left atrium.

1. Left atrium
2. Mass in left atrium
3. Left ventricle (LV)
4. RV
5. Right atrium

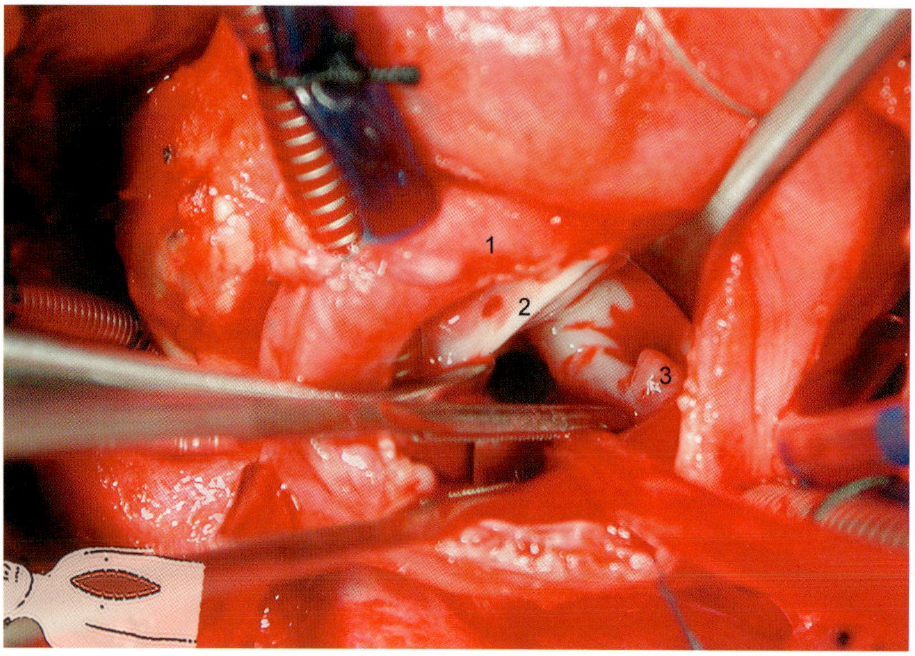

Figure 24.18. Intraoperative view of the patient whose echocardiogram is shown in Figure 24.17. The left atrium is accessed through a transseptal approach from the right atrium. The left atrial mass turned out to be an invaginated LAA.

1. Right atrial wall
2. Interatrial septum
3. Invaginated LAA

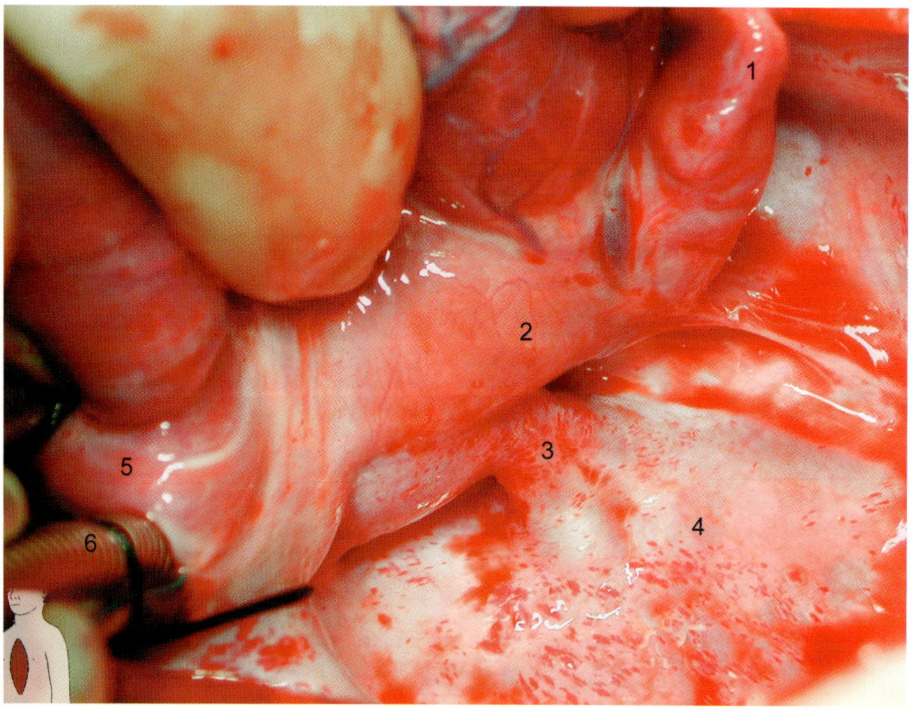

Figure 24.19. A median sternotomy view of an 11-month-old infant with pulmonary venous stenosis. The heart is retracted rightward to reveal the left-sided PVs as they enter the left atrium.

1. LAA
2. Left atrium
3. Left PVs
4. Left lung
5. Right atrium
6. IVC cannula

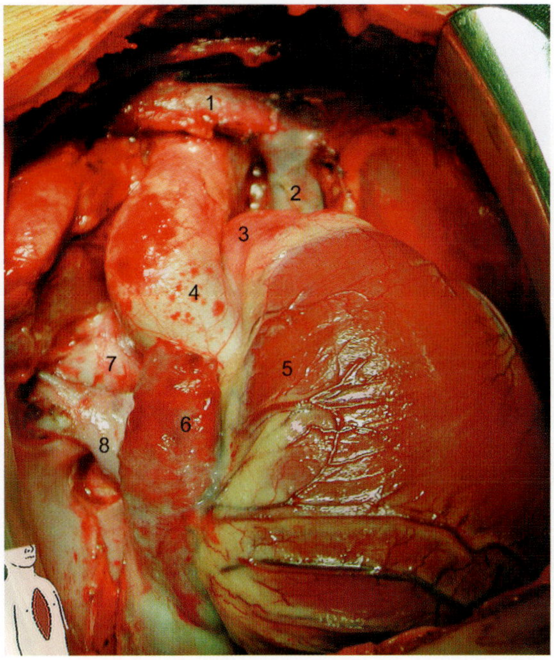

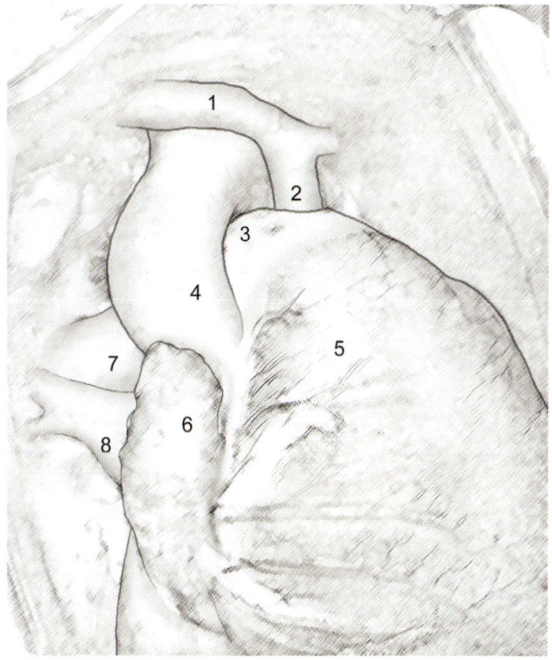

Figure 24.20 **Figure 24.21**

Median sternotomy view of an 18-month-old infant with pulmonary venous stenosis. The patient has visceral situs solitus, levocardia, left SVC to the CS, no right SVC, and a subaortic membrane. Note that the right PVs join each other to form a common PV (8) before entering the heart.

1. Innominate vein
2. SVC
3. MPA
4. Ascending aorta
5. RV
6. RAA
7. Right PA
8. Right PV

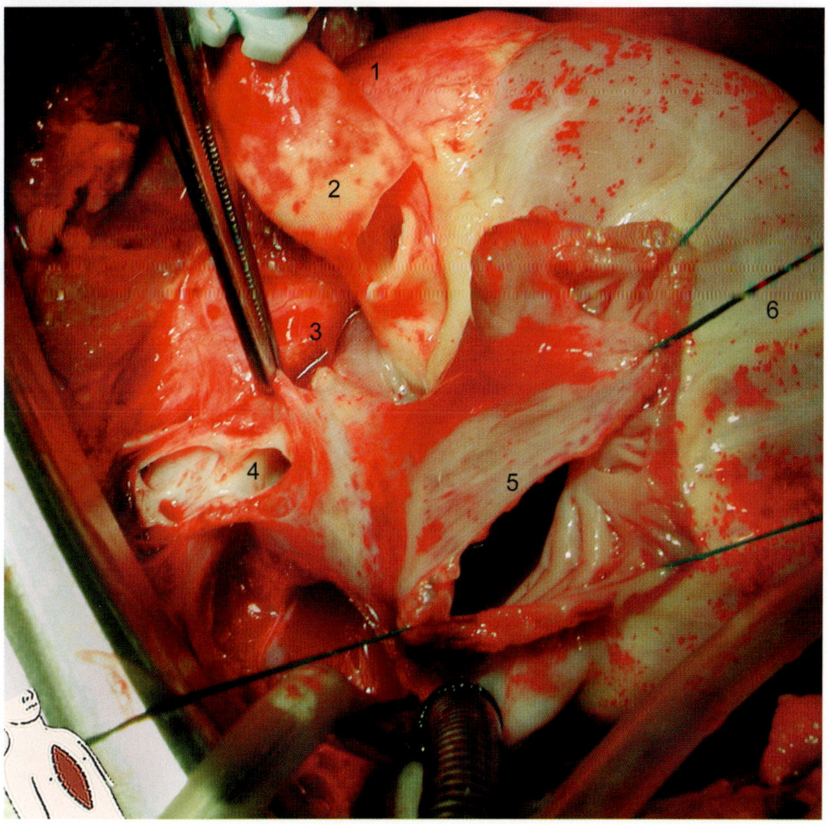

Figure 24.22. The same patient as in Figure 24.20. The right PV has been opened. A transverse ridge is seen in the lumen. An aortotomy has also been performed to access the subaortic membrane.

1. MPA
2. Ascending aorta
3. Right PA
4. Opened right PV
5. Right atrial wall
6. RV

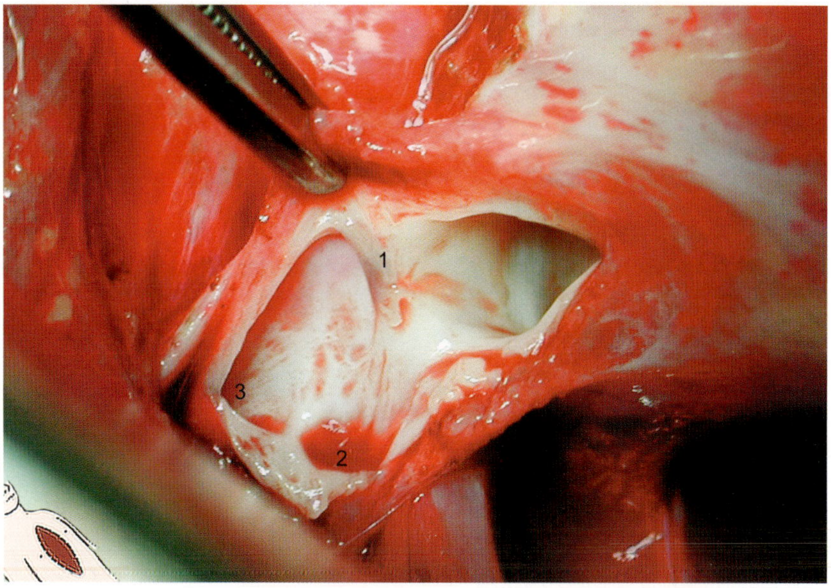

Figure 24.23. A close-up view of the right PV of the same patient as in Figures 24.20 to 24.22. The stenosis is partly because of a fibromuscular transverse ridge in the right common PV.

1. Transverse ridge
2. Right lower PV
3. Right upper PV

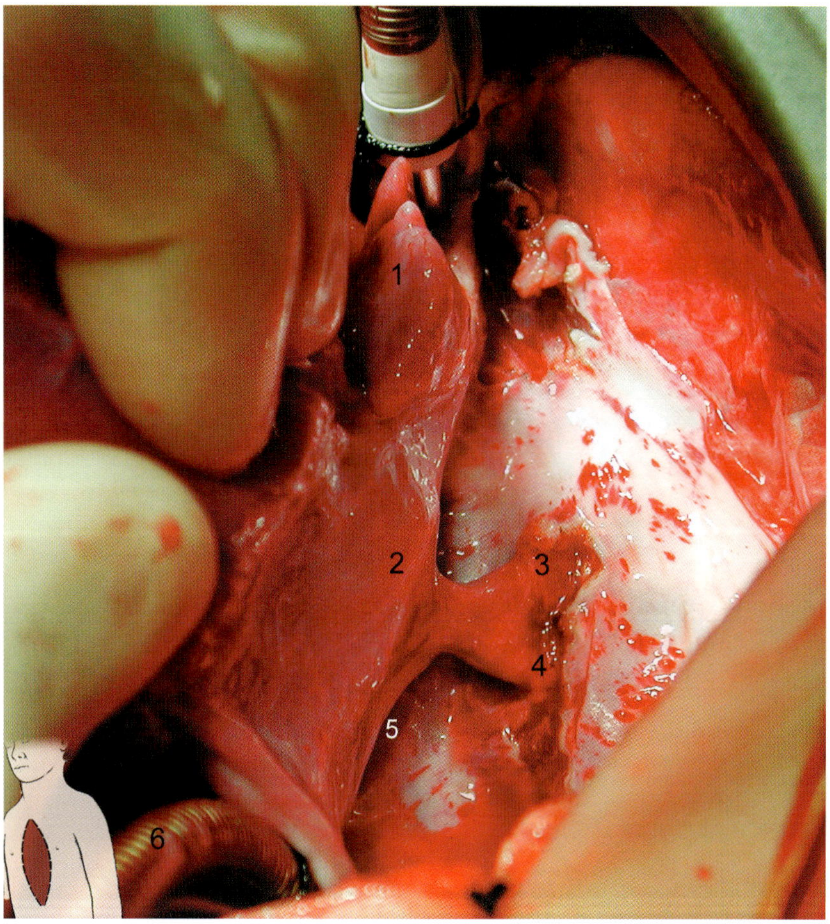

Figure 24.24. The left PVs of the same patient as in Figures 24.20 to 24.23. Similarly, the left PVs join each other to form a single vein that enters the left atrium.

1. LAA
2. Left atrium
3. Left upper PV
4. Left lower PV
5. Oblique pericardial sinus
6. IVC cannula

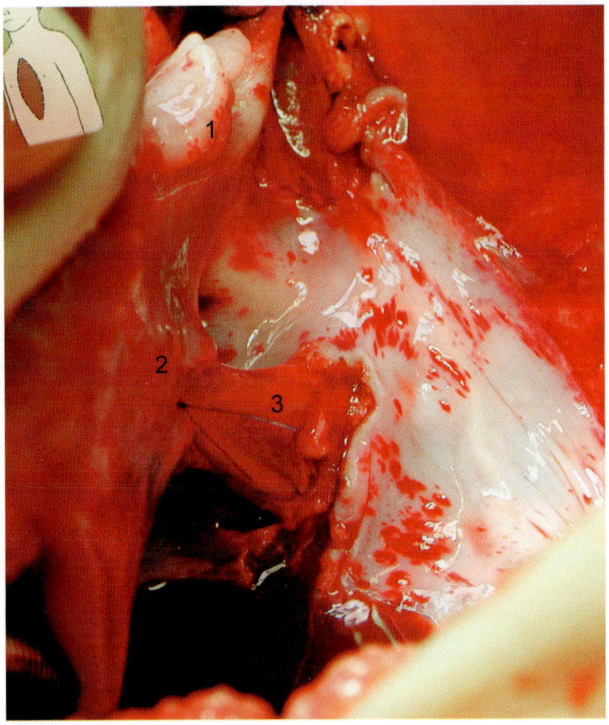

Figure 24.25. The same patient as in Figures 24.20 to 24.24 after repair. The left PVs are shown here, augmented with a patch of autologous pericardium.

1. LAA
2. Left atrium
3. Repaired left PVs

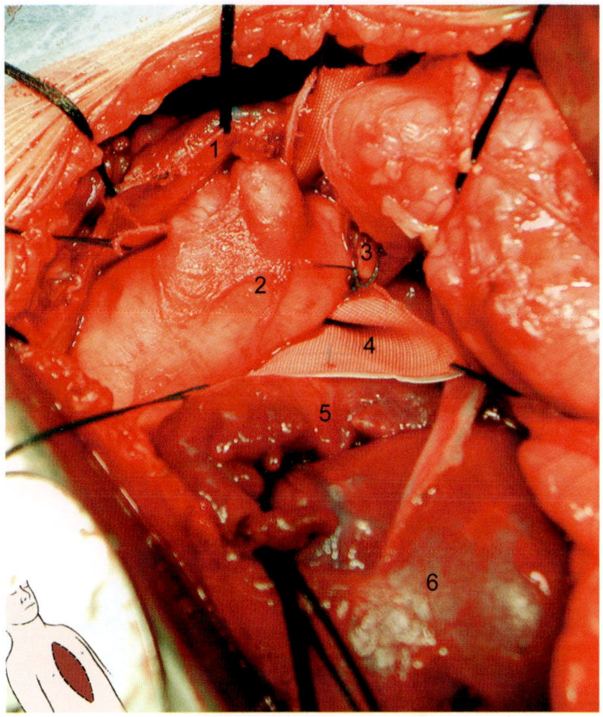

Figure 24.26. A median sternotomy view of a 3-month-old infant with dextrocardia, DORV, and pulmonary stenosis. The aorta is dilated and runs an almost horizontal course compressing the underlying trachea. A Dacron patch is being used to suspend the arch to the anterior chest wall (aortopexy).

1. Innominate vein
2. Transverse aortic arch
3. Ligated ductus arteriosus
4. Dacron patch
5. Left atrium
6. LV

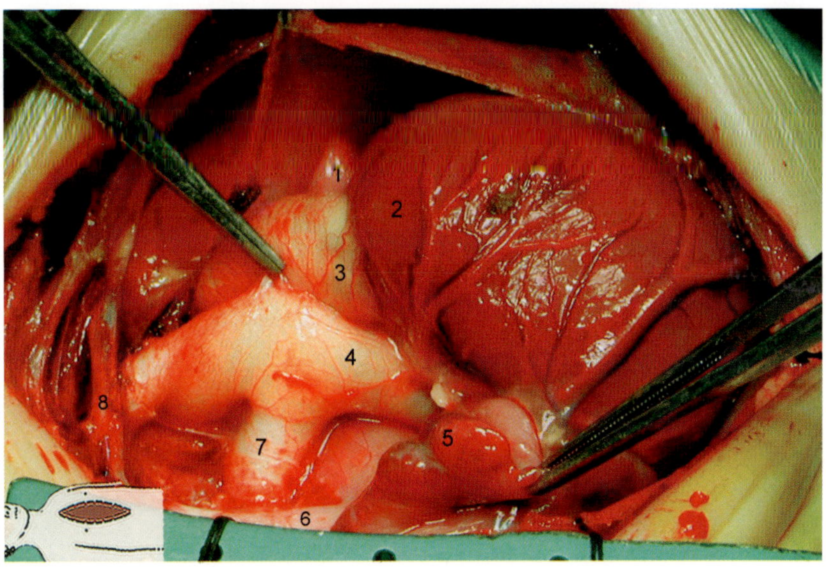

Figure 24.27. Median sternotomy view of a 1-month-old infant with anomalous origin of the right PA from the ascending aorta.

1. LAA
2. RV
3. MPA
4. Ascending aorta
5. RAA
6. SVC
7. Right PA
8. Innominate vein

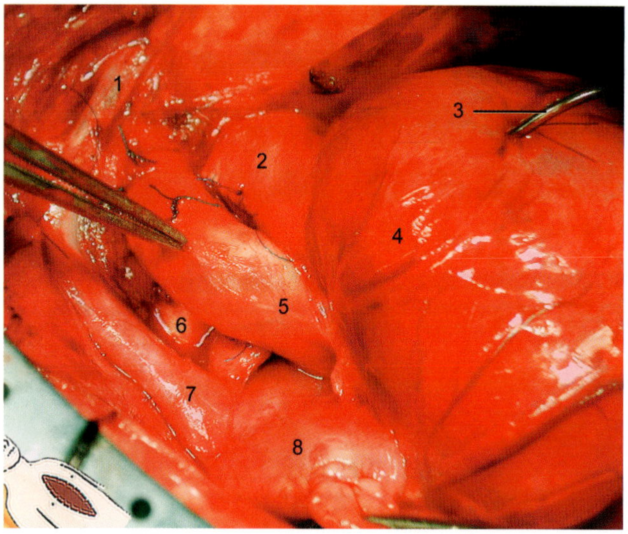

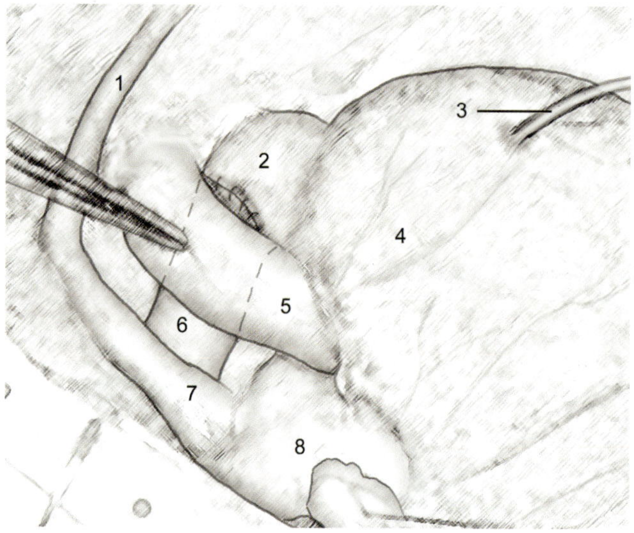

Figure 24.28 **Figure 24.29**

The same patient as in Figure 24.27 after repair. The right PA was detached from the aorta and was anastomosed to the MPA. The anterior part of the anastomosis was augmented with a patch of autologous pericardium. The defect in the aorta (not visible) was also closed with autologous pericardium.

1. Innominate vein
2. MPA
3. PA catheter
4. RV
5. Ascending aorta
6. Right PA
7. SVC
8. Right atrium

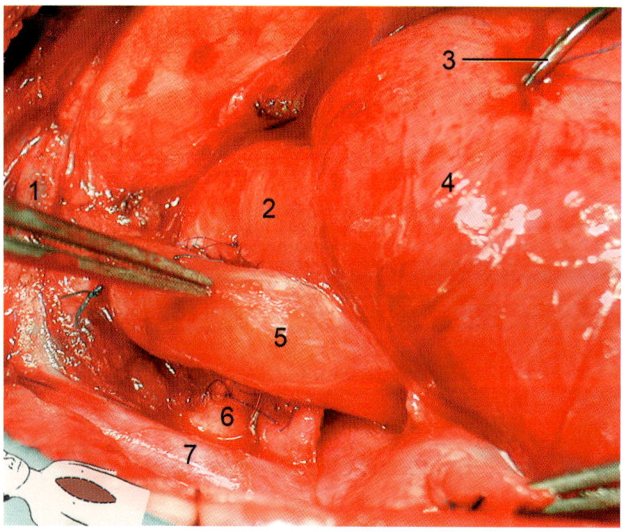

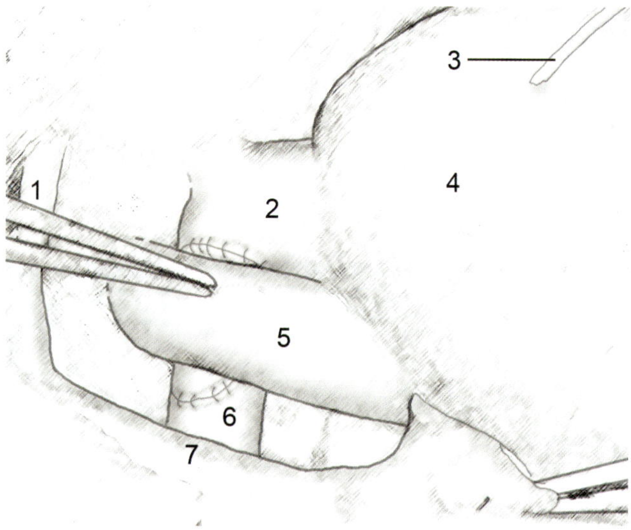

Figure 24.30 **Figure 24.31**

The same patient as in Figures 24.27 to 24.29 with the aorta retracted to show the patch used in the right PA angioplasty.

1. Innominate vein
2. MPA
3. PA catheter
4. RV
5. Ascending aorta
6. Right PA
7. SVC

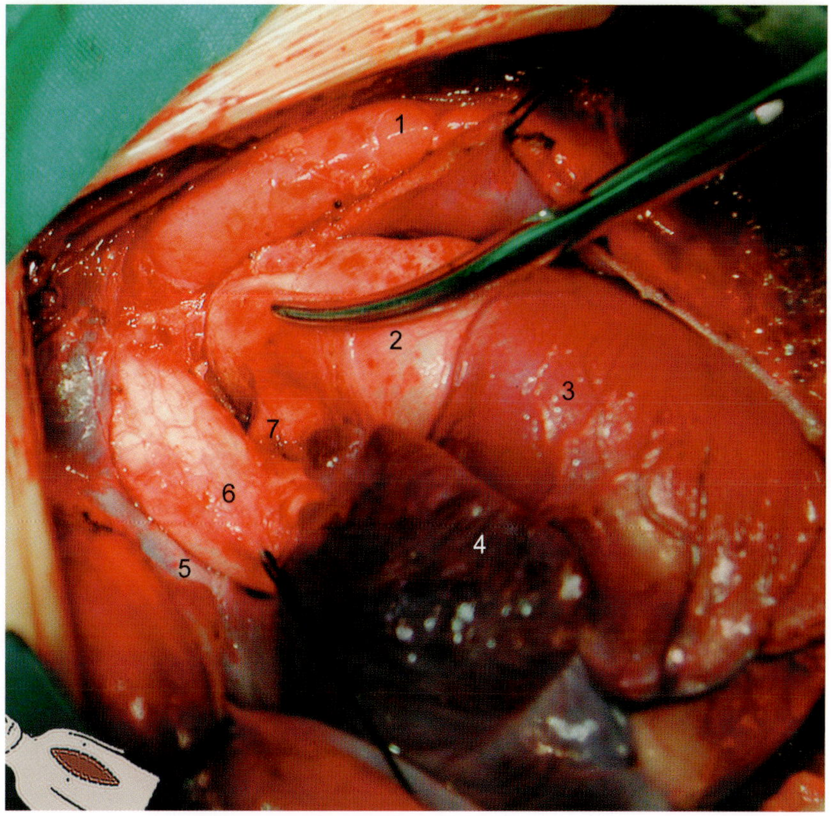

Figure 24.32. Median sternotomy view of a 10-month-old infant with VSD and hypoplastic right PA. Note the dilated MPA (caused by the VSD) and small right PA (7).

1. Left lung
2. MPA
3. RV
4. RAA
5. SVC
6. Ascending aorta
7. Right PA

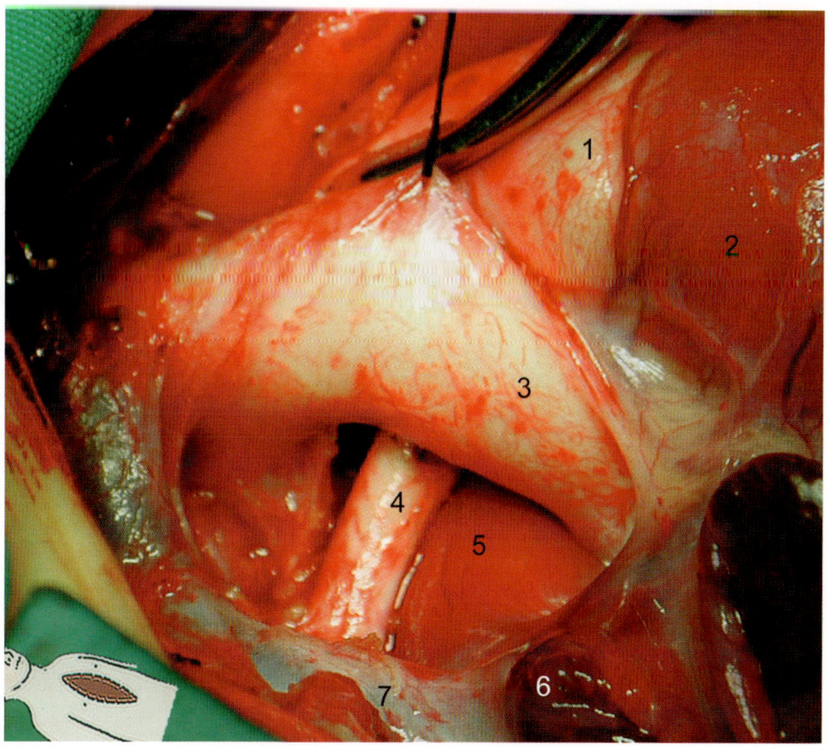

Figure 24.33. The same patient as in Figure 24.32. The aorta is retracted to reveal the right PA.

1. MPA
2. RV
3. Ascending aorta
4. Right PA
5. Left atrium
6. RAA
7. SVC

Figure 24.34. The same patient as in Figures 24.32 and 24.33 after repair. The right PA is augmented with a patch of xenograft pericardium.

1. RV
2. PA catheter
3. Right coronary artery
4. RAA
5. SVC
6. Repaired right PA
7. Ascending aorta
8. MPA

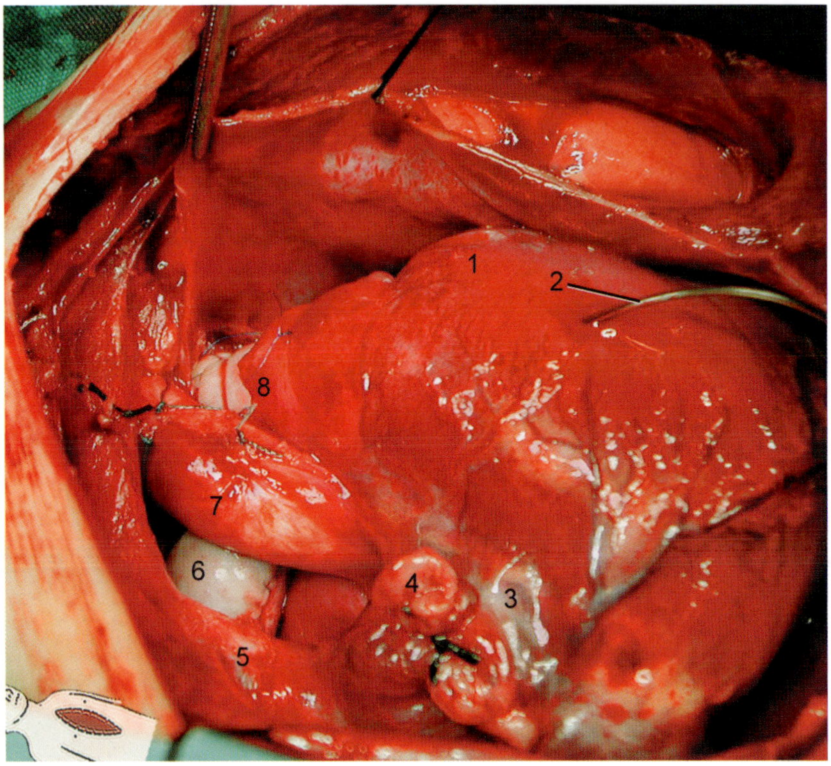

Figure 24.35. Median sternotomy view of a 1.5-year-old infant with unilateral agenesis of the right PA. The right lung is hypoplastic and is supplied by an aortopulmonary collateral artery. The heart is shifted to the right hemithorax, with its apex pointing down and slightly to the right. The RV is also hypoplastic.

1. Pericardium overlying left lung
2. LV
3. RV
4. MPA
5. Ascending aorta
6. Left PA

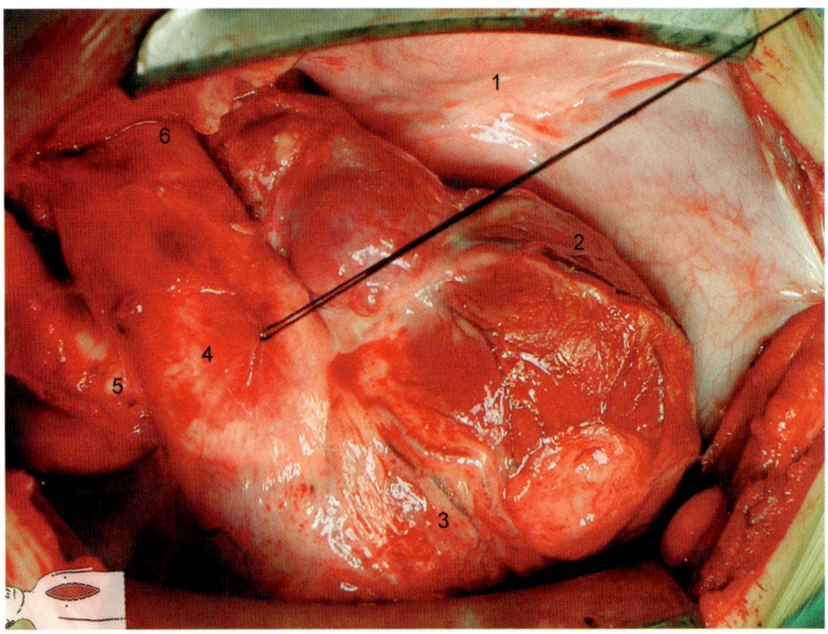

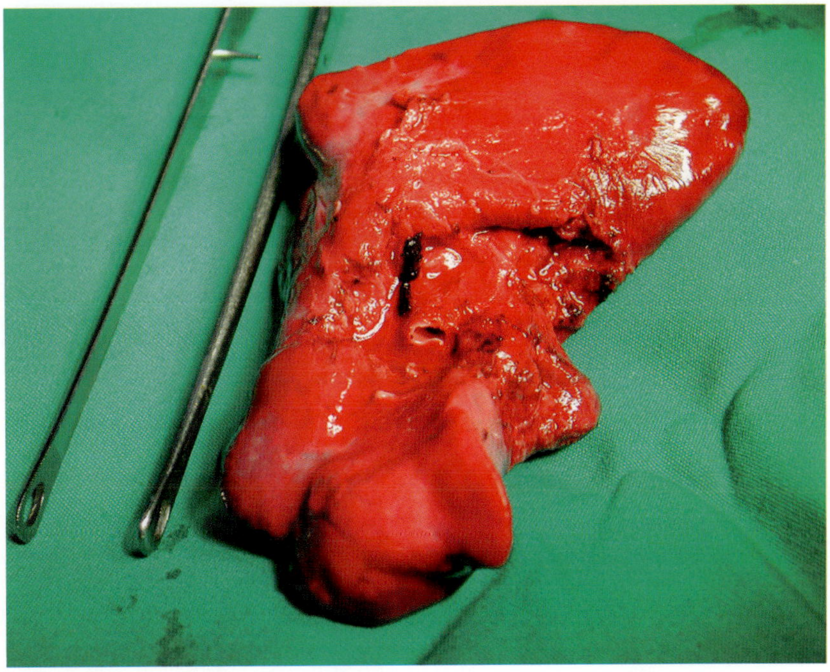

Figure 24.36. The excised, hypoplastic right lung of the patient shown in Figure 24.35.

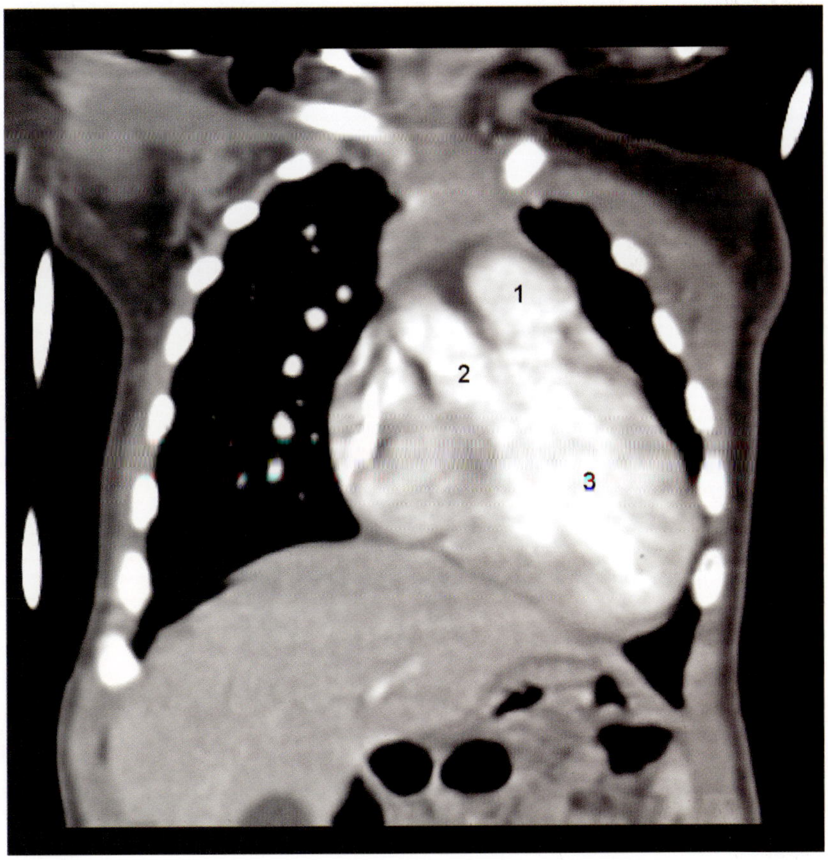

Figure 24.37. Computed tomography scan with contrast of a 4-month-old infant with DOLV. In this coronal section, both great arteries are seen side-by-side arising from the LV, a finding corroborated by echocardiography and intraoperative inspection (Figures 24.38 to 24.40).

1. MPA
2. Ascending aorta
3. LV

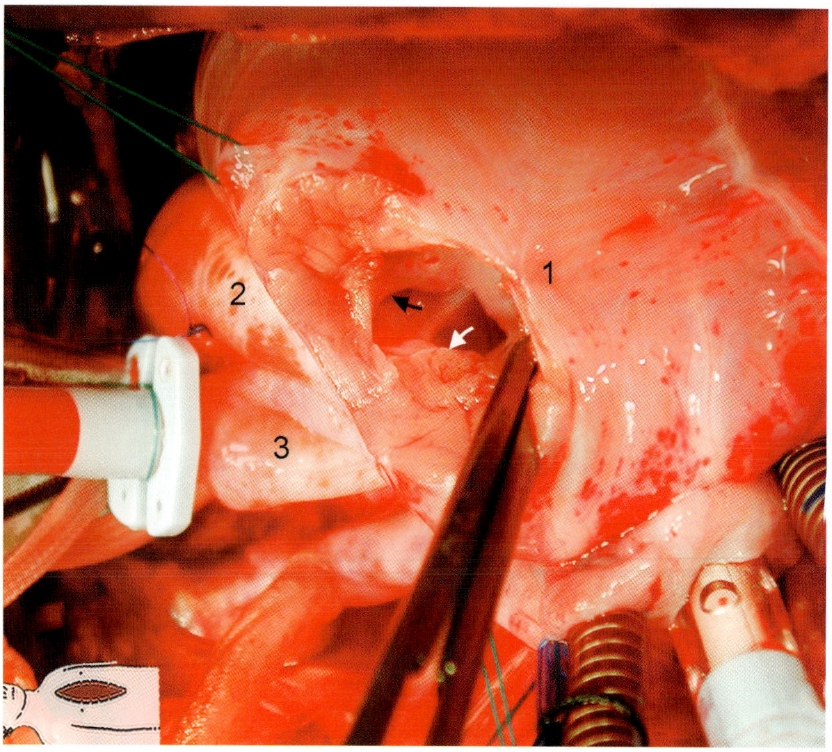

Figure 24.38. An intraoperative view of the patient shown in Figure 24.37. A right ventriculotomy has been performed, revealing a large VSD. Both outflows are seen through the VSD arising from the LV. The black arrow points to the pulmonary outflow, and the white arrow points to the aortic outflow.

1. RV
2. MPA
3. Ascending aorta

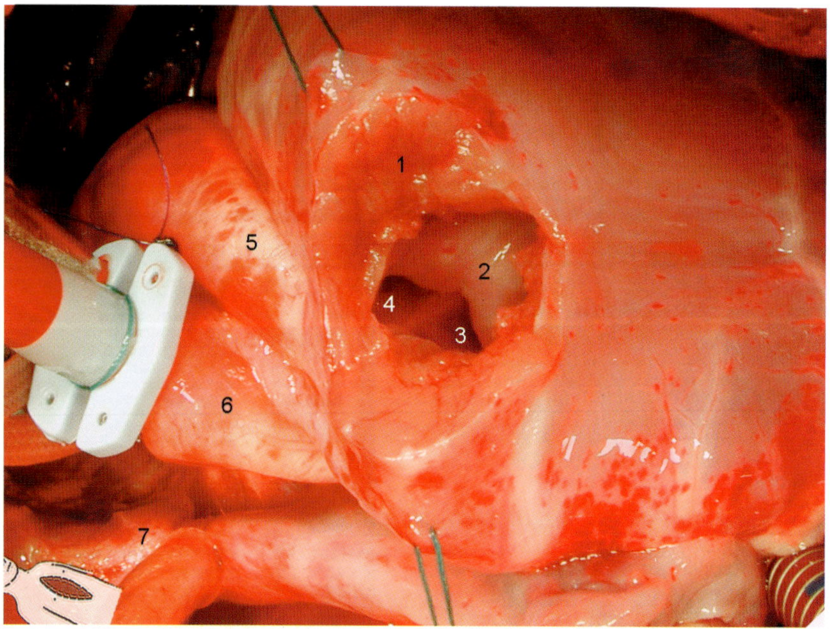

Figure 24.39. The same patient as in Figures 24.37 and 24.38. Both aortic and pulmonary valves are on the left side of the interventricular septum.

1. Right ventriculotomy incision
2. Interventricular septum
3. Aortic valve
4. Pulmonary valve
5. MPA
6. Ascending aorta
7. SVC

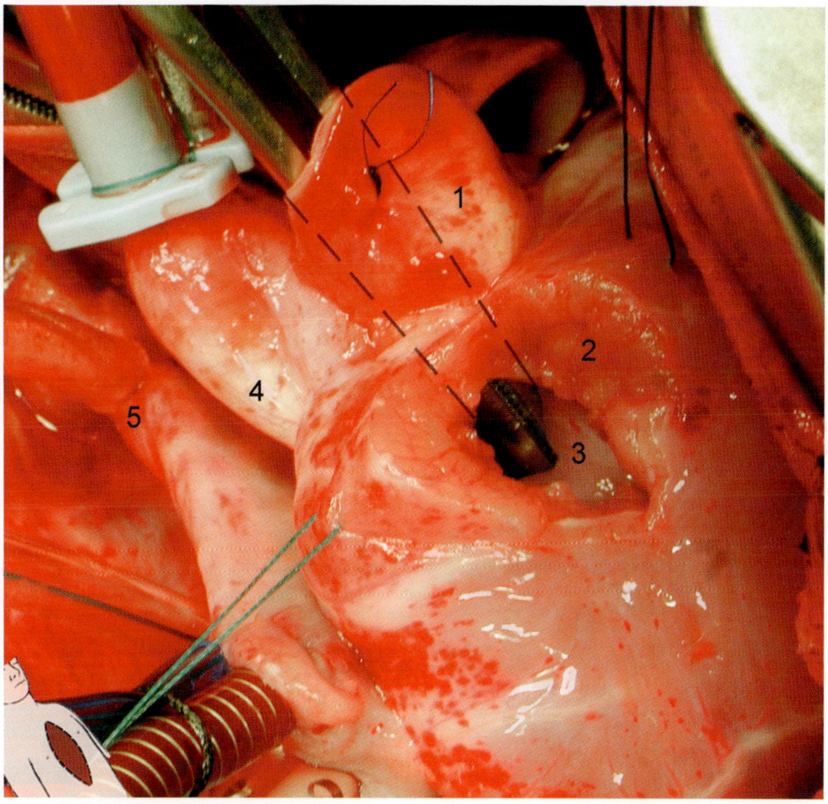

Figure 24.40. The same patient as in Figures 24.37 to 24.39. A pair of forceps is passed through the opened MPA. The tip of the forceps is unequivocally on the left of the interventricular septum.

1. MPA
2. Right ventriculotomy incision
3. Interventricular septum
4. Ascending aorta
5. SVC

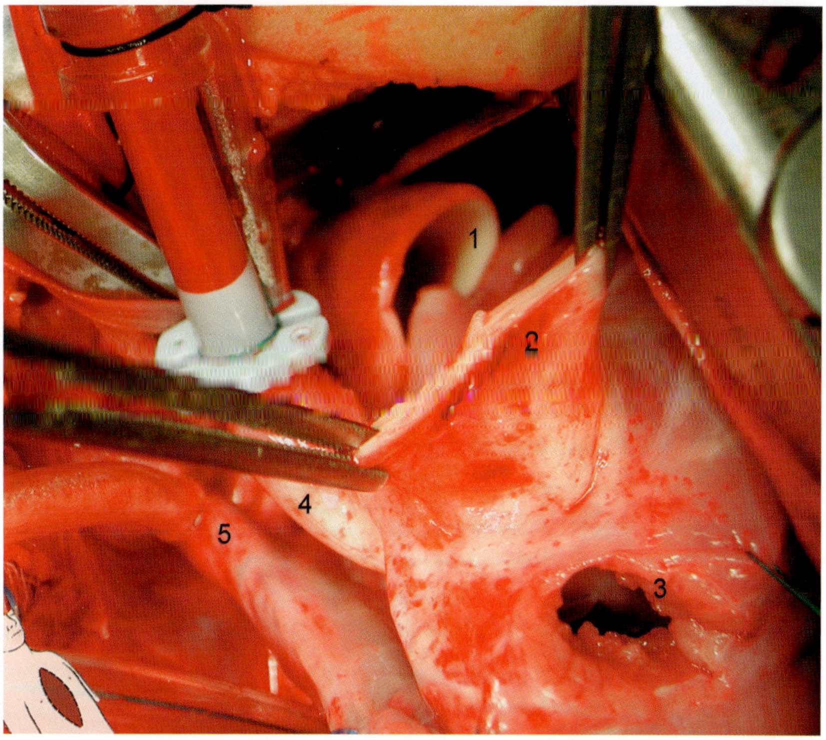

Figure 24.41. The same patient as in Figures 24.37 to 24.40. The proximal MPA will be oversewn.

1. Distal part of MPA
2. Proximal part of MPA
3. Right ventriculotomy incision
4. Ascending aorta
5. SVC

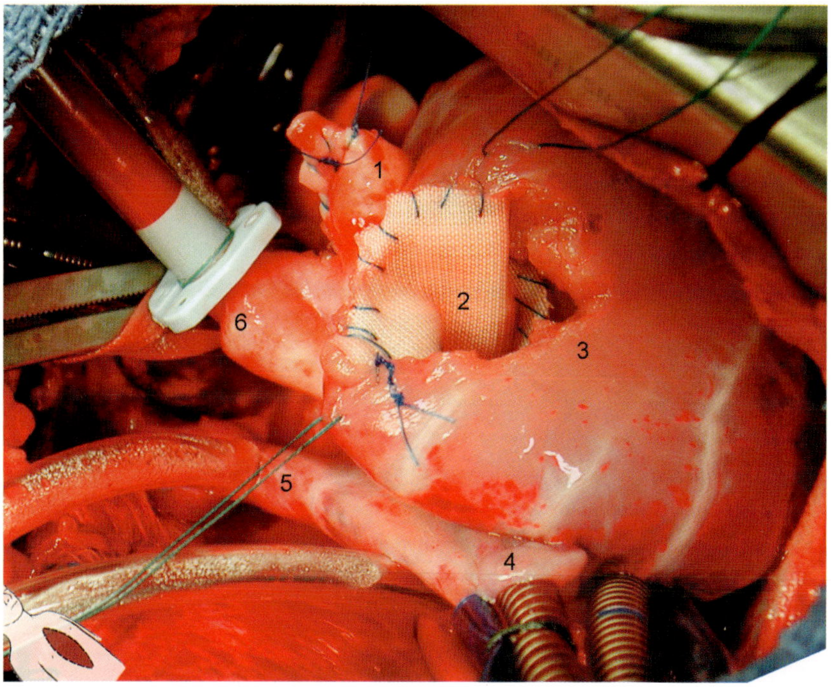

Figure 24.42. The same patient as in Figures 24.37 to 24.41. The proximal MPA stump has already been oversewn. The VSD has been closed using a Dacron patch so that both semilunar valves remain on the left. Because the VSD had no superior muscular rim, the upper part of the patch was sutured to the RV free wall directly.

1. Oversewn MPA
2. VSD patch (Dacron)
3. RV
4. RAA
5. SVC
6. Ascending aorta

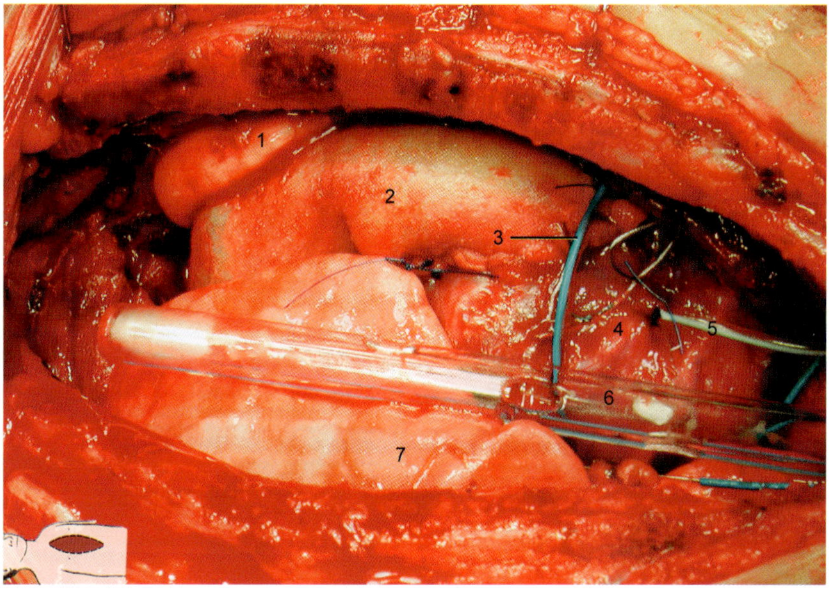

Figure 24.43. The completed operation of the patient shown in Figures 24.37 to 24.42, just before sternal closure. A bovine internal jugular vein graft (12 mm Contegra) was implanted between the RV and the PAs.

1. Left lung
2. RV-to-PA conduit (Contegra)
3. Temporary pacing wire
4. RV
5. PA catheter
6. Mediastinal chest tube
7. Right lung

REFERENCES

1. Pilati M, Luciani GB, Prioli MA, Puppini G. A neonate with cyanosis and tortuous great arteries. *Pediatr Cardiol.* 2009;30:1146–1149.
2. Fox MA, Fox JA, Davies MH. Budd–Chiari syndrome—a review of the diagnosis and management. *Acute Med.* 2011;10(1):5–9.
3. Latson L, Prieto L. Congenital and acquired pulmonary vein stenosis. *Circulation.* 2007;115:103–108.
4. Seale A, Webber S, Uemura H, et al. Pulmonary vein stenosis: the UK, Ireland and Sweden collaborative study. *Heart.* 2009;95;1944–1949.
5. Abu-Suliman RM, Hashmi A, McCrindle BW, Williams WG, Freedom RM. Anomalous origin of one pulmonary artery from the ascending aorta: 36 years' experience from one center. *Cardiol Young.* 1998;8:449–454.
6. Welch K, Hanley F, Johnston T, Cailes C, Shah MJ. Isolated unilateral absence of right proximal pulmonary artery: surgical repair and follow-up. *Ann Thorac Surg.* 2005;79(4):1399–1402.
7. Menon SC, Hagler DJ. Double-outlet left ventricle: diagnosis and management. *Curr Treat Options Cardiovasc Med.* 2008;10(5):448–452.

INDEX